# Bone Diseases: Diagnosis and Treatment

# Bone Diseases: Diagnosis and Treatment

Editor: Dan Heller

AMERICAN
MEDICAL PUBLISHERS
www.americanmedicalpublishers.com

AMERICAN
MEDICAL PUBLISHERS
www.americanmedicalpublishers.com

**Cataloging-in-Publication Data**

Bone diseases : diagnosis and treatment / edited by Dan Heller.
p. cm.
Includes bibliographical references and index.
ISBN 978-1-63927-939-5
1. Bones--Diseases. 2. Bones--Diseases--Diagnosis. 3. Bones--Diseases--Treatment. I. Heller, Dan.
RC930 .B66 2023
616.71--dc23



American Medical Publishers,
41 Flatbush Avenue,
1st Floor, New York,
NY 11217, USA

ISBN 978-1-63927-939-5 (Hardback)

# Contents

**Preface** ........ VII

Chapter 1 **CircCOG8 Downregulation Contributes to the Compression-Induced Intervertebral Disk Degeneration by Targeting miR-182-5p and FOXO3** ........ 1
Qian Xiang, Liang Kang, Kangcheng Zhao, Juntan Wang, Wenbin Hua, Yu Song, Xiaobo Feng, Gaocai Li, Saideng Lu, Kun Wang, Cao Yang and Yukun Zhang

Chapter 2 **Src Homology 2 Domain-Containing Protein Tyrosine Phosphatase Promotes Inflammation and Accelerates Osteoarthritis by Activating β-Catenin** ........ 17
Tenghui Tao, Danni Luo, Chenghao Gao, Hui Liu, Zehua Lei, Wenbin Liu, Chuankun Zhou, Dahu Qi, Zhenhan Deng, Xuying Sun and Jun Xiao

Chapter 3 **Communications Between Bone Marrow Macrophages and Bone Cells in Bone Remodeling** ........ 32
Kaixuan Chen, Yurui Jiao, Ling Liu, Mei Huang, Chen He, Wenzhen He, Jing Hou, Mi Yang, Xianghang Luo and Changjun Li

Chapter 4 **Low Dose BMP2-Doped Calcium Phosphate Graft Promotes Bone Defect Healing in a Large Animal Model** ........ 47
Tie Liu, Wen Fang, Gang Wu, Yining Li, Janak L. Pathak and Yuelian Liu

Chapter 5 **Multifaceted Functions and Novel Insight into the Regulatory Role of RNA $N^6$-Methyladenosine Modification in Musculoskeletal Disorders** ........ 60
Wenchao Zhang, Lile He, Zhongyue Liu, Xiaolei Ren, Lin Qi, Lu Wan, Wanchun Wang, Chao Tu and Zhihong Li

Chapter 6 **BMSC-Derived Exosomal miR-29a Promotes Angiogenesis and Osteogenesis** ........ 74
Guo-dong Lu, Peng Cheng, Ting Liu and Zhong Wang

Chapter 7 **Functions and Clinical Significance of Super-Enhancers in Bone-Related Diseases** ........ 84
Jian Qu, Zhanbo Ouyang, Wenqiang Wu, Guohua Li, Jiaojiao Wang, Qiong Lu and Zhihong Li

Chapter 8 **Medium-Intensity Treadmill Exercise Exerts Beneficial Effects on Bone Modeling Through Bone Marrow Mesenchymal Stromal Cells** ........ 96
Lingli Zhang, Yu Yuan, Wei Wu, Zhongguang Sun, Le Lei, Jing Fan, Bo Gao and Jun Zou

Chapter 9 **SLIT2 Overexpression in Periodontitis Intensifies Inflammation and Alveolar Bone Loss, Possibly via the Activation of MAPK Pathway** ........ 109
Liping Wang, Jing Zheng, Janak L. Pathak, Yunxin Chen, Dongliang Liang, Luxi Yang, Haobo Sun, Mei Zhong, Lihong Wu, Li Li, Shuhua Deng, Lingyun Zheng, Yongyong Yan, Dan Hou, Lijing Wang and Linhu Ge

Chapter 10 **Obesity and Bone Health: A Complex Link** ........ 125
Jing Hou, Chen He, Wenzhen He, Mi Yang, Xianghang Luo and Changjun Li

Chapter 11 **Conditional Knockout of PKC-δ in Osteoclasts Favors Bone Mass Accrual in Males Due to Decreased Osteoclast Function** ..... 141
Shangfu Li, Tianwei He, Depeng Wu, Liangming Zhang, Ruiqiang Chen, Bin Liu, Jinbo Yuan, Jennifer Tickner, An Qin, Jiake Xu and Limin Rong

Chapter 12 **The Role of Bone-Derived Exosomes in Regulating Skeletal Metabolism and Extraosseous Diseases** ..... 156
Huili Lyu, Ye Xiao, Qi Guo, Yan Huang and Xianghang Luo

Chapter 13 **A Novel Variant in *CLCN7* Regulates the Coupling of Angiogenesis and Osteogenesis** ..... 173
Hui Peng, Hong-Bo He and Ting Wen

Chapter 14 **Construction of a Five-Super-Enhancer-Associated-Genes Prognostic Model for Osteosarcoma Patients** ..... 184
Zhanbo Ouyang, Guohua Li, Haihong Zhu, Jiaojiao Wang, Tingting Qi, Qiang Qu, Chao Tu, Jian Qu and Qiong Lu

Chapter 15 **Moderate Fluid Shear Stress Regulates Heme Oxygenase-1 Expression to Promote Autophagy and ECM Homeostasis in the Nucleus Pulposus Cells** ..... 197
Sheng Chen, Lei Qin, Xiaohao Wu, Xuekun Fu, Sixiong Lin, Di Chen, Guozhi Xiao, Zengwu Shao and Huiling Cao

Chapter 16 **Positive Effect of Gushukang on Type-H Vessel and Bone Formation** ..... 211
Wantao Li, Xiaoqing Zhou, Tiejian Jiang, Hongbo He and Ting Wen

Chapter 17 **Human Umbilical Mesenchymal Stem Cells Display Therapeutic Potential in Rheumatoid Arthritis by Regulating Interactions Between Immunity and Gut Microbiota *via* the Aryl Hydrocarbon Receptor** ..... 220
Xiaoya Li, Cheng Lu, Danping Fan, Xiangchen Lu, Ya Xia, Hongyan Zhao, Huihui Xu, Yongliang Zhu, Jingtao Li, Honglin Liu and Cheng Xiao

**Permissions**

**List of Contributors**

**Index**

# Preface

A condition that affects the human skeletal system, making bones weaker and vulnerable to fractures is termed as a bone disease. There are several types of bone diseases including osteoporosis, metabolic bone diseases, fracture, stress fracture, bone cancer and scoliosis. Osteoporosis is one of most common bone conditions that cause a loss of bone due to weakened bones. Metabolic bone diseases lead to abnormal bone mass or structure caused by deficiency of a mineral or vitamin. Scoliosis is an abnormal condition in which there is side to side curvature of the spine that results in S- or C-shaped curvature when seen from behind. A number of factors such as age, occupation, environmental factors and genetics play a significant role in bone diseases. The risk of osteoporosis increases in people having low sun exposure and deficiency of vitamin D. The symptoms of these diseases include joint stiffness (arthritis), decreased range of motion, fatigue, and whole body symptoms (rheumatoid arthritis), etc. Physical activity can prove beneficial in the treatment and management of bone disease. From theories to research to practical applications, case studies related to all contemporary topics of relevance to bone diseases have been included in this book. It will provide comprehensive knowledge to the readers.

Significant researches are present in this book. Intensive efforts have been employed by authors to make this book an outstanding discourse. This book contains the enlightening chapters which have been written on the basis of significant researches done by the experts.

Finally, I would also like to thank all the members involved in this book for being a team and meeting all the deadlines for the submission of their respective works. I would also like to thank my friends and family for being supportive in my efforts.

**Editor**

# 1

# CircCOG8 Downregulation Contributes to the Compression-Induced Intervertebral Disk Degeneration by Targeting miR-182-5p and FOXO3

*Qian Xiang†, Liang Kang†, Kangcheng Zhao†, Juntan Wang, Wenbin Hua, Yu Song, Xiaobo Feng, Gaocai Li, Saideng Lu, Kun Wang, Cao Yang and Yukun Zhang**

*Department of Orthopaedics, Union Hospital, Tongji Medical College, Huazhong University of Science and Technology, Wuhan, China*

***Correspondence:**
*Yukun Zhang*
*zhangyukuncom@126.com*

*† These authors have contributed equally to this work*

Circular RNAs (circRNAs) have been increasingly demonstrated to play critical roles in the pathogenesis of various human diseases. Intervertebral disk degeneration (IDD) is recognized as the major contributor to lower back pain, and mechanical stress is a predominant trigger for IDD. However, little is known about the part that circRNAs play in the involvement of mechanical stress during IDD development. In the present study, we identified a novel circRNA and examined the role of this circRNA in a compression loading-induced IDD process. We detected the expression pattern of circCOG8 and observed its function in disk NP cells under mechanical stress. We conducted bioinformatics analysis, RNA immunoprecipitation experiment, and reporter gene assay to unveil the mechanism of the circCOG8 downregulation mediated IVD degeneration. Results showed that the circCOG8 expression was obviously down-regulated by the mechanical stress in disk NP cells. CircCOG8 attenuated NP cells apoptosis, intracellular ROS accumulation, and ECM degradation *in vitro* and *ex vivo*. CircCOG8 directly interacted with miR-182-5p and, thus, modulated the FOXO3 expression to affect the compression-induced IDD progression. Altogether, the present study revealed that the circCOG8/miR-182-5p/FOXO3 pathway was an important underlying mechanism in the involvement of compression during the IDD progression. Intervention of circCOG8 is a new therapeutic strategy for IDD treatment.

**Keywords: nucleus pulposus cell, intervertebral disk degeneration, mechanical stress, circular RNA, circCOG8, microRNA sponge**

## INTRODUCTION

Lower back pain is a global health problem with a high morbidity and it is the leading cause of job disability in the modern society (Hoy et al., 2014). Although there are various initiating contributors associated with lower back pain, it is widely accepted that the intervertebral disk degeneration (IDD) is the major reason (Hughes et al., 2012). However, the pathogenesis and etiology of IDD have not been explicitly clarified yet. Physiologically, the intervertebral disk (IVD) comprises the inner gelatinous nucleus pulposus (NP), the surrounding collagenous annulus fibrosus (AF), as well as the cartilaginous endplates (EP), and the disks act as the most important load-bearing structure of the spine (Roberts et al., 2006). Disk NP cells are in the center of IVD and play a crucial part in maintaining the balance between the NP extracellular matrix (ECM) catabolism and anabolism. The abundance of ECM, including the proteoglycans and type II collagen generated by the NP cells, make important contributions to the physiological structure and function of IVD (Roughley, 2004). And, IVD degeneration is typically characterized by the aberrant conditions of NP cells that the ECM catabolism exceeds anabolism, cell apoptosis rates are abnormally increased, and reactive oxygen species (ROS) generation and antioxidant defense get out of balance to cause oxidative stress (Zhao et al., 2007; Risbud and Shapiro, 2014; Feng et al., 2017). Deep research into the underlying mechanism of these aberrant activities of the NP cells can help clinicians get a better understanding of the IDD pathogenesis and, thus, provide new strategies for the IDD treatment (Hughes et al., 2012; Sakai and Grad, 2015).

Mechanical stress is a critical etiological factor that provokes IVD degeneration (Setton and Chen, 2006; Neidlinger-Wilke et al., 2014). The pressure of the human IVD ranges from 0.1 to 1.1 MPa *in vivo* depending on the postures and the disk is also subjected to various non-physiological mechanical loading, which, in return, contributes significantly to the disk damage (Wilke et al., 1999; Adams and Roughley, 2006). Studies have reported that mechanical loads could induce the ECM degradation via shifting the balance of the ECM metabolism homeostasis toward catabolism, accompanied by an elevated expression of catabolic genes, such as disintegrin and metalloproteinase with thrombospondin motifs (ADAMTS), as well as, matrix metalloproteinases (MMP) (Yurube et al., 2012; Holguin and Silva, 2018). Meanwhile, it was demonstrated that mechanical compression contributed to excessive ROS accumulation to promote oxidative stress in NP cells (Li et al., 2017). In our previous work, we elucidated that applying a static compression of 1.0 MPa to human NP cells obviously induced programmed cell death by which it was deeply involved in disk injury (Li et al., 2018). Furthermore, we also unveiled that mechanical loading could effectively induce various pathological responses of disk cells in an *ex vivo* organ-cultured rat IVD model (Wu et al., 2019).

Accumulating evidence have revealed that non-coding RNAs, including microRNAs (miRNAs) and circular RNAs (circRNAs), functionally participate in the pathophysiological process of IDD (Li et al., 2015, 2019). MiRNAs are highly conserved, short, and single stranded endogenous RNAs which can regulate the target mRNA expression via associating with AGO proteins (Bartel, 2004). For instance, miR-7 was found to be a critical contributor to the IDD by targeting GDF5 in disk NP cells, as reported in our previous work (W. Liu et al., 2016). In the present study, results revealed that miR-182-5p contributed to the compression-induced damage in NP cells which was obviously upregulated under compression stress. CircRNAs are another type of understudied non-coding RNAs and they have a closed continuous loop which enables them to be more stable compared to the linear RNAs and resistant to degradation by exonucleases or RNase R (Han et al., 2018). In regard to the biological function of circRNAs, evidence has claimed that a number of circRNAs can sequester miRNAs to indirectly regulate the corresponding target genes expression which was also called "miRNA sponge" (Memczak et al., 2013). The most representative miRNA sponge is that the Cdr1as, an antisense transcript of cerebellar degeneration-related protein 1, harbors 74 conserved binding sites for miR-7 (Hansen et al., 2013). It has been reported that circRNAs exerted significant effects on the initiation and development of degenerative disk diseases by functioning as competing endogenous RNAs and consequently modulating target mRNAs levels (Cheng et al., 2018; Song et al., 2018). However, little is known about the part circRNAs play in the IDD progression induced by mechanical stress. Therefore, this study was aimed to explore a possible role of circRNAs in the mechanisms leading to IDD by examining their expression in disk NP cells under mechanical stress. We identified a novel circular RNA circCOG8 based on the circRNA microarray and bioinformatics analysis and systemically investigated the role of this circRNA in the progression of compression-loading-induced IDD.

## RESULTS

### CircCOG8 Was Significantly Down Regulated in the Disk NP Cells Under Mechanical Stress

To uncover the potential role of circRNAs in the progression of IDD induced by mechanical loading, we examined the effects of compression on human disk NP cells in three different samples. Compression treatment significantly increased the NP cell apoptosis and intracellular ROS accumulation, increased the expression of Bax, ADAMTS-4, ADAMTS-5 as well as MMP-13, and inhibited the expression of Bcl-2, Aggrecan as well as Type II collagen (**Figures 1A–C**). It was suggested that the compression treatment resulted in elevated cell apoptosis, ROS accumulation, and ECM degradation in human disk NP cells. Then, we performed circRNAs microarray assays using three pairs of disk cells samples treated by 1.0 MPa mechanical loading for 36 h. Data revealed that a total of 1,784 circRNAs were significantly dysregulated, among which, 1,498 gene items were downregulated by mechanical loading compared with the control. **Figure 1D** showed the top 100 most significantly down-regulated circRNAs. Since most of the differentially expressed circRNAs were down-regulated in the compression treatment group, we then selected seven out of the top 100 remarkably down-regulated circRNAs for the validation in three different pairs of cell samples by real-time qPCR analysis and these seven circRNAs were all rich in miRNA binding sites. The log2 fold-changes of microarray data and RT-qPCR data were both calculated and we found that, of the seven circRNAs, the circCOG8 showed the highest fold-change (**Figure 1E**). As a result, the circCOG8 was chosen as the subject for further experiments. CircCOG8 (hsa_circ_0040060)

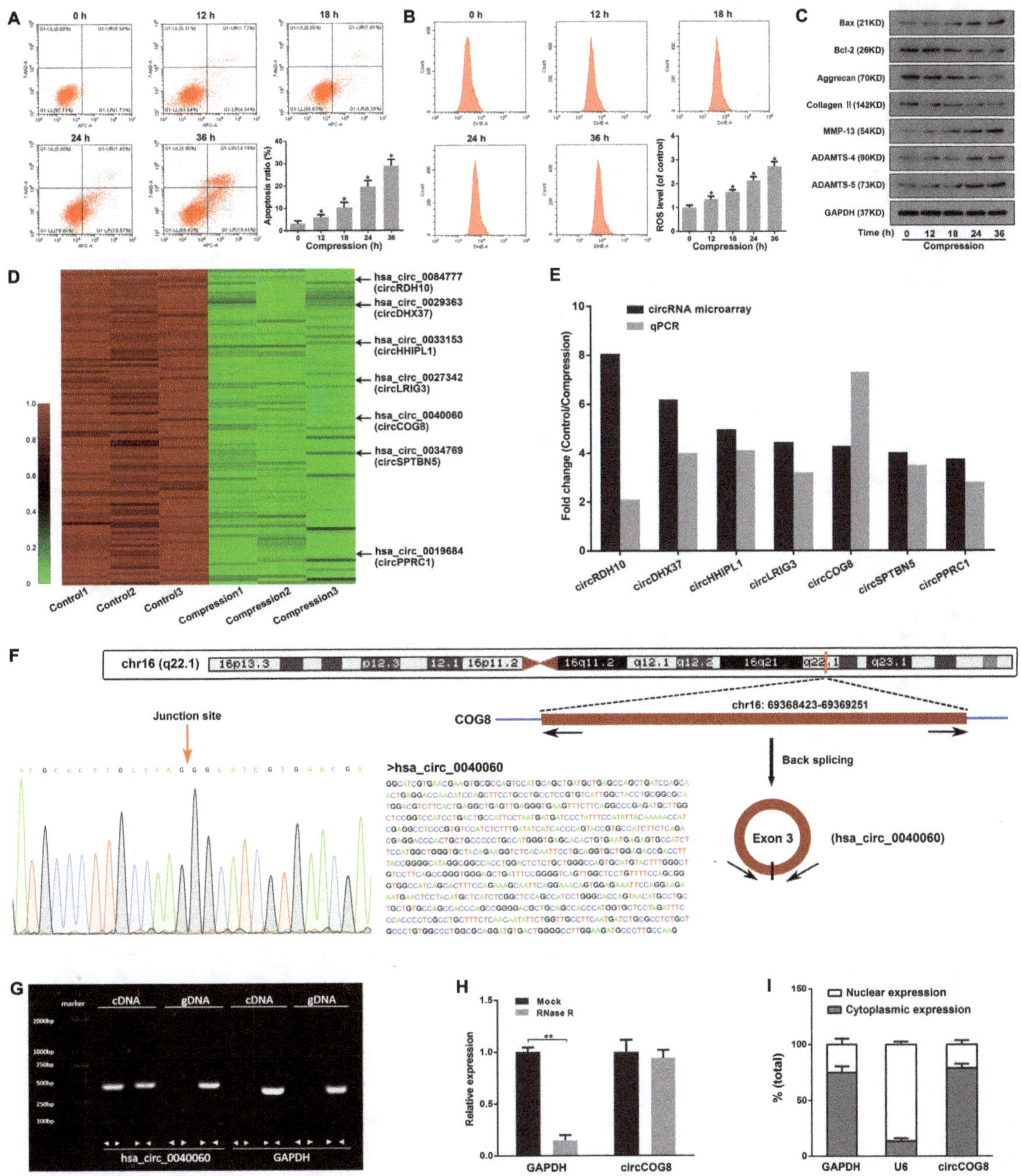

**FIGURE 1 |** CircCOG8 was significantly down-regulated in the compression-treated human NP cells. **(A)** The human NP cells were treated with 1 MPa compression for the indicated time points (0, 12, 18, 24, and 36 h), and the cell apoptosis was determined by the Annexin V-APC and 7-AAD double-staining with subsequent flow cytometry analysis. Data were represented as mean ± SD. 0 h group served as a control, $^{*}p < 0.05$ versus control, $n = 3$ (ANOVA with Tukey's post-test). **(B)** The intracellular ROS production of the NP cells with compression for indicated time points were examined by the ROS-specific fluorescent probe DHE and measured by the flow cytometry analysis. Data were represented as mean ± SD. 0 h group served as a control, $^{*}p < 0.05$ versus control, $n = 3$ (ANOVA with Tukey's post-test). **(C)** Western blot analysis was used to detect the protein expression level of ECM anabolism markers (Aggrecan, Type II collagen), ECM catabolism enzymes (MMP-13, ADAMTS-4, ADAMTS-5), and apoptosis-associated markers (Bax, Bcl-2). Data were normalized to the GAPDH control. The GAPDH band served as a common internal loading control for Bax, Bcl-2, Aggrecan, Type II collagen, MMP-13, ADAMTS-4, and ADAMTS-5. **(D)** Clustered heat map showed the top 100 significantly down-regulated circRNAs in three samples of the compression treated human NP cells and three control samples. The arrows indicated the seven candidate circRNAs which were further validated using a real-time qPCR analysis. **(E)** Comparison of the fold changes for the seven candidate circRNAs from the circRNA array and real-time qPCR validation. **(F)** The genomic loci of the COG8 gene and circCOG8. The expression of circCOG8 was validated by the Sanger sequencing. **(G)** The products amplified using the divergent or convergent primers were verified by agarose gel electrophoresis. Divergent primers were used to amplify circCOG8 in cDNA but not in genomic DNA (gDNA). Convergent primers could amplify both the circCOG8 and linear RNA GAPDH. **(H)** The RT-qPCR analysis of circCOG8 and linear control GAPDH mRNA after treatment with RNase R in the disk NP cells. $^{**}p < 0.05$, $n = 3$. **(I)** RT-qPCR assay in nuclear and cytoplasmic fractions showed the levels of nuclear control transcript (U6), cytoplasmic control transcript (GAPDH), and circCOG8.

is generated from back-spliced exon 3 of COG8 which is located on chromosome 16q22.1 (chr16:69368423-69369251), as annotated in the circBase online database using the human reference genome GRCh37/hg19 (**Figure 1F**). The length of the circCOG8 is 828 nt (nucleotide). The PCR assay suggested that divergent primers could amplify the circular circCOG8 in cDNA but not in gDNA, and convergent primers could amplify both the circCOG8 and linear control GAPDH (**Figure 1G**). Sanger sequencing was performed to confirm the amplified products using divergent primers, as shown in **Figure 1F**. CircCOG8 was resistant to RNase R exonuclease digestion, further supporting the notion that this type of RNA was circular (**Figure 1H**). Moreover, the circCOG8 was primarily distributed in the cytoplasm, as examined by the cytoplasmic and nuclear RNA isolation followed by RT-qPCR in disk NP cells (**Figure 1I**).

## Overexpression of CircCOG8 Protected Disk NP Cells From Mechanical Stress-Induced Cellular Damage

Next, we transfected the disk NP cells with the circCOG8 expression adenovirus vector to overexpress circCOG8, or with shRNA targeting the junction site of circCOG8 to knockdown circCOG8. As revealed in **Figure 2A**, the NP cells transfected with the circCOG8 overexpression vector showed a higher

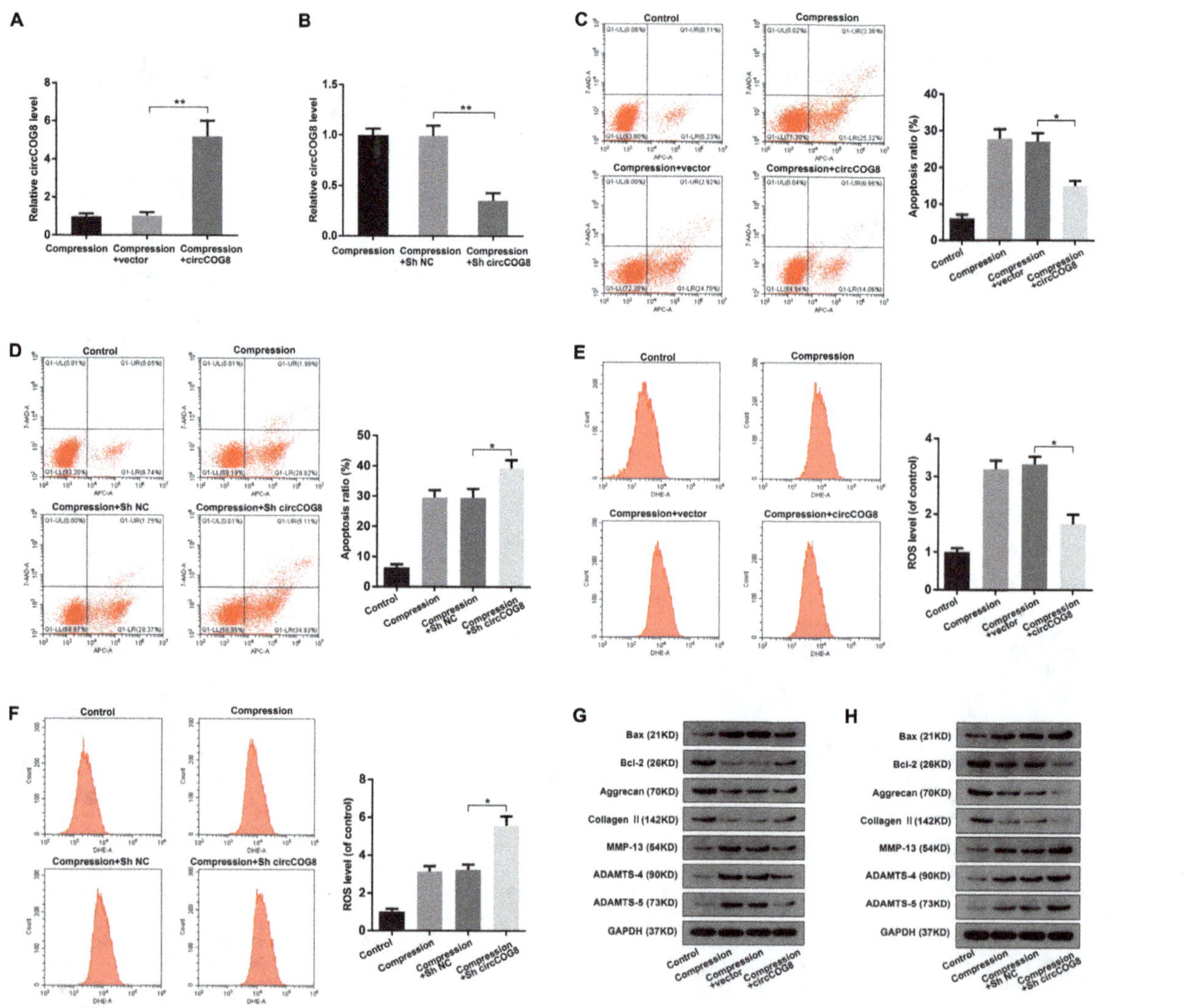


**FIGURE 2 |** Function of circCOG8 in disk NP cells under mechanical stress. **(A,B)** The human NP cells under compression treatment were transfected with the circCOG8 overexpression vector or circCOG8 shRNA, and the circCOG8 RNA level was examined using the RT-qPCR analysis. **(C,D)** The apoptosis ratio of the NP cells transfected with the circCOG8 overexpression vector or circCOG8 shRNA was determined by the flow cytometry analysis after the Annexin V-APC and 7-AAD double-staining. **(E,F)** The intracellular ROS levels of the NP cells transfected with the circCOG8 overexpression vector or circCOG8 shRNA were detected by DHE and measured by the flow cytometry analysis. **(G,H)** Human NP cells under compression were treated with the circCOG8 overexpression or circCOG8 shRNA, and the protein levels of Bax, Bcl-2, Aggrecan, Type II collagen, MMP-13, ADAMTS-4, and ADAMTS-5 were determined by the western blot analysis. The corresponding GAPDH band served as a common internal loading control for Bax, Bcl-2, Aggrecan, Type II collagen, MMP-13, ADAMTS-4, and ADAMTS-5. Data were represented as mean ± SD. $^{*}p < 0.05$, $^{**}p < 0.01$, $n = 3$ (Student's *t*-test).

circCOG8 expression level under the compression treatment. In contrast, the circCOG8 shRNA obviously resulted in the circCOG8 downregulation (**Figure 2B**). Then, we used flow cytometry analysis by Annexin V/PI dual staining to evaluate the circCOG8's effect on the NP cells apoptosis under compression. We found that the circCOG8 overexpression obviously decreased the apoptosis incidence of NP cells (**Figure 2C**) and circCOG8 knockdown increased the apoptosis rate of NP cells under compression (**Figure 2D**). The intracellular ROS level were examined using the fluorescent probe DHE and flow cytometry which indicated that circCOG8 could markedly inhibit the ROS production of NP cells (**Figure 2E**) and the circCOG8 shRNA could promote the ROS production of disk NP cells induced by mechanical loading (**Figure 2F**). Western blot analysis suggested that the circCOG8 knockdown increased the protein level of ADAMTS-4, ADAMTS-5, MMP-13 as well as Bax and decreased the expression of Type II collagen, aggrecan as well as Bcl-2 while the circCOG8 overexpression partially counteracted the effects of mechanical loading on these gene expression (**Figures 2G,H**). The results above demonstrated that circCOG8 could alleviate the effect of mechanical stress on disk NP cells.

## CircCOG8 Functioned as miR-182-5p Sponge to Inhibit Its Expression

Considering the circular RNAs can interact with microRNAs to function as microRNA sponges, circCOG8 might target a critical microRNA to regulate its activity. Firstly, we used the StarBase online tool and Circular RNA Interactome online database to predict the targeting miRNAs of circCOG8, and found that there were eight candidate miRNAs identified by overlapping the predicting results from these two databases (**Figure 3A**). Then, we used real-time qPCR analysis to determine whether these predicted miRNAs were dysregulated in the disk NP cells under mechanical stress. Results showed that the miR-182-5p was the only significantly upregulated miRNA with a fold change $> 2$ (**Figure 3B**). According to the StarBase online database, there was a potential binding site between the circCOG8 and miR-182-5p seed region (**Figure 3C**). Next, we performed the subsequent experiments to investigate the ability of the circCOG8 to directly interact with the miR-182-5p in disk NP cells. We transfected the disk NP cells with the circCOG8 shRNA to inhibit the circCOG8 expression, with the results proving that the miR-182-5p level was obviously enhanced after the circCOG8 knockdown (**Figure 3D**). Then, we conducted the Argonaute-2 (AGO2) immunoprecipitation by RT-qPCR to examine whether the AGO2 was associated with the miR-182-5p transcripts which could bind circCOG8. We found that both the circCOG8 and miR-182-5p were highly enriched by the anti-AGO2 antibodies (**Figure 3E**). Furthermore, the pMIR-REPORT luciferase reporter plasmids with mutant (MUT) or wild type (WT) circCOG8 fragment which possessed miR-182-5p complementary binding sequence were co-transfected to the HEK293T cells with miR-182-5p. Results revealed that the relative Luc/R-luc ratio of WT luciferase reporter was obviously lower in the miR-182-5p mimic group compared to the negative control (**Figure 3F**). In summary, the above data demonstrated that circCOG8 functioned as an miR-182-5p sponge to suppress its expression in the disk NP cells.

## MiR-182-5p Facilitated Mechanical Stress-Induced Cellular Damage of Disk NP Cells

Since miR-182-5p is the circCOG8-targeted microRNA, we speculated that miR-182-5p could have crucial regulating effects on the disk NP cells with compression loading. To test our hypothesis, we carried out the following experiments. Using the RT-qPCR assay, we found that miR-182-5p was elevated in the disk NP cells after the compression stimulation; the miR-182-5p expression was markedly inhibited after the miRNA inhibitor treatment and increased after the miRNA mimic treatment (**Figures 4A,E**). As revealed in **Figures 4B–D**, the miR-182-5p inhibitor markedly inhibited the up-regulation of apoptosis rate, ROS production, and ECM degradation in disk NP cells induced by mechanical stress. Conversely, these changes in NP cells induced by compression stress were enhanced when co-treated with the miR-182-5p overexpression (**Figures 4F–H**). The above data revealed the critical role of miR-182-5p in promoting cell apoptosis, oxidative stress, and ECM degradation in the disk NP cells under mechanical stress.

## MiR-182-5p Functioned in Disk NP Cells via Interacting With FOXO3

It has been reported that the transcription factors of the Forkhead box O class (FOXOs) played important regulating roles in the intervertebral disk maturation and homeostasis (Alvarez-Garcia et al., 2018; Penolazzi et al., 2018). Using the TargetScan online tool, we found that the Forkhead box O3 (FOXO3) possessed complementary sequence to the miR-182-5p seed region (**Figure 5A**). Then, we performed the luciferase analysis to validate that the miR-182-5p could directly target FOXO3. Luciferase reporter vector with mutant (MUT) or wild type (WT) FOXO3 3′-UTR, which possessed the miR-182-5p binding sites, were transfected to the HEK293T cells treated with miR-182-5p. As expected, miR-182-5p markedly suppress the luciferase activity of the WT-FOXO3 3′-UTR reporter while there was no significant difference in the MUT-FOXO3 3′-UTR reporter activity between the miR-182-5p mimic and control group (**Figure 5B**). Next, we performed the western blotting analysis in the disk NP cells to further validate the above findings. It was illustrated that miR-182-5p markedly suppressed the FOXO3 protein level (**Figure 5C**). Conversely, the miR-182-5p knockdown dramatically promoted the FOXO3 protein level (**Figure 5D**). The above results suggested that miR-182-5p could bind to FOXO3 3′-UTR to repress its expression. Then, we carried out the western blot analysis to explore the role of interaction between miR-182-5p and FOXO3 in the disk NP cells under mechanical stress. It was suggested that the level of FOXO3 protein was obviously decreased under the compression loading (**Figures 5E,F**). Overexpressing miR-182-5p could facilitate the inhibitive effect of mechanical stress on FOXO3 expression (**Figure 5E**) and the miR-182-5p inhibitor could mitigate the inhibitive effect of compression on the FOXO3 protein level

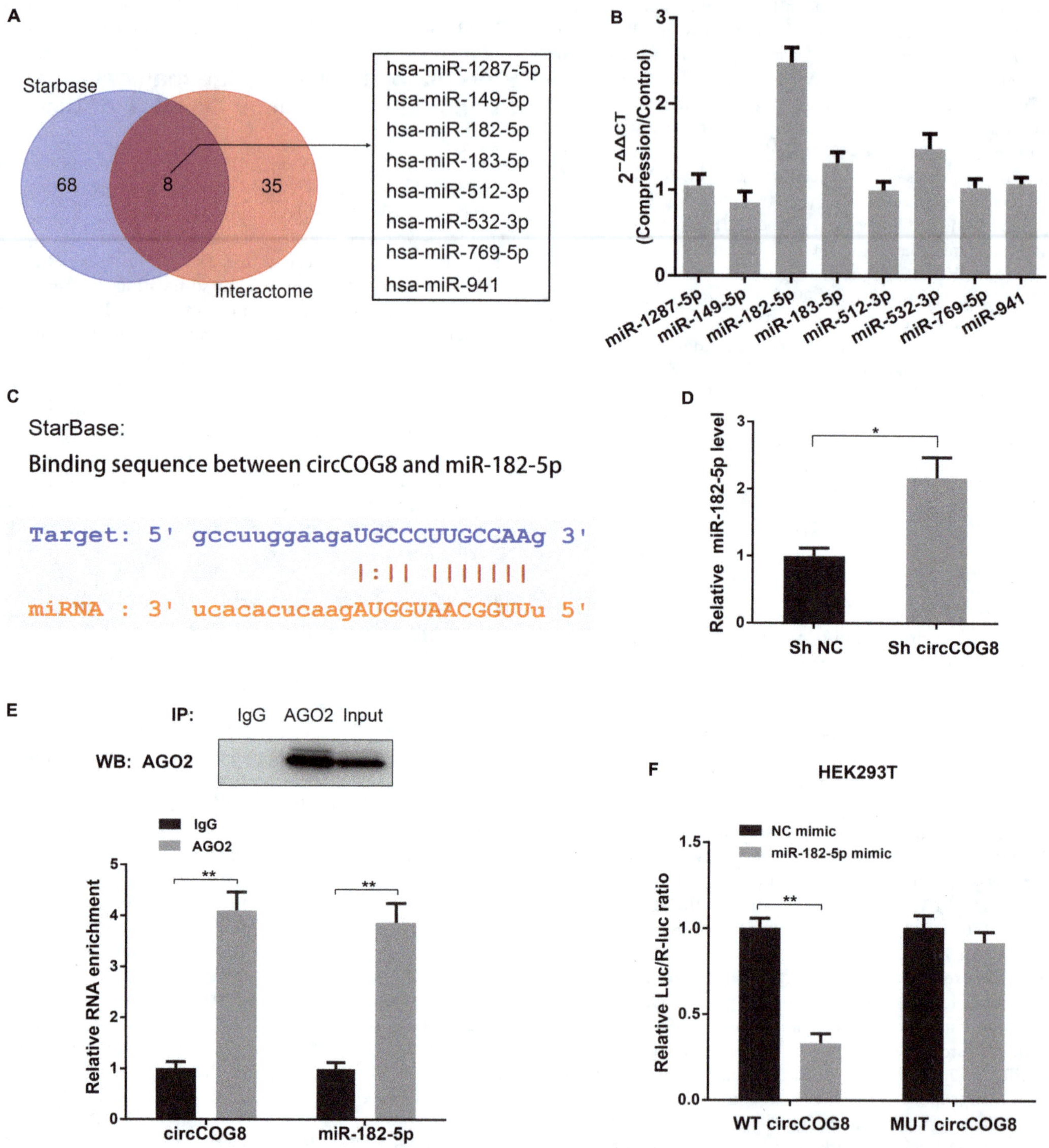


**FIGURE 3 |** CircCOG8 acted as a sponge for miR-182-5p to inhibit its expression. **(A)** The Veen diagram revealed the eight candidate circCOG8-targeting miRNAs identified using the StarBase online tool and the Circular RNA Interactome online database. **(B)** The expression pattern of these eight candidate miRNAs in the disk NP cells under mechanical stress were determined by the real-time qPCR analysis. The upregulated magnitudes of these eight miRNAs were shown as fold changes of the compression treated cell samples to control cell samples. **(C)** Schematic of the binding sequence between circCOG8 and miR-182-5p based on the StarBase online database. **(D)** The expression level of miR-182-5p in the disk NP cells transfected with the circCOG8 shRNA or control was examined by the real-time qPCR analysis. **(E)** The RNA immunoprecipitation (RIP) assay was used to detect circCOG8 and miR-182-5p enrichment. The AGO2 protein level was examined by the IP-western blot analysis (upper) and co-precipitated circCOG8 and miR-182-5p RNA levels were examined using the qRT-PCR analysis (lower). **(F)** Wild-type (WT) or mutant (MUT) circCOG8 luciferase reporter vectors were co-transfected with the miR-182-5p mimic or NC mimic into HEK-293T cells. The relative luciferase activity was determined as the ratio of firefly luciferase/Renilla luciferase (Luc/R-luc). Data were represented as mean ± SD. $^{*}p < 0.05$, $^{**}p < 0.01$, $n = 3$ (Student's $t$-test).

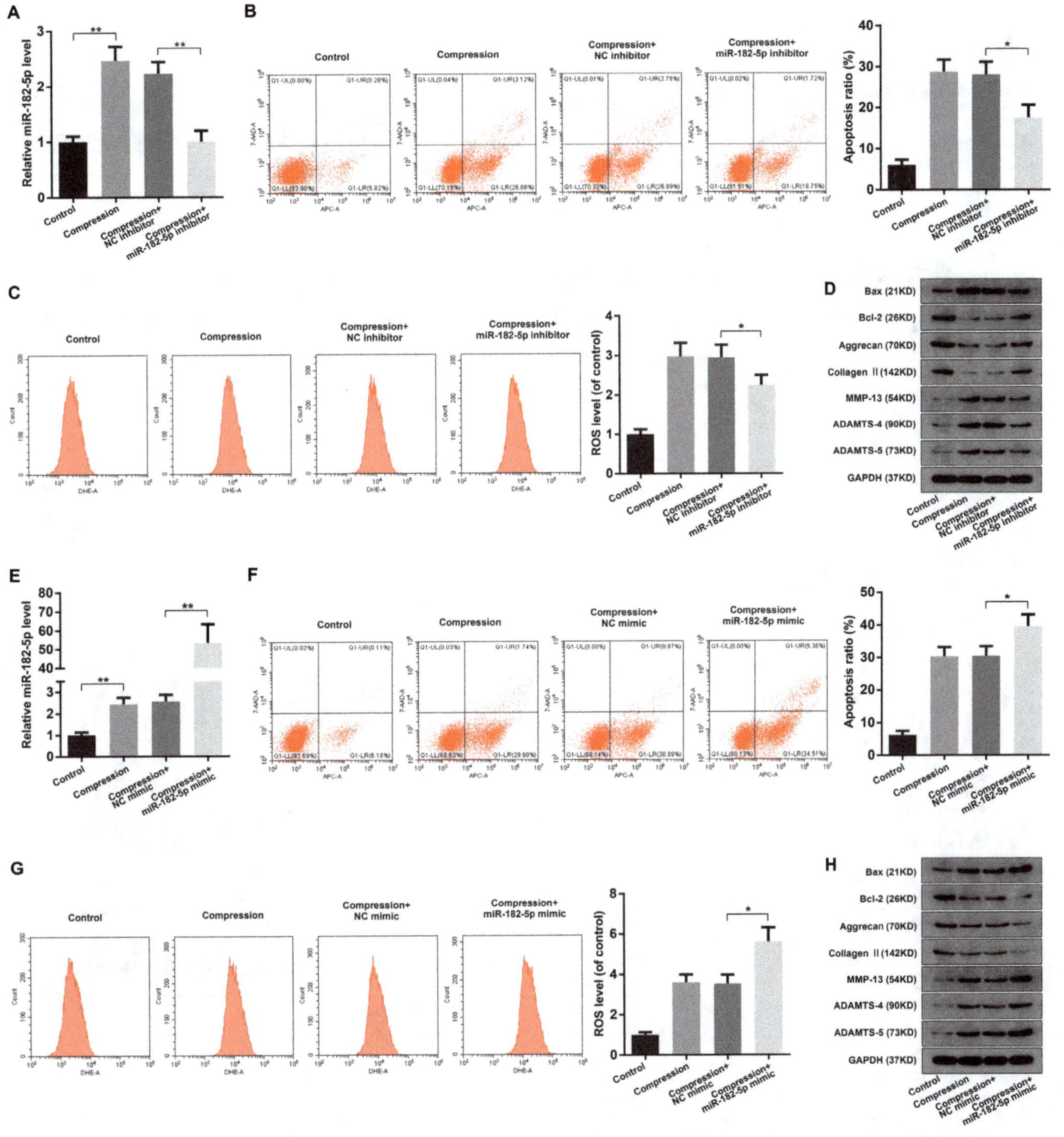


**FIGURE 4 |** Function of miR-182-5p in disk NP cells under mechanical stress. **(A)** The human NP cells under compression were transfected with the miR-182-5p inhibitor and the miR-182-5p expression level was examined using the RT-qPCR analysis. **(B)** The apoptosis ratio of the NP cells with the miR-182-5p inhibitor treatment was evaluated using the Annexin V-APC and 7-AAD double-staining with subsequent flow cytometry analysis. **(C)** The intracellular ROS accumulation of the NP cells with the miR-182-5p inhibitor treatment were detected by DHE and measured by the flow cytometry analysis. **(D)** The protein expression levels of Bax, Bcl-2, Aggrecan, Type II collagen, MMP-13, ADAMTS-4, and ADAMTS-5 were determined by the western blot analysis. The GAPDH band served as a common internal loading control for Bax, Bcl-2, Aggrecan, Type II collagen, MMP-13, ADAMTS-4, and ADAMTS-5. **(E)** The human NP cells under compression were transfected with the miR-182-5p mimic and the miR-182-5p level was determined by the RT-qPCR analysis. **(F)** The apoptosis ratio of the NP cells with miR-182-5p mimic treatment. **(G)** The intracellular ROS levels of the NP cells transfected with the miR-182-5p mimic. **(H)** The protein levels of Bax, Bcl-2, Aggrecan, Type II collagen, MMP-13, ADAMTS-4, and ADAMTS-5 were determined by the western blot analysis. The GAPDH band served as a common internal loading control for Bax, Bcl-2, Aggrecan, Type II collagen, MMP-13, ADAMTS-4, and ADAMTS-5. Data were represented as mean ± SD. $^{*}p < 0.05$, $^{**}p < 0.01$, $n = 3$ (Student's $t$-test).

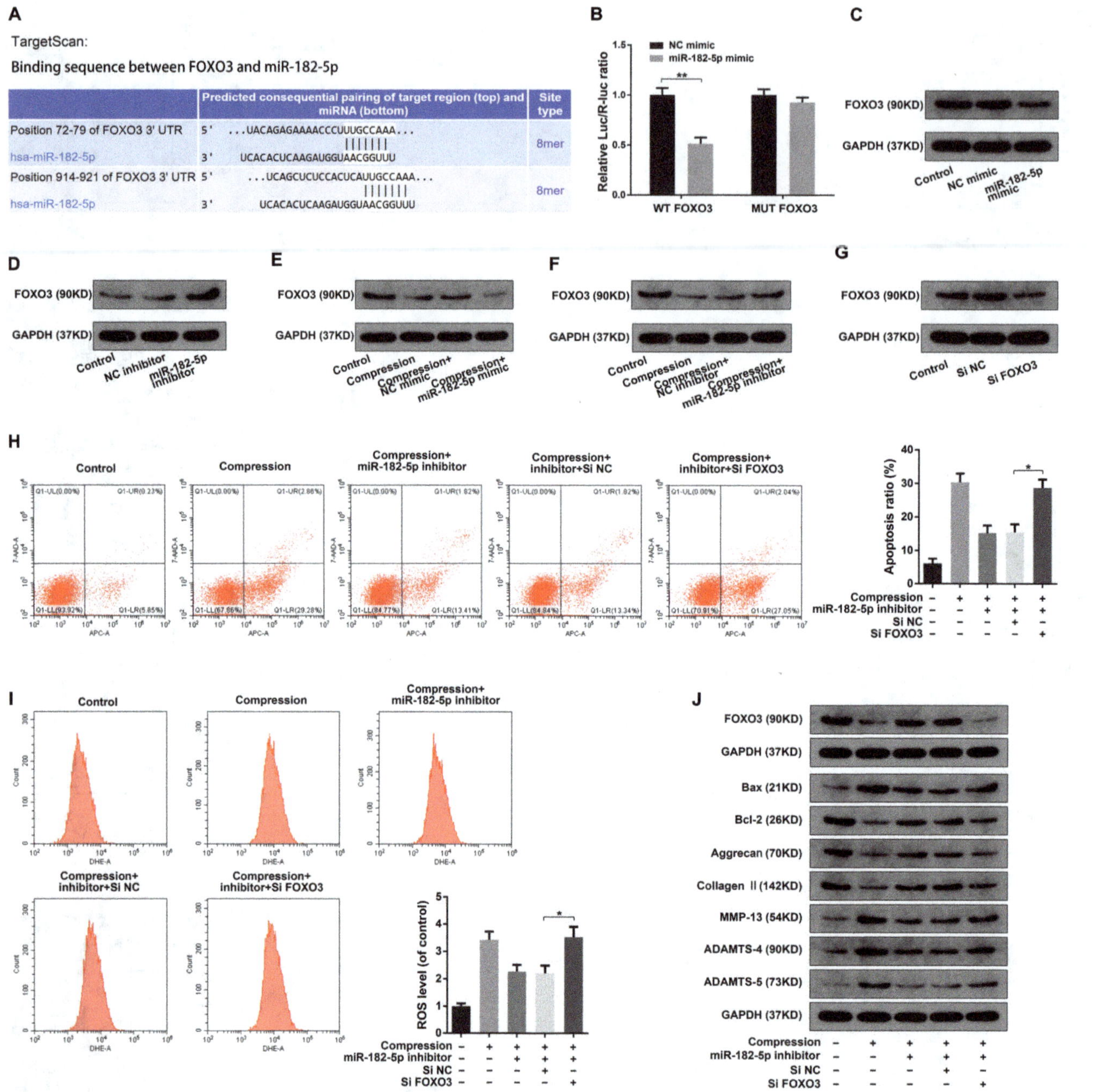


**FIGURE 5** | MiR-182-5p functioned in disk NP cells via targeting FOXO3. **(A)** Schematic of the binding sequence between the 3′ UTR of FOXO3 and miR-182-5p based on the TargetScan online database. **(B)** WT or MUT FOXO3 luciferase reporter vectors were co-transfected into the HEK-293T cells with the miR-182-5p mimic or NC mimic, and the luciferase reporter activity was presented as the relative Luc/R-Luc ratio. **(C,D)** The human NP cells were transfected with the miR-182-5p mimic or miR-182-5p inhibitor, the FOXO3 expression level was were determined by the western blot analysis. **(E,F)** The human NP cells under the compression treatment were transfected with the miR-182-5p mimic or miR-182-5p inhibitor, the FOXO3 expression level was were determined by the western blot analysis. **(G)** The FOXO3 protein expression level in the disk NP cells treated with the FOXO3 siRNA or siNC. **(H)** The Annexin V-APC and 7-AAD double-staining results indicating the apoptosis ratio of the NP cells. **(I)** The intracellular ROS levels in the NP cells were detected by DHE with the flow cytometry analysis. **(J)** The protein levels of FOXO3, Bax, Bcl-2, Aggrecan, Type II collagen, MMP-13, ADAMTS-4, and ADAMTS-5 were determined by the western blot analysis. The upper GAPDH band served as an internal loading control for FOXO3; the lower GAPDH band served as a common internal loading control for Bax, Bcl-2, Aggrecan, Type II collagen, MMP-13, ADAMTS-4, and ADAMTS-5. Data were represented as mean ± SD. $^{*}p < 0.05$, $^{**}p < 0.01$, $n = 3$ (Student's $t$-test).

(**Figure 5F**). Subsequently, the FOXO3 siRNA was used to further validate the critical role of FOXO3 (**Figure 5G**). It was revealed that the FOXO3 siRNA could partially counteract the effect of the miR-182-5p knockdown on human NP cells (**Figures 5H–J**). The above results demonstrated that miR-182-5p functioned in the disk NP cells through interacting with FOXO3.

## CircCOG8 Functioned in Disk NP Cells via Targeting miR-182-5p and FOXO3

To further examine the effects of circCOG8 on the FOXO3 expression with the involvement of miR-182-5p, we then carried out the following experiments. The luciferase activity assay revealed that miR-182-5p markedly repressed the WT-FOXO3 luciferase activity while circCOG8 could partially reverse this inhibitory effect (**Figure 6A**). Western blotting analysis also revealed that the repressive function of miR-182-5p on the FOXO3 expression level could be neutralized by the circCOG8 upregulation (**Figure 6B**). It was suggested that circCOG8 could function as the miR-182-5p sponge to modulate the FOXO3 expression. Subsequently, we found that the up-regulation of cell death rate, ROS production as well as the ECM catabolic activity in the disk NP cells caused by miR-182-5p could be counteracted by the circCOG8 overexpression (**Figures 6C–E**). Moreover, using the siRNA-mediated FOXO3 knockdown, we found that the absence of FOXO3 evidently abolished the protective effect of the circCOG8 overexpression in the disk NP cells under mechanical stress (**Figures 6F–H**). The above results revealed that circCOG8 exerted its functions by targeting miR-182-5p and FOXO3.

## CircCOG8 Overexpression Attenuated Compression-Induced IDD *ex vivo*

To further test the function of circCOG8 exhibited on the compression-induced IDD progression, we established the *ex vivo* organ-cultured rat disk model. The modeled rat IVDs *ex vivo* were injected with the adenovirus circCOG8 or control vector. Then, the IVD specimens were harvested and subjected to histopathological analysis (**Figures 7A,B**). In the control groups, the round-shaped NP tissues occupied more than half area of the disk as examined by the HE staining, and abundant proteoglycan matrix was confirmed in the NP area as indicated by the Safranin-O staining (**Figure 7A**). In the compression-induced IDD groups, the NP tissues area in the disk was obviously smaller with the collapsed disk height and the proteoglycan matrix volume was markedly decreased. Conversely, the circCOG8 overexpression could alleviate these disk degenerative changes induced by the compression when comparing with the IDD groups. The statistical data also suggested that the histological grades in the IDD groups were higher than that in the circCOG8 overexpression groups (**Figure 7B**). The TUNEL assay showed that the NP cell apoptosis ratio was elevated in the compression-induced IDD groups and markedly decreased after co-treatment of the circCOG8 overexpression (**Figures 7C,D**). Furthermore, compared to the IDD groups, the ROS level in IVD tissues indicated by $H_2O_2$ content was obviously decreased in the circCOG8 overexpression groups (**Figure 7E**). Lastly, the western blot analysis revealed that circCOG8 could alleviate the FOXO3 reduction, ECM degradation, and apoptotic response in the *ex vivo* organ-cultured model (**Figure 7F**). Collectively, the above results indicated that the circCOG8 overexpression could attenuate the compression-induced IDD *ex vivo*.

## DISCUSSION

Previous studies have demonstrated that IVD degeneration was a complicated disease involving numerous pathologic processes during which the nucleus pulposus cells residing in the IVD center has played a key role (Sakai et al., 2012). The impairment of the structural and functional integrity of the NP is a classical character of IDD progression, including the imbalanced metabolism of the ECM, NP cell apoptosis, and excessive ROS accumulation (Roberts et al., 2006; Zhao et al., 2007; Feng et al., 2017). The IVD is an important load-bearing structure and it is under various degrees of mechanical stress during which the NP could counteract and distribute the mechanical loads in the spine (Wilke et al., 1999; Gilchrist et al., 2011). Accumulating evidences have corroborated that mechanical stress was a predominant initiating factor for IDD and abnormal mechanical stress induced various pathological cellular responses within the IVD (MacLean et al., 2005; Li S. et al., 2018). Recently, research demonstrated that the compression treatment on NP cells could lead to the activation of the NF-κB pathway, MAPK pathway, and the deactivation of the PI3K/Akt pathway (Jiang et al., 2018; Li et al., 2018; Glaeser et al., 2020; Huang et al., 2020), which provided new insights into the association between mechanical stress and IDD. In this study, we found that applying a static mechanical load of 1.0 MPa could induce ECM degradation, cell apoptosis, and excessive ROS production in NP cells, which was consistent with the previous findings (Li et al., 2017; Lin et al., 2017; Chen et al., 2018; Wu et al., 2019). Moreover, we also applied an *ex vivo* IDD model induced by mechanical stress in this study. Compared with the *in vitro* analysis, the *ex vivo* system provided a better model to uncover the pathogenesis of IDD, with the intervertebral disk structure and native ECM intact, which were important to further investigate the involvement of mechanical loading in IVD degeneration (Lee et al., 2006; Koerner et al., 2016; Wu et al., 2019). In the *ex vivo* model, the imbalance between the ECM deposition and degradation, the increased NP cell apoptosis, and overproduction of ROS were also detected. However, the precise molecular mechanism of the involvement of mechanical stress during IDD progression remains unclear and more efforts should be made to develop novel therapeutic targets for IDD.

Recently, evidence increasingly reported that circRNAs played crucial roles during the physiology and pathology of various human diseases (Zhao and Shen, 2017; Chen et al., 2018; Kleaveland et al., 2018; Liu et al., 2018). CircRNAs are single-stranded non-coding RNA molecules without 5′–3′ polarities and polyadenylated tails as a result of the circular structure generated by back splicing of introns, exons, or intergenic regions. With the following characteristics including the exceptional stability, conservation across species, and cell and tissue-specific expression patterns, circRNAs have been found involved in many crucial cellular processes and the dysregulation of circRNAs resulted in the initiation and development of a broad range of diseases. CircRNAs could directly bind to microRNAs and sequester them from the cytoplasm and, thus, counteract the inhibitory effect of miRNAs on their targeting mRNA (Li et al., 2018). The most representative circRNA Cdr1as

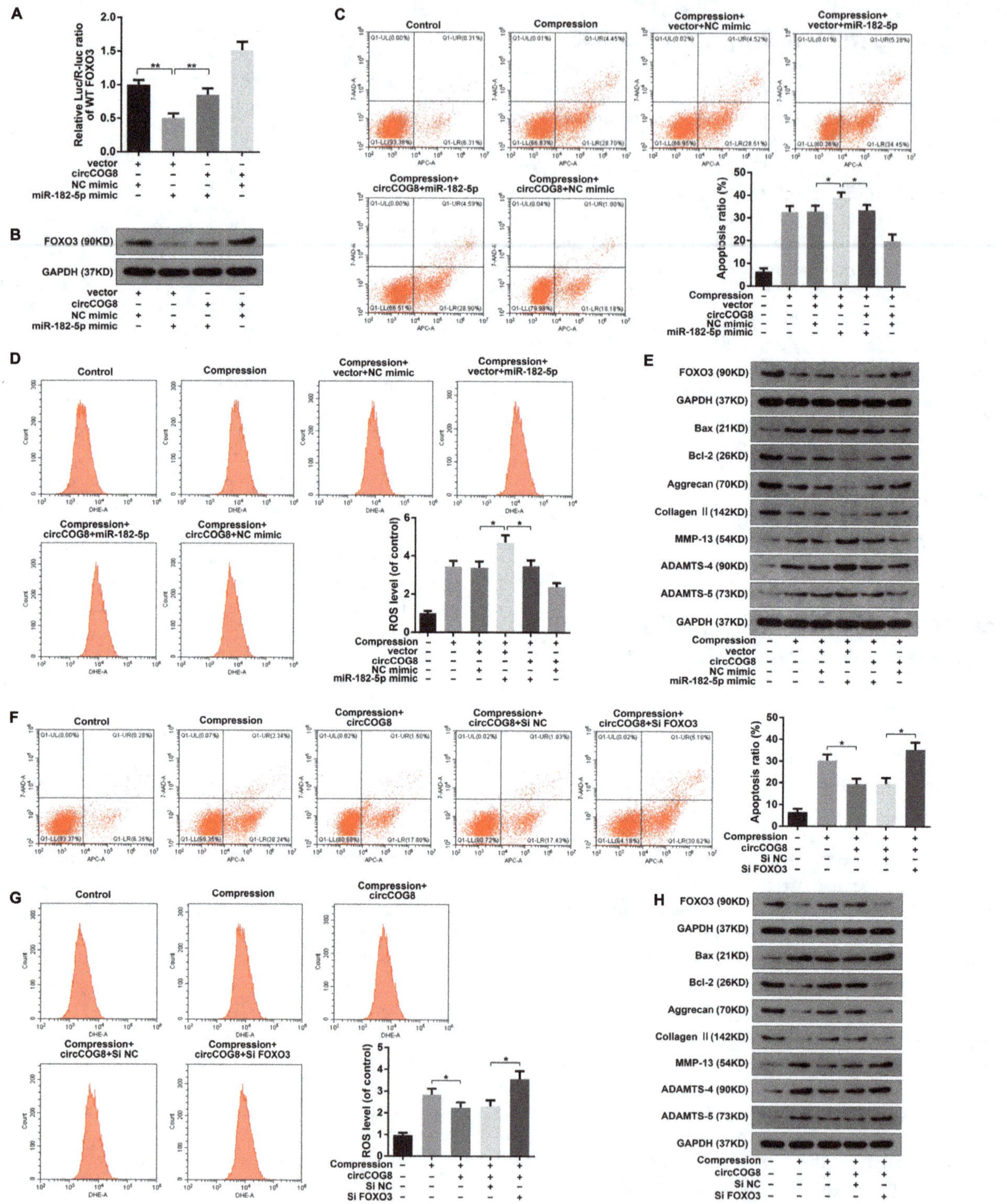


**FIGURE 6 |** CircCOG8 functioned in the disk NP cells by targeting miR-182-5p and FOXO3. **(A)** WT FOXO3 luciferase reporter vector was co-transfected into the HEK-293T cells with the miR-182-5p mimic or NC mimic, thecircCOG8 overexpression or control vector, and the luciferase reporter activity was presented as the relative Luc/R-Luc ratio. **(B)** The FOXO3 protein expression levels of the human NP cells under compression in corresponding groups were examined by the western blot analysis. **(C)** The apoptosis ratio in the NP cells was detected by Annexin V-APC and 7-AAD double-staining. **(D)** The intracellular ROS levels in the NP cells were detected by DHE with the flow cytometry analysis. **(E)** The protein levels of FOXO3, Bax, Bcl-2, Aggrecan, Type II collagen, MMP-13, ADAMTS-4, and ADAMTS-5 were determined by the western blot analysis. The upper GAPDH band served as an internal loading control for FOXO3; the lower GAPDH band served as a common internal loading control for Bax, Bcl-2, Aggrecan, Type II collagen, MMP-13, ADAMTS-4, and ADAMTS-5. **(F)** The Annexin V-APC and 7-AAD double-staining results indicating the apoptosis ratio of the NP cells. **(G)** The intracellular ROS production in the NP cells was detected by DHE with flow cytometry analysis. **(H)** The protein levels of FOXO3, Bax, Bcl-2, Aggrecan, Type II collagen, MMP-13, ADAMTS-4, and ADAMTS-5 were examined by the western blot analysis. The upper GAPDH band served as an internal loading control for FOXO3; the lower GAPDH band served as a common internal loading control for Bax, Bcl-2, Aggrecan, Type II collagen, MMP-13, ADAMTS-4, and ADAMTS-5. Data were represented as mean ± SD. $^{*}p < 0.05$, $^{**}p < 0.01$, $n = 3$ (Student's $t$-test).

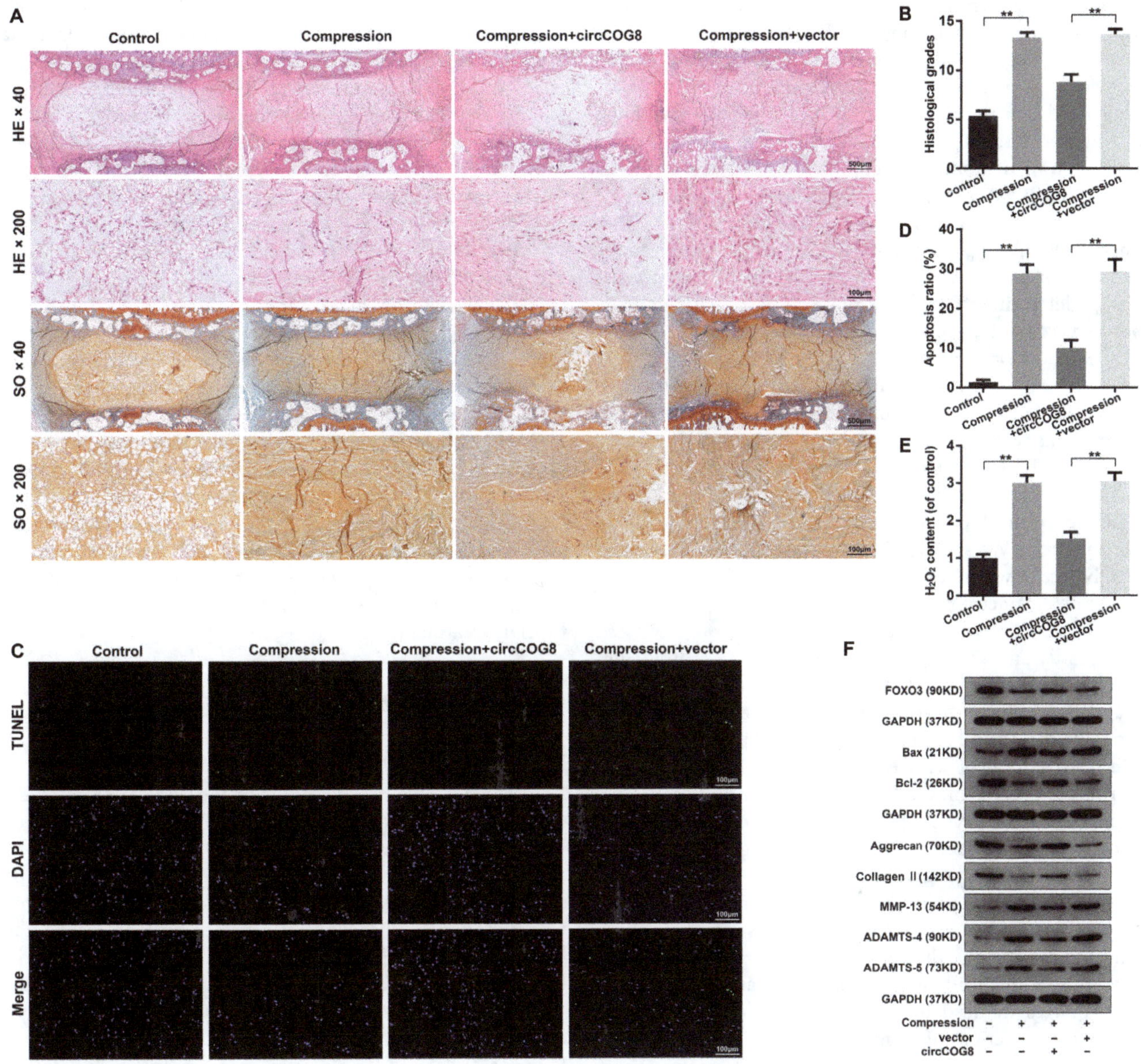


**FIGURE 7 |** CircCOG8 overexpression attenuated the compression-induced IDD *ex vivo*. **(A)** Representative photograph of the rat IVD tissues stained with HE and SO. The images were scanned at × 40 magnification (scale bar = 500 μm) and × 200 magnification (scale bar = 100 μm). **(B)** The histological grades of the disk samples evaluated by the histological grading scale. **(C)** Representative photograph of the TUNEL analysis to examine the NP cell apoptosis (scale bar = 100 μm). **(D)** Quantitative analysis of the TUNEL-positive cells indicating the apoptosis ratio. **(E)** The $H_2O_2$ content in the IVD tissues indicating the ROS level. **(F)** Western blot analysis was used to determine the protein expression level of FOXO3, Bax, Bcl-2, Aggrecan, Type II collagen, MMP-13, ADAMTS-4, and ADAMTS-5. The upper GAPDH band served as an internal loading control for FOXO3; the middle GAPDH band served as a common internal loading control for Bax and Bcl-2; the lower GAPDH band served as a common internal loading control for Aggrecan, Type II collagen, MMP-13, ADAMTS-4, and ADAMTS-5. Data were represented as mean ± SD. $^{*}p < 0.05$, $^{**}p < 0.01$, $n = 6$ IVDs per group (Student's *t*-test).

possesses more than 70 miR-7-binding sites and emerging evidence indicates that the interactions between Cdr1as and its targeting miRNAs are closely associated with the pathology of some human diseases, such as neuropsychiatric disorders, melanoma invasion and metastasis, and β-cell dysfunction in diabetic conditions (Piwecka et al., 2017; Stoll et al., 2018; Hanniford et al., 2020). A previous research by Liu et al. (2017) reported that a dysregulated circular RNA named circRNA-MSR participated in the chondrocyte ECM degradation through binding to miRNAs and, thus, regulating the TNF-α expression during osteoarthritis progression. Emerging evidence has shown several upregulated or downregulated circRNAs in the degenerated disks played an important part in the IDD pathogenesis. For example, a circular RNA hsa_circ_001653 was upregulated in the degenerated disk tissues with close relation to the IVD degeneration degrees. This circRNA could inhibit the NP cell proliferation and ECM synthesis through targeting miR-486-3p to modulate CEMIP, which contributed significantly to the IDD development (Cui and Zhang, 2020). It was reported that a critical circRNA named circVMA21 was downregulated during IDD. CircVMA21 obviously inhibited inflammatory cytokines-induced disk cells apoptosis and ECM degradation by functioning as competing endogenous RNAs to bind to miR-200c and, thus, regulate the targeting gene XIAP (Cheng et al., 2018). There were also several other identified circRNAs reported to participate in the pathogenesis of IDD in the past few years (Li et al., 2019). However, it remains undetermined how circRNAs play a part functionally in the involvement of mechanical loads during the IVD degeneration development.

Although an increasing number of circRNAs have been identified across different eukaryotic species from microorganisms to animals, only a minor fraction of them have been researched for the biological implications (Conn et al., 2015). The circRNA identified in this study was a novel circRNA which played a critical role during the IDD progression involving mechanical stress. We showed that the circCOG8 expression in the disk NP cells was markedly downregulated by mechanical loading as determined by the microarray and RT-qPCR assays. CircCOG8 overexpression significantly alleviated the NP cell ECM degradation, cell apoptosis, and ROS accumulation induced by compression. And, downregulating circCOG8 could aggravate these effects of compression on the disk NP cells. Functionally, the critical microRNA miR-182-5p might mediate the effects of circCOG8 exerted on the disk cells. Using the bioinformatics prediction, the RNA immunoprecipitation assay and reporter gene analysis, we unveiled that circCOG8 could directly interact with miR-182-5p. Interestingly, miR-182-5p was found markedly upregulated in the disk NP cells under mechanical loading in this study. We showed that miR-182-5p facilitated the elevated apoptosis, oxidative stress as well as ECM degradation in the disk NP cells induced by mechanical loading. Inhibiting miR-182-5p markedly attenuated these cellular damages induced by compression loading. Generally, the regulatory function of a microRNA mainly is achieved by interacting with 3′-UTR of targeting mRNA to negatively regulate the gene expression. Using the online miRNA binding predicting tool, we found FOXO3 was an important miR-182-5p targeting gene and we further verified the interaction between them. FOXO3, known as FOXO3a or FKHR-L1, is among the Forkhead box O (FOXO) family of transcription factors which plays a crucial part in the normal physiological structure and function of IVD (Alvarez-Garcia et al., 2018). Previous study revealed that the FOXO3 expression level was obviously downregulated in severe degenerated human IVDs, contributing to the major histopathological changes during IDD progression (Penolazzi et al., 2018). In the present study, we observed that the FOXO3 expression in the NP cells was repressed by compression loading. FOXO3 was identified as the key targeting gene for miR-182-5p and their interaction accounted for a crucial part in the involvement of compression during IVD degeneration. Moreover, circCOG8 evidently neutralized the repressive function of miR-182-5p exerted on FOXO3, suggesting the role of circCOG8 as an miR-182-5p sponge to modulate the FOXO3 expression. We further validated that the absence of FOXO3 could counteract the protective effect of circCOG8 on human NP cells under compression loading by using the siRNA-mediated FOXO3 knockdown. However, the underlying mechanism by which circCOG8 and miR-182-5p could respond to mechanical stress still needed further investigation. Taken together, this study revealed that circCOG8 attenuated the mechanical stress induced damage in NP cells via restoring the FOXO3 expression achieved by sponging the miR-182-5p.

Collectively, the major findings from our study can be summarized as the following. (1) CircCOG8, derived from the third exon of COG8 gene, is a novel identified circRNA that functionally participates in the involvement of mechanical stress during IDD progression. (2) CircCOG8 can directly interact with miR-182-5p and, thus, modulate the FOXO3 expression in NP cells. (3) Compression-induced circCOG8 downregulation is an important underlying mechanism in the NP cell ECM degradation, cell apoptosis, and ROS accumulation via regulating the miR-182-5p/FOXO3 axis. In conclusion, the present study suggested that targeting the circCOG8/miR-182-5p/FOXO3 pathway provides a new therapeutic strategy for IDD treatment.

## MATERIALS AND METHODS

### Patient Samples

The present study was supervised by the Clinical Research Ethics Committee of Tongji Medical College, Huazhong University of Science and Technology, and all methods were used in strict adherence with the approved guidelines. The IVD tissue specimens were obtained from patients with idiopathic scoliosis who underwent spinal surgery. Informed consents were obtained from all subjects. Patients' medical records were collected and the IVD degeneration degrees were assessed by the Pfirrmann MRI-grading system (Pfirrmann et al., 2001). Generally, six disk tissue specimens were collected from two males and four females, aged 17–26 years old (mean: 21.3 years). The Pfirrmann grades of these disk samples were generally evaluated as Grade I or II. Among these specimens, three NP tissues were used to isolate the disk NP cells for the circRNA microarray assay and the other three were used for further *in vitro* experiments.

### Primary Cells Culture

The disk NP tissue samples were dissected and digested using 0.25% pronase for 0.5 h and 0.2% type II collagenase for 4 h at 37°C. After filtering through a 70 μm pore size mesh, the NP cells were transferred to Dulbecco's modified Eagle medium (DMEM; Gibco, United States) with 15% fetal bovine serum (FBS; Gibco, United States), streptomycin (100 mg/ml; Gibco, United States) as well as penicillin (100 units/ml; Gibco, United States). The NP cells were cultured at 37°C in a $CO_2$ incubator with a controlled humidified atmosphere composed of 95% air and 5% $CO_2$. The culture medium was replaced every 3 days. The second-generation cells were used in this study. For the compression treatment, the disk NP cells were treated by a previously described compression device to provide 1 MPa static mechanical loading (Wu et al., 2019). Briefly, the stainless pressure vessel allowed for pumping compressed gas into it to form a closed high-pressure environment which was monitored with a barometer. The pressure vessel was pumped into the mixed 0.5% $CO_2$ and 99.5% compressed air and the cells were placed in cell culture plates under humidified atmosphere at 37°C. Unless otherwise specified in the figures, the NP cells were treated under mechanical stress for 36 h.

## Western Blotting

Samples were lysed by a radio immunoprecipitation lysis buffer and their protein contents were determined by an Enhanced BCA Protein Assay Kit (Beyotime, China). After centrifugation, the lysates were run by sodium dodecyl sulfate-polyacrylamide gel electrophoresis gels and transferred onto the polyvinylidene fluoride membranes. Then, the membranes were blocked for 1 h at 25°C with 5% non-fat dried milk in TBST, incubated overnight at 4°C with primary antibody. The membranes were subsequently incubated with the HRP-conjugated secondary antibody (dilution 1:2,000; Abcam). Protein bands were detected with enhanced chemiluminescence reagents (Amersham). The primary antibodies used are as follows: Bax (ab32503, Abcam), Bcl-2 (ab196495, Abcam), ADAMTS-4 (ab185722, Abcam), ADAMTS-5 (ab41037, Abcam), MMP-13 (ab39012, Abcam), aggrecan (13880-1-AP, Proteintech), Type II collagen (ab34712, Abcam), and FOXO3 (ab23683, Abcam). GAPDH (#5174, Cell Signaling Technology) was used as controls.

## Flow Cytometry Analysis

The NP cell samples after various treatments were harvested and the apoptosis rates were examined by the dual-staining with Annexin V-APC and 7-AAD (KeyGen Biotech). Cell samples were washed twice by PBS and resuspended with the binding buffer then doubly stained with annexin-V and 7-AAD. And, the intracellular ROS production were examined by an ROS-specific fluorescent probe dihydroethidium (DHE, Beyotime). The stained cells from each experiment were analyzed by the FACSCalibur flow cytometer (Becton Dickinson).

## RNA Extraction and qPCR Assay

Total cellular RNA extraction was performed with the TRIzol method following the merchant guide. The NE-PER Nuclear and Cytoplasmic Extraction Reagents (Thermo Scientific) were applied to isolate the nuclear and cytoplasmic fractions, following manufacturer's protocols. The first-strand cDNA was obtained from total RNA via a PrimeScript RT reagent kit (Takara Bio). The qPCR was carried out using SYBR Green Supermix (BioRad) and All-in-One miRNA RT-qPCR Kit (GeneCopoeia, Inc.). GAPDH was used as the internal control for mRNA and circRNA, and U6 was used to normalize miRNA level. Primers used in this study are as follows: *circCOG8* F, TTCAATGATCTGCGCCTCTG; *circCOG8* R, TTGGTCCTCAGTTGCTGGAT; *GAPDH* F, GTCTTCACCACCATGGAGAA; *GAPDH* R, TAAGC AGTTGGTGGTGCAG; *U6* F, CTCGCTTCGGCAGCACA; *U6* R, AACGCTTCACGAATTTGCGT; *MiR-182-5p stem-loop primer*, GTCGTATCCAGTGCAGGGTC CGAGGTATTCGCACTGGATACGACAGTGTG. *Divergent-circCOG8* F, ATGCTCATCTCGGCTCCAG; *Divergent-circCOG8* R, AGGAATGGCAGTCAGGATGG; *Convergent-circCOG8* F, CCATCCTGACTGCCATTCCT; *Convergent-circCOG8* R, CTGGAGCCGAGATGAGCAT; *Divergent-GAPDH* F, CACTTTGTCAAGCTCATTTCC; *Divergent-GAPDH* R, TTGGCAGTGGGGACACGGAAG; *Convergent-GAPDH* F, TCCATGCCATCACTGCCAC; and *Convergent-GAPDH* R, GTGGTCGTTGAGGGCAATG.

## Circular RNA Microarray and Bioinformatics Analysis

Total cellular RNA from mechanical loading treated the disk NP cells or corresponding control cells was isolated to carry out the microarray assay. And, the circRNAs microarray assay was performed by the CapitalBio Corporation (Beijing, China) according to standard procedures. The GeneSpring GX software was used to analyze the microarray data. The thresholds were set as follows: fold change > 2, $P$-value < 0.05 evaluated using the Student's $t$-test. Clustered heat map was made to present the significantly down-regulated gene items in mechanical loading treated disk cells. The targeting miRNA of circCOG8 was predicted using the StarBase online database[1] and the Circular RNA Interactome online database[2]. And, the targeting genes of miR-182-5p were predicted based on the TargetScan online tool[3] as well as the miRDB[4]. Microarray raw data used in this study were available from the corresponding author upon reasonable request.

## RNase R Treatment

Total cellular RNA (2 μg) extracted from the human disk NP cells was treated with 3 unit/μg of RNase R and the samples were incubated for 0.5 h at 37°C. GAPDH mRNA was used as the linear control group. Three independent experiments were performed with triplicate samples.

## Luciferase Reporter Assay

The HEK-293T cells were cultured in 24-well plates to 60% confluence. Then, the cells were co-transfected with a luciferase reporter construct and miR-182-5p overexpression construct. The corresponding reporter construct of the WT pMIR-REPORT-circCOG8 as well as the MUT pMIR-REPORT-circCOG8 and the WT pMIR-REPORT-FOXO3-3′ UTR as well as the MUT

[1] http://starbase.sysu.edu.cn
[2] http://circinteractome.nia.nih.gov
[3] http://www.targetscan.org
[4] http://www.mirdb.org

pMIR-REPORT-FOXO3-3'UTR were obtained from the Obio Technology, Corp. 48 h after the transfection by lipofectamine 3000, the cells were assayed with the dual-luciferase reporter assay system (Promega), and measurements were performed on the Beckman–Coulter DTX880. Relative luciferase activity was presented as the Luc/R-Luc ratio by dividing the firefly luciferase (Luc) value by the *Renilla* luciferase (R-Luc) value.

## RNA-Binding Protein Immunoprecipitation (RIP)

The RIP analysis was carried out by using a Magna RIP RNA-Binding Protein Immunoprecipitation Kit (EMD Millipore Corporation, Billerica, MA, United States) combined with the human anti-AGO2 antibody (#2897, Cell signaling), according to the merchant guide. Briefly, after pelleting and re-suspending by RIP lysis buffer, the cells extract was treated with the RIP buffer containing A/G magnetic beads conjugated with an anti-AGO2 antibody or corresponding control IgG. Co-precipitated circCOG8, as well as miR-182-5p, was subsequently examined using the RT-qPCR assay.

## Cell Transfection

For the circCOG8 overexpression, exon 3 of human COG8 gene (828 bp) with approximate 1 kb flanking introns containing complementary Alu elements were amplified to construct the recombinant adenovirus vector (Obio Technology, Shanghai, China), as described previously (Zhang et al., 2014). For the lentiviral circCOG8 shRNA construction, oligonucleotides with the circCOG8 targeting sequences were inserted to the pLKD-CMV-G&PR-U6-shRNA vector (Obio Technology, Shanghai, China). Targeting sequence for circCOG8: CCAAGGGCATCGTGAACGA, negative control sequence: TTCTCCGAACGTGTCACGT. MiR-182-5p mimic, miR-182-5p inhibitor, as well as their corresponding negative controls, were produced by the GenePharma, Corp. FOXO3 siRNA (targeting sequence: GCATGTTCAATGGGAGCTTGGA) and its control siRNA was purchased from the Obio Technology, Corp. The NP cells were cultured with six-well plates to 70–80% confluence and then, the cell transfection was achieved by the Lipofectamine 3000 transfection reagent (Invitrogen, United States), according to the merchant guide.

## IVD Organ Model Culture

Rat IVDs of Co6/7 and Co7/8 were collected from Sprague-Dawley rats of 3 months, with an approval from the Animal Experimentation Committee of Huazhong University of Science and Technology. Interact disks were meticulously isolated and cultured by the DMEM (Gibco, United States) with 15% FBS (Gibco, United States), streptomycin (100 mg/ml; Gibco, United States) as well as penicillin (100 units/ml; Gibco, United States), according to our previous study (Wu et al., 2019). The IVDs were cultured at 37°C and the medium was replaced every 3 days. For the compression treatment, the IVD organ model was placed on the culture plates in the compression device which could provide 1 MPa static compression, as described above. According to the classic air-pressure principle, the custom-made compression apparatus was applied, as previously described, to expose the IVDs to static high pressure (Hutton et al., 1999; Wu et al., 2019). And, the IVDs were treated under continuous mechanical loading except for the time when the culture medium was replaced.

## CircRNA Injection Into *ex vivo* Cultured IVD Models

The adeno-associated virus (AAV) vector overexpressing circCOG8 and the control vector were constructed and packaged by the Obio Technology (Shanghai, China). The *ex vivo* IVD organs were randomly divided into four groups: control group ($n$ = 6), compression group ($n$ = 6), circCOG8 injection with compression group ($n$ = 6), and control vector injection with compression group ($n$ = 6). The *ex vivo* disks were injected with a 2 μl solution containing the experimental virus vector overexpressing circCOG8 or the control virus vector by using the 33-G needle. Then, the cultured IVDs were treated under a static mechanical loading for 4 weeks.

## Histological Evaluation, TUNEL Staining, and ROS Measurement in *ex vivo* Cultured IVD Models

The rat disk tissues were collected and rinsed using PBS. Disk samples were fixed by formalin and decalcified using EDTA. Then, the disks were embedded in paraffin, sectioned, and stained using the hematoxylin-eosin, as well as the safranin O. Histological evaluation grades were determined according to a previous study (Mao et al., 2011). The *in situ* apoptotic activity was examined by the TUNEL Apoptosis Assay Kit (C1088, Beyotime, China). The specimens were overlaid by the Vectashield Hard Set mounting medium containing DAPI. TUNEL positive cells were counted from three different fields of disk NP and the ratio of positive cells relative to total was determined. The ROS level in IVD tissues was measured by the Hydrogen Peroxide assay kit (NJJCbio, Nanjing, China), following the merchant guide.

## Statistical Analysis

The data were expressed as a mean value ± standard deviation (SD). Each experiment was repeated independently for three times, unless otherwise indicated. All data in the study were processed by the GraphPad Prism 7.0 software. Statistical significance was analyzed using the Student's $t$-test for two-group comparisons, one-way analysis of variance (ANOVA) with Tukey's post-test for multiple group comparisons. Significance levels were set as $^{*}p < 0.05$, $^{**}p < 0.01$.

## ETHICS STATEMENT

The animal study was reviewed and approved by the Animal Experimentation Committee of Huazhong University of Science and Technology.

## AUTHOR CONTRIBUTIONS

QX and LK designed the study protocol. QX, LK, KZ, JW, WH, YS, XF, and SL performed the experiments. KZ, GL, and KW collected and analyzed data. QX, LK, and KZ wrote the manuscript. CY and YZ reviewed and revised the manuscript. YZ supported and supervised the study. All authors contributed to the article and approved the submitted version.

## REFERENCES


Adams, M. A., and Roughley, P. J. (2006). What is intervertebral disc degeneration, and what causes it? *Spine* 31, 2151–2161. doi: 10.1097/01.brs.0000231761.73859.2c

Alvarez-Garcia, O., Matsuzaki, T., Olmer, M., Miyata, K., Mokuda, S., Sakai, D., et al. (2018). FOXO are required for intervertebral disk homeostasis during aging and their deficiency promotes disk degeneration. *Aging Cell* 17:e12800. doi: 10.1111/acel.12800

Bartel, D. P. (2004). MicroRNAs: genomics, biogenesis, mechanism, and function. *Cell* 116, 281–297.

Chen, B., Wei, W., Huang, X., Xie, X., Kong, Y., Dai, D., et al. (2018). circEPSTI1 as a prognostic marker and mediator of triple-negative breast cancer progression. *Theranostics* 8, 4003–4015. doi: 10.7150/thno.24106

Chen, S., Lv, X., Hu, B., Zhao, L., Li, S., Li, Z., et al. (2018). Critical contribution of RIPK1 mediated mitochondrial dysfunction and oxidative stress to compression-induced rat nucleus pulposus cells necroptosis and apoptosis. *Apoptosis* 23, 299–313. doi: 10.1007/s10495-018-1455-x

Cheng, X., Zhang, L., Zhang, K., Zhang, G., Hu, Y., Sun, X., et al. (2018). Circular RNA VMA21 protects against intervertebral disc degeneration through targeting miR-200c and X linked inhibitor-of-apoptosis protein. *Ann. Rheum. Dis.* 77, 770–779. doi: 10.1136/annrheumdis-2017-212056

Conn, S. J., Pillman, K. A., Toubia, J., Conn, V. M., Salmanidis, M., Phillips, C. A., et al. (2015). The RNA binding protein quaking regulates formation of circRNAs. *Cell* 160, 1125–1134. doi: 10.1016/j.cell.2015.02.014

Cui, S., and Zhang, L. (2020). circ_001653 silencing promotes the proliferation and ECM synthesis of NPCs in IDD by downregulating miR-486-3p-mediated CEMIP. *Mol. Ther. Nucleic Acids* 20, 385–399. doi: 10.1016/j.omtn.2020.01.026

Feng, C., Yang, M., Lan, M., Liu, C., Zhang, Y., Huang, B., et al. (2017). ROS: crucial intermediators in the pathogenesis of intervertebral disc degeneration. *Oxid. Med. Cell. Longev.* 2017:5601593. doi: 10.1155/2017/5601593

Gilchrist, C. L., Darling, E. M., Chen, J., and Setton, L. A. (2011). Extracellular matrix ligand and stiffness modulate immature nucleus pulposus cell-cell interactions. *PLoS One* 6:e27170. doi: 10.1371/journal.pone.0027170

Glaeser, J. D., Salehi, K., Kanim, L. E. A., NaPier, Z., Kropf, M. A., Cuéllar, J. M., et al. (2020). NF-κB inhibitor, NEMO-binding domain peptide attenuates intervertebral disc degeneration. *Spine J.* 20, 1480–1491. doi: 10.1016/j.spinee.2020.04.025

Han, B., Chao, J., and Yao, H. (2018). Circular RNA and its mechanisms in disease: from the bench to the clinic. *Pharmacol. Ther.* 187, 31–44. doi: 10.1016/j.pharmthera.2018.01.010

Hanniford, D., Ulloa-Morales, A., Karz, A., Berzoti-Coelho, M. G., Moubarak, R. S., Sánchez-Sendra, B., et al. (2020). Epigenetic silencing of CDR1as drives IGF2BP3-mediated melanoma invasion and metastasis. *Cancer Cell* 37, 55.e15–70.e15. doi: 10.1016/j.ccell.2019.12.007

Hansen, T. B., Jensen, T. I., Clausen, B. H., Bramsen, J. B., Finsen, B., Damgaard, C. K., et al. (2013). Natural RNA circles function as efficient microRNA sponges. *Nature* 495, 384–388. doi: 10.1038/nature11993

Holguin, N., and Silva, M. J. (2018). In-vivo nucleus pulposus-specific regulation of adult murine intervertebral disc degeneration via Wnt/Beta-catenin signaling. *Sci. Rep.* 8:11191. doi: 10.1038/s41598-018-29352-3

Hoy, D. G., Smith, E., Cross, M., Sanchez-Riera, L., Buchbinder, R., Blyth, F. M., et al. (2014). The global burden of musculoskeletal conditions for 2010: an overview of methods. *Ann. Rheum. Dis.* 73:982. doi: 10.1136/annrheumdis-2013-204344

Huang, D., Peng, Y., Ma, K., Qing, X., Deng, X., Li, Z., et al. (2020). Puerarin relieved compression-induced apoptosis and mitochondrial dysfunction in human nucleus pulposus mesenchymal stem cells via the PI3K/Akt pathway. *Stem Cells Int.* 2020:7126914. doi: 10.1155/2020/7126914

Hughes, S. P., Freemont, A. J., Hukins, D. W., McGregor, A. H., and Roberts, S. (2012). The pathogenesis of degeneration of the intervertebral disc and emerging therapies in the management of back pain. *J. Bone Joint Surg. Br.* 94, 1298–1304. doi: 10.1302/0301-620x.94b10.28986

Hutton, W. C., Elmer, W. A., Boden, S. D., Hyon, S., Toribatake, Y., Tomita, K., et al. (1999). The effect of hydrostatic pressure on intervertebral disc metabolism. *Spine* 24:1507. doi: 10.1097/00007632-199908010-00002

Jiang, Y., Dong, G., and Song, Y. (2018). Nucleus pulposus cell senescence is alleviated by resveratrol through regulating the ROS/NF-κB pathway under high-magnitude compression. *Biosci. Rep.* 38:BSR20180670. doi: 10.1042/bsr20180670

Kleaveland, B., Shi, C. Y., Stefano, J., and Bartel, D. P. (2018). A network of noncoding regulatory RNAs acts in the mammalian brain. *Cell* 174, 350.e17–362.e17. doi: 10.1016/j.cell.2018.05.022

Koerner, J. D., Markova, D. Z., Schroeder, G. D., Rihn, J. A., Hilibrand, A. S., Vaccaro, A. R., et al. (2016). The effect of substance p on an intervertebral disc rat organ culture model. *Spine* 41, 1851–1859. doi: 10.1097/brs.0000000000001676

Lee, C. R., Iatridis, J. C., Poveda, L., and Alini, M. (2006). In vitro organ culture of the bovine intervertebral disc: effects of vertebral endplate and potential for mechanobiology studies. *Spine* 31, 515–522. doi: 10.1097/01.brs.0000201302.59050.72

Li, P., Hou, G., Zhang, R., Gan, Y., Xu, Y., Song, L., et al. (2017). High-magnitude compression accelerates the premature senescence of nucleus pulposus cells via the p38 MAPK-ROS pathway. *Arthritis Res. Ther.* 19:209. doi: 10.1186/s13075-017-1384-z

Li, S., Hua, W., Wang, K., Gao, Y., Chen, S., Liu, W., et al. (2018). Autophagy attenuates compression-induced apoptosis of human nucleus pulposus cells via MEK/ERK/NRF1/Atg7 signaling pathways during intervertebral disc degeneration. *Exp. Cell Res.* 370, 87–97. doi: 10.1016/j.yexcr.2018.06.012

Li, X., Yang, L., and Chen, L. L. (2018). The biogenesis, functions, and challenges of circular RNAs. *Mol. Cell.* 71, 428–442. doi: 10.1016/j.molcel.2018.06.034

Li, Z., Chen, X., Xu, D., Li, S., Chan, M. T. V., and Wu, W. K. K. (2019). Circular RNAs in nucleus pulposus cell function and intervertebral disc degeneration. *Cell. Prolif.* 52:e12704. doi: 10.1111/cpr.12704

Li, Z., Yu, X., Shen, J., Chan, M. T., and Wu, W. K. (2015). MicroRNA in intervertebral disc degeneration. *Cell. Prolif.* 48, 278–283. doi: 10.1111/cpr.12180

Lin, H., Ma, X., Wang, B. C., Zhao, L., Liu, J. X., Pu, F. F., et al. (2017). Edaravone ameliorates compression-induced damage in rat nucleus pulposus cells. *Life Sci.* 189, 76–83. doi: 10.1016/j.lfs.2017.09.024

Liu, G., Huang, K., Jie, Z., Wu, Y., Chen, J., Chen, Z., et al. (2018). CircFAT1 sponges miR-375 to promote the expression of Yes-associated protein 1 in osteosarcoma cells. *Mol. Cancer* 17:170. doi: 10.1186/s12943-018-0917-7

Liu, Q., Zhang, X., Hu, X., Yuan, L., Cheng, J., Jiang, Y., et al. (2017). Emerging roles of circRNA related to the mechanical stress in human cartilage degradation of osteoarthritis. *Mol. Ther. Nucleic Acids* 7, 223–230. doi: 10.1016/j.omtn.2017.04.004

Liu, W., Zhang, Y., Xia, P., Li, S., Feng, X., Gao, Y., et al. (2016). MicroRNA-7 regulates IL-1beta-induced extracellular matrix degeneration by targeting GDF5 in human nucleus pulposus cells. *Biomed. Pharmacother.* 83, 1414–1421. doi: 10.1016/j.biopha.2016.08.062

MacLean, J. J., Lee, C. R., Alini, M., and Iatridis, J. C. (2005). The effects of short-term load duration on anabolic and catabolic gene expression in the rat tail intervertebral disc. *J. Orthop. Res.* 23, 1120–1127. doi: 10.1016/j.orthres.2005.01.020

Mao, H. J., Chen, Q. X., Han, B., Li, F. C., Feng, J., Shi, Z. L., et al. (2011). The effect of injection volume on disc degeneration in a rat tail model. *Spine* 36, E1062–E1069. doi: 10.1097/BRS.0b013e3182027d42

Memczak, S., Jens, M., Elefsinioti, A., Torti, F., Krueger, J., Rybak, A., et al. (2013). Circular RNAs are a large class of animal RNAs with regulatory potency. *Nature* 495, 333–338. doi: 10.1038/nature11928

Neidlinger-Wilke, C., Galbusera, F., Pratsinis, H., Mavrogonatou, E., Mietsch, A., Kletsas, D., et al. (2014). Mechanical loading of the intervertebral disc: from the macroscopic to the cellular level. *Eur. Spine J.* 23(Suppl. 3), S333–S343. doi: 10.1007/s00586-013-2855-9

Penolazzi, L., Lambertini, E., Bergamin, L. S., Roncada, T., De Bonis, P., Cavallo, M., et al. (2018). MicroRNA-221 silencing attenuates the degenerated phenotype of intervertebral disc cells. *Aging* 10, 2001–2015. doi: 10.18632/aging.101525

Pfirrmann, C. W., Metzdorf, A., Zanetti, M., Hodler, J., and Boos, N. (2001). Magnetic resonance classification of lumbar intervertebral disc degeneration. *Spine* 26, 1873–1878. doi: 10.1097/00007632-200109010-00011

Piwecka, M., Glažar, P., Hernandez-Miranda, L. R., Memczak, S., Wolf, S. A., Rybak-Wolf, A., et al. (2017). Loss of a mammalian circular RNA locus causes miRNA deregulation and affects brain function. *Science* 357:eaam8526. doi: 10.1126/science.aam8526

Risbud, M. V., and Shapiro, I. M. (2014). Role of cytokines in intervertebral disc degeneration: pain and disc content. *Nat. Rev. Rheumatol.* 10, 44–56. doi: 10.1038/nrrheum.2013.160

Roberts, S., Evans, H., Trivedi, J., and Menage, J. (2006). Histology and pathology of the human intervertebral disc. *J. Bone Joint Surg. Am.* 88(Suppl. 2), 10–14. doi: 10.2106/jbjs.F.00019

Roughley, P. J. (2004). Biology of intervertebral disc aging and degeneration: involvement of the extracellular matrix. *Spine* 29, 2691–2699. doi: 10.1097/01.brs.0000146101.53784.b1

Sakai, D., and Grad, S. (2015). Advancing the cellular and molecular therapy for intervertebral disc disease. *Adv. Drug Deliv. Rev* 84, 159–171. doi: 10.1016/j.addr.2014.06.009

Sakai, D., Nakamura, Y., Nakai, T., Mishima, T., Kato, S., Grad, S., et al. (2012). Exhaustion of nucleus pulposus progenitor cells with ageing and degeneration of the intervertebral disc. *Nat. Commun.* 3:1264. doi: 10.1038/ncomms2226

Setton, L. A., and Chen, J. (2006). Mechanobiology of the intervertebral disc and relevance to disc degeneration. *J. Bone Joint Surg. Am.* 88(Suppl. 2), 52–57. doi: 10.2106/jbjs.F.00001

Song, J., Wang, H. L., Song, K. H., Ding, Z. W., Wang, H. L., Ma, X. S., et al. (2018). CircularRNA_104670 plays a critical role in intervertebral disc degeneration by functioning as a ceRNA. *Exp. Mol. Med.* 50:94. doi: 10.1038/s12276-018-0125-y

Stoll, L., Sobel, J., Rodriguez-Trejo, A., Guay, C., Lee, K., Venø, M. T., et al. (2018). Circular RNAs as novel regulators of β-cell functions in normal and disease conditions. *Mol. Metab.* 9, 69–83. doi: 10.1016/j.molmet.2018.01.010

Wilke, H. J., Neef, P., Caimi, M., Hoogland, T., and Claes, L. E. (1999). New in vivo measurements of pressures in the intervertebral disc in daily life. *Spine* 24, 755–762. doi: 10.1097/00007632-199904150-00005

Wu, X., Liao, Z., Wang, K., Hua, W., Liu, X., Song, Y., et al. (2019). Targeting the IL-1beta/IL-1Ra pathways for the aggregation of human islet amyloid polypeptide in an ex vivo organ culture system of the intervertebral disc. *Exp. Mol. Med.* 51:110. doi: 10.1038/s12276-019-0310-7

Yurube, T., Takada, T., Suzuki, T., Kakutani, K., Maeno, K., Doita, M., et al. (2012). Rat tail static compression model mimics extracellular matrix metabolic imbalances of matrix metalloproteinases, aggrecanases, and tissue inhibitors of metalloproteinases in intervertebral disc degeneration. *Arthritis Res. Ther.* 14:R51. doi: 10.1186/ar3764

Zhang, X. O., Wang, H. B., Zhang, Y., Lu, X., Chen, L. L., and Yang, L. (2014). Complementary sequence-mediated exon circularization. *Cell* 159, 134–147. doi: 10.1016/j.cell.2014.09.001

Zhao, C. Q., Wang, L. M., Jiang, L. S., and Dai, L. Y. (2007). The cell biology of intervertebral disc aging and degeneration. *Ageing Res. Rev.* 6, 247–261. doi: 10.1016/j.arr.2007.08.001

Zhao, Z. J., and Shen, J. (2017). Circular RNA participates in the carcinogenesis and the malignant behavior of cancer. *RNA Biol.* 14, 514–521. doi: 10.1080/15476286.2015.1122162

2

# Src Homology 2 Domain-Containing Protein Tyrosine Phosphatase Promotes Inflammation and Accelerates Osteoarthritis by Activating β-Catenin

*Tenghui Tao[1], Danni Luo[1], Chenghao Gao[1], Hui Liu[1], Zehua Lei[1], Wenbin Liu[1], Chuankun Zhou[1], Dahu Qi[1], Zhenhan Deng[2], Xuying Sun[1]* and Jun Xiao[1]**

*[1] Department of Orthopedics, Tongji Hospital, Tongji Medical College, Huazhong University of Science and Technology, Wuhan, China, [2] Department of Sports Medicine, The First Affiliated Hospital of Shenzhen University, Shenzhen Second People's Hospital, Shenzhen, China*

***Correspondence:**
*Xuying Sun*
*Xuying_Sun@hust.edu.cn*
*Jun Xiao*
*Jun_Xiao@hust.edu.cn*

Osteoarthritis (OA) is a chronic articular disease characterized by cartilage degradation, subchondral bone remodeling and osteophyte formation. Src homology 2 domain-containing protein tyrosine phosphatase (SHP2) has not been fully investigated in the pathogenesis of OA. In this study, we found that SHP2 expression was significantly increased after interleukin-1β (IL-1β) treatment in primary mouse chondrocytes. Inhibition of SHP2 using siRNA reduced MMP3, MMP13 levels, but increased AGGRECAN, COL2A1, SOX9 expression *in vitro*. On the contrary, overexpression of SHP2 exerted the opposite results and promoted cartilage degradation. Mechanistically, SHP2 activated Wnt/β-catenin signaling possibly through directly binding to β-catenin. SHP2 also induced inflammation through activating Mitogen-activated protein kinase (MAPK) and nuclear factor κB (NF-κB) pathways. Our *in vivo* studies showed that SHP2 knockdown effectively delayed cartilage destruction and reduced osteophyte formation in the mouse model of OA induced by destabilization of the medial meniscus (DMM). Altogether, our study identifies that SHP2 is a novel and potential therapeutic target of OA.

**Keywords: SHP2, osteoarthritis, chondrocytes, β-catenin, MAPK, NF-κB**

## INTRODUCTION

Osteoarthritis (OA) is the most common chronic joint disorder characterized by increased pain and joint dysfunction. It was once regarded as a disease of purely mechanical cartilage degradation. However, increased research and knowledge have revealed it to be a complex condition affecting the whole joint (Glyn-Jones et al., 2015). The pathology of OA includes the loss of articular cartilage, hypertrophic differentiation of chondrocytes, subchondral bone remodeling, synovial inflammation, and osteophyte formation (Li et al., 2018). In such inflammatory condition, terminally differentiated hypertrophic chondrocytes abnormally release several kinds of growth factors, cathepsins, and matrix metalloproteases (MMPs), which disturb the coordinated coupling between osteoclastogenesis and matrix remodeling at the chondro-osseous front, leading to cartilage degradation (Naski et al., 1998; Uusitalo et al., 2000; Stickens et al., 2004; Nakashima et al., 2011). The most well-known mechanisms of OA include the increased expression of matrix-degrading enzymes like MMPs, a disintegrin and metalloproteinases (ADAMTS), and the degradation of COL2A1 (collagen, type II, alpha 1) and AGGRECAN (Hollander et al., 1995; Lark et al., 1995; Neuhold et al., 2001; Glasson et al., 2005). Recently, an increasing amount of new molecules have been reported to be responsible for the degeneration of articular cartilage, such as tyrosine kinase Fyn, complement C5, Yes-associated protein, and hypoxia-inducible factor-2α. Dysregulation of these proteins is correlated with abnormal signaling pathways, such as the Wnt, Mitogen-activated protein kinase (MAPK), and nuclear factor κB (NF-κB) pathway (Wang et al., 2011; Deng et al., 2018; Li et al., 2018). However, the exact molecular mechanisms crucial for OA remain to be fully elucidated, because there is still a lack of effective targets for the treatment of such disease. Exploring new pathogenic factors and accurate signaling pathways will pave the way and provide new strategies for developing novel medications for the disease.

SHP2, encoded by *Ptpn11*, is a ubiquitously expressed Src homology 2 domain-containing protein tyrosine phosphatase, which has been proved to be involved in several kinds of bone diseases (Kamiya et al., 2014). Mesenchymal stem cell (MSC)-specific SHP2 knock-out mice develop a distinct increased number of terminally differentiated chondrocytes, accompanied by severe chondrodysplasia and completely blocked osteogenesis, resulting in various skeletal defects including postnatal growth retardation, delayed closure of the skull, pectus carinatum, and limb deformity. Consistently, the MAPK and protein kinase B (Akt) signal pathways are also suppressed (Lapinski et al., 2013). Conditional knockout of SHP2 in osteoclasts significantly suppresses receptor activator of nuclear factor (NF)-κB ligand (RANKL)-mediated signaling and impairs osteoclast (OCL) precursor cells differentiation or maturation (Zhou et al., 2015). These studies strongly indicate the vital role of SHP2 in bone remodeling. Besides, several studies have been conducted about SHP2 in OA. For example, one study revealed that long non-coding RNA named MM2P can prevent SHP2-mediated dephosphorylation of STAT3, the activation of which promotes transcription of chondrocyte-specific protein *Sox9* and contributes to cartilage repairment (Bai et al., 2020). Recently, Keisuke reported that the *Ptpn11* gene is up-regulated in fibroblast-like synoviocytes of rheumatoid arthritis (RA) compared to that of OA (Maeshima et al., 2016). However, the effect of SHP2 on OA progress remains elusive.

In our study, we found SHP2 is accumulated in the primary chondrocytes after IL-1β stimulation. We further investigated the role of SHP2 in OA by regulating SHP2 expression both *in vitro* and *in vivo*. The results demonstrated that inhibition of SHP2 alleviated the cartilage destruction in chondrocytes by targeting β-catenin signaling. Consistently, SHP2 knockdown delayed cartilage degradation in OA animal model. This study provided a potential novel therapeutic target for treating OA.

# MATERIALS AND METHODS

## Reagents and Antibodies

Recombinant mouse IL-1β was purchased from R&D Systems (Minneapolis, MN, United States). Lipofectamine 3000 reagent was obtained from Invitrogen (Waltham, MA, United States). Anti-SHP2, β-catenin, p38, p-p38, extracellular signal-regulated kinase (ERK), p-ERK, c-Jun N-terminal kinase (JNK), p-JNK, p65, p-p65, IκBα, p-IκBα, IκB kinase (IKK)-β and p-IKKα/β antibodies were supplied by Cell Signaling Technology (Beverly, MA, United States). MMP3, MMP13 and p-β-catenin(Y142) antibodies were obtained from Abcam (Cambridge, United Kingdom). p-β-catenin(S33/37/141), COL2A1, and AGGRECAN antibodies were purchased from Abclonal (Wuhan, China). GAPDH antibody was purchased from Boster (Wuhan, China) and secondary antibodies were obtained from the Jackson lab.

## Isolation and Culture of Primary Chondrocytes

Knee joint cartilages were dissected from newborn mice (5-days-old) to harvest the primary chondrocytes. After digestion with 0.2% trypsin for 30 min, cartilage pieces were purified and digested with 0.25% collagenase II dissolved in Dulbecco's Modified Eagle Medium (DMEM)/F12 (Hyclone, United States) culture medium at 37℃ for 6–8 h. The released chondrocytes were resuspended and cultured in DMEM/F12 supplemented with 10% fetal bovine serum (FBS) (Gibco, Waltham, United States), 100 units/ml penicillin and 100 μg/ml streptomycin at 37°C in an incubator. Cells were plated onto 10 cm plates and grown to approximately 80% confluences before each experiment.

## Small Interfering RNA and Plasmid Transfections

Transfections were performed using Lipofectamine 3000 reagent. Chondrocytes were plated onto six-well plates. For siRNA transfection, 50 pM siRNA (RiboBio, Guangzhou, China) or scrambled siRNAs, 5 μL of Lipofectamine 3000, 250 μL of Opti-MEM, and 2 mL of complete medium were mixed and added to each well. The siRNA (sequence 5′-GAACCTTCATTGTGATTGA-3′) targeting mouse SHP2 was purchased from RiboBio (Guangzhou, China). For SHP2 or active form of β-catenin (β-cat-S33Y) overexpression, chondrocytes were transfected with 1 μg SHP2 overexpression plasmids (OriGene, Rockville, MD, United States) or β-cat-S33Y in 2 mL complete medium, added with 5 μL Lipofectamine 3000 and 250 μL Opti-MEM. 48 h after transfection, chondrocytes were harvested and subjected to different experiments. The efficiency of knockdown or overexpression was confirmed by RT-qPCR and western blot.

## Cell Proliferation Analysis

Primary chondrocytes were plated onto 96-well plates for SHP2 siRNA or over-expressed plasmid transfection and then were stimulated with IL-1β for 24 h. All tests were performed in triplicate and cell proliferation was measured by Cell Counting Kit-8 Assay (CCK-8, TargetMol). To measure the proliferation rate, cells were cultured in the CCK-8 culture medium for 1 h, and then were subjected to absorbance measurement at 450 nm using a microplate reader (Bio Tek, United States).

## Flow Cytometry

An Annexin V-FITC Apoptosis Detection Kit (Keygentec, China) was applied to determine the apoptosis rates following the manufacturer's instructions. Briefly, Collected chondrocytes were suspended in binding buffer in a concentration of $1 \times 10^5$ cells/ml and were stained with 5 μl Annexin V-FITC and 10 μl PI for 15 min in the darkroom. The results were analyzed using a flow cytometer (Becton Dickinson, United States).

## Cell Migration Assay

A two-well Ibidi silicone culture insert (Ibidi, Martinsried, Germany) was set onto the middle of the well in 12-well plates, and 70 μL chondrocyte suspension with $5 \times 10^5$ cells were seeded onto each well of the chamber. After cell attachment, the silicone insert was carefully removed, leaving a 500-μm cell-free gap. The chondrocytes were incubated for 24 h in the presence or absence of IL-1β, and images were captured at different time points using Nikon inverted microscope (Nikon, Tokyo, Japan).

## Animal Model

Animals were purchased from the Experimental Animal Center of Tongji Hospital, Huazhong University of Science and Technology. All the experiments were approved by the Ethics Committee on Animal Experimentation of the hospital. 12-weeks-old male C57BL/6J mice were used to induce OA by the destabilized medial meniscus (DMM) surgery which was performed as previously described (Glasson et al., 2007). To conduct animal experiments, a total of forty-eight mice were randomly divided into four groups: (1) Sham group: sham-operated mice administered with Ad-shControl adenoviruses ($n$ = 6 for both 8 and 12 weeks); (2) Sham + Ad-shSHP2 group: sham-operated mice treated with Ad-shSHP2 adenoviruses ($n$ = 6 for both 8 and 12 weeks); (3) DMM + Ad-shControl group: DMM-operated mice administered with Ad-shControl adenoviruses ($n$ = 6 for both 8 and 12 weeks); (4) DMM + Ad-shSHP2 group: DMM-operated mice administered with Ad-shSHP2 adenoviruses ($n$ = 6 for both 8 and 12 weeks). Half of the mice were sacrificed 8 weeks after surgery, and the other half were sacrificed 12 weeks after surgery. To perform the surgery, the mice were anesthetized and the right knee was prepared before surgery. Then, the joint capsule was opened and the fat pad was removed to expose the medial menisco-tibial ligament under the microscope. The ligament was cut before suturing the joint capsule and skin wound. In sham-operated groups, only the joint capsule was opened, while other tissues remained intact. The knees were dissected at 8 or 12 weeks after surgery, respectively after sacrificing. To knock down SHP2 *in vivo*, shRNA was designed and mixed by Vigene Biosciences Inc. (Shandong, China). 10 μL Ad-shSHP2 or Ad-shControl adenoviruses ($1 \times 10^9$ plaque-forming units [PFUs]) were injected into the right knee joint cavity 1 week after DMM surgery using a 33G needle (Hamilton, Bonaduz, GR, Switzerland) once a week for 8 or 12 weeks after surgery.

## RNA Extraction and RT-qPCR

Total RNA was extracted from cultured chondrocytes using TRIzol reagent (Takara Bio, Japan) according to the manufacturer's descriptions. 0.5–1 μg RNA was used to synthesize cDNA using Revert Aid First Strand cDNA synthesis Kit (Toyobo, Osaka, Japan). Templates were amplified using the SYBR Green Quantitative PCR Protocol (TaKaRa, Shiga, Japan) to determine mRNA levels. All primer sequences used are listed below: *Shp2*, 5′-AGAGGGAAGAGCAAATGTGTCA –3′ (sense), 5′-CTGTGTTTCCTTGTCCGACCT-3′ (antisense); *Axin2*, 5′-ATGAGTAGCGCCGTGTTAGTG-3′ (sense), 5′-GG GCATAGGTTTGGTGGACT-3′ (antisense); *Lef1*, 5′-GCCA CCGATGAGATGATCCC-3′ (sense), 5′-TTGATGTCGGCTA AGTCGCC-3′ (antisense); *Tcf4*, 5′-GATGGGACTCCCT ATGACCAC-3′ (sense), 5′-GAAAGGGTTCCTGGATTGCCC-3′ (antisense); *Aggrecan*, 5′-AGGTGTCGCTCCCCAACTAT-3′ (sense), 5′-CTTCACAGCGGTAGATCCCAG-3′ (antisense); *Col2a1*, 5′-CTTCACAGCGGTAGATCCCAG-3′ (sense), 5′-ACCAGGGGAACCACTCTCAC (antisense); *Mmp3*, 5′-ACTC CCTGGGACTCTACCAC-3′ (sense), 5′-GGTACCACGAGGA CATCAGG-3′ (antisense); *Mmp13*, 5′-TGATGGACCTTCT GGTCTTCTGG-3′ (sense), 5′-CATCCACATGGTTGGGAAGT TCT-3′ (antisense); *Gapdh*, 5′-CTCCCACTCTTCCACCTTCG-3′ (sense), 5′-TTGCTGTAGCCGTATTCATT-3′ (antisense); *Sox9*, 5′-CAGCCCCTTCAACCTTCCTC-3′ (sense), 5′-TGATGGTCAGCGTAGTCGTATT-3′ (antisense); *Col10a1*, 5′-T TCTGCTGCTAATGTTCTTGACC-3′ (sense), 5′-GGGATGAA GTATTGTGTCTTGGG-3′ (antisense). The relative mRNA levels of target genes were calculated using the $2^{-\Delta\Delta Cq}$ method.

## Western Blotting Analysis

Cultured chondrocytes were lysed by ice-cold RIPA lysis buffer (Boster, Wuhan) containing 1% protease and phosphatase inhibitor for 30 min. Then, the cell lysates were immediately configurated at 10,000 g at 4°C for 30 min. Equal amounts of protein were loaded on SDS-PAGE (10–15%) for electrophoresis, and then the proteins were transferred to polyvinylidene fluoride (PVDF) membranes. Each membrane was blocked with 5% non-fat milk in Tris-buffered saline with 0.1% Tween 20 buffer (TBST) for 1 h and then incubated with primary antibodies overnight at 4°C on a shaker. After incubation with horseradish peroxidase-conjugated secondary antibodies for 1 h, proteins were visualized by an enhanced chemiluminescence kit (Thermo Fisher Scientific, Waltham, MA, United States) in the ChemiDoc XRS System (Bio-Rad Laboratories, Hercules, CA, United States). Proteins were quantified using Image lab software and the targeted protein levels were normalized to GAPDH or relative total proteins.

## Co-immunoprecipitation

The interactions of SHP2 with β-catenin proteins were detected in primary chondrocytes. Cells were lysed in lysis buffer (20 mM Tris, pH 7.5, 150 mM NaCl, 1% Triton, and 10% glycerol) containing 1% protease and phosphatase inhibitor. Lysates were pre-cleared with the control IgG for 1 h to remove any proteins that bind non-specifically to immunoprecipitation components. Then, the primary antibodies or relative IgG, and the protein A/G beads were added to the lysates, and the mixture was incubated overnight at 4°C for immunoprecipitation. After being rinsed five times with lysis buffer, the immunoprecipitates were boiled in the loading buffer and then were subjected to western blotting.

### Micro-Computed Tomography

After euthanasia, the right knee joints of the mice were harvested and fixed in 4% formaldehyde for 48 h. High-resolution micro-computed tomography (μCT, Scanco Medical, Bassersdorf, Switzerland) was used to analyze the subchondral bone structures at 15 μm resolution, 70 kVP and 112 μA x-ray energy. The three-dimensional images were reconstructed according to the manufacturer's instructions. The parameters of Bone volume per unit total volume (BV/TV), Trabecular number (Tb.N), trabecular separation (Tb.Sp) and trabecular thickness (Tb.Th) were evaluated using the μCT system software.

### Histopathological and Immunocytochemical Analysis

After scanning, the tissues were fixed in 4% paraformaldehyde for 2 days and decalcified in 10% EDTA (pH 7.4) for 4 weeks. Subsequently, the tissues were embedded in paraffin and sectioned continuously at 5 μm thickness for hematoxylin and eosin (HE), toluidine blue and Safranin O/Fast Green staining. The images were taken and scored for degree of articular cartilage damage according to the Osteoarthritis Research Association (OARSI) histopathology scoring system in a blind manner (Glasson et al., 2010). For DAB or immunofluorescence staining, sections were deparaffinized, hydrated, and blocked with BSA containing 0.1% Triton X-100 for 1 h at room temperature. After incubation with primary antibodies against MMP3 (1:100), MMP13 (1:100), SHP2 (1:100), COL2A1 (1:200), AGGRECAN (1:100) overnight at 4°C, the sections were incubated with HRP-conjugated secondary antibodies and counterstained with hematoxylin or corresponded fluorescence secondary antibodies. Finally, all the images were taken under a microscope.

### Immunofluorescence

The co-expression analysis of SHP2 and β-catenin in chondrocytes were performed by immunofluorescence staining. After being fixed in 4% paraformaldehyde and permeabilized in 0.2% Triton X-100, the chondrocytes were incubated with primary antibodies against β-catenin (1:100) and SHP2 (1:100) overnight at 4°C. The cells were subsequently incubated with anti-mouse and anti-rabbit secondary antibodies for 1 h. Finally, all images were captured using a fluorescence microscope.

### Statistical Analysis

All data were presented as means ± SEM. Statistical analyses were conducted using GraphPad Prism v. 5.0 (Graphpad Software Inc., San Diego, CA, United States). All experiments were independently repeated at least three times. One-way ANOVA followed by LSD's *post hoc* tests were used to test the differences among groups. The student's *t*-test was used to assess statistically significant differences in the data between groups. Values of $P < 0.05$ were considered statistically significant.

## RESULTS

### SHP2 Expression Is Increased in Primary Chondrocytes After IL-1β Treatment and in Mouse OA Cartilage

To investigate the role of SHP2 in OA, cultured chondrocytes were exposed to different concentrations of IL-1β (0, 1, 5, 10, 20 ng/ml) to mimic OA model *in vitro*. Matrix-degrading enzyme MMP13 and MMP3 were gradually increased, while Col2a1 level was decreased upon IL-1β treatment in a dose-dependent manner, indicating a successful induction of inflammation in chondrocytes. Subsequently, SHP2 was elevated gradually by IL-1β (**Figure 1A**). Besides, the mRNA levels of *Shp2* were also increased after 5 and 20 ng/ml IL-1β treatment for 24 h although no obvious significance was observed at 1 and 10 ng/ml after IL-1β treatment (**Figure 1B**). We thus treated chondrocytes using 5 ng/ml IL-1β for different time points. Results showed MMP13 level increased within 24 h exposure but was slightly decreased at 48 h, SHP2 expression showed the same trend, MMP3 level elevated while COL2A1 decreased time-dependently within 48 h of treatment (**Figure 1C**). The mRNA level of *Shp2* was up-regulated in a time-dependently manner but was statistically significant at 24 and 48 h after IL-1β treatment (**Figure 1D**). Furthermore, we assessed the expression of SHP2 in the articular cartilage of DMM and Sham-operated mice by immunofluorescence staining, and the result revealed that SHP2 was strongly elevated in OA cartilage compared with the sham-operated mice (**Figure 1E**). Our data demonstrated that SHP2 was up-regulated both *in vivo* and *in vitro* in OA pathogenesis.

### SHP2 Regulates IL-1β–Induced Chondrocyte Destruction *in vitro*

To further investigate the effect of SHP2 on IL-1β–induced chondrocyte destruction, SHP2 was knocked down using siRNA or overexpressed using plasmid in mice chondrocytes. The efficiency of SHP2 knockdown and overexpression was verified by qPCR and western blotting (**Figures 2A,B,I,J**). Subsequently, we performed CCK8 assays, flow cytometry and cell migration assays to test cell function. Results showed chondrocytes stimulated with IL-1β (5 ng/ml) for 24 h markedly increased the apoptotic rates which was not significantly influenced by SHP2 knockdown or overexpression (**Supplementary Figures 1A–D**). Furthermore, SHP2 knockdown or overexpression has no effect on chondrocyte viability (**Supplementary Figures 1E,F**). Cell migration assays showed scratch distances were not altered in SHP2 knockdown or overexpressed chondrocytes (**Supplementary Figures 1G–J**). These results suggested SHP2 had no significant effect on chondrocyte apoptosis, proliferation or migration. We then evaluated the role of SHP2 in IL-1β–induced chondrocyte degeneration. Downregulation of SHP2 decreased the elevation of MMP3 and MMP13 induced by IL-1β in both protein and mRNA levels (**Figures 2A,C,D**). *Aggrecan*, *Col2a1*, *Sox9*, and *Col10a1* levels were also tested by qPCR. The results showed that SHP2 knockdown increased *Aggrecan*, *Col2a1* and *Sox9* mRNA level, but decreased *Col10a1* mRNA level after IL-1β treatment in chondrocytes (**Figures 2E–H**). Furthermore, SHP2 overexpression distinctly increased the elevation of levels

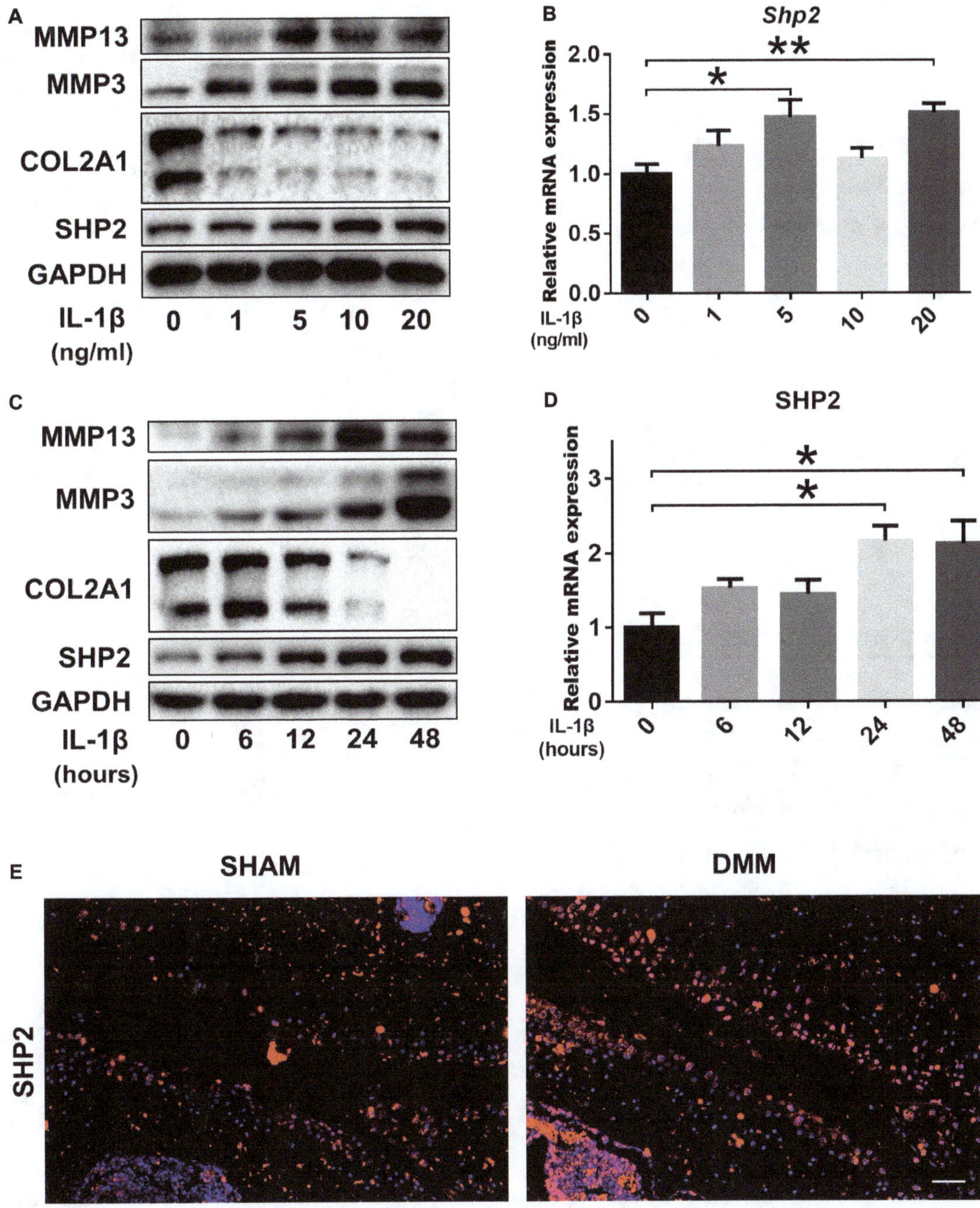


**FIGURE 1 |** SHP2 expression is increased in primary chondrocytes after IL-1β treatment and in mouse OA cartilage. **(A)** Representative western blot of MMP3, MMP13, COL2A1, SHP2, and **(B)** mRNA level of *Shp2* determined by qRT-PCR in chondrocytes after stimulation with various doses of IL-1β for 24 h. **(C)** Representative western blot of MMP3, MMP13, COL2A1, SHP2, and **(D)** mRNA level of *Shp2* determined by qRT-PCR in chondrocytes after stimulation with 5 ng/ml IL-1β for different time points. $^{*}P < 0.05$, $^{**}P < 0.01$ versus chondrocytes without IL-1β treatment. **(E)** Representative immunofluorescence images of SHP2 in articular cartilage in DMM and Sham mice, scale bar = 100 μm.

of MMP3 and MMP13 induced by IL-1β in protein and mRNA (**Figures 2I,K,L**). Consistently, *Aggrecan*, *Col2a1*, *Sox9* mRNA levels were reduced and *Col10a1* mRNA level was increased in chondrocytes exposed to IL-1β (**Figures 2M–P**). In short, our data displayed that SHP2 aggravated IL-1β–induced chondrocyte destruction *in vitro*.

## SHP2 Interacts With β-Catenin in Chondrocytes and Activates Wnt/β-Catenin Pathway

Accumulating data identified that canonical Wnt/β-catenin signaling plays an important role in modulating the pathogenesis

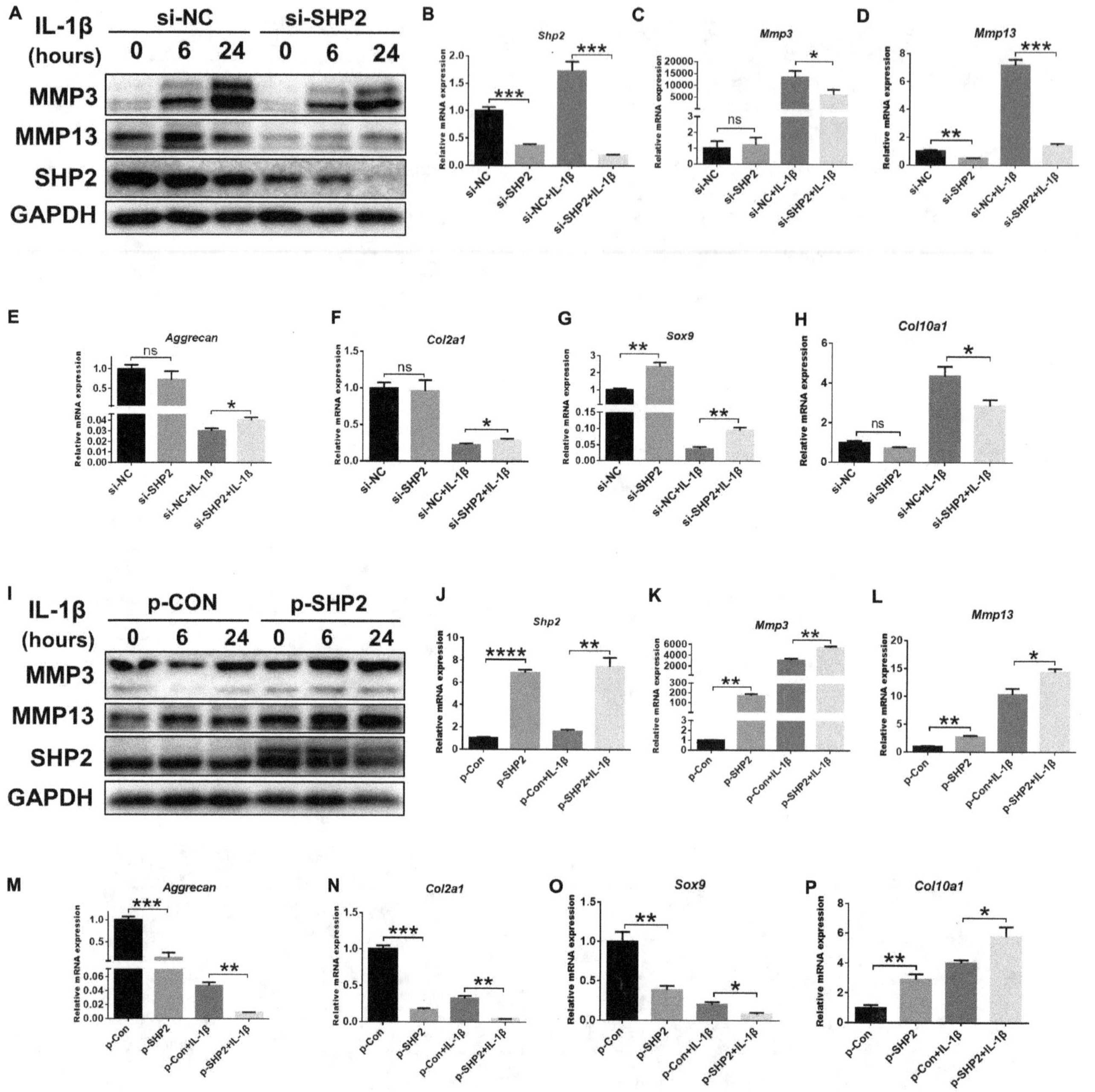


**FIGURE 2 |** SHP2 regulates IL-1β–induced cartilage destruction *in vitro*. **(A)** Representative western blot of MMP3, MMP13 and SHP2 after chondrocytes were transfected with si-NC or si-SHP2 for 48 h and then were treated with IL-1β (5 ng/ml) for indicated time points. **(B–H)** mRNA levels of *Shp2*, *Mmp3*, *Mmp13*, *Aggrecan*, *Col2a*, *Sox9,* and *Col10a1* were shown in chondrocytes that were transfected with si-NC or si-SHP2 for 48 h and then were treated with IL-1β (5 ng/mL) for 24 h. $^*P < 0.05$, $^{**}P < 0.01$, $^{***}P < 0.001$ versus si-NC transfected chondrocytes. **(I)** Representative western blot of MMP3, MMP13 and SHP2 after chondrocytes transfected with control plasmid (p-CON) or SHP2 (p-SHP2) overexpressed plasmid for 48 h and then incubated with or without IL-1β (5 ng/ml) for indicated time points. **(J–P)** mRNA levels of *Shp2*, *Mmp3*, *Mmp13*, *Aggrecan*, *Col2a1*, *Sox9,* and *Col10a1* were shown in chondrocytes transfected with p-CON or p-SHP2 plasmids for 48 h and then stimulated with IL-1β (5 ng/mL) for 24 h. $^*P < 0.05$, $^{**}P < 0.01$, $^{***}P < 0.001$, $^{****}P < 0.0001$ versus p-CON transfected chondrocytes.

of OA (Wu et al., 2010; Bouaziz et al., 2015; Zhou et al., 2017). Activation of β-catenin resulted in the development of an OA-like phenotype (Zhu et al., 2009), while inhibition of β-catenin signaling in articular chondrocytes contributes to cartilage destruction (Zhu et al., 2008). Other studies found that SHP2 and β-catenin proteins can form a complex and SHP2 increased β-catenin accumulation by inhibiting glycogen synthase kinase 3β (GSK-3β)–mediated β-catenin degradation in liver cancer (Biswas et al., 2006; Xiang et al., 2017). To unveil the possible mechanism by which SHP2 promotes OA progression, we treated primary chondrocytes with IL-1β and found that IL-1β suppressed phosphorylated β-catenin at S33/37/141 sites, induced β-catenin phosphorylation at Y142, and increased total β-catenin expression at 6 and 12 h after IL-1β treatment. Although the expression of total β-catenin was slightly decreased 24 h after IL-1β treatment (**Figure 3A**). Downregulation of SHP2 by siRNA remarkably reduced β-catenin expression at 6 and 24 h after IL-1β treatment. However, the phosphorylated site at Y142 of β-catenin was not significantly changed in SHP2-downregulated cells after IL-1β treatment, indicating that SHP2 did not specifically dephosphorylate this site (**Figure 3B**). On the contrary, SHP2 overexpression promoted the expression of β-catenin (**Figure 3D**). To confirm SHP2 induced overexpression of matrix-degrading enzymes was indeed through β-catenin, we transfected mouse chondrocytes with plasmids expressing an active form of β-catenin with a mutation on the S33 site (β-cat-S33Y) (Ming et al., 2012). Overexpression of β-cat-S33Y prominently reversed the downregulation of MMP13 and MMP3 caused by SHP2 knockdown at 24 h after IL-1β treatment (**Figure 3C**). Additionally, the interaction of SHP2 and β-catenin in the primary chondrocytes was identified by co-immunoprecipitation (CO-IP) (**Figures 4A,B**). Besides, double staining for β-catenin and SHP2 was also performed and SHP2 colocalized with β-catenin in chondrocytes (**Figure 4C**). We further examined the target genes of the canonical Wnt/β-catenin pathway such as *Axin2*, *Lef1*, and *Tcf4*. In accordance with the β-catenin expression, the mRNA levels of these genes were attenuated by knocking down SHP2, but were increased significantly after SHP2 overexpression in chondrocytes (**Figures 4D,E**). Together, our results suggested that SHP2 activated Wnt/β-catenin signaling in chondrocytes.

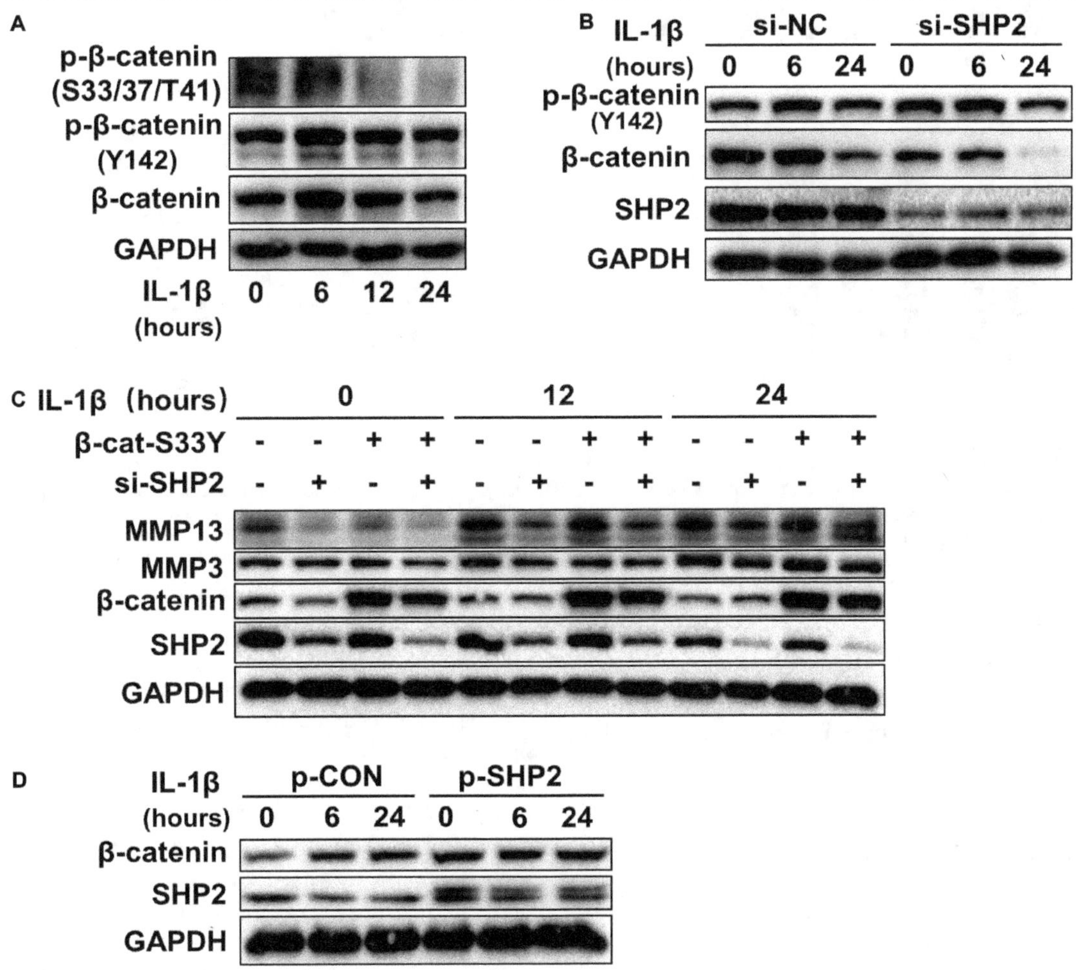


**FIGURE 3 |** SHP2 activates Wnt/β-catenin in chondrocytes. **(A)** Representative western blot of p-β-catenin (S33/37/T41), p-β-catenin (Y142) and β-catenin, in chondrocytes incubated with IL-1β of 5 ng/ml for the indicated time points. **(B)** Representative western blot of p-β-catenin (Y142), β-catenin and SHP2 in chondrocytes incubated with IL-1β (5 ng/ml) for indicated time points after si-NC or si-SHP2 transfection for 48 h. **(C)** Representative western blot of MMP3, MMP13, β-catenin, and SHP2 in chondrocytes incubated with IL-1β (5 ng/ml) for indicated time points after siRNA or active form of β-catenin (β-cat-S33Y) transfection with for 48 h. **(D)** Representative western blot of β-catenin and SHP2 in chondrocytes incubated with IL-1β (5 ng/ml) for the indicated time points after p-CON or p-SHP2 transfection for 48 h.

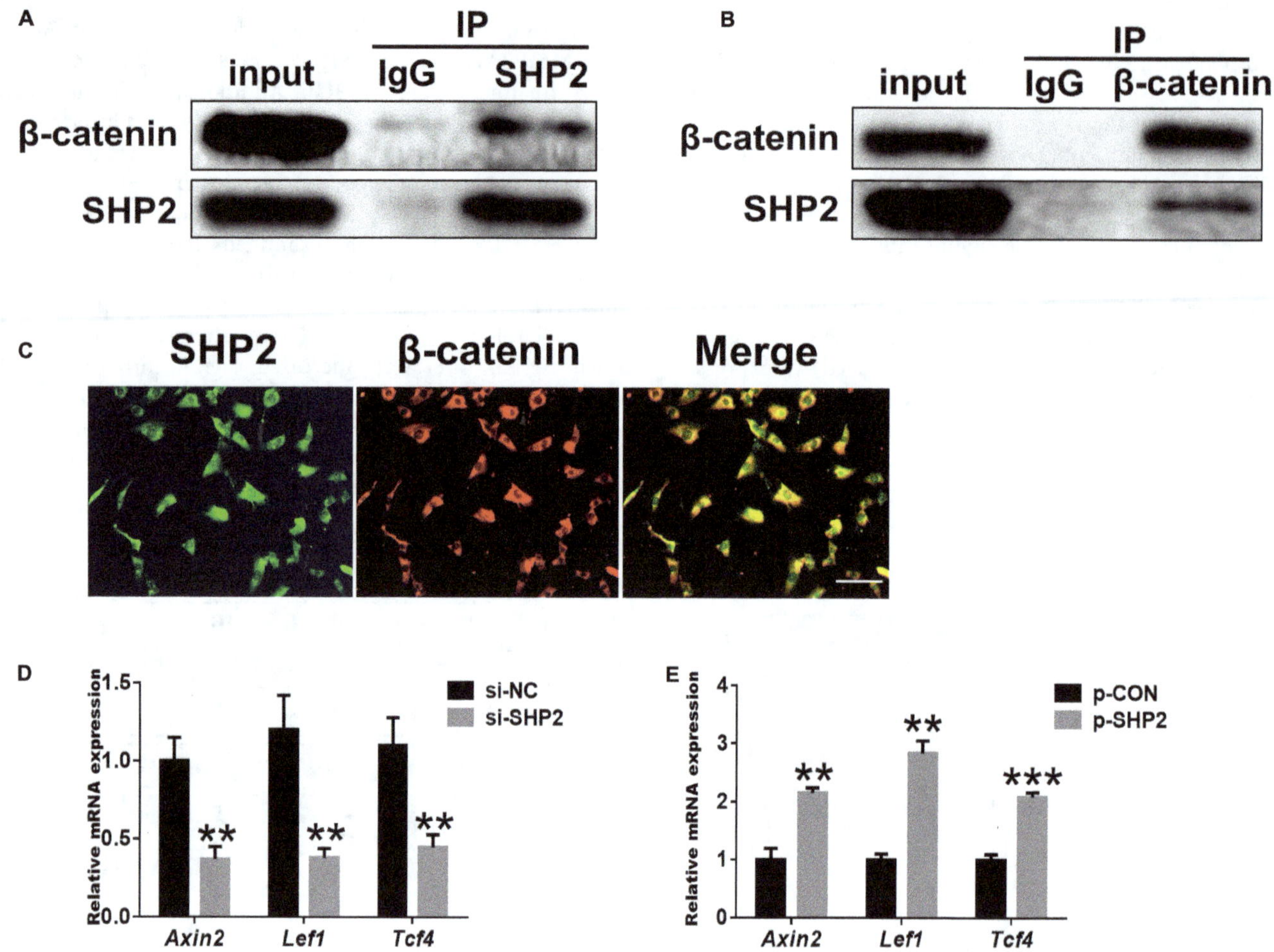


**FIGURE 4 |** SHP2 interacts with β-catenin and activates Wnt/β-catenin target genes. **(A)** β-catenin was co-immunoprecipitated with an anti-SHP2 antibody and **(B)** SHP2 was co-immunoprecipitated with an anti-β-catenin antibody in chondrocytes. **(C)** Immunofluorescence image for SHP2 and β-catenin cellular localization in chondrocytes. Scale bar, 100 μm. **(D)** Relative mRNA levels of three Wnt/β-catenin targets *Axin2*, *Lef1*, and *Tcf4* in chondrocytes after si-NC or si-SHP2 transfection. **(E)** Relative mRNA levels of three Wnt/β-catenin targets *Axin2*, *Lef1*, and *Tcf4* in chondrocytes after p-CON or p-SHP2 transfection. $n = 3$, $^{**}P < 0.01$, $^{***}P < 0.001$ versus si-NC or p-CON transfected chondrocytes.

## SHP2 Promotes MAPK and NF-κB Signaling Pathways

The MAPK and NF-κB signaling pathways, widely involved in OA pathophysiology through various effects, are activated in osteoarthritic chondrocytes during aging and inflammation (Chang et al., 2019; Wongwichai et al., 2019). Hence, to investigate whether SHP2 influences IL-1β induced cartilage degradation via NF-κB and MAPK signaling pathways, we examined the phosphorylation levels of components of the MAPK and NF-κB pathways in chondrocytes. As shown in **Figures 5A,B**, the phosphorylated JNK, ERK, p38 protein levels were diminished in IL-1β stimulated chondrocytes following SHP2 siRNA transfection. The NF-κB pathway-related proteins were also tested. Phosphorylated IKKβ, p65 and IκBα were apparently decreased (**Figures 5C,D**). In contrast, overexpression of SHP2 significantly elevated the level of phosphorylated JNK, ERK, and p38 induced by IL-1β (**Figures 6A,B**). Phosphorylated IKKβ, p65, and IκBα were also increased after SHP2 overexpression (**Figures 6C,D**). These results implicated that SHP2 induced inflammation by activating MAPK and NF-κB signaling pathways.

## Knockdown of SHP2 Attenuates Cartilage Degradation in DMM Model

To explore the possible association between SHP2 and OA *in vivo*, the mice OA model was induced by destabilized medial meniscus (DMM) surgery. A week after surgery, mice were intra-articular injected weekly with Ad-shControl or Ad-shSHP2 adenovirus both in sham-operated and DMM groups. Eight or twelve weeks after surgery, hematoxylin and eosin (HE), Safranin O/Fast Green, Toluidine blue staining and Immuno-histochemical staining were performed to assess the histomorphology differences among these groups. The efficiency of SHP2 knockdown in the cartilage was confirmed

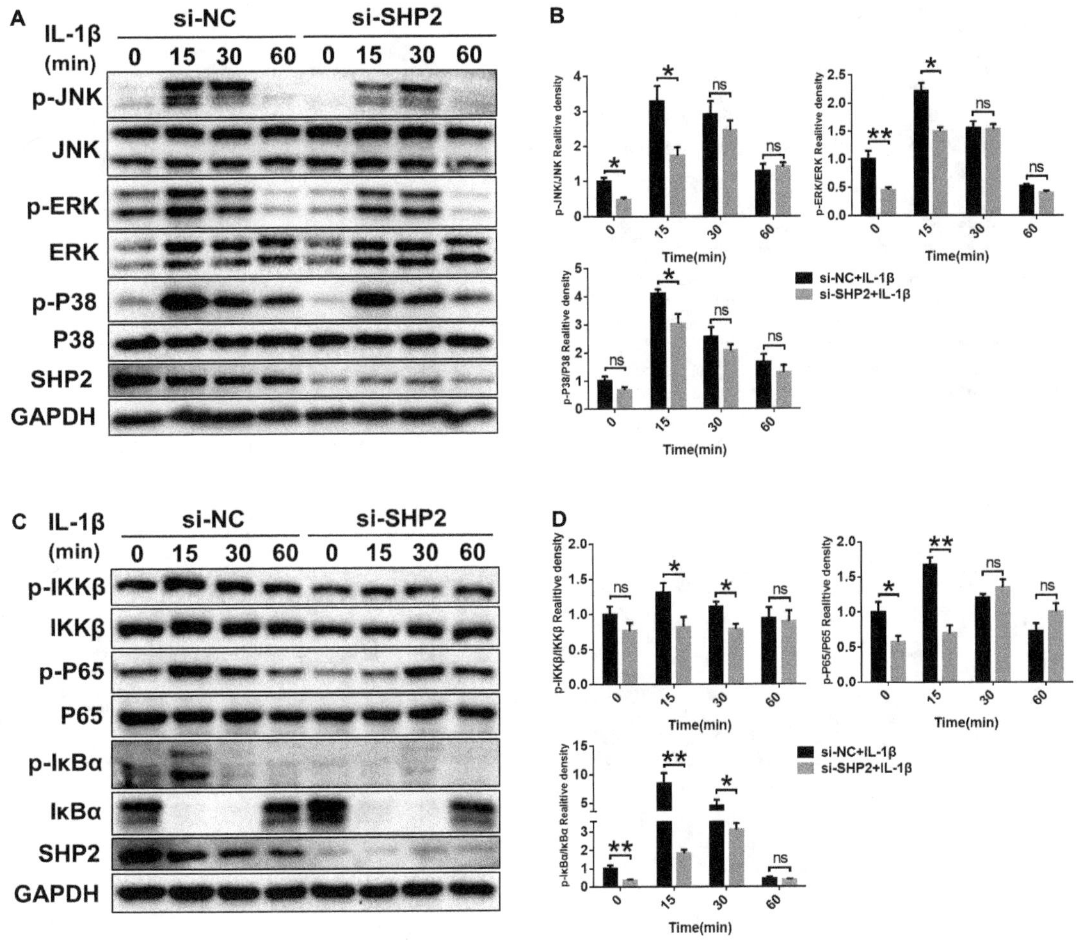


**FIGURE 5 |** SHP2 knockdown inhibits MAPK and NF-κB signaling pathways. Chondrocytes were transfected with siRNA for 48 h, and then stimulated with IL-1β for indicated time points. **(A)** Representative western blot and **(B)** quantification of the effect of SHP2 silencing on phosphorylated p38, JNK, ERK in chondrocytes. **(C)** Representative western blot and **(D)** quantification of the effect of SHP2 silencing on phosphorylated p65, IKKβ, and IκBα in chondrocytes. $^{*}P < 0.05$, $^{**}P < 0.01$ versus cells transfected with si-NC and without IL-1β treatment.

by SHP2 staining (**Figure 7A**). Data showed DMM group developed moderate cartilage destruction at 8 weeks after surgery. However, knockdown of SHP2 (Ad-shSHP2) dramatically alleviated cartilage degradation as demonstrated by Safranin O and Toluidine blue staining, with significantly lower OARSI grades at 8 weeks after DMM surgery (**Figures 7B,C**). In addition, the expression of MMP3 and MMP13 were significantly decreased in the DMM + shSHP2 group compared with the DMM + shControl group, while the levels of COL2A1 and AGGRECAN were significantly increased (**Figures 7D,E**). μCT was applied to view the osteophyte formation and determine the effects of SHP2 on the structure of tibial subchondral bone in these mice. More osteophytes were seen in DMM + Ad-shControl group, and SHP2 depletion reduced osteophyte formation at 8 weeks after surgery (**Figure 7F**). Also, we tested the effect of SHP2 in DMM model 12 weeks after surgery. Although osteophyte formation at 12 weeks seems to be less pronounced than that at 8 weeks after surgery in DMM + Ad-shControl group, SHP2 knockdown still ameliorated osteophyte formation and osteoarthritis progress (**Figures 8A–F**). The parameters of BV/TV, Tb.Th, and Tb.Sp were evaluated. Interestingly, SHP2 knockdown remarkably decreased BV/TV in sham-operated mice both at 8 and 12 weeks after surgery in subchondral bone, but no differences were seen in Tb.N, Tb.Th, and Tb.Sp. However, the difference in BV/TV was not observed between DMM + Ad-shSHP2 and DMM + Ad-shControl groups at 8 and 12 weeks after surgery (**Supplementary Figure 2**). The above results illustrated that inhibition of SHP2 reversed cartilage degradation and osteophyte formation *in vivo* without significantly affecting tibial subchondral bone remodeling in mice.

## DISCUSSION

Degeneration of the articular cartilage is the main pathological feature of OA joints, which leads to cartilage damage, subchondral bone remodeling, and osteophyte formation (Loeser et al., 2012). To date, there is still no effective treatment

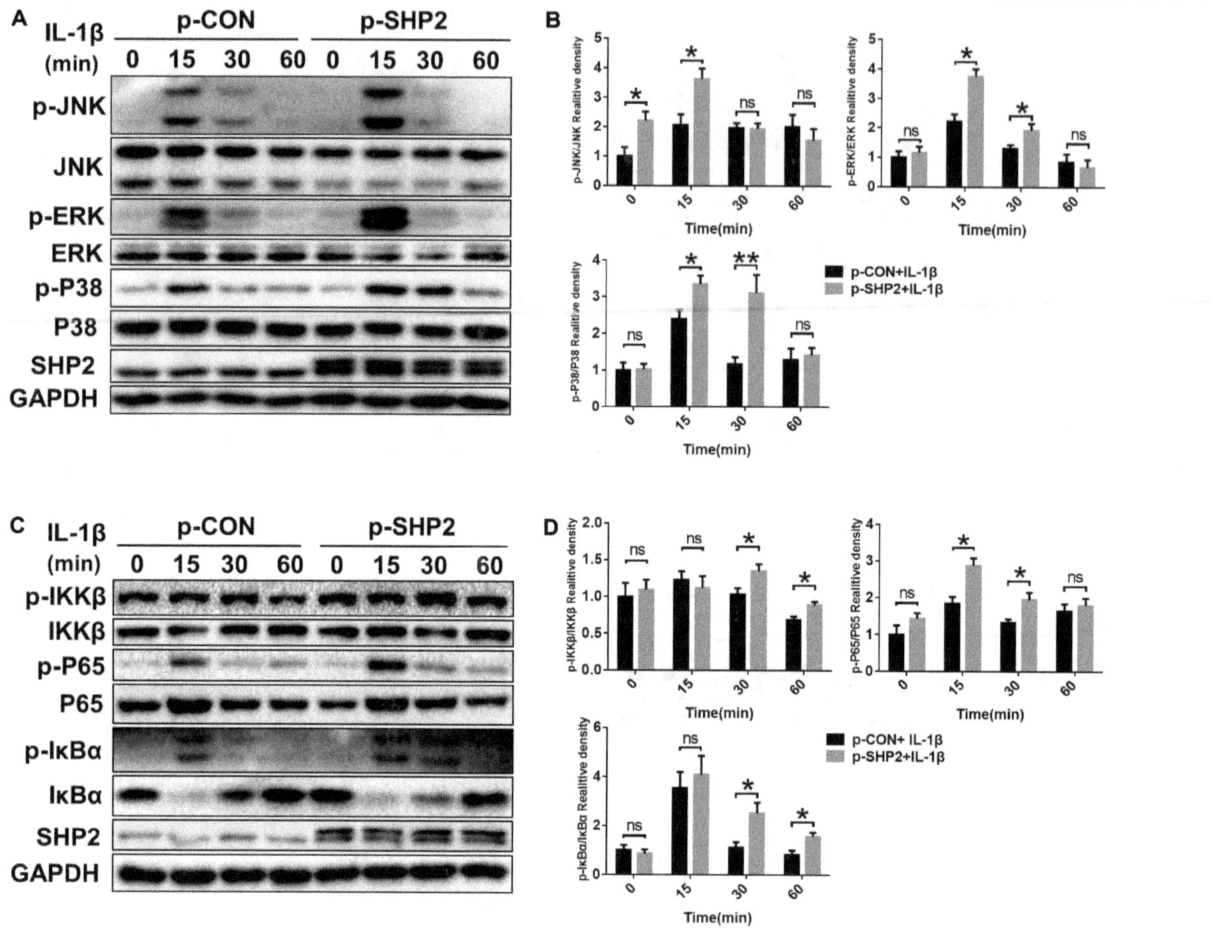


**FIGURE 6 |** SHP2 overexpression activates MAPK and NF-κB Signaling Pathways. Chondrocytes were transfected with p-CON or p-SHP2 overexpression plasmid for 48 h, and then stimulated with IL-1β for indicated time points. **(A)** Representative western blot and **(B)** quantification of the effect of SHP2 overexpression on phosphorylated p38, JNK, ERK in chondrocytes. **(C)** Representative western blot and **(D)** quantification of the effect of SHP2 overexpression on phosphorylated p65, IKKβ, and IκBα in chondrocytes. $^{*}P < 0.05$, $^{**}P < 0.01$ versus cells transfected with p-CON and without IL-1β treatment.

for OA. In the past 20 years, SHP2 has been reported to participate in developmental diseases, such as Noonan syndrome, metachondromatosis, and malignancies such as juvenile myelomonocytic leukemia (Zhang et al., 2015). For example, two studies focused on the upregulation of SHP2 in cancer and concomitant enhancement in tumor invasion (Chauhan et al., 2000; Sturla et al., 2011). Therefore, we aim to identify the association between SHP2 and OA. In the present study, we found SHP2 expression was significantly induced by IL-1β treatment. By loss-of-function and gain-of-function studies in chondrocytes, we found that SHP2 apparently affected MMP3, MMP13, AGGRECAN, COL2A1, SOX9, and COL10A1 expression. These results strongly suggested SHP2 play an important role in cartilage degeneration. However, we found SHP2 had no significant effect on chondrocyte apoptosis, proliferation or migration, indicating the effect of SHP2 on cartilage degeneration was not through influencing chondrocyte function.

The canonical Wnt/β-catenin signal axis has been involved in the pathogenesis of OA (Corr, 2008). Researchers concluded that activation of the Wnt/β-catenin pathway resulted in articular chondrocytes degradation toward catabolism and loss of structure and function. Several studies demonstrated the relation between SHP2 and β-catenin. Ilse Timmerman et al. reported that SHP2 regulated the restoration of endothelial cell adhesion junctions by regulating β-catenin phosphorylation (Timmerman et al., 2012). However, how SHP2 regulate β-catenin was not studied in cartilage. Our data recognized a targeted β-catenin in OA progression. SHP2 knockdown reduced β-catenin level accompanied by decreased levels of target genes such as *Axin2*, *LEF1*, and *TCF4*. The interaction of SHP2 and β-catenin was identified by co-immunoprecipitation and double immune-staining. Besides, constitute activation of β-catenin reversed the decrease of catabolic enzymes MMP3 and MMP13 induced by knockdown of SHP2 after IL-1β stimulation in primary chondrocytes, showing that β-catenin was a direct target of SHP2 to induce chondral degeneration. Notably, as SHP2 is a protein tyrosine phosphatase, we found p-β-catenin (Y142) was not altered by SHP2. Therefore, we speculated Y142 site of β-catenin may not be the specific dephosphorylated site for SHP2 to interact

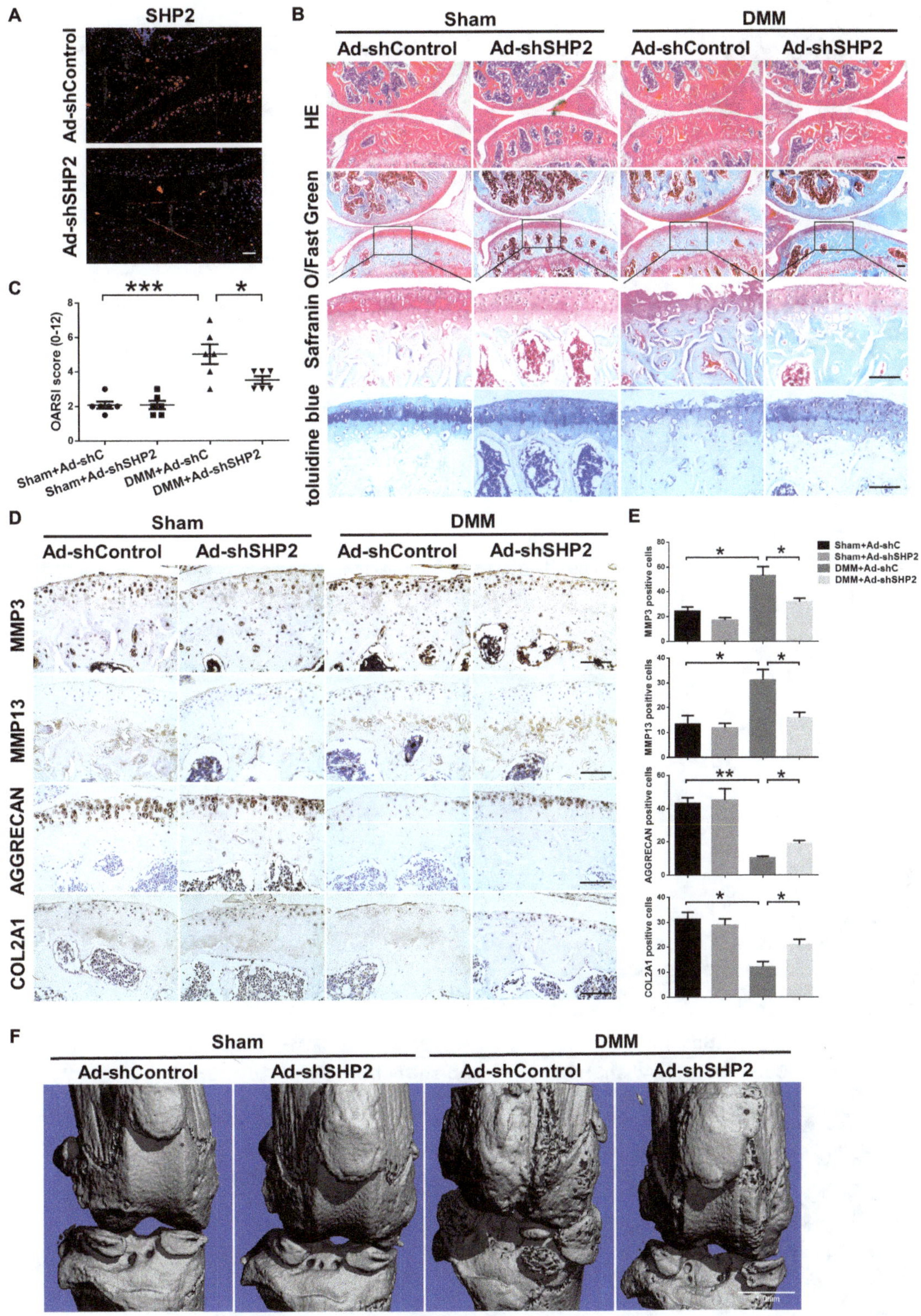


**FIGURE 7 |** Knockdown of SHP2 prevents cartilage destruction at 8 weeks after DMM surgery. **(A)** Immunofluorescence image of SHP2 after mice were intra-articular injected with Ad-shControl and Ad-shSHP2 virus 8 weeks after DMM surgery, scale bar = 100 μm. **(B)** HE, Safranin O/Fast Green, and toluidine blue staining and **(C)** OARSI grades of knee joints from Ad-shControl and Ad-shSHP2 mice at 8 weeks after DMM surgery. Scale bars, 100 μm, $^{*}P < 0.05$, $^{***}P < 0.001$ versus Sham + Ad-shC or DMM + Ad-shC group. **(D,E)** Immunostaining images and quantification of MMP3, MMP13, AGGRECAN, and COL2A1 in the joint cartilage of control and SHP2 knockdown mice at 8 weeks after DMM surgery. $^{*}P < 0.05$, $^{**}P < 0.01$ versus Sham + Ad-shC or DMM + Ad-shC group. $n = 6$. Scale bars, 100 μm. **(F)** Representative micro-CT images of the knee joints in each group. $n = 6$. Scale bar, 1.0 mm.

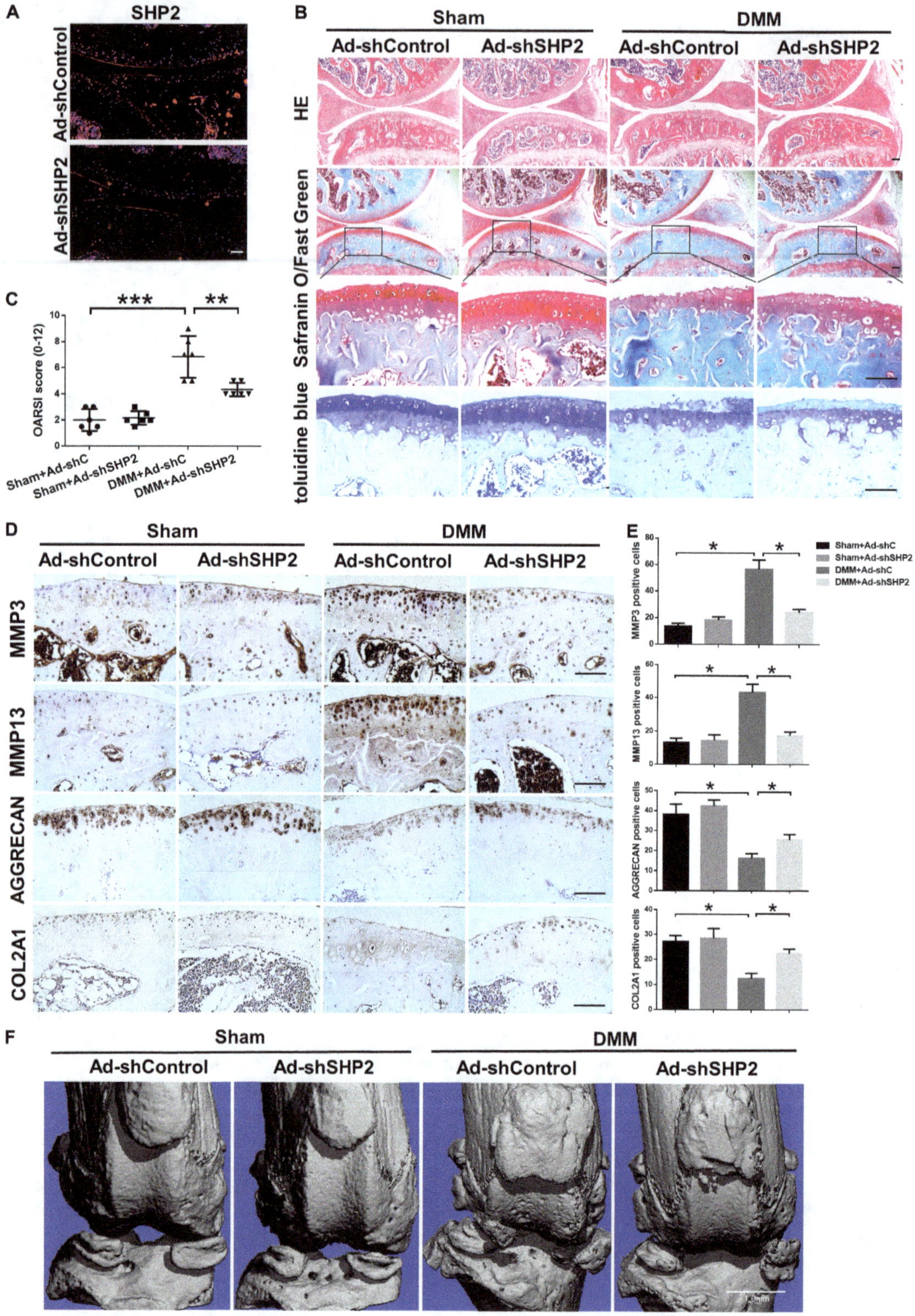


**FIGURE 8 |** Knockdown of SHP2 prevents cartilage destruction at 12 weeks after DMM surgery. **(A)** Immunofluorescence image of SHP2 after mice were intra-articular injected with Ad-shControl and Ad-shSHP2 virus 12 weeks after DMM surgery, scale bar = 100 μm. **(B)** HE, Safranin O/Fast Green, and toluidine blue staining and **(C)** OARSI grades of knee joints from Ad-shControl and Ad-shSHP2 mice at 12 weeks after DMM surgery. Scale bars, 100 μm, $^{**}P < 0.01$, $^{***}P < 0.001$ versus Sham + Ad-shC or DMM + Ad-shC group. **(D,E)** Immunostaining images and quantification of MMP3, MMP13, AGGRECAN, and COL2A1 in the joint cartilage of control and SHP2 knockdown mice at 12 weeks after DMM surgery. $^{*}P < 0.05$ versus Sham + Ad-shC or DMM + Ad-shC group. $n = 6$. Scale bars, 100 μm. **(F)** Representative u-CT images of the knee joints in each group. $n = 6$. Scale bar, 1.0 mm.

with. Further investigations need to be performed to recognize the specific dephosphorylation site of SHP2 on β-catenin.

The inflammation status in cartilage or periarticular tissues is mostly attributed to MAPK and NF-κB pathways whose hyperactivation directly initiate and target articular cartilage and subchondral bone, causing cartilage degeneration and subchondral bone formation. Previous studies have shown SHP2 mediated MAPK and NF-κB activation (Zou et al., 2007; Heun et al., 2019; Niogret et al., 2019; Liu et al., 2020). However, whether SHP2 regulated these signaling in OA pathogenesis was not fully elucidated. Our data found that inhibition of SHP2 impaired MAPK and NF-κB pathways while overexpression of SHP2 significantly activated MAPK and NF-κB pathways after IL-1β exposure, indicated SHP2 indeed regulate inflammation status *in vitro*. This may be one of the mechanisms for a better understanding of the potential role of SHP2 in OA initiation and progression. Surprisingly, SHP2 knockdown or overexpression, have a significant impact on cartilage degeneration such as altered MMP3, MMP13 level and downstream MAPK, NF-κB pathways without IL-1β treatment (see IL-1β 0 h treatment). This may attribute to that SHP2 knockdown or overexpression already affected β-catenin signaling at baseline levels (**Figures 3B,D**). Altered β-catenin further affect downstream OA-like phenotype (**Figure 2A**) and MAPK, NF-κB pathways (**Figures 5A–D**). The similar phenomenon was not seen in our DMM models, where knockdown of SHP2 by intra-articular injection of Ad-shSHP2 robustly prevented cartilage degradation compared with the control both at 8 and 12 weeks after DMM surgery, but not in sham-operated mice. Since *in vivo* researches are much more complicated than *in vitro*, it is normal to see some of the inconsistency in different models. Accordingly, MMP3 and MMP13 levels decreased in Ad-shSHP2 injected mice confirmed its role in catabolic enzymes, the increased AGGRECAN and COL2A1 levels further proved its protective role in OA pathogenesis after SHP2 knockdown.

Interestingly, osteophyte formation was not so obvious as 8 weeks results, this maybe explained that the osteophyte formation rate was alleviated as time went by in all groups but SHP2 knockdown still has a beneficial effect on osteophyte formation at 12 weeks after surgery. Unlike cartilage degeneration process, most degenerated chondrocytes are hypertrophic differentiated and are kind of "irreversible" in OA pathogenesis. Osteophyte formation was a result of sclerosis of the subchondral bone, which should be faster to be alleviated. The current study found the subchondral bone mass was not significantly altered after SHP2 reduction as shown by μCT although SHP2 knockdown remarkably decreased BV/TV in sham-operated mice both at 8 and 12 weeks after surgery in subchondral bone, no differences were seen in Tb.N, Tb.Th, and Tb.Sp. Collectively, our results indicated that increased SHP2 is important for the initiation and progression of OA, SHP2 knockdown ameliorated cartilage degeneration.

Consistent with *in vitro* studies, there were some limitations of this study. First, the effect of overexpressing SHP2 *in vivo* was not detected although the *in vitro* results were shown in the present study, future researches will be conducted to see these results. Second, it would be more convincing if chondrocytes-specific SHP2 deletion mice can be used. However, since the construction and breeding of these mice are very time-consuming, we will extend this to animal models in the future.

Given the facts above, our study identified that SHP2 played a vital role in the degeneration of articular cartilage in OA. SHP2 knockdown protected cartilage from degradation during OA pathogenesis via suppressing the Wnt/β-catenin pathway, MAPK and NF-κB signaling pathways. These proved SHP2 might be a promising therapeutic target for OA.

## ETHICS STATEMENT

The animal study was reviewed and approved by the Ethics Committee on Animal Experimentation of Tongji Hospital, Huazhong University of Science and Technology. Written informed consent was obtained from the owners for the participation of their animals in this study.

## AUTHOR CONTRIBUTIONS

JX and XS designed the study. TT performed most of the experiments. DL, CG, HL, and ZL helped with the DMM surgery. WL, CZ, and DQ helped inject the mice. ZD analyzed some of the data. All authors provided editorial comments.

## ACKNOWLEDGMENTS

We thank Dr. Ke Chen in Department of Urology, Tonji Hospital, Tongji Medical College, Huazhong University of Science and Technology for providing β-cat-S33Y plasmid.

**Supplementary Figure 1 |** The impact of SHP2 on cell migration, proliferation and apoptosis. Chondrocytes were seeded onto each well after transfection for 48 h, and then chondrocytes were incubated with or without IL-1β (5 ng/mL) for 24 h. **(A,B)** An apoptosis detection kit was used to detect chondrocytes apoptosis by flow cytometry after si-NC or si-SHP2 transfection. Data are means ± SEM of three independent experiments; $^{*}P < 0.05$ versus the control group. **(C,D)** Chondrocytes apoptosis by flow cytometry after p-Con or p-SHP2 transfection. Data are means ± SEM of three independent experiments; $^{*}P < 0.05$ versus the control group. **(E,F)** The proliferation of chondrocytes was detected by CCK-8 assay. **(G–J)** The scratch-wound assay and Quantitative data revealed the impacts of transfection with SHP2 siRNA or overexpression plasmid on the migration of chondrocytes. Scale bar, 100 μm. Data are means ± SEM of three independent experiments; $*P < 0.05$ versus the control group.

**Supplementary Figure 2** | The effect of SHP2 on subchondral bone quality in mice. **(A)** μCT parameters of BV/TV, Tb. N, Tb. Th and Tb. Sp of subchondral bone in each group of mice 8 weeks after DMM surgery. $n = 6$, $*P < 0.05$ versus Sham+Ad−shControl group. **(B)** uCT parameters of BV/TV, Tb. N, Tb. Th and Tb. Sp of subchondral bone in each group of mice 12 weeks after DMM surgery. $n = 6$, $*P < 0.05$ versus Sham+Ad−shControl group.

## REFERENCES


Bai, J., Zhang, Y., Zheng, X., Huang, M., Cheng, W., Shan, H., et al. (2020). LncRNA MM2P-induced, exosome-mediated transfer of Sox9 from monocyte-derived cells modulates primary chondrocytes. *Cell Death Dis.* 11:763. doi: 10.1038/s41419-020-02945-5

Biswas, P., Canosa, S., Schoenfeld, D., Schoenfeld, J., Li, P., Cheas, L. C., et al. (2006). PECAM-1 affects GSK-3beta-mediated beta-catenin phosphorylation and degradation. *Am. J. Pathol.* 169, 314–324. doi: 10.2353/ajpath.2006.051112

Bouaziz, W., Funck-Brentano, T., Lin, H., Marty, C., Ea, H. K., Hay, E., et al. (2015). Loss of sclerostin promotes osteoarthritis in mice via beta-catenin-dependent and -independent Wnt pathways. *Arthritis Res. Ther.* 17:24. doi: 10.1186/s13075-015-0540-6

Chang, S. H., Mori, D., Kobayashi, H., Mori, Y., Nakamoto, H., Okada, K., et al. (2019). Excessive mechanical loading promotes osteoarthritis through the gremlin-1-NF-kappaB pathway. *Nat. Commun.* 10:1442. doi: 10.1038/s41467-019-09491-5

Chauhan, D., Pandey, P., Hideshima, T., Treon, S., Raje, N., Davies, F. E., et al. (2000). SHP2 mediates the protective effect of interleukin-6 against dexamethasone-induced apoptosis in multiple myeloma cells. *J. Biol. Chem.* 275, 27845–27850. doi: 10.1074/jbc.M003428200

Corr, M. (2008). Wnt-beta-catenin signaling in the pathogenesis of osteoarthritis. *Nat. Clin. Pract. Rheumatol.* 4, 550–556. doi: 10.1038/ncprheum0904

Deng, Y., Lu, J., Li, W., Wu, A., Zhang, X., Tong, W., et al. (2018). Reciprocal inhibition of YAP/TAZ and NF-kappaB regulates osteoarthritic cartilage degradation. *Nat. Commun.* 9:4564. doi: 10.1038/s41467-018-07022-2

Glasson, S. S., Askew, R., Sheppard, B., Carito, B., Blanchet, T., Ma, H. L., et al. (2005). Deletion of active ADAMTS5 prevents cartilage degradation in a murine model of osteoarthritis. *Nature* 434, 644–648.

Glasson, S. S., Blanchet, T. J., and Morris, E. A. (2007). The surgical destabilization of the medial meniscus (DMM) model of osteoarthritis in the 129/SvEv mouse. *Osteoarthritis Cartilage* 15, 1061–1069. doi: 10.1016/j.joca.2007.03.006

Glasson, S. S., Chambers, M. G., Van Den Berg, W. B., and Little, C. B. (2010). The OARSI histopathology initiative - recommendations for histological assessments of osteoarthritis in the mouse. *Osteoarthritis Cartilage* 18(Suppl. 3), S17–S23. doi: 10.1016/j.joca.2010.05.025

Glyn-Jones, S., Palmer, A. J. R., Agricola, R., Price, A. J., Vincent, T. L., Weinans, H., et al. (2015). Osteoarthritis. *Lancet* 386, 376–387. doi: 10.1016/s0140-6736(14)60802-3

Heun, Y., Pircher, J., Czermak, T., Bluem, P., Hupel, G., Bohmer, M., et al. (2019). Inactivation of the tyrosine phosphatase SHP-2 drives vascular dysfunction in sepsis. *EBioMedicine* 42, 120–132. doi: 10.1016/j.ebiom.2019.03.034

Hollander, A. P., Pidoux, I., Reiner, A., Rorabeck, C., Bourne, R., and Poole, A. R. (1995). Damage to type II collagen in aging and osteoarthritis starts at the articular surface, originates around chondrocytes, and extends into the cartilage with progressive degeneration. *J. Clin. Invest.* 96, 2859–2869.

Kamiya, N., Kim, H. K., and King, P. D. (2014). Regulation of bone and skeletal development by the SHP-2 protein tyrosine phosphatase. *Bone* 69, 55–60. doi: 10.1016/j.bone.2014.08.015

Lapinski, P. E., Meyer, M. F., Feng, G. S., Kamiya, N., and King, P. D. (2013). Deletion of SHP-2 in mesenchymal stem cells causes growth retardation, limb and chest deformity, and calvarial defects in mice. *Dis. Model Mech.* 6, 1448–1458. doi: 10.1242/dmm.012849

Lark, M. W., Bayne, E. K., and Lohmander, L. S. (1995). Aggrecan degradation in osteoarthritis and rheumatoid arthritis. *Acta Orthop. Scand. Suppl.* 266, 92–97.

Li, K., Zhang, Y., Zhang, Y., Jiang, W., Shen, J., Xu, S., et al. (2018). Tyrosine kinase fyn promotes osteoarthritis by activating the beta-catenin pathway. *Ann. Rheum. Dis.* 77, 935–943. doi: 10.1136/annrheumdis-2017-212658

Liu, Y. N., Guan, Y., Shen, J., Jia, Y. L., Zhou, J. C., Sun, Y., et al. (2020). Shp2 positively regulates cigarette smoke-induced epithelial mesenchymal transition by mediating MMP-9 production. *Respir. Res.* 21:161. doi: 10.1186/s12931-020-01426-9

Loeser, R. F., Goldring, S. R., Scanzello, C. R., and Goldring, M. B. (2012). Osteoarthritis: a disease of the joint as an organ. *Arthritis Rheum.* 64, 1697–1707.

Maeshima, K., Stanford, S. M., Hammaker, D., Sacchetti, C., Zeng, L. F., Ai, R., et al. (2016). Abnormal PTPN11 enhancer methylation promotes rheumatoid arthritis fibroblast-like synoviocyte aggressiveness and joint inflammation. *JCI Insight* 1:e86580. doi: 10.1172/jci.insight.86580

Ming, M., Wang, S., Wu, W., Senyuk, V., Le Beau, M. M., Nucifora, G., et al. (2012). Activation of Wnt/β-catenin protein signaling induces mitochondria-mediated apoptosis in hematopoietic progenitor cells. *J. Biol. Chem.* 287, 22683–22690. doi: 10.1074/jbc.M112.342089

Nakashima, T., Hayashi, M., Fukunaga, T., Kurata, K., Oh-Hora, M., Feng, J. Q., et al. (2011). Evidence for osteocyte regulation of bone homeostasis through RANKL expression. *Nat. Med.* 17, 1231–1234. doi: 10.1038/nm.2452

Naski, M. C., Colvin, J. S., Coffin, J. D., and Ornitz, D. M. (1998). Repression of hedgehog signaling and BMP4 expression in growth plate cartilage by fibroblast growth factor receptor 3. *Development* 125, 4977–4988.

Neuhold, L. A., Killar, L., Zhao, W., Sung, M. L., Warner, L., Kulik, J., et al. (2001). Postnatal expression in hyaline cartilage of constitutively active human collagenase-3 (MMP-13) induces osteoarthritis in mice. *J. Clin. Invest.* 107, 35–44.

Niogret, C., Miah, S. M. S., Rota, G., Fonta, N. P., Wang, H., Held, W., et al. (2019). Shp-2 is critical for ERK and metabolic engagement downstream of IL-15 receptor in NK cells. *Nat. Commun.* 10:1444. doi: 10.1038/s41467-019-09431-3

Stickens, D., Behonick, D. J., Ortega, N., Heyer, B., Hartenstein, B., Yu, Y., et al. (2004). Altered endochondral bone development in matrix metalloproteinase 13-deficient mice. *Development* 131, 5883–5895. doi: 10.1242/dev.01461

Sturla, L. M., Zinn, P. O., Ng, K., Nitta, M., Kozono, D., Chen, C. C., et al. (2011). Src homology domain-containing phosphatase 2 suppresses cellular senescence in glioblastoma. *Br. J. Cancer* 105, 1235–1243. doi: 10.1038/bjc.2011.345

Timmerman, I., Hoogenboezem, M., Bennett, A. M., Geerts, D., Hordijk, P. L., and van Buul, J. D. (2012). The tyrosine phosphatase SHP2 regulates recovery of endothelial adherens junctions through control of beta-catenin phosphorylation. *Mol. Biol. Cell* 23, 4212–4225. doi: 10.1091/mbc.E12-01-0038

Uusitalo, H., Hiltunen, A., Soderstrom, M., Aro, H. T., and Vuorio, E. (2000). Expression of cathepsins B, H, K, L, and S and matrix metalloproteinases 9 and 13 during chondrocyte hypertrophy and endochondral ossification in mouse fracture callus. *Calcif. Tissue Int.* 67, 382–390. doi: 10.1007/s002230001152

Wang, Q., Rozelle, A. L., Lepus, C. M., Scanzello, C. R., Song, J. J., Larsen, D. M., et al. (2011). Identification of a central role for complement in osteoarthritis. *Nat. Med.* 17, 1674–1679. doi: 10.1038/nm.2543

Wongwichai, T., Teeyakasem, P., Pruksakorn, D., Kongtawelert, P., and Pothacharoen, P. (2019). Anthocyanins and metabolites from purple rice inhibit IL-1beta-induced matrix metalloproteinases expression in human articular chondrocytes through the NF-kappaB and ERK/MAPK pathway. *Biomed. Pharmacother.* 112:108610. doi: 10.1016/j.biopha.2019.108610

Wu, Q., Zhu, M., Rosier, R. N., Zuscik, M. J., O'Keefe, R. J., and Chen, D. (2010). Beta-catenin, cartilage, and osteoarthritis. *Ann. N. Y. Acad. Sci.* 1192, 344–350. doi: 10.1111/j.1749-6632.2009.05212.x

Xiang, D., Cheng, Z., Liu, H., Wang, X., Han, T., Sun, W., et al. (2017). Shp2 promotes liver cancer stem cell expansion by augmenting beta-catenin signaling and predicts chemotherapeutic response of patients. *Hepatology* 65, 1566–1580. doi: 10.1002/hep.28919

Zhang, J., Zhang, F., and Niu, R. (2015). Functions of Shp2 in cancer. *J. Cell. Mol. Med.* 19, 2075–2083. doi: 10.1111/jcmm.12618

Zhou, Y., Mohan, A., Moore, D. C., Lin, L., Zhou, F. L., Cao, J., et al. (2015). SHP2 regulates osteoclastogenesis by promoting preosteoclast fusion. *FASEB J.* 29, 1635–1645. doi: 10.1096/fj.14-260844

Zhou, Y., Wang, T., Hamilton, J. L., and Chen, D. (2017). Wnt/beta-catenin signaling in osteoarthritis and in other forms of arthritis. *Curr. Rheumatol. Rep.* 19:53. doi: 10.1007/s11926-017-0679-z

Zhu, M., Chen, M., Zuscik, M., Wu, Q., Wang, Y. J., Rosier, R. N., et al. (2008). Inhibition of beta-catenin signaling in articular chondrocytes results in articular cartilage destruction. *Arthritis Rheum.* 58, 2053–2064. doi: 10.1002/art.23614

Zhu, M., Tang, D., Wu, Q., Hao, S., Chen, M., Xie, C., et al. (2009). Activation of beta-catenin signaling in articular chondrocytes leads to osteoarthritis-like phenotype in adult beta-catenin conditional activation mice. *J. Bone Miner. Res.* 24, 12–21. doi: 10.1359/jbmr.080901

Zou, G. M., Hu, W. Y., and Wu, W. (2007). TNF family molecule LIGHT regulates chemokine CCL27 expression on mouse embryonic stem cell-derived dendritic cells through NF-kappaB activation. *Cell. Signal.* 19, 87–92. doi: 10.1016/j.cellsig.2006.05.025

# 3

# Communications Between Bone Marrow Macrophages and Bone Cells in Bone Remodeling

*Kaixuan Chen*[1], *Yurui Jiao*[1], *Ling Liu*[1], *Mei Huang*[1], *Chen He*[1], *Wenzhen He*[1], *Jing Hou*[1], *Mi Yang*[1], *Xianghang Luo*[1,2,3] *and Changjun Li*[1,2,3*]

[1] Department of Endocrinology, Endocrinology Research Center, The Xiangya Hospital of Central South University, Changsha, China, [2] National Clinical Research Center for Geriatric Disorders, Xiangya Hospital, Changsha, China, [3] Key Laboratory of Organ Injury, Aging and Regenerative Medicine of Hunan Province, Changsha, China

***Correspondence:**
Changjun Li
lichangjun@csu.edu.cn

The mammalian skeleton is a metabolically active organ that continuously undergoes bone remodeling, a process of tightly coupled bone resorption and formation throughout life. Recent studies have expanded our knowledge about the interactions between cells within bone marrow in bone remodeling. Macrophages resident in bone (BMMs) can regulate bone metabolism via secreting numbers of cytokines and exosomes. This review summarizes the current understanding of factors, exosomes, and hormones that involved in the communications between BMMs and other bone cells including mensenchymal stem cells, osteoblasts, osteocytes, and so on. We also discuss the role of BMMs and potential therapeutic approaches targeting BMMs in bone remodeling related diseases such as osteoporosis, osteoarthritis, rheumatoid arthritis, and osteosarcoma.

**Keywords: macrophages, intracellular communication, macrophage-derived exosome, bone remodeling, bone diseases**

## INTRODUCTION

Macrophages are diverse, multifunctional, and plastic cells that regulate tissue homeostasis under physiological conditions and in various pathophysiological processes according to the surrounding environment.

Macrophages can be divided into circulating and resident macrophages. During embryonic development, macrophages are also the first emerged cells of the nascent immune system and they would infiltrate various developing organs to differentiate into tissue-resident macrophages, such as bone-resident macrophages (Wynn et al., 2013). Current knowledge of bone-resident macrophages (Michalski and McCauley, 2017) is limited. Osteal macrophages are a subset of bone-resident macrophages and are f4/80 positive and trap negative. Close to the bone surface, osteal macrophages are adjacent to osteoblasts, regulate bone formation, and are closely related to the osteogenic differentiation of mesenchymal stem cells. One characteristic of this group of myeloid cells is that although they share a common precursor with osteoclasts, they have different markers on their surfaces from osteoclasts. Communications between macrophages and other bone cells play an important role in bone tissue homeostasis and new bone formation. In this review, we focus primarily on the effects of macrophages on other bone cells. Extracellular vesicles are a group of cell-derived heterogeneous membranous structures that facilitate cell-cell communications. Hence, we discussed the potential contribution of the new-found microRNAs and alarmins contained in macrophage-derived extracellular vesicles in maintaining bone homeostasis in the context of bone stromal regulation. In the end, we further explained the role of macrophages in bone remodeling-related bone diseases and described the relationship between macrophages and bone tumors such as osteosarcoma.

This review focuses on the presence of macrophages in endosseous tissue, revealing the important role of macrophages in bone physiology and pathology.

## MACROPHAGES

### The Occurrence and Function of Macrophages

Since Elie Metchnikoff first translated macrophages into Greek "big eaters," macrophages are primarily known for their phagocytosis in inflammation and immunity (Gordon, 2008). Macrophages are differentiated immune cells with heterogeneity and plasticity. They are activated under different environmental signals and participate in diverse functions (Das et al., 2014, 2015; Jafarnezhad-Ansariha et al., 2018). Macrophage is often referred to as polarization. Different subtypes of macrophages have been derived from the simple M1/M2 classification, according to the environment, transcription factors, and cytokines secreted by macrophages. According to the expression of marker in macrophage surface, M1/M2 are currently also called "M1-like" and "M2-like" (Biswas and Mantovani, 2010), but in this review, we still only use M1 and M2 to represent.

M1 or classical activation of macrophages is an important inflammatory responser. Polarized M1 can produce high levels of reactive oxygen species (ROS), nitric oxide (NO), and pro-inflammatory cytokines such as interleukin IL-1, IL-2, IL-6, IL-12, TNF-α, and IFN-γ, which are involved in enhancing the host's defense response (Mosser, 2003; Genin et al., 2015). However, excessive stimulation of M1 macrophages can lead to tissue damage and autoimmune diseases (Mosser and Edwards, 2008). M2 macrophages mainly present in the subsiding phase of inflammation and are responsible for the production of anti-inflammatory cytokines and the clearance of apoptotic cells. Exposure to anti-inflammatory cytokines (IL-4, IL-10, and IL-13) or IL-1 receptor ligands or immune complexes and toll-like receptors (TLRs) can lead to M2 macrophage polarization (Mantovani et al., 2004; Guihard et al., 2012; Woo et al., 2015). M2 can produce anti-inflammatory cytokines such as chemokines ligands 18 (CCL-18), CCL-22, IL-10, and a small amount of IL-12 family members (Mosser and Edwards, 2008; Guo et al., 2019). In addition, M2 macrophages can produce a large number of osteogenic growth factors such as BMP-2 bone morphogenetic protein-2, a subclass of the TGF-β family and a potent promoter to osteogenic differentiation of MSCs (Champagne et al., 2002; Li et al., 2018), TGF-β (Assoian et al., 1987), osteopontin (Takahashi et al., 2004), and 1,25-dihydroxy-vitamin D3 (Kreutz et al., 1993). M2 can be further subdivided into M2a, M2c, and M2d by different signal activation, cell surface markers, and their functions (**Figure 1**) (Mosser and Edwards, 2008; Jetten et al., 2014; Murray et al., 2014; Roszer, 2015; Ogle et al., 2016; Arora et al., 2018).

Moreover, macrophages can also be divided into circulating and tissue-resident types. Tissue-resident macrophages are a diverse family of cells found in most organs (such as liver kupffer cells and alveolar macrophages in the lungs). Based on the origin, tissue-resident macrophages can be divided into two subsets. One derives from the yolk sac and another population originates from hematopoietic progenitors and circulating monocytes (**Figure 1**) (Heideveld and van den Akker, 2017). Tissue-resident macrophages express a large number of cell surface receptors, growth factors, proinflammatory and anti-inflammatory cytokines, and many other cell products (Jamalpoor et al., 2018). Most damage-related factors are first sensed by the resident macrophages, which become tense and recruit more macrophages when activated. Resident and recruited macrophages respond to their local environment and activate specific transcriptional programs that drive macrophages to a range of different phenotypes, from pro-inflammatory M1 macrophages to anti-inflammatory M2 macrophages (Xue et al., 2014; Juhas et al., 2018). Tissue damage caused by external (damage, chemicals, infection) and internal triggers (DNA damage, immune response) or by lack (nutrients, oxygen) and excess (sugar, cholesterol) factors may induce macrophage activation, sequentially lead to a disruption of the delicate balance between bone formation and resorption.

### One Subset of Bone-Resident Macrophages—Osteal Macrophages

Bone macrophage includes bone marrow macrophage (erythroblastic island macrophage, hematopoietic stem cell niche macrophage), osteoclast and osteal macrophages which also named osteomacs. Osteal macrophages were found in both periosteum and endosseous tissue, which support osteoblastic function and maintain bone homeostasis (Winkler et al., 2010; Cho et al., 2014b; Raggatt et al., 2014; Miron et al., 2016; Michalski and McCauley, 2017). Osteal macrophages account for about one sixth of the total cells in bone tissue (Chang et al., 2008), they present in resting bone tissue and increase in active bone anabolism sites. Osteal macrophages are a unique subset of bone-resident macrophages, close to the bone surface, f4/80 positive and trap-negative (Geissmann et al., 2010), adjacent to bone-forming cells (osteoblasts), dormant cells, and osteoclasts. The osteoblasts on the inner surface of cortical bone were mostly covered by $f4/80^+$, $CD68^+$, $mac\text{-}3^+$, and trap-macrophages and be regulated by osteomacs (Chang et al., 2008; Batoon et al., 2019).

CSF-1 (colony stimulating factor 1) and various molecular markers are required for the proliferation and differentiation of mononuclear phagocyte progenitor cells to monocytes, osteal macrophages, and osteoclasts. Previous studies have shown that osteomacs on and in the periosteum are highly expressed with the mature macrophage marker CD169, which can be distinguished from osteoclasts (Mohsenzadegan et al., 2015; Batoon et al., 2019). So far, there is no unique marker between osteal cells and other bone macrophage subsets, but it is known osteal cells that in endosteum do not express ER-HR3 antigen which can be distinguished (Wu et al., 2016; Kaur et al., 2017).

## COMMUNICATIONS BETWEEN MACROPHAGES AND BONE CELLS

Bone is a kind of mineralized connective tissue, which plays the role of movement, support, and protection of soft tissues, storage of calcium and phosphorus, and preservation of bone marrow

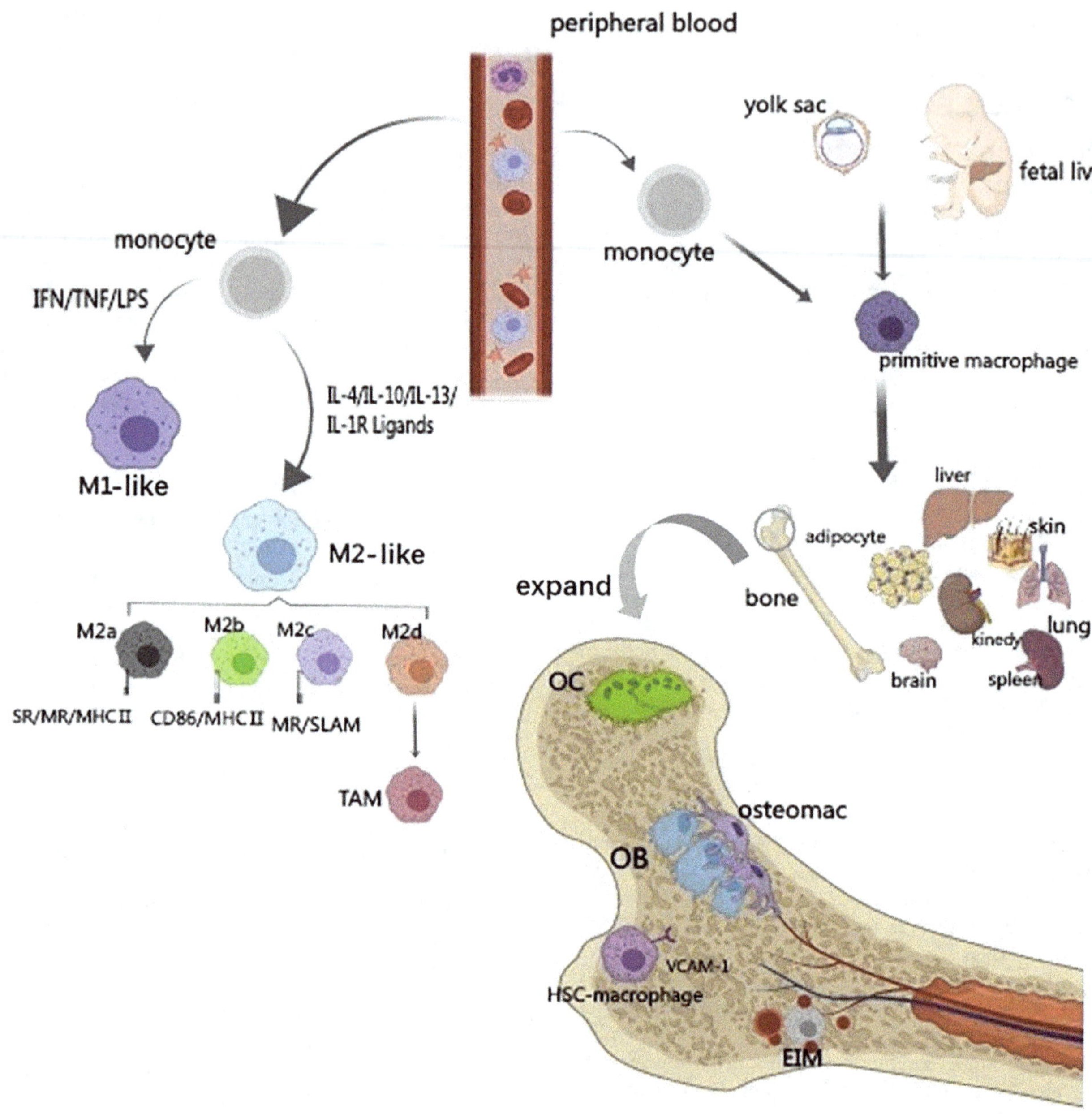


**FIGURE 1 |** Origin and classification of macrophages. The diagram illustrates the source and classification of macrophages. Circulating macrophages are classified into M1 and M2 types according to their activators and functions. M2-type can be further subdivided into M2a, M2c, and M2d by different signal activation, cell surface markers and their functions. Based on the origin, tissue-resident macrophages can be divided into two subsets. One derives from the yolk sac and another population originates from hematopoietic progenitors and circulating monocytes. Bone macrophage includes bone marrow macrophage (erythroblastic island macrophage, hematopoietic stem cell niche macrophage), osteoclast and osteal macrophages (osteomacs).

(Robling et al., 2006; Datta et al., 2008). Bone tissue is composed of roughly two parts: the dense layer and the spongy layer. The dense layer consists primarily of bone cells that make up the outermost layer of bone and functions primarily to support structural stability of the body and movement. The spongy layer is a trabecular, highly vascularized network of bone that houses the red and white marrow and is a hotbed of hematopoietic blood (Le et al., 2017). Despite bone is inert in appearance, it is a highly dynamic organ, constantly absorbed by osteoclasts and regenerated by osteoblasts, by which old bone is replaced by new bone. The equilibrium state of bone resorption and formation is regulated by local and systemic factors including cells, hormones,

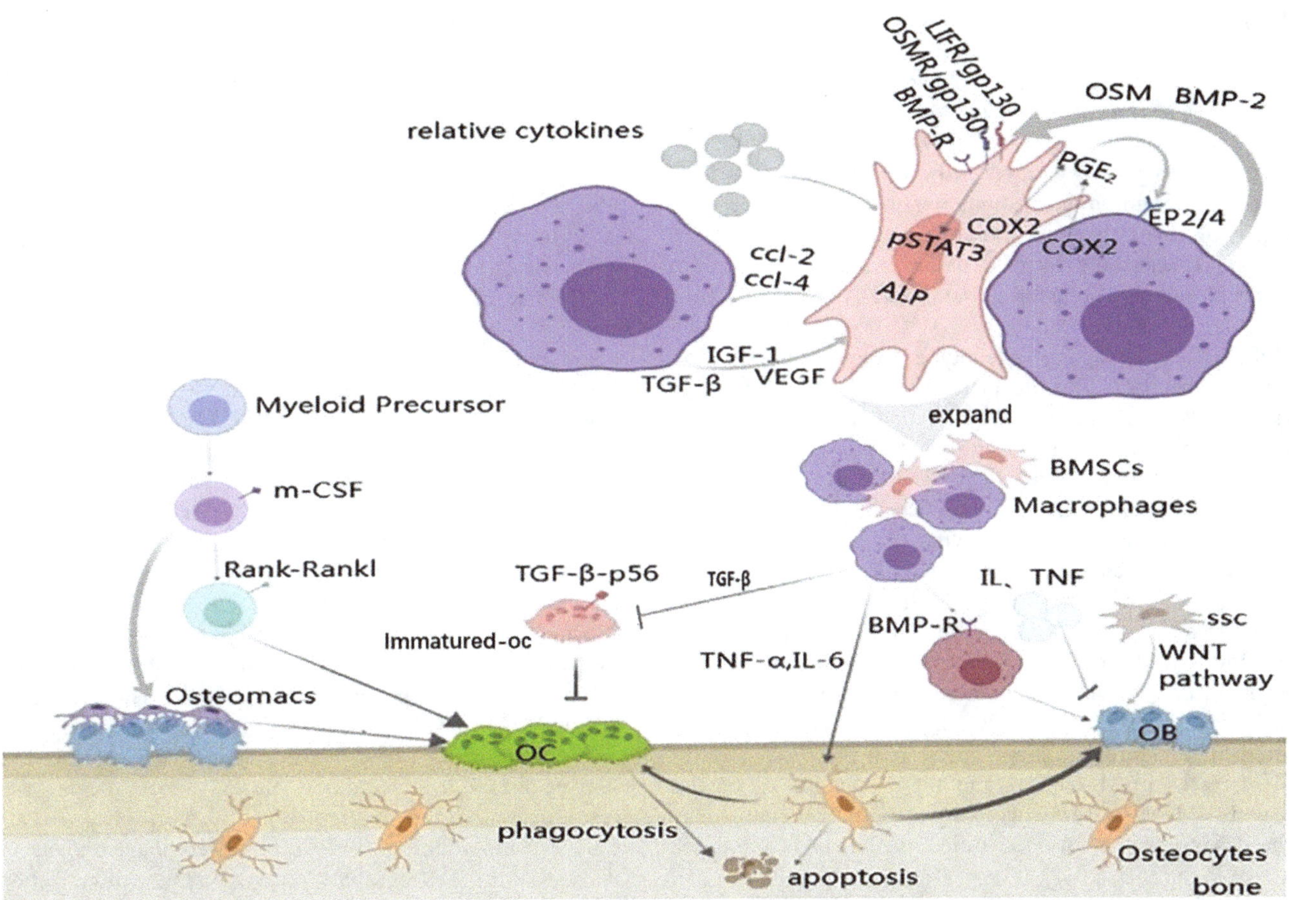


**FIGURE 2 |** Communications between macrophages and bone remodeling cells. Arrow represents "stimulatory modification;" the gray triangle means "enlarged display;" the arrow with a line means "suppress." Cell-cell communication between MSCs and macrophages results in the production of PGE2 and through the EP2/4 receptors to produce OSM. OSM acts on the MSCs via the gp130 receptors to activate STAT3 phosphorylation. Macrophage can also release BMP-2 to active the osteoblast differentiation genes, such as ALP, via the BMP-R in MSCs. MSCs can produce CCL-2 and CCL-4 to regulate macrophages and in reverse, this process is under the control of the macrophages; The differentiation of osteoblasts is regulated by variety of aspects including macrophages, osteocytes, inflammatory mediators and MSCs; Osteoclasts and osteomacs can derive from the same myeloid precursor, but it's unknown if the osteomac is a kind of the osteoclast precursors. Besides, macrophages mediate the growth of osteoclasts through various cytokines; Osteocytes apoptosis is under the regulation of macrophages.

cytokines, etc. Here we focus on the relationship between bone derived macrophages and bone remodeling related cells.

## Macrophage and BMSCs

Champagne is the first one to propose the mechanism by which macrophages contribute to osteogenic differentiation of bone marrow mesenchymal stem cells (BMSCs). In their study, the conditioned medium of the inactive J774A.1 mouse macrophage cell line was used for experiments, and it was found that the activity of alkaline phosphatase in human bone marrow mesenchymal stem cells was enhanced by the mediation of BMP-2 (**Figure 2**) (Champagne et al., 2002; Jamalpoor et al., 2018). A subsequent study co-cultured inactive human monocytes and human bone marrow mesenchymal stem cells (hbMSCs) and found that monocytes promoted MSC proliferation and increased expression of osteocalcin and osteopontin (Pirraco et al., 2013). Osteomacs regulate maintenance and proliferation of Nestin-positive MSC. These MSC express a variety of HSC retention factors and it is thought that macrophages talk to MSC via unknown secreted factors, excluding IL-1, IL-10, TNF-α, and insulin like growth factor 1 (IGF-1) (Heideveld and van den Akker, 2017). Nicolaidou et al. found that the number of macrophages in culture was positively correlated with bone formation when they co-culture human peripheral blood mononuclear cells (PBMCs) with hbMSCs (Nicolaidou et al., 2012). This process requires direct cell-cell contact to produce a soluble factor that induces STAT3 phosphorylation, known as oncostatin M (OSM). OSM is bound by two receptor complexes, consisting of a gp130 subunit and a leukemia suppressor receptor (LIFR). OSM gene deletion altered bone healing in the tibial injury model in mice. *In vitro* studies have described the stimulating effect of OSM produced by macrophages on the mineralization activity and differentiation of osteoblasts (Sims and Quinn, 2014). This process also depends on prostaglandin E2 (PGE2) and cox-2 (COX2) (Nicolaidou et al., 2012). Cell-cell contact between MSCs and macrophages produces PGE2 and induces OSM production through EP2/4 receptor on macrophages. Then OSM activates STAT3 phosphorylation through OSM and LIF receptors (**Figure 2**) (Nicolaidou et al., 2012; Horwood, 2016). Guihard also found the OSM signaling pathway. However, when hbMSCs were cultured in the conditioned medium of mononuclear cells treated with IL-4 or IL-10, there was no enhanced osteogenesis found and no OSM secretion detected (Guihard et al., 2012). Found in the study of inducing bone formation through bone Ti implants, the osteogenic differentiation of BMSCs could be changed by shifting the macrophage phenotype. Excessive polarization in the M1 direction leads to prolonged inflammation, while excessive polarization in the M2 direction leads to enhanced osteogenesis around Ti implants greatly (Wang et al., 2018). In contrast to the above studies, the effects of M0, M1, and M2 mouse bone marrow macrophages on osteogenic differentiation of mouse bone marrow mesenchymal stem cells have been studied. It was noted that all the macrophage subtypes could promote bone formation, and the M1-type macrophages had the greatest effect on bone formation (Lu et al., 2017). Studies have found that M1 macrophages increase the early and middle osteogenesis of MSCs, but do not increase matrix mineralization, while M2 macrophages co-culture can lead to increasing matrix mineralization. Moreover, it was found that the production of OSM increased in M1 culture and the production of BMP-2 increased in M2 co-culture, suggesting that different factors may be the driving factors for MSC differentiation in M1 and M2 cultures (Zhang et al., 2017).

In the co-culture model, MSCs significantly inhibited the production of LPS-induced pro-inflammatory cytokines (TNF-α, IL-1β, and IL-6) through iNOS and COX2-dependent pathways, and increased the secretion of IL-10 in macrophages by enhancing the production of PGE2 (Maggini et al., 2010). Experiments have proved that co-culture of MSCs and macrophages can significantly inhibit M1-macrophage polarization and induce M2 polarization (Kim and Hematti, 2009; Cho et al., 2014a). Human and mouse bone marrow mesenchymal stem cells secrete a large number of chemokines, including CCL-2 and CCL-4 (Seebach et al., 2014), which are the main chemokines for monocytes and macrophages (Mantovani et al., 2004). Combining INF-γ with another pro-inflammatory cytokine (TNF-β, IL-1β) activates bone marrow mesenchymal stem cells in damaged or inflammatory tissue, leading to increased secretion of various chemokines (**Figure 2**) (Ren et al., 2008). This MSC-mediated macrophage recruitment and macrophage phenotypic regulation may promote tissue regeneration (Bernardo and Fibbe, 2013).

## Macrophage and Osteoblasts

The purest form of bone formation is intramembrane ossification, in which the bone matrix is formed and deposited directly by osteoblasts. *In vivo*, osteal cells occur in multiple stages of intramembranous bone healing and form a unique canopy structure on mature osteoblasts. Osteal cells are in direct contact with stromal production and mineralized osteoblasts. Moreover, osteomacs promoted osteoblast differentiation, through the OSM-mediated tyrosine phosphorylation and interaction between the STAT3 and Yes-associated protein 1 (YAP1) (Wang et al., 2020). Depletion of osteomacs significantly inhibited the formation of new bone, however, specific enlargement of osteomacs resulted in a significant increase in new mineralized substrates (Raggatt et al., 2014). In MAFIA mice (a macrophage Fas-induced apoptosis mouse model), the bone transformation rate is significantly reduced (Cho et al., 2014b). TNF-α released by activated macrophages can stimulate osteoblast chemotactic effect *in vitro*, and can inhibit osteoblast differentiation in rheumatoid arthritis patients (Sun et al., 2018). IL-6 inhibits osteoblast differentiation and disrupts the balance of normal bone turnover (Harmer et al., 2018). Osteoblasts are derived from a subtype of skeleton stem cells (SSC) which belongs to bone marrow mesenchymal stem cells (Fierro et al., 2017). The WNT pathway is a major pathway for the transformation of SSC into osteoblasts. Macrophage-derived BMP-2 plays a critical role in inducing ossification by inducing alkaline phosphatase production through the signaling cascade of Wnt and Wnt/LRP5 in osteoblasts (Rawadi et al., 2003; Jamalpoor et al., 2018). Treatment of macrophages with BMP-2 antibody can prevent osteogenesis (Champagne et al., 2002). The conditioned medium collected from the BMP-2-stimulated macrophages also accelerated the osteogenic differentiation of the BMSC (Wei et al., 2018). In addition, BMP-2 affects the migration, recruitment and the differentiation of macrophages (Pardali et al., 2018).In addition to WNT, the macrophage derived-BMP can bind to the BMP receptor, which causes the dimerization of BMP-R and the phosphorylation of Smad proteins. Then, the phosphorylated molecule activates Runx2 to up-regulate OB activity and differentiation (**Figure 2**) (Kawabata et al., 1998). In a study of xenografts about deproteinized bovine bone matrix (DBBM), it was found that IL-10 released by macrophages can promote the osteogenic response of osteoblasts induced by macrophages (Shi et al., 2018).

## Macrophage and Osteoclasts

Osteal macrophages and osteoclasts are derived from myeloid progenitor cell precursors and can be stimulated by many of the same cytokines to function. But it must be emphasized that the osteomacs are not osteoclasts, because osteoclasts do not contain F4/80 Ag at all. Osteoclasts activated by pro-inflammatory stimuli may produce pre-osteoclast cytokines, including IL-6 and IL-1, which can promote the differentiation and/or function of osteoclasts. Therefore, osteoporosis may provide some candidate cellular mechanisms to explain why chronic inflammation and systemic infection often lead to osteopenia/osteoporosis (Chang et al., 2008). The generation of macrophage-derived osteoclasts can be activated by M-CSF and RANKL, and the blocking of the RANKL signaling pathway may prevent the progression of osteoporosis in mice (Jin et al., 2019). Macrophages can produce TGF-β1, which is essential for bone metabolism. NF-kB, composed of subunits such as p65, is a downstream transcription factor of the RANKL-RANKL signaling pathway (Park et al.,

**TABLE 1** | Macrophage-derived exosomes in bone metabolism.

| Cell of origin | Types | Mediators | Main biological effects | References |
|---|---|---|---|---|
| Bone marrow macrophage | Exosomes | Undetected | Promote osteogenesis | Wei et al., 2019 |
| | MicroRNAs | mir-21 | Promote tendon cell formation and fibrosis by decreasing Smad7 | Cui et al., 2019 |
| | | | Interfere the PTEN/PI3K/AKT signaling pathway to regulate the biological behavior of cells | Zheng et al., 2017; Yang et al., 2018 |
| | | mir-155 | Promote the secretion of inflammatory cytokines | Stanczyk et al., 2008; Heymans et al., 2013; Ying et al., 2017 |
| | | mir-5106 | Inhibit the genes SIK2 and SIK3 to promote bone formation | Xiong et al., 2020 |
| | Alarmins | Annexins | Induce bone resorption and help macrophages to work | Li et al., 2005; D'Souza et al., 2012; Stukes et al., 2016; McArthur et al., 2020; Xia et al., 2020; Xiong et al., 2020 |
| | | Galectins | Act on the differentiation of various bone cells | Andersen et al., 2003; Shimura et al., 2005; Nakajima et al., 2014; Weilner et al., 2016; Simon et al., 2017; Iacobini et al., 2018 |
| | | HSP; fibronectin | Functions through osteoblasts and osteoclasts. | Moursi et al., 1996; Koh et al., 2009; Gramoun et al., 2010; Notsu et al., 2016; Nakamura et al., 2019 |

2017). Nuclear factor of activated T cells cytoplasmic 1 (NFATc1) is a master regulator of osteoclast differentiation (Okamoto and Takayanagi, 2011). Some studies have shown that TGF-β1 directly down-regulates NFATc1 activity by blocking the p65 in the receptor activator and then inhibits the generation and bone resorption of osteoclasts (**Figure 2**) (Tokunaga et al., 2020). Recently, the role of the NEMO protein (a core component of the NF-kB signaling pathway) in mouse bone marrow macrophages was investigated that if the lysine-270 (NEMO-Lys270) in NEMO protein was mutated to Ala, the NF-kB signal in bone marrow macrophages would lose control, leading to the accelerated production of osteoclasts (Adapala et al., 2020). What's more, studies have found that the overexpression of cr6 interaction factor-1 (Crif1) in mouse BMSCs can increase the secretion of RANKL through the cAMP/PKA pathway, and then combine with RANK on macrophages to promote the formation of osteoclasts *in vitro* (Xiang et al., 2020).

## Macrophage and Osteocytes

Osteocytes account for 90–95% of all bone cells and are the most abundant and long-lived cells (Franz-Odendaal et al., 2006). Activated macrophages can induce the production of pro-inflammatory cytokines such as IL-1, IL-6, and TNF-α, which may play a significant role in inflammatory bone loss. Activated fibroblast growth factor-23 secreted by osteocytes after activation induced by IL-1 and TNF-α may cause hypophosphatemia during sepsis. TNF-α attracts osteoclasts by inducing osteocyte apoptosis (Tan et al., 2006). IL-1 may cause the decrease of bone cell activity through the NF-kB/RANKL signaling pathway, and soluble IL-6 can increase osteocyte-mediated osteoclastic differentiation by activating JAK2 and RANKL during normal bone growth and bone remodeling (Wu et al., 2017; Yang and Yang, 2019). It was reported that purified osteocytes can express a much higher amount of RANKL, which bind with mouse bone marrow macrophage and support osteoclast differentiation (Elango et al., 2018). Inflammation is thought to be highly correlated with bone cell apoptosis. If macrophages in part of the femoral head are polarized to the M1 phenotype and up-regulate a large number of inflammatory mediators, they can promote bone cell apoptosis and accelerate femoral head necrosis (**Figure 2**) (Jin et al., 2020).

In summary, bone formation relies on the interaction of a variety of cells which reminded above and other cytokines including HIF-1α (Karshovska et al., 2020)and CSF-1 (Alexander et al., 2011; Raggatt et al., 2014)to maintain the dynamic balance of the skeletal environment.

# MACROPHAGE-DERIVED EXOSOMES (VESICLES) REGULATE BONE METABOLISM

Intercellular communication is a key biological process that enables cells to coordinate their responses spatially and temporally to physiological changes. A fresh member of the intercellular communication system is the extracellular vesicle (EVs) (Théry, 2011) which is a small membrane derived phospholipid bilayer with a diameter between 30 and 2,000 nm. A vital class of EVs is exosomes (released by exocytosis, 30–150 nm diameter) (Colombo et al., 2014), has gained closely attention.

Recent studies have shown that macrophage-derived EVs play an important role in maintaining stability of the bone environment and bone remodeling (**Table 1**). In the study of BMP-2/macrophage-derived exosomes implantation of titanium nanotube, BMP2/macrophage-derived exosomes dramatically increased the expression of osteogenesis-related genes (ALP, osteopontin, Runx2, BMP-2, and BMP-7). Furthermore,

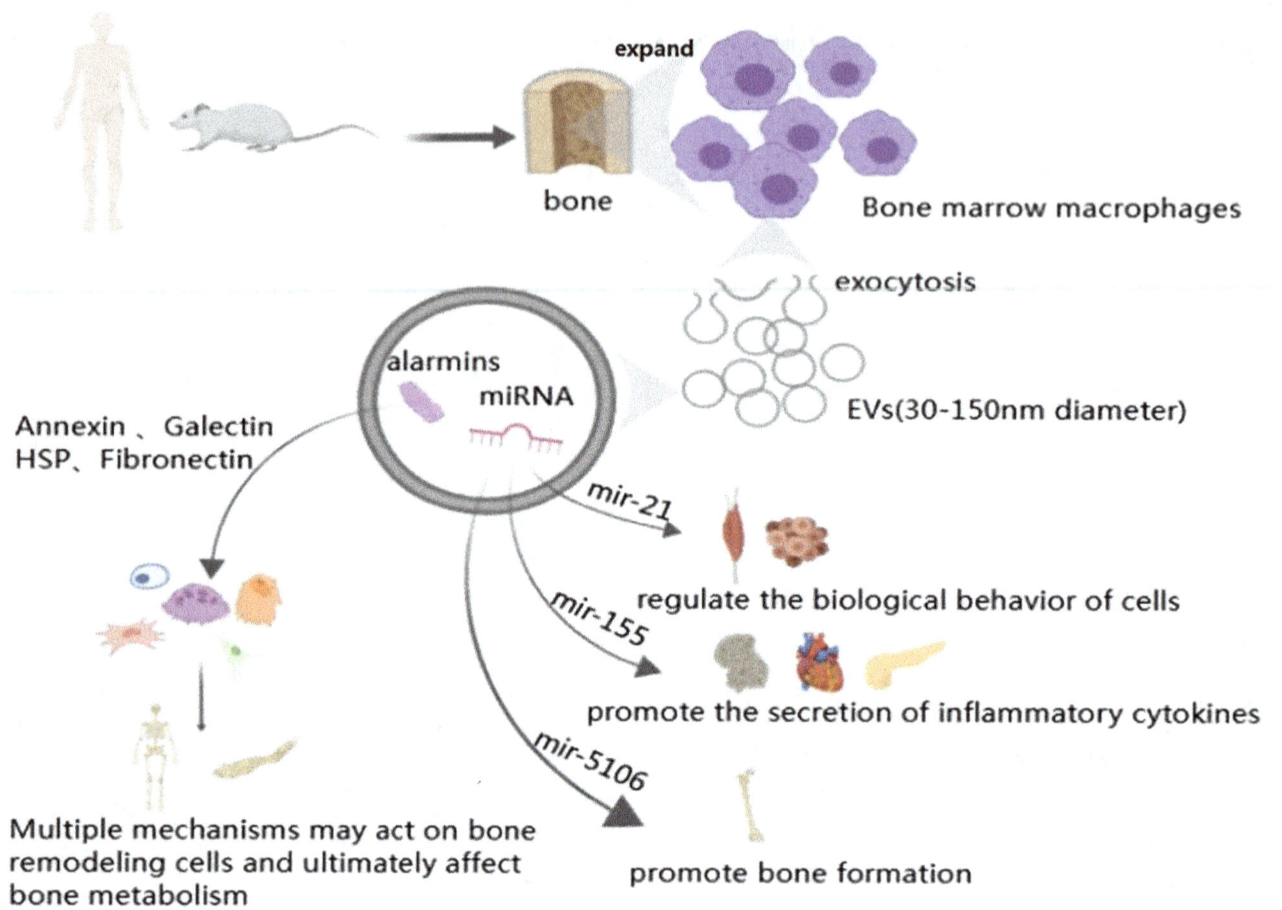


**FIGURE 3 |** Macrophage-derived exosomes in bone metabolism. Arrow represents "stimulatory modification;" the gray triangle means "enlarged display." The structure of macrophage derived exosomes is phospholipid bilayer with a diameter between 30 and 150 nm. Macrophage derived exosomes contain miRNAs (such as mir-21, mir-155, and mir-5106) and alarmins (such as Annexin, Galectin, HSP, and Fibronectin), all of them can through diverses signal pathways or release relative cytokines to participate in variety organs metabolism, including bone remodeling.

exosome-encapsulated nanotubes activated autophagy of hBMSCs and altered the secretion of cytokines associated with bone remodeling. All of these indicate the pro-osteogenic role of the BMP-2/macrophage-derived exosomes (Wei et al., 2019). And studies have found that after tendon injury, the development of the fibrotic healing response impairs the function of the tendon and restricts the movement of the tendon. MicroRNAs are a same category of small, single-stranded non-coding RNAs discovered in diverse organisms, which can regulate the expression of mRNAs (Yang et al., 2017). Studies have found that exosome miR-21-5p secreted by bone marrow macrophages activates and promotes tendon cell fibrosis fiber formation by inhibiting the expression of Smad7 (Cui et al., 2019). After induction into M2 macrophages, murine bone marrow derived macrophages can secrete miR-21, interfere with the normal signal of the PTEN/PI3K/AKT signaling pathway, and thus regulate the biological behavior of a variety of tumors, including osteosarcoma (**Figure 3**) (Zheng et al., 2017; Yang et al., 2018). This finding serves as a potential target for the prevention and treatment of tendon adhesion and bone tumors. Bone marrow macrophage-derived miR-155 can be induced to release by the activators of pro-inflammatory M1 phenotype macrophages (LPS, IFN-α) and promote the secretion of inflammatory cytokines such as TNF-α, IL-12, thereby aggravating the inflammatory response in RA (Stanczyk et al., 2008), diabetes (Ying et al., 2017), and heart disease (**Figure 3**) (Heymans et al., 2013). The latest studies found that M2-type macrophages derived from mouse bone marrow macrophages enriched miR-5106. M2D-Exo containing miR-5106 can promote osteogenic differentiation of bone marrow mesenchymal stem cells and accelerate fracture healing *in vivo* by inhibiting the expression of osteogenic related genes SIK2 and SIK3 (**Figure 3**) (Xiong et al., 2020). Unexpectedly, compared to exosomes from M0 and M2, exosomes from M1 have a stronger stimulating effect on the proliferation, osteogenesis, and adipogenic differentiation of BMSCS and all three types of exosomes had an adverse effect on the chondrogenic differentiation of BMMSCs (Xia et al., 2020). The above findings indicate that the exact mechanisms of

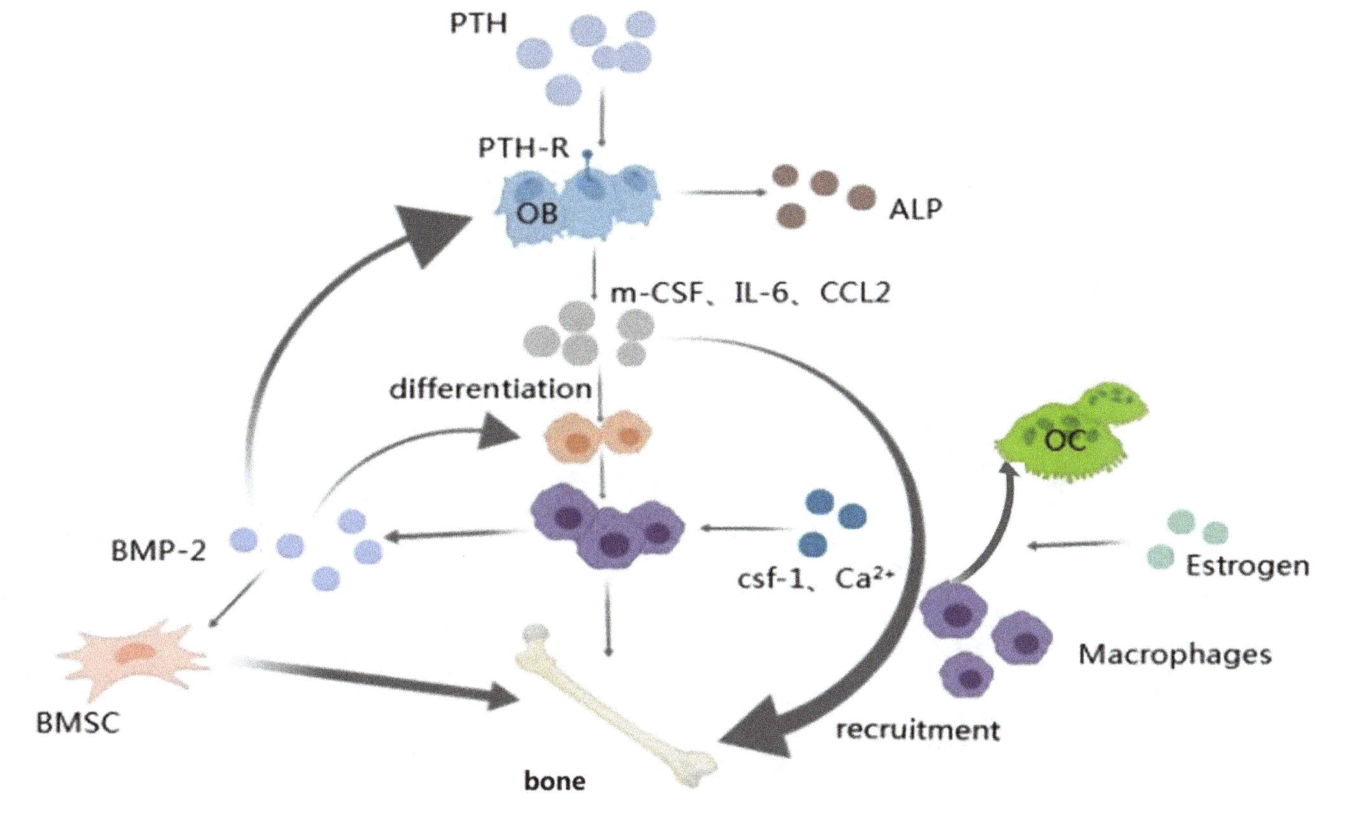


**FIGURE 4 |** Macrophage and regulatory hormones and factors. Arrow represents "stimulatory modification;" the gray triangle means "enlarged display." Macrophages play a part in the anabolic response to intermittent PTH therapy via osteoblasts which can secrete factors (IL-6, etc.) that promote the differentiation and recruitment of macrophages; Worthy to be mentioned the work of CSF-1 and $Ca^{2+}$ on macrophages; Macrophage-derived BMP-2 has effect on BMSCs, osteoblasts and macrophages via BMP-R to accelerate the osteogenic differentiation so as to make bone metabolism balance; Estrogen regulates bone homeostasis mainly through osteoblasts and osteoclasts. Estrogen mainly affects the activity of macrophages by interfering with the macrophage-mediated osteoclast formation process.

the macrophage-derived EVs still need to be further investigated and could be used as an effective therapeutic strategy for tissue regeneration.

Proteomic studies have shown that macrophage-derived EVs contain a large number of alarmins (one of endogenous molecules) (**Figure 3**). Annexins can stimulate bone resorption (Li et al., 2005), improve the phagocytic efficiency of macrophage (Stukes et al., 2016), which is related to Multiple myeloma (MM) (D'Souza et al., 2012) and play an auxiliary role of macrophages in infected tissues (Silva et al., 2019; McArthur et al., 2020; Sanches et al., 2020). Galectins mainly affect the differentiation of bone marrow stromal cells (Andersen et al., 2003), osteoblast, osteoclast (Shimura et al., 2005; Nakajima et al., 2014; Simon et al., 2017; Iacobini et al., 2018) and the osteogenesis of mesenchymal stem cells (Weilner et al., 2016). What's more, HSP-60 (Koh et al., 2009), HSP-70 (Notsu et al., 2016; Nakamura et al., 2019) and fibronectin are also primarily concerned with osteoblasts (Moursi et al., 1996) and osteoclasts (Gramoun et al., 2010) to come into play (**Table 1**).

Macrophages play a critical role in bone remodeling as a source of vehicle-carried alarmins. In conclusion, future studies should be more detailed to determine the contribution of the macrophage-derived exosomes.

The body's regulatory agents are complex and poorly understood, and future efforts would be made to unravel them (**Figure 4**).

## MACROPHAGE AND BONE REMODELING-RELATED BONE DISEASES

Tissue homeostasis requires a tight tissue system of various cell types to maintain. If the balance is disrupted, the progression of abnormal disease states may continue. Macrophages are involved in the development of many diseases with various phenotypes, but the direct link between macrophage function and bone-related diseases has not been thoroughly studied.

### Osteoporosis

Osteoporosis is a common disease characterized by the destruction of bone mass and microstructure, resulting in brittle fractures. The characterize of age-related osteoporosis is reduced bone formation and increased marrow fat accumulation (Li et al., 2015). People with osteoporosis are under a 40% lifetime risk of fractures, most often in the spine, hip or wrist. As the aging of the population, postmenopausal osteoporosis, in particular,

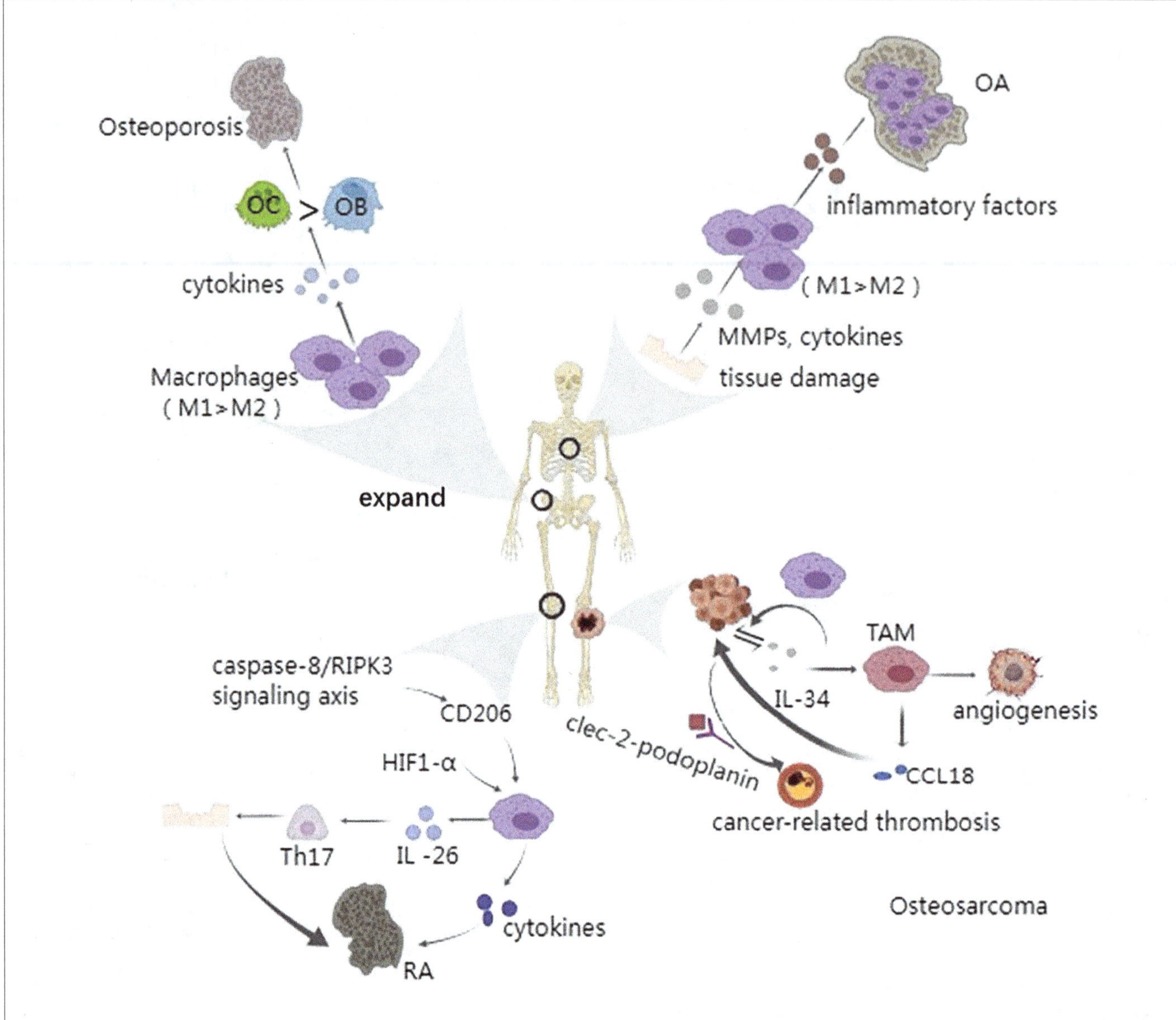


**FIGURE 5 |** Macrophage and bone remodeling related diseases. Arrow represents "stimulatory modification;" the gray triangle means "enlarged display." Osteoporosis is an age-related bone disease to some extent. The release and accumulation of proinflammatory cytokines can active osteoclasts and thus greatly accelerate the process of osteoporosis; The patients of osteoarthritis have a vital inducer that is tissue damage which can release various cytokines, leading to the imbalance between M1 and M2 macrophages. Usually, the quantity of M1 prevails, leading to the aggravation of OA; Caspase-8/RIPK3 signaling pathway and HIF1-α have been found to play a role in regulating macrophages, through CD206 and glycolysis, respectively. Besides, macrophages can secret IL-26, an inducer of Th17 cells which can cause autoimmune tissue damage; Osteosarcoma always occurs in the metaphyseal region of the long bone and the growth and metastasis of tumor cells have a closely relationship with IL-34 and CCL18. Moreover, tumor cell-derived IL-34 stimulates the angiogenesis of TAM. Cancer-related thrombosis could be made by the interaction of clec-2-podoplanin and the ectopic expression of podoplanin in patient's macrophages is the inducer, leading to the severe complications.

will further increase (Rachner et al., 2011). In addition, the 12-month mortality rate for osteoporotic hip and spinal fractures is up to 20%, and the incidence of fracture complications such as pneumonia or thromboembolic disease increases due to chronic fixation (Center et al., 1999).

Aging is usually accompanied by an irreversible recession in physiological functions. Age-associated metabolic dysfunction includes, but is not limited to, increased fat mass accumulation and insulin sensitivity deterioration (Huang et al., 2020). Aging is usually accompanied by a decrease in M2-type macrophages and an increase in proinflammatory factors, which promote the M1 transformation of the macrophage phenotype to aggravate the symptom. A study of transplanted bone marrow from 4-week-old mice into 12-month-old mice found improved fracture healing in older mice, which was attributed to younger inflammatory cells participating in the repair process (Xing et al., 2010). Cytokines secreted by macrophages related to osteoclasts including IL-1, IL-6, IL-18,

IL-23, IL-27, and TNF-α may promote osteoclast differentiation and activation in an inflammatory state (**Figure 5**) (Yang and Yang, 2019). As mentioned, macrophages regulate osteoclasts and osteoblasts mainly through inflammatory cytokines to mediate the occurrence of osteoporosis.

In addition to inflammatory response, latest studies have identified new regulatory mechanisms of macrophages in osteoporosis. They employed mice BMMs modified for over expression or inhibition of miR-128 levels to determine its effect on osteoclast differentiation. *In vitro* experiments showed that miR-128 may play a regulatory role in BMMs through miR-128/SIRT1/NF-kB signaling axis, and over expression or inhibition of miR-128 can significantly increase or decrease the occurrence of macrophage-derived osteoclasts, respectively (Shen et al., 2020). Further studies found that miR-506-3p can selectively inhibit NFATc1 in RANKL-induced activated rat BMMs, further reduce the release of bone resorption enzymes, thus relieving osteolysis (Dinesh et al., 2020). What's more, both the smo-GLI1/2 axis (Hh ligands permitting the activation of Hh signal transducer smoothened (SMO) and transmitting intracellular signaling through transcription factors of the GLI family)in the Hedgehog (Hh) signaling pathway (Kohara et al., 2020) and delphinidin (Imangali et al., 2020) can mediate the regulation of osteoclasts by macrophages.

The new studies provide an important basis for the treatment of senile osteoporosis by preventing osteoclast formation which derived from macrophages, but the exact mechanism of macrophages in osteoporosis has yet to be investigated.

## Osteoarthritis

Osteoarthritis (Murray et al., 2014), the most common form of joint disease, is characterized by cartilage destruction, synovial fibrosis, osteophyte (osteophyte at the edge of the joint) formation and pain, and sometimes swelling of certain joints such as the knee, hip, hand, and spine (Hügle and Geurts, 2017). Depending on the world health organization (WHO), the prevalence of OA worldwide exceeds 150 million (Harrell et al., 2019). The exact mechanism of OA appears to be the result of complex interactions among mechanical, cellular, and immune factors. Synovitis has turned out to be found in the early and late stages of most patients with OA (Sellam and Berenbaum, 2010), and the accumulation of macrophages in the synovium is a feature of synovitis (Sun et al., 2016).

The high proportion of M2 macrophages in the synovial tissues has certain clinical diagnostic significance for OA (Chen et al., 2020), and the pro-inflammatory M1 macrophages are also increased significantly (Sun et al., 2017). Some studies have confirmed that macrophages play an important role in the occurrence of OA through inflammatory factors, cytokines and proteins, whether it is inflammatory or mechanical injury (Bondeson et al., 2010). Since M1 macrophages are considered to be pro-inflammatory while M2 macrophages are anti-inflammatory, the degree of imbalance between M1 and M2 macrophages in OA is related to the severity of OA (Xue et al., 2019). In OA, potential mediators (MMPs, cytokines, and growth factors due to cartilage injury) leak into synovial fluid through damaged cartilage and activate synovial macrophages. Subsequently, the proinflammatory cytokines, catabolism, and anabolic factors are released, which induce osteophyte formation (**Figure 5**) (Liu-Bryan, 2013). OA was induced by intra articular injection of collagenase (collagenase-induced osteoarthritis (CIOA) and surgical medial meniscus instability (DMM) and the result showed that compared with M2 macrophages, M1 polarization of synovial macrophages was increased in the CIOA and DMM circu;amodels (Zhang et al., 2018). All above studies indicate that M1 macrophages are potential therapeutic targets for OA therapy.

## Rheumatoid Arthritis

Rheumatoid arthritis (RA) is a chronic immune-mediated inflammatory disease that affects nearly 1% of the world's population. It mainly affects synovial tissue, cartilage, and bone, leading to delayed joint damage, pain, swelling, and stiffness (McInnes and Schett, 2011). RA patients are at a higher risk of serious infection, respiratory disease, osteoporosis, cardiovascular disease, cancer, and death than the general population.

The exact pathogenesis of RA is unknown, but the activated macrophages play an important role in the pathogenesis. Caspase-8 is a promoter of apoptosis and an inhibitor of cell necrosis. Studies have found that the caspase-8/RIPK3 signaling axis is involved in maintaining stability of macrophages in synovial tissues, thereby limiting arthritis. The lack of caspase-8 in mouse synovium macrophage reduces the expression of CD206, resulting the inadequate of caspase-8-deficient macrophages to endocytosis of cellular debris caused by joint inflammation, thereby failing to control subsequent inflammation (**Figure 5**) (Dominguez et al., 2017). IL-34 is a pleiotropic cytokine and it's expression is associated with inflammatory diseases involving excessive proliferation of monocytes/macrophages (Ushach and Zlotnik, 2016). The plasma concentration of IL-34 in synovial fluid and serum is low (Nandi et al., 2012; Tian et al., 2013), but in rheumatoid arthritis, the content of IL-34 is dramatically increased, hence it's level is a useful biomarker for predicting the progression of rheumatoid arthritis (Ding et al., 2015; Liu et al., 2018; Ge et al., 2019). IL-34 and CSF-1R act in combination on mononuclear cell line (THP-1) can through a series of reactions to promote the production of helper T (Th17) cells, which is the main driver of autoimmune tissue damage, especially RA (Kuwabara et al., 2017). Additional data indicated that mononuclear/macrophage-derived IL−26 stimulation is also an important inducer of Th17 cells in RA (**Figure 5**) (Kragstrup et al., 2018). In addition, scientists have found that increasing the amount of anti-inflammatory macrophages by decreasing FLIP (flice-like inhibitory protein, highly expressed in RA synovial macrophages) in macrophages may be an effective treatment for suppressing inflammation (Huang et al., 2017). What's more, it is now becoming clear that metabolic pathways are the characteristic of rheumatoid arthritis and they may be the potential therapeutic targets (Sanchez-Lopez et al., 2019). Glycolysis is the preferred source of ATP under anoxic conditions (Epstein et al., 2017). Inflammatory joints are usually in a severe hypoxia environment, which results in the synovial fluid hypoxia inducing factor 1 α (HIF1-α) generation increases. The HIF1-α can inhibit the progression of glycolysis to stimulate the production of IL-1 and other pro-inflammatory cytokines by macrophages (**Figure 5**) (Tannahill et al., 2013), thus to accelerate the incidence of RA, increase oxidative damage and cartilage erosion (Hua and Dias, 2016).

## Osteosarcoma

Osteosarcoma is the most common primary malignant bone tumor. It can occur in any bone but most seen in the metaphyseal region of the long bone, and initially presents as progressive pain and/or swelling. Risk factors are various (Harrison and Schwartz, 2017) and this tumor tend to involve the lung (Kelleher and O'Sullivan, 2017).

Both cancer cells and immune cells can secrete various interleukins such as IL-34 (Franzè et al., 2020), which can increase the recruitment of M2 macrophages and promote the growth and metastasis of osteosarcoma (Ségaliny et al., 2015). There is increasing evidences that IL-34 promotes tumorigenesis through autocrine and paracrine mechanisms. In the autocrine pathway, IL-34 interacts with the M-CSF receptor on cancer cells to activate signaling pathways, stimulate the growth, and spread of cancer cells and increase their resistance to chemotherapy drugs (**Figure 5**) (Baghdadi et al., 2016). In the paracrine pathway, IL-34 produced by tumor cells and/or immune cells triggers M-CSF1-R signaling in tumor-associated macrophages (TAMs), thereby promoting recruitment of TAM to the tumor area, facilitating the formation of new blood vessels and the exosmosis of immunosuppressive cells (**Figure 5**) (Mantovani et al., 2017). CCL-18 (c-c motif chemokine ligand 18) is an element secreted by TAM. Studies have shown that CCL-18 can be the activator of the EP300/UCA1/Wnt/hy-catenin pathway and promote the proliferation and migration of OS cells (**Figure 5**) (Su et al., 2019). Patients with cancer have an increased risk of thromboembolism. Platelet-activated receptor c-type lectin-like receptor 2 (clec-2) is almost specifically expressed in human platelets/megakaryocytes. The endogenous ligand podoplanin is a membrane protein. Patients with osteosarcoma may have ectopic expression of podoplanin in macrophages, and the interaction of clec-2-podoplanin stimulates the formation of cancer-related thrombosis, thus aggravating the patient's condition (**Figure 5**) (Suzuki-Inoue, 2019). The exact mechanism of osteosarcoma is still unknown, but recent studies on macrophages may provide new methods for clinical treatment and prevention of complications in patients with osteosarcoma.

Bisphosphonates, PTH, estrogen, or selective estrogen receptor modulators (SERMs) and calcitonin have been used to treat osteoporosis. Non-steroidal anti-inflammatory drugs are commonly used in rheumatoid. Moreover, surgical treatment is considered the first choice for the treatment of OA and osteosarcoma. But long-term use of PTH/bisphosphonates can increase the risk of severe side effects (osteosarcoma, mandibular necrosis, and atypical femoral fractures). Surgical treatment is unsuitable for the patients who cannot tolerate it. Thus, it seems that new treatments for common bone diseases are especially important in terms of conservative treatment. At present, we have known that bone tissue macrophages can communicate with a variety of cells in the bone by secreting a series of hormones, cytokines, and exosomes. They mediate bone remodeling in various aspects and provides a new direction for clinical treatments.

## CONCLUSIONS AND FUTURE DIRECTIONS

Current knowledge of macrophages has been outlined, including their polarization, support for bone formation, potential role in bone biology, and regulation of bone metastasis. Osteal macrophages construct the cell canopy structure at the bone reconstruction site, anabolic cytokines promote bone formation and coordinate the coupling between osteoclasts and osteoblasts. However, the study of osteal macrophages is a relatively new research field, and many important and puzzling research problems still exist. The identification of specific markers of osteal macrophages remains to be explored, and the mice with specific Cre expression in BMMs/osteal macrophages is also expected to provide greater convenience for scientific research.

The potential role of microRNAs and protein profiles in exosomes, secreted by bone-resident macrophages, remains the critical issues. The prospect of improving patient outcomes and designing new therapeutic approaches are the eventual goals by better understanding the change of macrophages in the state of aging and figuring out the effects of the change on bone remodeling related diseases. Presently, new treatments targeting macrophages mainly focus on mediating the inflammatory response while lack the specific methods targeting the communications of bone-resident macrophages and other cells. Thus, validation of the role of macrophages in human bone disease requires further investigation. Targeting bone-resident macrophages may be a powerful tool for the treatment of bone remodeling related diseases.

## AUTHOR CONTRIBUTIONS

CL conceived the presented idea and supervised the written of this work. KC wrote the manuscript with supports from CL, XL, MH, YJ, CH, WH, JH, LL, and MY. All authors discussed the results and contributed to the final manuscript.

## REFERENCES

Adapala, N. S., Swarnkar, G., Arra, M., Shen, J., Mbalaviele, G., Ke, K., et al. (2020). Inflammatory osteolysis is regulated by site-specific ISGylation of the scaffold protein NEMO. *Elife.* 9:e56095. doi: 10.7554/eLife.56095

Alexander, K. A., Chang, M. K., Maylin, E. R., Kohler, T., Müller, R., Wu, A. C., et al. (2011). Osteal macrophages promote *in vivo* intramembranous bone healing in a mouse tibial injury model. *J. Bone Miner. Res.* 26, 1517–1532. doi: 10.1002/jbmr.354

Andersen, H., Jensen, O. N., Moiseeva, E. P., and Eriksen, E. F. (2003). A proteome study of secreted prostatic factors affecting osteoblastic activity: galectin-1 is involved in differentiation of human bone marrow stromal cells. *J. Bone Miner. Res.* 18, 195–203. doi: 10.1359/jbmr.2003.18.2.195

Arora, S., Dev, K., Agarwal, B., Das, P., and Syed, M. A. (2018). Macrophages: their role, activation and polarization in pulmonary diseases. *Immunobiology* 223, 383–396. doi: 10.1016/j.imbio.2017.11.001

Assoian, R. K., Fleurdelys, B. E., Stevenson, H. C., Miller, P. J., Madtes, D. K., Raines, E. W., et al. (1987). Expression and secretion of type beta transforming growth factor by activated human macrophages. *Proc. Natl. Acad. Sci. U.S.A.* 84, 6020–6024. doi: 10.1073/pnas.84.17.6020

Baghdadi, M., Wada, H., Nakanishi, S., Abe, H., Han, N., Putra, W. E., et al. (2016). Chemotherapy-induced IL34 enhances immunosuppression by tumor-associated macrophages and mediates survival of chemoresistant lung cancer cells. *Cancer Res.* 76, 6030–6042. doi: 10.1158/0008-5472.CAN-16-1170

Batoon, L., Millard, S. M., Wullschleger, M. E., Preda, C., Wu, A. C., Kaur, S., et al. (2019). $CD169^+$ macrophages are critical for osteoblast maintenance and promote intramembranous and endochondral ossification during bone repair. *Biomaterials* 196, 51–66. doi: 10.1016/j.biomaterials.2017.10.033

Bernardo, M. E., and Fibbe, W. E. (2013). Mesenchymal stromal cells: sensors and switchers of inflammation. *Cell Stem Cell* 13, 392–402. doi: 10.1016/j.stem.2013.09.006

Biswas, S. K., and Mantovani, A. (2010). Macrophage plasticity and interaction with lymphocyte subsets: cancer as a paradigm. *Nat. Immunol.* 11, 889–896. doi: 10.1038/ni.1937

Bondeson, J., Blom, A. B., Wainwright, S., Hughes, C., Caterson, B., and van den Berg, W. B. (2010). The role of synovial macrophages and macrophage-produced mediators in driving inflammatory and destructive responses in osteoarthritis. *Arthritis Rheum.* 62, 647–657. doi: 10.1002/art.27290

Center, J. R., Nguyen, T. V., Schneider, D., Sambrook, P. N., and Eisman, J. A. (1999). Mortality after all major types of osteoporotic fracture in men and women: an observational study. *Lancet* 353, 878–882. doi: 10.1016/S0140-6736(98)09075-8

Champagne, C. M., Takebe, J., Offenbacher, S., and Cooper, L. F. (2002). Macrophage cell lines produce osteoinductive signals that include bone morphogenetic protein-2. *Bone* 30, 26–31. doi: 10.1016/S8756-3282(01)00638-X

Chang, M. K., Raggatt, L. J., Alexander, K. A., Kuliwaba, J. S., Fazzalari, N. L., Schroder, K., et al. (2008). Osteal tissue macrophages are intercalated throughout human and mouse bone lining tissues and regulate osteoblast function *in vitro* and *in vivo*. *J. Immunol.* 181, 1232–1244. doi: 10.4049/jimmunol.181.2.1232

Chen, Z., Ma, Y., Li, X., Deng, Z., Zheng, M., and Zheng, Q. (2020). The immune cell landscape in different anatomical structures of knee in osteoarthritis: a gene expression-based study. *Biomed. Res. Int.* 2020:9647072. doi: 10.1155/2020/9647072

Cho, D. I., Kim, M. R., Jeong, H. Y., Jeong, H. C., Jeong, M. H., Yoon, S. H., et al. (2014a). Mesenchymal stem cells reciprocally regulate the M1/M2 balance in mouse bone marrow-derived macrophages. *Exp. Mol. Med.* 46:e70. doi: 10.1038/emm.2013.135

Cho, S. W., Soki, F. N., Koh, A. J., Eber, M. R., Entezami, P., Park, S. I., et al. (2014b). Osteal macrophages support physiologic skeletal remodeling and anabolic actions of parathyroid hormone in bone. *Proc. Natl. Acad. Sci. U.S.A.* 111, 1545–1550. doi: 10.1073/pnas.1315153111

Colombo, M., Raposo, G., and Théry, C. (2014). Biogenesis, secretion, and intercellular interactions of exosomes and other extracellular vesicles. *Annu. Rev. Cell Dev. Biol.* 30, 255–289. doi: 10.1146/annurev-cellbio-101512-122326

Cui, H., He, Y., Chen, S., Zhang, D., Yu, Y., and Fan, C. (2019). Macrophage-derived miRNA-containing exosomes induce peritendinous fibrosis after tendon injury through the miR-21-5p/Smad7 pathway. *Mol. Ther. Nucl. Acids* 14, 114–130. doi: 10.1016/j.omtn.2018.11.006

Das, A., Ganesh, K., Khanna, S., Sen, C. K., and Roy, S. (2014). Engulfment of apoptotic cells by macrophages: a role of microRNA-21 in the resolution of wound inflammation. *J. Immunol.* 192, 1120–1129. doi: 10.4049/jimmunol.1300613

Das, A., Sinha, M., Datta, S., Abas, M., Chaffee, S., Sen, C. K., and Roy, S. (2015). Monocyte and macrophage plasticity in tissue repair and regeneration. *Am. J. Pathol.* 185, 2596–2606. doi: 10.1016/j.ajpath.2015.06.001

Datta, H. K., Ng, W. F., Walker, J. A., Tuck, S. P., and Varanasi, S. S. (2008). The cell biology of bone metabolism. *J. Clin. Pathol.* 61, 577–587. doi: 10.1136/jcp.2007.048868

Dinesh, P., Kalaiselvan, S., Sujitha, S., and Rasool, M. (2020). miR-506-3p alleviates uncontrolled osteoclastogenesis via repression of RANKL/NFATc1 signaling pathway. *J. Cell. Physiol.* 235, 9497–9509. doi: 10.1002/jcp.29757

Ding, R., Li, P., Song, D., Zhang, X., and Bi, L. (2015). Predictors of response to TNF-α antagonist therapy in Chinese rheumatoid arthritis. *Clin. Rheumatol.* 34, 1203–1210. doi: 10.1007/s10067-015-2973-3

Dominguez, S., Montgomery, A. B., Haines, G. K. 3rd, Bloomfield, C. L., and Cuda, C. M. (2017). The caspase-8/RIPK3 signaling axis in antigen presenting cells controls the inflammatory arthritic response. *Arthritis Res. Ther.* 19:224. doi: 10.1186/s13075-017-1436-4

D'Souza, S., Kurihara, N., Shiozawa, Y., Joseph, J., Taichman, R., Galson, D. L., et al. (2012). Annexin II interactions with the annexin II receptor enhance multiple myeloma cell adhesion and growth in the bone marrow microenvironment. *Blood* 119, 1888–1896. doi: 10.1182/blood-2011-11-393348

Elango, J., Sanchez, C., de Val, J., Henrotin, Y., Wang, S., Motaung, K., et al. (2018). Cross-talk between primary osteocytes and bone marrow macrophages for osteoclastogenesis upon collagen treatment. *Sci. Rep.* 8:5318. doi: 10.1038/s41598-018-23532-x

Epstein, T., Gatenby, R. A., and Brown, J. S. (2017). The Warburg effect as an adaptation of cancer cells to rapid fluctuations in energy demand. *PLoS ONE* 12:e0185085. doi: 10.1371/journal.pone.0185085

Fierro, F. A., Nolta, J. A., and Adamopoulos, I. E. (2017). Concise review: stem cells in osteoimmunology. *Stem Cells* 35, 1461–1467. doi: 10.1002/stem.2625

Franzè, E., Stolfi, C., Troncone, E., Scarozza, P., and Monteleone, G. (2020). Role of interleukin-34 in cancer. *Cancers* 12:252. doi: 10.3390/cancers12010252

Franz-Odendaal, T. A., Hall, B. K., and Witten, P. E. (2006). Buried alive: how osteoblasts become osteocytes. *Dev. Dyn.* 235, 176–190. doi: 10.1002/dvdy.20603

Ge, Y., Huang, M., and Yao, Y. M. (2019). Immunomodulation of interleukin-34 and its potential significance as a disease biomarker and therapeutic target. *Int. J. Biol. Sci.* 15, 1835–1845. doi: 10.7150/ijbs.35070

Geissmann, F., Manz, M. G., Jung, S., Sieweke, M. H., Merad, M., and Ley, K. (2010). Development of monocytes, macrophages, and dendritic cells. *Science* 327, 656–661. doi: 10.1126/science.1178331

Genin, M., Clement, F., Fattaccioli, A., Raes, M., and Michiels, C. (2015). M1 and M2 macrophages derived from THP-1 cells differentially modulate the response of cancer cells to etoposide. *BMC Cancer* 15:577. doi: 10.1186/s12885-015-1546-9

Gordon, S. (2008). Elie Metchnikoff: father of natural immunity. *Eur. J. Immunol.* 38, 3257–3264. doi: 10.1002/eji.200838855

Gramoun, A., Azizi, N., Sodek, J., Heersche, J. N., Nakchbandi, I., and Manolson, M. F. (2010). Fibronectin inhibits osteoclastogenesis while enhancing osteoclast activity via nitric oxide and interleukin-1β-mediated signaling pathways. *J. Cell. Biochem.* 111, 1020–1034. doi: 10.1002/jcb.22791

Guihard, P., Danger, Y., Brounais, B., David, E., Brion, R., Delecrin, J., et al. (2012). Induction of osteogenesis in mesenchymal stem cells by activated monocytes/macrophages depends on oncostatin M signaling. *Stem Cells.* 30, 762–772. doi: 10.1002/stem.1040

Guo, Y., Cao, W., and Zhu, Y. (2019). Immunoregulatory functions of the IL-12 family of cytokines in antiviral systems. *Viruses* 11:772. doi: 10.3390/v11090772

Harmer, D., Falank, C., and Reagan, M. R. (2018). Interleukin-6 interweaves the bone marrow microenvironment, bone loss, and multiple myeloma. *Front. Endocrinol.* 9:788. doi: 10.3389/fendo.2018.00788

Harrell, C. R., Markovic, B. S., Fellabaum, C., Arsenijevic, A., and Volarevic, V. (2019). Mesenchymal stem cell-based therapy of osteoarthritis: current knowledge and future perspectives. *Biomed. Pharmacother.* 109, 2318–2326. doi: 10.1016/j.biopha.2018.11.099

Harrison, D. J., and Schwartz, C. L. (2017). Osteogenic sarcoma: systemic chemotherapy options for localized disease. *Curr. Treat. Options Oncol.* 18:24. doi: 10.1007/s11864-017-0464-2

Heideveld, E., and van den Akker, E. (2017). Digesting the role of bone marrow macrophages on hematopoiesis. *Immunobiology* 222, 814–822. doi: 10.1016/j.imbio.2016.11.007

Heymans, S., Corsten, M. F., Verhesen, W., Carai, P., van Leeuwen, R. E., Custers, K., et al. (2013). Macrophage microRNA-155 promotes cardiac hypertrophy and failure. *Circulation* 128, 1420–1432. doi: 10.1161/CIRCULATIONAHA.112.001357

Horwood, N. J. (2016). Macrophage polarization and bone formation: a review. *Clin. Rev. Allergy Immunol.* 51, 79–86. doi: 10.1007/s12016-015-8519-2

Hua, S., and Dias, T. H. (2016). Hypoxia-inducible factor (HIF) as a target for novel therapies in rheumatoid arthritis. *Front. Pharmacol.* 7:184. doi: 10.3389/fphar.2016.00184

Huang, Q. Q., Birkett, R., Doyle, R. E., Haines, G. K., Perlman, H., Shi, B., et al. (2017). Association of increased F4/80(high) macrophages with suppression of serum-transfer arthritis in mice with reduced FLIP in myeloid cells. *Arthritis Rheumatol.* 69, 1762–1771. doi: 10.1002/art.40151

Huang, Y., Xiao, Y., Liu, Y., Guo, M., Guo, Q., Zhou, F., et al. (2020). MicroRNA-188 regulates aging-associated metabolic phenotype. *Aging Cell.* 19:e13077. doi: 10.1111/acel.13077

Hügle, T., and Geurts, J. (2017). What drives osteoarthritis?-synovial versus subchondral bone pathology. *Rheumatology* 56, 1461–1471. doi: 10.1093/rheumatology/kew389

Iacobini, C., Blasetti Fantauzzi, C., Bedini, R., Pecci, R., Bartolazzi, A., Amadio, B., et al. (2018). Galectin-3 is essential for proper bone cell differentiation and activity, bone remodeling and biomechanical competence in mice. *Metab. Clin. Exp.* 83, 149–158. doi: 10.1016/j.metabol.2018.02.001

Imangali, N., Phan, Q. T., Mahady, G., and Winkler, C. (2020). The dietary anthocyanin delphinidin prevents bone resorption by inhibiting Rankl-induced differentiation of osteoclasts in a medaka (Oryzias latipes) model of osteoporosis. *J. Fish Biol.* doi: 10.1111/jfb.14317. [Epub ahead of print].

Jafarnezhad-Ansariha, F., Yekaninejad, M. S., Jamshidi, A. R., Mansouri, R., Vojdanian, M., Mahmoudi, M., et al. (2018). The effects of β-D-mannuronic acid (M2000), as a novel NSAID, on COX1 and COX2 activities and gene expression in ankylosing spondylitis patients and the murine monocyte/macrophage, J774 cell line. *Inflammopharmacology* 26, 375–384. doi: 10.1007/s10787-017-0386-4

Jamalpoor, Z., Asgari, A., Lashkari, M. H., Mirshafiey, A., and Mohsenzadegan, M. (2018). Modulation of macrophage polarization for bone tissue engineering applications. *Iran. J. Allergy Asthma Immunol.* 17, 398–408. doi: 10.18502/ijaai.v17i5.298

Jetten, N., Verbruggen, S., Gijbels, M. J., Post, M. J., De Winther, M. P., and Donners, M. M. (2014). Anti-inflammatory M2, but not pro-inflammatory M1 macrophages promote angiogenesis *in vivo*. *Angiogenesis* 17, 109–118. doi: 10.1007/s10456-013-9381-6

Jin, H., Yao, L., Chen, K., Liu, Y., Wang, Q., Wang, Z., et al. (2019). Evodiamine inhibits RANKL-induced osteoclastogenesis and prevents ovariectomy-induced bone loss in mice. *J. Cell. Mol. Med.* 23, 522–534. doi: 10.1111/jcmm.13955

Jin, S., Meng, C., He, Y., Wang, X., Zhang, Q., Wang, Z., et al. (2020). Curcumin prevents osteocyte apoptosis by inhibiting M1-type macrophage polarization in mice model of glucocorticoid-associated osteonecrosis of the femoral head. *J. Orthop. Res.* 38, 2020–2030. doi: 10.1002/jor.24619

Juhas, M., Abutaleb, N., Wang, J. T., Ye, J., Shaikh, Z., Sriworarat, C., Qian, Y., and Bursac, N. (2018). Incorporation of macrophages into engineered skeletal muscle enables enhanced muscle regeneration. *Nat. Biomed. Eng.* 2, 942–954. doi: 10.1038/s41551-018-0290-2

Karshovska, E., Wei, Y., Subramanian, P., Mohibullah, R., Geißler, C., Baatsch, I., et al. (2020). HIF-1α (hypoxia-inducible factor-1α) promotes macrophage necroptosis by regulating miR-210 and miR-383. *Arterioscler. Thromb. Vasc. Biol.* 40, 583–596. doi: 10.1161/ATVBAHA.119.313290

Kaur, S., Raggatt, L. J., Batoon, L., Hume, D. A., Levesque, J. P., and Pettit, A. R. (2017). Role of bone marrow macrophages in controlling homeostasis and repair in bone and bone marrow niches. *Semin. Cell Dev. Biol.* 61, 12–21. doi: 10.1016/j.semcdb.2016.08.009

Kawabata, M., Imamura, T., and Miyazono, K. (1998). Signal transduction by bone morphogenetic proteins. *Cytokine Growth Factor Rev.* 9, 49–61. doi: 10.1016/S1359-6101(97)00036-1

Kelleher, F. C., and O'Sullivan, H. (2017). Monocytes, macrophages, and osteoclasts in osteosarcoma. *J. Adolesc. Young Adult Oncol.* 6, 396–405. doi: 10.1089/jayao.2016.0078

Kim, J., and Hematti, P. (2009). Mesenchymal stem cell-educated macrophages: a novel type of alternatively activated macrophages. *Exp. Hematol.* 37, 1445–1453. doi: 10.1016/j.exphem.2009.09.004

Koh, J. M., Lee, Y. S., Kim, Y. S., Park, S. H., Lee, S. H., Kim, H. H., et al. (2009). Heat shock protein 60 causes osteoclastic bone resorption via toll-like receptor-2 in estrogen deficiency. *Bone* 45, 650–660. doi: 10.1016/j.bone.2009.06.007

Kohara, Y., Haraguchi, R., Kitazawa, R., Imai, Y., and Kitazawa, S. (2020). Hedgehog inhibitors suppress osteoclastogenesis in *in vitro* cultures, and deletion of smo in macrophage/osteoclast lineage prevents age-related bone loss. *Int. J. Mol. Sci.* 21:2745. doi: 10.3390/ijms21082745

Kragstrup, T. W., Andersen, T., Heftdal, L. D., Hvid, M., Gerwien, J., Sivakumar, P., et al. (2018). The IL-20 cytokine family in rheumatoid arthritis and spondyloarthritis. *Front. Immunol.* 9:2226. doi: 10.3389/fimmu.2018.02226

Kreutz, M., Andreesen, R., Krause, S. W., Szabo, A., Ritz, E., and Reichel, H. (1993). 1,25-dihydroxyvitamin D3 production and vitamin D3 receptor expression are developmentally regulated during differentiation of human monocytes into macrophages. *Blood* 82, 1300–1307. doi: 10.1182/blood.V82.4.1300.1300

Kuwabara, T., Ishikawa, F., Kondo, M., and Kakiuchi, T. (2017). The role of IL-17 and related cytokines in inflammatory autoimmune diseases. *Mediators Inflamm.* 2017:3908061. doi: 10.1155/2017/3908061

Le, B. Q., Nurcombe, V., Cool, S. M., van Blitterswijk, C. A., de Boer, J., and LaPointe, V. L. S. (2017). The components of bone and what they can teach us about regeneration. *Materials* 11:14. doi: 10.3390/ma11010014

Li, C. J., Cheng, P., Liang, M. K., Chen, Y. S., Lu, Q., Wang, J. Y., et al. (2015). MicroRNA-188 regulates age-related switch between osteoblast and adipocyte differentiation. *J. Clin. Invest.* 125, 1509–1522. doi: 10.1172/JCI77716

Li, C. J., Xiao, Y., Yang, M., Su, T., Sun, X., Guo, Q., et al. (2018). Long noncoding RNA Bmncr regulates mesenchymal stem cell fate during skeletal aging. *J. Clin. Invest.* 128, 5251–5266. doi: 10.1172/JCI99044

Li, F., Chung, H., Reddy, S. V., Lu, G., Kurihara, N., Zhao, A. Z., et al. (2005). Annexin II stimulates RANKL expression through MAPK. *J. Bone Miner. Res.* 20, 1161–1167. doi: 10.1359/JBMR.050207

Liu, Q., Fan, J., Bai, J., Peng, L., Zhang, T., Deng, L., et al. (2018). IL-34 promotes foam cell formation by enhancing CD36 expression through p38 MAPK pathway. *Sci. Rep.* 8:17347. doi: 10.1038/s41598-018-35485-2

Liu-Bryan, R. (2013). Synovium and the innate inflammatory network in osteoarthritis progression. *Curr. Rheumatol. Rep.* 15:323. doi: 10.1007/s11926-013-0323-5

Lu, L. Y., Loi, F., Nathan, K., Lin, T. H., Pajarinen, J., Gibon, E., et al. (2017). Pro-inflammatory M1 macrophages promote osteogenesis by mesenchymal stem cells via the COX-2-prostaglandin E2 pathway. *J. Orthop. Res.* 35, 2378–2385. doi: 10.1002/jor.23553

Maggini, J., Mirkin, G., Bognanni, I., Holmberg, J., Piazzón, I. M., Nepomnaschy, I., et al. (2010). Mouse bone marrow-derived mesenchymal stromal cells turn activated macrophages into a regulatory-like profile. *PLoS ONE* 5:e9252. doi: 10.1371/journal.pone.0009252

Mantovani, A., Marchesi, F., Malesci, A., Laghi, L., and Allavena, P. (2017). Tumour-associated macrophages as treatment targets in oncology. *Nat. Rev. Clin. Oncol.* 14, 399–416. doi: 10.1038/nrclinonc.2016.217

Mantovani, A., Sica, A., Sozzani, S., Allavena, P., Vecchi, A., and Locati, M. (2004). The chemokine system in diverse forms of macrophage activation and polarization. *Trends Immunol.* 25, 677–686. doi: 10.1016/j.it.2004.09.015

McArthur, S., Juban, G., Gobbetti, T., Desgeorges, T., Theret, M., Gondin, J., et al. (2020). Annexin A1 drives macrophage skewing to accelerate muscle regeneration through AMPK activation. *J. Clin. Invest.* 130, 1156–1167. doi: 10.1172/JCI124635

McInnes, I. B., and Schett, G. (2011). The pathogenesis of rheumatoid arthritis. *N. Engl. J. Med.* 365, 2205–2219. doi: 10.1056/NEJMra1004965

Michalski, M. N., and McCauley, L. K. (2017). Macrophages and skeletal health. *Pharmacol. Ther.* 174, 43–54. doi: 10.1016/j.pharmthera.2017.02.017

Miron, R. J., Zohdi, H., Fujioka-Kobayashi, M., and Bosshardt, D. D. (2016). Giant cells around bone biomaterials: osteoclasts or multi-nucleated giant cells? *Acta Biomater.* 46, 15–28. doi: 10.1016/j.actbio.2016.09.029

Mohsenzadegan, M., Fayazi, M. R., Abdolmaleki, M., Bakhshayesh, M., Seif, F., and Mousavizadeh, K. (2015). Direct immunomodulatory influence of IFN-β on human astrocytoma cells. *Immunopharmacol. Immunotoxicol.* 37, 214–219. doi: 10.3109/08923973.2015.1014559

Mosser, D. M. (2003). The many faces of macrophage activation. *J. Leukoc. Biol.* 73, 209–212. doi: 10.1189/jlb.0602325

Mosser, D. M., and Edwards, J. P. (2008). Exploring the full spectrum of macrophage activation. *Nat. Rev. Immunol.* 8, 958–969. doi: 10.1038/nri2448

Moursi, A. M., Damsky, C. H., Lull, J., Zimmerman, D., Doty, S. B., Aota, S., et al. (1996). Fibronectin regulates calvarial osteoblast differentiation. *J. Cell Sci.* 109, 1369–1380.

Murray, P. J., Allen, J. E., Biswas, S. K., Fisher, E. A., Gilroy, D. W., Goerdt, S., et al. (2014). Macrophage activation and polarization: nomenclature and experimental guidelines. *Immunity* 41, 14–20. doi: 10.1016/j.immuni.2014.06.008

Nakajima, K., Kho, D. H., Yanagawa, T., Harazono, Y., Gao, X., Hogan, V., et al. (2014). Galectin-3 inhibits osteoblast differentiation through notch signaling. *Neoplasia* 16, 939–949. doi: 10.1016/j.neo.2014.09.005

Nakamura, M., Notsu, K., and Nakagawa, M. (2019). Heat shock protein 60 negatively regulates the biological functions of ubiquitin-like protein MNSFβ in macrophages. *Mol. Cell. Biochem.* 456, 29–39. doi: 10.1007/s11010-018-3487-5

Nandi, S., Gokhan, S., Dai, X. M., Wei, S., Enikolopov, G., Lin, H., et al. (2012). The CSF-1 receptor ligands IL-34 and CSF-1 exhibit distinct developmental brain expression patterns and regulate neural progenitor cell maintenance and maturation. *Dev. Biol.* 367, 100–113. doi: 10.1016/j.ydbio.2012.03.026

Nicolaidou, V., Wong, M. M., Redpath, A. N., Ersek, A., Baban, D. F., Williams, L. M., et al. (2012). Monocytes induce STAT3 activation in human mesenchymal stem cells to promote osteoblast formation. *PLoS ONE* 7:e39871. doi: 10.1371/journal.pone.0039871

Notsu, K., Nakagawa, M., and Nakamura, M. (2016). Ubiquitin-like protein MNSFβ noncovalently binds to molecular chaperone HSPA8 and regulates osteoclastogenesis. *Mol. Cell. Biochem.* 421, 149–156. doi: 10.1007/s11010-016-2795-x

Ogle, M. E., Segar, C. E., Sridhar, S., and Botchwey, E. A. (2016). Monocytes and macrophages in tissue repair: implications for immunoregenerative biomaterial design. *Exp. Biol. Med.* 241, 1084–1097. doi: 10.1177/1535370216650293

Okamoto, K., and Takayanagi, H. (2011). Regulation of bone by the adaptive immune system in arthritis. *Arthritis Res. Ther.* 13:219. doi: 10.1186/ar3323

Pardali, E., Makowski, L. M., Leffers, M., Borgscheiper, A., and Waltenberger, J. (2018). BMP-2 induces human mononuclear cell chemotaxis and adhesion and modulates monocyte-to-macrophage differentiation. *J. Cell. Mol. Med.* 22, 5429–5438. doi: 10.1111/jcmm.13814

Park, J. H., Lee, N. K., and Lee, S. Y. (2017). Current understanding of RANK signaling in osteoclast differentiation and maturation. *Mol. Cells* 40, 706–713. doi: 10.14348/molcells.2017.0225

Pirraco, R. P., Reis, R. L., and Marques, A. P. (2013). Effect of monocytes/macrophages on the early osteogenic differentiation of hBMSCs. *J. Tissue Eng. Regen. Med.* 7, 392–400. doi: 10.1002/term.535

Rachner, T. D., Khosla, S., and Hofbauer, L. C. (2011). Osteoporosis: now and the future. *Lancet* 377, 1276–1287. doi: 10.1016/S0140-6736(10)62349-5

Raggatt, L. J., Wullschleger, M. E., Alexander, K. A., Wu, A. C., Millard, S. M., Kaur, S., et al. (2014). Fracture healing via periosteal callus formation requires macrophages for both initiation and progression of early endochondral ossification. *Am. J. Pathol.* 184, 3192–3204. doi: 10.1016/j.ajpath.2014.08.017

Rawadi, G., Vayssière, B., Dunn, F., Baron, R., and Roman-Roman, S. (2003). BMP-2 controls alkaline phosphatase expression and osteoblast mineralization by a Wnt autocrine loop. *J. Bone Miner. Res.* 18, 1842–1853. doi: 10.1359/jbmr.2003.18.10.1842

Ren, G., Zhang, L., Zhao, X., Xu, G., Zhang, Y., Roberts, A. I., et al. (2008). Mesenchymal stem cell-mediated immunosuppression occurs via concerted action of chemokines and nitric oxide. *Cell Stem Cell* 2, 141–150. doi: 10.1016/j.stem.2007.11.014

Robling, A. G., Castillo, A. B., and Turner, C. H. (2006). Biomechanical and molecular regulation of bone remodeling. *Annu. Rev. Biomed. Eng.* 8, 455–498. doi: 10.1146/annurev.bioeng.8.061505.095721

Roszer, T. (2015). Understanding the mysterious M2 macrophage through activation markers and effector mechanisms. *Mediators Inflamm.* 2015:816460. doi: 10.1155/2015/816460

Sanches, J. M., Branco, L. M., Duarte, G. H. B., Oliani, S. M., Bortoluci, K. R., Moreira, V., et al. (2020). Annexin A1 regulates NLRP3 inflammasome activation and modifies lipid release profile in isolated peritoneal macrophages. *Cells* 9:926. doi: 10.3390/cells9040926

Sanchez-Lopez, E., Cheng, A., and Guma, M. (2019). Can metabolic pathways be therapeutic targets in rheumatoid arthritis? *J. Clin. Med.* 8:753. doi: 10.3390/jcm8050753

Seebach, E., Freischmidt, H., Holschbach, J., Fellenberg, J., and Richter, W. (2014). Mesenchymal stroma cells trigger early attraction of M1 macrophages and endothelial cells into fibrin hydrogels, stimulating long bone healing without long-term engraftment. *Acta Biomater.* 10, 4730–4741. doi: 10.1016/j.actbio.2014.07.017

Ségaliny, A. I., Mohamadi, A., Dizier, B., Lokajczyk, A., Brion, R., Lanel, R., et al. (2015). Interleukin-34 promotes tumor progression and metastatic process in osteosarcoma through induction of angiogenesis and macrophage recruitment. *Int. J. Cancer* 137, 73–85. doi: 10.1002/ijc.29376

Sellam, J., and Berenbaum, F. (2010). The role of synovitis in pathophysiology and clinical symptoms of osteoarthritis. *Nat. Rev. Rheumatol.* 6, 625–635. doi: 10.1038/nrrheum.2010.159

Shen, G., Ren, H., Shang, Q., Zhang, Z., Zhao, W., Yu, X., et al. (2020). miR-128 plays a critical role in murine osteoclastogenesis and estrogen deficiency-induced bone loss. *Theranostics* 10, 4334–4348. doi: 10.7150/thno.42982

Shi, M., Wang, C., Wang, Y., Tang, C., Miron, R. J., and Zhang, Y. (2018). Deproteinized bovine bone matrix induces osteoblast differentiation via macrophage polarization. *J. Biomed. Mater. Res. A* 106, 1236–1246. doi: 10.1002/jbm.a.36321

Shimura, T., Takenaka, Y., Fukumori, T., Tsutsumi, S., Okada, K., Hogan, V., et al. (2005). Implication of galectin-3 in Wnt signaling. *Cancer Res.* 65, 3535–3537. doi: 10.1158/0008-5472.CAN-05-0104

Silva, J. M. D., Silva, H., Zelenski, C., Souza, J. A. M., Hueb, M., and Damazo, A. S. (2019). Analysis of macrophage subtypes and annexin A1 expression in lesions of patients with cutaneous leishmaniasis. *Rev. Soc. Bras. Med. Trop.* 52:e20190361. doi: 10.1590/0037-8682-0361-2019

Simon, D., Derer, A., Andes, F. T., Lezuo, P., Bozec, A., Schett, G., et al. (2017). Galectin-3 as a novel regulator of osteoblast-osteoclast interaction and bone homeostasis. *Bone* 105, 35–41. doi: 10.1016/j.bone.2017.08.013

Sims, N. A., and Quinn, J. M. (2014). Osteoimmunology: oncostatin M as a pleiotropic regulator of bone formation and resorption in health and disease. *Bonekey Rep.* 3:527. doi: 10.1038/bonekey.2014.22

Stanczyk, J., Pedrioli, D. M., Brentano, F., Sanchez-Pernaute, O., Kolling, C., Gay, R. E., et al. (2008). Altered expression of MicroRNA in synovial fibroblasts and synovial tissue in rheumatoid arthritis. *Arthritis Rheum.* 58, 1001–1009. doi: 10.1002/art.23386

Stukes, S., Coelho, C., Rivera, J., Jedlicka, A. E., Hajjar, K. A., and Casadevall, I. (2016). The membrane phospholipid binding protein annexin A2 promotes phagocytosis and nonlytic exocytosis of cryptococcus neoformans and impacts survival in fungal infection. *J Immunol.* 197, 1252–61. doi: 10.4049/jimmunol.1501855

Su, Y., Zhou, Y., Sun, Y. J., Wang, Y. L., Yin, J. Y., Huang, Y. J., et al. (2019). Macrophage-derived CCL18 promotes osteosarcoma proliferation and migration by upregulating the expression of UCA1. *J. Mol. Med.* 97, 49–61. doi: 10.1007/s00109-018-1711-0

Sun, A. R., Friis, T., Sekar, S., Crawford, R., Xiao, Y., and Prasadam, I. (2016). Is synovial macrophage activation the inflammatory link between obesity and osteoarthritis? *Curr. Rheumatol. Rep.* 18:57. doi: 10.1007/s11926-016-0605-9

Sun, A. R., Panchal, S. K., Friis, T., Sekar, S., Crawford, R., Brown, L., et al. (2017). Obesity-associated metabolic syndrome spontaneously induces infiltration of pro-inflammatory macrophage in synovium and promotes osteoarthritis. *PLoS ONE* 12:e0183693. doi: 10.1371/journal.pone.0183693

Sun, W., Meednu, N., Rosenberg, A., Rangel-Moreno, J., Wang, V., Glanzman, J., et al. (2018). B cells inhibit bone formation in rheumatoid arthritis by suppressing osteoblast differentiation. *Nat. Commun.* 9:5127. doi: 10.1038/s41467-018-07626-8

Suzuki-Inoue, K. (2019). Platelets and cancer-associated thrombosis: focusing on the platelet activation receptor CLEC-2 and podoplanin. *Blood* 134, 1912–1918. doi: 10.1182/blood.2019001388

Takahashi, F., Takahashi, K., Shimizu, K., Cui, R., Tada, N., Takahashi, H., et al. (2004). Osteopontin is strongly expressed by alveolar macrophages in the lungs of acute respiratory distress syndrome. *Lung* 182, 173–185. doi: 10.1007/s00408-004-0309-1

Tan, S. D., Kuijpers-Jagtman, A. M., Semeins, C. M., Bronckers, A. L., Maltha, J. C., Von den Hoff, J. W., et al. (2006). Fluid shear stress inhibits TNFalpha-induced osteocyte apoptosis. *J. Dent. Res.* 85, 905–909. doi: 10.1177/154405910608501006

Tannahill, G. M., Curtis, A. M., Adamik, J., Palsson-McDermott, E. M., McGettrick, A. F., Goel, G., et al. (2013). Succinate is an inflammatory signal that induces IL-1β through HIF-1α. *Nature* 496, 238–242. doi: 10.1038/nature11986

Théry, C. (2011). Exosomes: secreted vesicles and intercellular communications. *F1000 Biol. Rep.* 3:15. doi: 10.3410/B3-15

Tian, Y., Shen, H., Xia, L., and Lu, J. (2013). Elevated serum and synovial fluid levels of interleukin-34 in rheumatoid arthritis: possible association with disease progression via interleukin-17 production. *J. Interferon Cytokine Res.* 33, 398–401. doi: 10.1089/jir.2012.0122

Tokunaga, T., Mokuda, S., Kohno, H., Yukawa, K., Kuranobu, T., Oi, K., et al. (2020). TGFβ1 Regulates human RANKL-induced osteoclastogenesis via suppression of NFATc1 expression. *Int. J. Mol. Sci.* 21:800. doi: 10.3390/ijms21030800

Ushach, I., and Zlotnik, A. (2016). Biological role of granulocyte macrophage colony-stimulating factor (GM-CSF) and macrophage colony-stimulating factor (M-CSF) on cells of the myeloid lineage. *J. Leukoc. Biol.* 100, 481–489. doi: 10.1189/jlb.3RU0316-144R

Wang, J., Meng, F., Song, W., Jin, J., Ma, Q., Fei, D., et al.(2018). Nanostructured titanium regulates osseointegration via influencing macrophage polarization in the osteogenic environment. *Int J Nanomedicine.* 13, 4029–4043. doi: 10.2147/IJN.S163956

Wang, J., Zheng, Z., Huang, B., Wu, H., Zhang, X., Chen, Y., et al. (2020). Osteal Tissue macrophages are involved in endplate osteosclerosis through the OSM-STAT3/YAP1 signaling axis in modic changes. *J. Immunol.* 205, 968–980. doi: 10.4049/jimmunol.1901001

Wei, F., Li, M., Crawford, R., Zhou, Y., and Xiao, Y. (2019). Exosome-integrated titanium oxide nanotubes for targeted bone regeneration. *Acta Biomater.* 86, 480–492. doi: 10.1016/j.actbio.2019.01.006

Wei, F., Zhou, Y., Wang, J., Liu, C., and Xiao, Y. (2018). The immunomodulatory role of BMP-2 on macrophages to accelerate osteogenesis. *Tissue Eng. A* 24, 584–594. doi: 10.1089/ten.tea.2017.0232

Weilner, S., Keider, V., Winter, M., Harreither, E., Salzer, B., Weiss, F., et al. (2016). Vesicular Galectin-3 levels decrease with donor age and contribute to the reduced osteo-inductive potential of human plasma derived extracellular vesicles. *Aging* 8, 16–33. doi: 10.18632/aging.100865

Winkler, I. G., Sims, N. A., Pettit, A. R., Barbier, V., Nowlan, B., Helwani, F., et al. (2010). Bone marrow macrophages maintain hematopoietic stem cell (HSC) niches and their depletion mobilizes HSCs. *Blood* 116, 4815–4828. doi: 10.1182/blood-2009-11-253534

Woo, S. R., Corrales, L., and Gajewski, T. F. (2015). Innate immune recognition of cancer. *Annu. Rev. Immunol.* 33, 445–474. doi: 10.1146/annurev-immunol-032414-112043

Wu, A. C., He, Y., Broomfield, A., Paatan, N. J., Harrington, B. S., Tseng, H. W., et al. (2016). $CD169^{+}$ macrophages mediate pathological formation of woven bone in skeletal lesions of prostate cancer. *J. Pathol.* 239, 218–230. doi: 10.1002/path.4718

Wu, Q., Zhou, X., Huang, D., Ji, Y., and Kang, F. (2017). IL-6 enhances osteocyte-mediated osteoclastogenesis by promoting JAK2 and RANKL activity *in vitro*. *Cell. Physiol. Biochem.* 41, 1360–1369. doi: 10.1159/000465455

Wynn, T. A., Chawla, A., and Pollard, J. W. (2013). Macrophage biology in development, homeostasis and disease. *Nature* 496, 445–455. doi: 10.1038/nature12034

Xia, Y., He, X. T., Xu, X. Y., Tian, B. M., An, Y., and Chen, F. M. (2020). Exosomes derived from M0, M1 and M2 macrophages exert distinct influences on the proliferation and differentiation of mesenchymal stem cells. *PeerJ.* 8:e8970. doi: 10.7717/peerj.8970

Xiang, L. X., Ran, Q., Chen, L., Xiang, Y., Li, F. J., Zhang, X. M., et al. (2020). CR6-interacting factor-1 contributes to osteoclastogenesis by inducing receptor activator of nuclear factor κB ligand after radiation. *World J. Stem Cells* 12, 222–240. doi: 10.4252/wjsc.v12.i3.222

Xing, Z., Lu, C., Hu, D., Miclau, T. 3rd, and Marcucio, R. S. (2010). Rejuvenation of the inflammatory system stimulates fracture repair in aged mice. *J. Orthop. Res.* 28, 1000–1006. doi: 10.1002/jor.21087

Xiong, Y., Chen, L., Yan, C., Zhou, W., Yu, T., Sun, Y., et al. (2020). M2 Macrophagy-derived exosomal miRNA-5106 induces bone mesenchymal stem cells towards osteoblastic fate by targeting salt-inducible kinase 2 and 3. *J. Nanobiotechnol.* 18:66. doi: 10.1186/s12951-020-00622-5

Xue, J., Schmidt, S. V., Sander, J., Draffehn, A., Krebs, W., Quester, I., et al. (2014). Transcriptome-based network analysis reveals a spectrum model of human macrophage activation. *Immunity* 40, 274–288. doi: 10.1016/j.immuni.2014.01.006

Xue, Y. Z. B., Niu, Y. M., Tang, B., and Wang, C. M. (2019). PCL/EUG scaffolds with tunable stiffness can regulate macrophage secretion behavior. *Prog. Biophys. Mol. Biol.* 148, 4–11. doi: 10.1016/j.pbiomolbio.2019.05.006

Yang, D. H., and Yang, M. Y. (2019). The role of macrophage in the pathogenesis of osteoporosis. *Int. J. Mol. Sci.* 20:2093. doi: 10.3390/ijms20092093

Yang, J., Zou, Y., and Jiang, D. (2018). Honokiol suppresses proliferation and induces apoptosis via regulation of the miR-21/PTEN/PI3K/AKT signaling pathway in human osteosarcoma cells. *Int. J. Mol. Med.* 41, 1845–1854. doi: 10.3892/ijmm.2018.3433

Yang, M., Li, C. J., Sun, X., Guo, Q., Xiao, Y., Su, T., et al. (2017). MiR-497∼195 cluster regulates angiogenesis during coupling with osteogenesis by maintaining endothelial Notch and HIF-1α activity. *Nat. Commun.* 8:16003. doi: 10.1038/ncomms16003

Ying, W., Riopel, M., Bandyopadhyay, G., Dong, Y., Birmingham, A., Seo, J. B., et al. (2017). Adipose tissue macrophage-derived exosomal miRNAs can modulate *in vivo* and *in vitro* insulin sensitivity. *Cell* 171, 372–384.e12. doi: 10.1016/j.cell.2017.08.035

Zhang, H., Lin, C., Zeng, C., Wang, Z., Wang, H., Lu, J., et al. (2018). Synovial macrophage M1 polarisation exacerbates experimental osteoarthritis partially through R-spondin-2. *Ann. Rheum. Dis.* 77, 1524–1534. doi: 10.1136/annrheumdis-2018-213450

Zhang, Y., Böse, T., Unger, R. E., Jansen, J. A., Kirkpatrick, C. J., and van den Beucken, J. (2017). Macrophage type modulates osteogenic differentiation of adipose tissue MSCs. *Cell Tissue Res.* 369, 273–286. doi: 10.1007/s00441-017-2598-8

Zheng, P., Chen, L., Yuan, X., Luo, Q., Liu, Y., Xie, G., et al. (2017). Exosomal transfer of tumor-associated macrophage-derived miR-21 confers cisplatin resistance in gastric cancer cells. *J. Exp. Clin. Cancer Res.* 36:53. doi: 10.1186/s13046-017-0528-y

# 4

# Low Dose BMP2-Doped Calcium Phosphate Graft Promotes Bone Defect Healing in a Large Animal Model

*Tie Liu [1,2†], Wen Fang [2,3†], Gang Wu [4], Yining Li [2,5], Janak L. Pathak [6*] and Yuelian Liu [4*]*

*[1] Department of Oral Implantology, The Affiliated Hospital of Stomatology, School of Stomatology, Zhejiang University School of Medicine, Hangzhou, China, [2] Key Laboratory of Oral Biomedical Research of Zhejiang Province, Hangzhou, China, [3] Department of Periodontology, The Affiliated Hospital of Stomatology, School of Stomatology, Zhejiang University School of Medicine, Hangzhou, China, [4] Department of Oral Implantology and Prosthetic Dentistry, Academic of Dentistry Amsterdam (ACTA), VU Universiteit Amsterdam and University of Amsterdam, Amsterdam, Netherlands, [5] Department of Oral Pathology, The Affiliated Hospital of Stomatology, School of Stomatology, Zhejiang University School of Medicine, Hangzhou, China, [6] Guangzhou Key Laboratory of Basic and Applied Research of Oral Regenerative Medicine, Affiliated Stomatology Hospital of Guangzhou Medical University, Guangzhou, China*

***Correspondence:***
*Janak L. Pathak*
*j.pathak@gzhmu.edu.cn*
*Yuelian Liu*
*y.liu@acta.nl*

*† These authors have contributed equally to this work and share first authorship*

**Background:** Bone grafts are in high demand due to the increase in the cases of bone defects mainly caused by trauma, old age, and disease-related bone damages. Tissue-engineered calcium phosphate (CaP) biomaterials match the major inorganic contents of bone, thereby could be the potential bone graft substitute. However, CaP-bone grafts lack the osteoinductivity that is vital for effective bone regeneration. In this study, we aimed to test the bone defect healing potential of biomimetically fabricated low dose BMP2-doped CaP (BMP2.BioCaP) grafts in a large animal model.

**Methods:** Low dose BMP2 was doped internally (BMP2-int.BioCaP) or on the surface of CaP (BMP2-sur.BioCaP) grafts during the fabrication process. Our previous study showed the robust bone regenerative potential of BMP2-int.BioCaP and BMP2-sur.BioCaP grafts in the rat ectopic model. In this study, we investigated the bone defect healing potential of BMP2.BioCaP grafts in sheep humerus/femoral defects, as well as compared with that of autologous bone graft and clinically used deproteinized bovine bone (DBB) xenograft.

**Results:** Different ways of BMP2 doping did not affect the surface morphology and degradation properties of the graft materials. Micro-CT and histology results showed robustly higher bone defect-healing potential of the BMP2.BioCaP grafts compared to clinically used DBB grafts. The bone defect healing potential of BMP2.BioCaP grafts was as effective as that of the autologous bone graft. Although, BMP2-int.BioCaP doped half the amount of BMP2 compared to BMP2-sur.BioCaP, its' bone defect healing potential was even robust. The BMP2.BioCaP grafts showed less immunogenicity compared to BioCaP or DBB grafts. The volume density of blood vessel-like and bone marrow-like structures in both BMP2.BioCaP graft groups were in a similar extent to the autologous group. Meticulous observation of higher magnification histological images showed active bone regeneration and remodeling during bone defect healing in BMP2.BioCaP graft groups.

**Conclusion:** The robust bone regenerative potential of BMP2.BioCaP grafts in the ectopic model and *in-situ* bone defects in small and large animals warrant the pre-clinical studies on large animal critical-sized segmental bone defects.

**Keywords: bone regeneration, BioCaP graft, BMP2, osteoinduction, bone defect healing**

## INTRODUCTION

Large bone defects caused by trauma, fracture, tumor resection, infection, and congenital malformation substantially impact patient health and quality of life (Greenwald et al., 2001; Huang et al., 2016; Kumar et al., 2016). The global bone graft substitutes market was valued at US$ 2.9 Bn in 2019 and is anticipated to expand at a Compound Annual Growth Rate of ~3% from 2020 to 2030 (Transperancy Market Research Report, 2020). Bone defect reconstruction is a complex biological process that involves proper bone grafts, a supply of precursor cells and growth factors, vascularization, immunomodulation, and osteogenesis (Greenwald et al., 2001; Huang et al., 2016). Therefore, the reconstruction of large bone defects is still a challenge for orthopedic and craniomaxillofacial surgeons. To treat a large bone defect, a functional bone graft must be implanted. Autografts are regarded as the gold standard for repairing bone defects; (Jung et al., 2003; Ferreira et al., 2013) however, their application is limited due to low graft availability and donor site morbidity (Nkenke et al., 2004). Alternative bone grafts such as allografts and xenografts are clinically used for critical size bone defect healing. Limited source, immunotoxicity, and risk of infection are the main limitations of these alternative bone grafts (Van Der Stok et al., 2011; Sun et al., 2019). Bone tissue engineering approaches are focused on developing novel biomaterials that address the limitations of conventional autogenic, allogenic, or xenogenic bone grafts.

The tissue-engineered ideal bone graft should be biocompatible, osteoconductive, osteoinductive, angiogenic, non-immunogenic, and biodegradable (Haugen et al., 2019). Recent advances in bone tissue engineering had developed 3D-prinetd biomaterial-based patient-specific scaffolds with enhanced biological and mechanical properties (Zhang et al., 2019). Synthetic scaffolds in combination with bioactive molecules or stem cells has shown promising potential for large size bone defect healing (Ho-Shui-Ling et al., 2018). Bone ingrowth pattern in synthetic scaffold directly correlates with the pore scale morphology and physical properties of the scaffolds (Jones et al., 2009). The primary inorganic component of bone is calcium phosphate (CaP), mainly the hydroxyapatite. CaP-based biomaterials including hydroxyapatite and beta-tricalcium phosphate had shown promising potential to be used as a bone graft (Samavedi et al., 2013). So far developed CaP-based bone grafts are reported to be biocompatible and osteoconductive, but they lack osteoinductivity. Doping osteogenic and/or angiogenic growth factors such as BMP2, VEGF, or FGF in biomaterials improves the bone regenerative potential of the bone grafts (Chim et al., 2013; Chen R. et al., 2016). Emerging pieces of literature had reported a robust bone defect healing potential of BMP2-loaded biomaterials (Selvig et al., 2002; Rao et al., 2013; Oortgiesen et al., 2014; Halloran et al., 2020). Although the Food and Drug Administration (FDA) approved usage of recombinant human BMP-2 (rhBMP-2) during spinal fusion surgery, tibial shaft repair, and maxillary sinus reconstructive surgery, series of systemic adverse effects were experienced during clinical application (Zhang et al., 2015; Halloran et al., 2020). Such systemic adverse effects of BMP2 applied for bone regeneration are mainly due to the burst released high dose BMP2 (James et al., 2016). Reducing the dose of doped BMP2 in graft materials and maintaining the slow and sustained release of low dose BMP2 in the defect site could minimize the systemic adverse effects of the BMP2. Moreover, the traditional CaP bone graft materials lack biomimicry and physicochemical properties required for bone defect healing (Fernandez-Yague et al., 2015). To overcome the above-mentioned issues, we had developed the BMP2-doped biomimetic CaP (BMP2.BioCaP) granules as a bone graft substitute with a robust bone defect healing potential (Liu et al., 2017; Wang et al., 2019).

The bone defect healing potential of the majority of the artificial bone grafts is usually tested in small animal models, which cannot represent the exact bone remodeling and bone properties in the human body. Large animal models, including sheep, dogs, and pigs, provide insights on the bone defect healing potential of artificial bone grafts in tibial and femoral bone defects with relevant clinical similarities to human bone defects (Weigand et al., 2017; Mcgovern et al., 2018). However, the differences in types of bone defects, animal models, surgical methods, and fixation procedures used in literature to test bone defect healing potential of bone grafts make it difficult to draw conclusions for clinical translation (Reichert et al., 2012). Among the large animal models, sheep bone properties and bone-remodeling rate are comparatively close to the human bone (Mcgovern et al., 2018; Hettwer et al., 2019). Moreover, sheep are less aggressive and easy to handle and house (Pearce et al., 2007; Reichert et al., 2012; Ingavle et al., 2019). Our previous studies had shown the bone defect healing potential of BMP2.BioCaP grafts alone or in combination with DBB in ectopic and critical size bone defects in murine models (Liu et al., 2014; Wang et al., 2017, 2019). Interestingly, BMP2.BioCaP grafts in the combination of DBB healed sheep humeral/femoral bone defect as effectively as the autologous bone graft (Liu et al., 2017). However, the bone defect healing potential of BMP2.BioCaP bone grafts alone in a large animal model has not been investigated yet.

Different methods of BMP2-doping incorporate the distinctive concentrations of BMP2 in bone grafts and affect the bioactivity of the grafts contrarily. We had developed BioCaP with an internal or surface biomimetic coating of BMP2. The

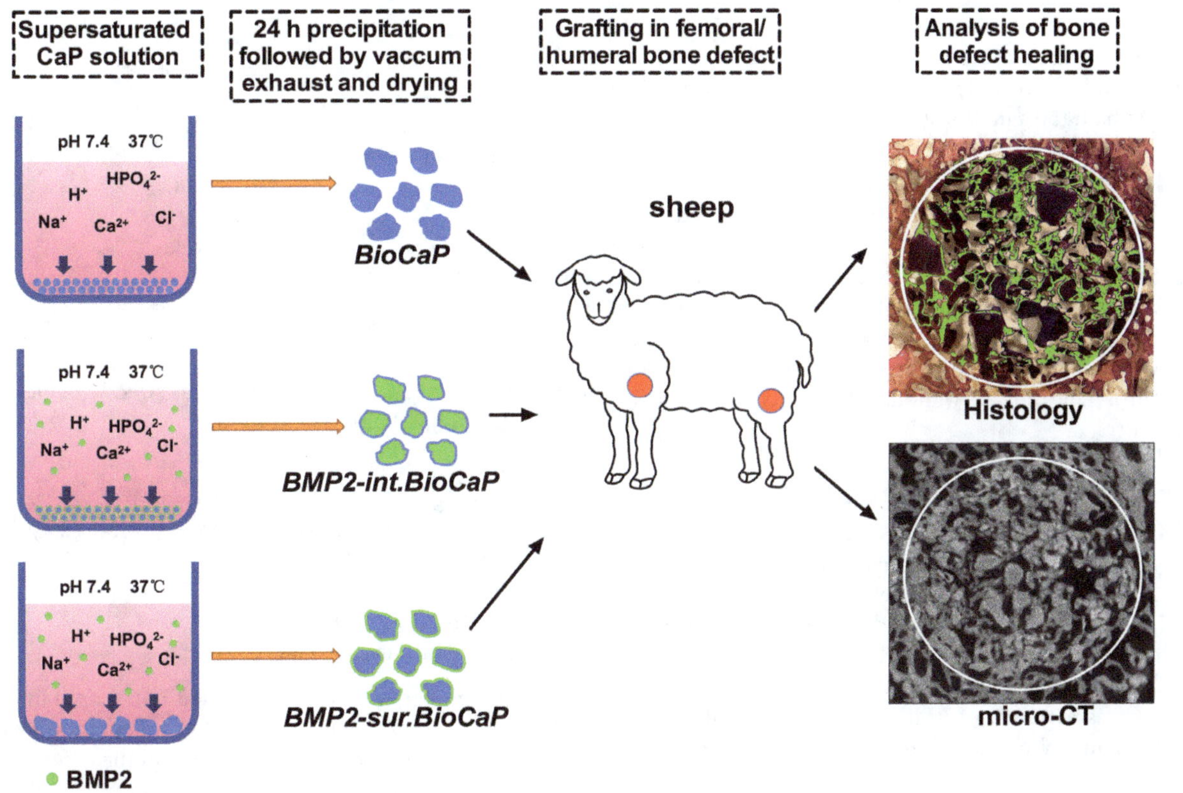


**FIGURE 1** | Scheme of BMP2.BioCaP preparation and sheep femoral/humeral bone defect healing potential analysis.

internal or surface biomimetic coating of BMP2 osteogenically functionalizes the BioCaP grafts as indicated by the robust bone regeneration in ectopic transplantation (Liu et al., 2014). Moreover, BMP2 release from the bone graft is mainly controlled by the cellular activity around the graft. In this study, we aimed to further investigate the bone defect healing potential of BMP2.BioCaP grafts in a large animal model (sheep) as indicated in **Figure 1**. We also compared the bone defect-repairing efficacy of BMP2.BioCaP grafts with that of autologous bone graft and clinically used deproteinized bovine bone (DBB) xenograft. BMP2.BioCaP grafts (BMP2 internally or on surface coating) promoted bone defect healing in sheep as effectively as the autologous graft.

# MATERIALS AND METHODS

## Fabrication of Biomimetic Calcium Phosphate (BioCaP) Granules

Since the incubation of biomaterials in 5-fold concentrated simulated body fluid can deposit a CaP layer resembling the *in vivo* surface structure, this method is named as a biomimetic coating (Lin et al., 2020). BioCaP granule was fabricated by refining a well-established biomimetic mineralization process (Wang et al., 2019). Briefly, a CaP solution (200 mM HCl, 20 mM $CaCl_2{\cdot}2H_2O$, 680 mM NaCl, and 10 mM $Na_2HPO_4$) buffered by TRIS (250 mM) to a pH of 7.4 was incubated in a shaking water bath (50 agitations/min) at 37°C for 24 h. For sterilization, the CaP solution was filtered with the vacuum filter (0.22-μm pore) before buffering. Precipitation was retrieved and gently washed by Milli-Q water, strongly filtered and compressed to a block using a vacuum exhaust filtering method with a vacuum filter (0.22-μm pore, Corning, NY, USA) and an air pump. After drying in air circulation at room temperature for 2 h, the hardened block was ground and filtered through metallic mesh filters to obtain BioCaP granules with a size of 0.25–1.0 mm. All the procedures were performed under aseptic conditions.

## Biomimetic Coating to Fabricate BMP2.BioCaP Grafts

BioCaP granules are osteoconductive but lack osteoinductive properties. A low dose of BMP2 was incorporated in BioCaP granules to obtain osteoconductive and osteoinductive BMP2.BioCaP graft materials. BMP-2 (INFUSE® Bone Graft, Medtronic, USA) was introduced into the CaP solution at a final concentration of 0.2 μg/ml before buffering and co-precipitated into the interior of BioCaP (BMP2-int.BioCaP), viz. the internally-incorporation mode. The doses of BMP2 and CaP solution were determined based on the results of our previous studies (Liu et al., 2014; Wei et al., 2019).

The superficial BMP2 coating was deposited on BioCaP granules according to the well-established biomimetic mineralization approach to obtain BMP2-sur.BioCaP (Liu et al., 2014). Briefly, 0.58 g of BioCaP granules (size: 0.25–1 mm) was incubated in the coating solution [40 mM HCl, 4 mM $CaCl_2 \cdot 2H_2O$, 136 mM NaCl, 2 mM $Na_2HPO_4$, and 50 mM TRIS (pH 7.4); total volume of 150 ml] containing 1 μg/ml BMP2 in a shaking water bath (50 agitations/min) at 37°C for 24 h.

## Quantification of Incorporated BMP-2

The amount of incorporated BMP-2 was determined by a commercially available BMP2 enzyme-linked immunosorbent assay (ELISA) kit (PeproTech, London, UK). BMP2-int.BioCaP and BMP2-sur.BioCaP (0.05 g/sample) were dissolved in 1 ml 0.5 M EDTA (pH 8.0) for 10 min in a 100-rpm stirrer. The ELISA assay was performed according to the manufacturer's instructions ($n = 6$/group). The BioCaP without BMP2 incorporation was used as a control.

## Surface Characteristics and Protein Distribution in BioCaP Grafts

The morphology and surface characteristics of BMP2.BioCaP grafts were visualized in a scanning electron microscope (SEM, XL20, FEI Company, the Netherlands), under an accelerating voltage of 10 kV using sputter-coated with gold. To analyze the pattern of BMP2 protein distribution in BMP2.BioCaP, FITC-BSA was used as a mimic of BMP2 to incorporate in BioCaP and visualized under a fluorescence microscope as described previously (Liu et al., 2014).

## *In vivo* BMP2.BioCaP Grafting in Bone Defect of Large Animal Model

Twelve Australian sheep (4 years old female, 40–50 kg body weight) were purchased from the Military Veterinary Institute, Quartermaster University of PLA, Changchun, China and housed at the Animal facility of Zhejiang University, Zhejiang, China. This study adapted the 4 years age sheep and defect model based on the previous literature (Nuss et al., 2006; Kobayashi et al., 2010; Liu et al., 2017). Sheep were anesthetized by administering Sumianxin II (0.3 ml/kg,) with the addition of penicillium ($5 \times 10^4$ U/kg) and atropine (0.03 mg/kg) at 30 min before surgery. Local anesthesia (1% lidocaine with 1:100,000 adrenaline) and skin disinfection (0.5% iodophor solution) were applied to the proximal part of femoral diaphysis or proximal diaphysis of humerus or distal epiphysis of humerus. Six implantation sites/sheep were randomly chosen. Cylindrical defects (8 mm diameter and 13 mm deep) were created in the cancellous bone anatomical sites (proximal part of femoral diaphysis or proximal diaphysis of humerus or distal epiphysis of humerus) as described previously (Nuss et al., 2006; Liu et al., 2017). These implantation sites were assigned to the six experiment groups according to a randomization protocol (Wang et al., 2012). A total of 72 defect areas were used in this study with 36 each for 4 and 8 weeks (6 defects/group). This study was approved by the Ethical Committee of the School of Stomatology, Zhejiang University. All the animal experiments were carried out according to the ethics laws and regulations of P.R. China. Throughout the study, the sheep were treated following the ARRIVE guidelines. The following six groups were established to analyze the critical-sized bone defect healing potential of BMP2.BioCaP grafts.

**TABLE 1** | Graft materials implanted in different experimental groups.

| Group | Graft material (volume/graft) | Loaded BMP2/graft |
|---|---|---|
| (i) No graft | - | - |
| (ii) Autologous bone | 0.65 cc | |
| (iii) DBB | 0.65 cc (0.35 g) | - |
| (iv) BioCaP | 0.65 cc (0.58 g) | - |
| (v) BMP2-sur.BioCaP | 0.65 cc (0.58 g) | 19.28 μg |
| (vi) BMP2-int.BioCaP | 0.65 cc (0.58 g) | 9.95 μg |

(i) No graft (Negative control)
(ii) Autologous bone graft (Positive control)
(iii) DBB graft, bovine bone (Bio-Oss®) (Clinical standard control)
(iv) BioCaP graft
(v) BMP2-sur.BioCaP graft
(vi) BMP2-int.BioCaP graft

The amount of graft and incorporated BMP2 used in each group is elaborated in **Table 1**. In the case of autograft, the autologous bone was harvested during the creation of the defect and minced to 0.25–1 mm chips using a rongeur. After implantation of grafts, the Geistlich Bio-Gide® membrane (Geistlich Biomaterials, Wolhuser, Switzerland) was used to cover the defect. All sheep were allowed to walk in the confined plain grassland. One week after surgery all the sheep showed normal mobility. All the sheep exhibited good health and all the surgical implant sites healed well without any significant wound complication. No visual signs of inflammation or adverse host tissue reaction were observed. After 4 or 8 weeks of grafting, sheep were sacrificed by an overdose of intramuscular veterinary Sumianxin II (Jilin Huamu Animal Health Product, Jilin Province, China) injection. Bone grafts with surrounding tissues were retrieved and processed for histological and micro-CT analysis.

## Micro Computed Tomography (Micro CT) Imaging and Quantification

Retrieved grafts with surrounding tissues were fixed in a 10% neutral buffered formalin solution and embedded into an MMA block as described previously (Liu et al., 2005; Wu et al., 2011). Three-dimensional distribution of BMP2.BioCaP graft with bone tissues in the bone defects was measured with a high-resolution micro CT system (μCT 40, Scanco Medical AG, Brüttisellen, Switzerland). Each specimen of the bone defect cylinder was positioned vertically and scanned with an isotropic spatial resolution of 18 μm and the beam energy 70 kV source voltage, 113 μA current, and an 18 μm isotropic voxel size. The specimens were mounted in cylindrical specimen holders (polyetherimide; outer diameter: 35.0 mm, wall thickness: 1.0 mm) and secured with synthetic foam to make sure the bone defect cylinder was vertical. The integration time of 750 ms was used to minimize noise. The system was equipped

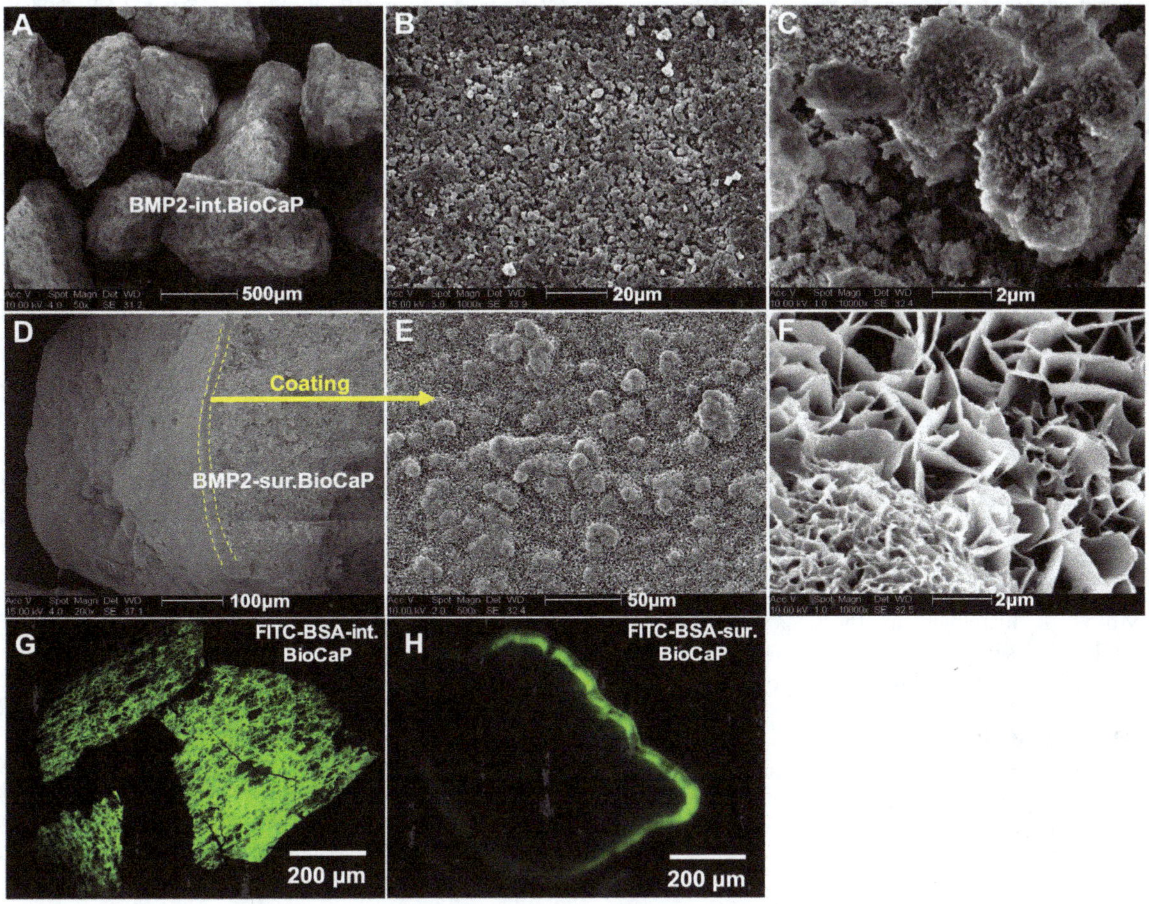


**FIGURE 2 |** Surface characteristic and morphology of BMP2.BioCaP grafts. Representative SEM images of BMP2-int.BioCaP **(A–C)** and BMP2-sur.BioCaP **(D–F)** from lower to higher magnification. Representative fluorescence images of FITC-BSA-int.BioCaP **(G)**, and FITC-BSA-sur.BioCaP **(H)**, showing the protein loading and distribution pattern.

with an aluminum filter and a correction algorithm to minimize beam-hardening artifacts (Mulder et al., 2006).

The gray values of each specimen, which depends on the radiopacity of the scanned material were converted into the degree of mineralization with the analysis software (Scanco Medical AG). Newly formed bone was distinguished from bone graft materials using the novel "onion-peeling" algorithm (Scanco Medical AG) (Schulten et al., 2013). Briefly, a low threshold of 560 mg hydroxyapatite (HA)/cm$^3$ was used to discriminate bone tissue from connective tissue and bone marrow. The gray values were scaled from 1 to 1,000 and the threshold was set at 200 to distinguish bone graft materials from newly formed bone tissue. These two thresholds were calculated by averaging the thresholds resolved in three slices of three samples by two blinded observers. Using this approach, we measured the bone volume/total volume in the bone grafts.

## Histological Procedures

Retrieved grafts with surrounding tissues were fixed and embedded into an MMA block as described previously (Liu et al., 2005; Wu et al., 2011). The tissue embedded blocks were trimmed and sawn vertically to the long axis into 10–12 slices of 600 μm thickness at an interval of 1 mm applying a systematic random-sampling strategy (Gundersen and Jensen, 1987). Slices of each sample were separately mounted on plexiglass holders and polished. The slices were surface-stained with McNeal's tetrachrome, basic fuchsine, and toluidine blue (Wu et al., 2011) and examined with a light microscope with a digital camera (Leica, Wetzlar, Germany).

## Histomorphometric Analysis

In addition to a subjective histological description, 10 slices of each graft were used for quantitative histomorphometric analysis including the volume of newly formed bone, bone marrow-like structure, remaining BioCaP, and the volume density of multinucleated giant cells (MGCs). The surface area (S) of a component per slice was obtained by two blinded observers using the point-counting technique in the whole area of 8 mm diameter of each slice (Cruz-Orive and Weibel, 1990). The interval between the two slices was 1 mm. Therefore, the volume (V) of a component is defined as $V = \sum_{n=1}^{10} (Sn \times 1)$.

**TABLE 2** | Amount of BMP2 loaded in two type of BMP2.BioCaP grafts.

| Sample number | Loaded BMP2 in BMP2-sur.BioCaP/graft (μg) | Loaded BMP2 in BMP2-int.BioCaP/graft (μg) |
|---|---|---|
| 1 | 19.89 | 10.03 |
| 2 | 19.90 | 9.40 |
| 3 | 20.08 | 11.35 |
| 4 | 19.10 | 9.30 |
| 5 | 18.84 | 8.20 |
| 6 | 17.90 | 11.40 |
| Average | **19.28** | **9.95** |

The volume density of MGCs was normalized to the volume of BioCaP or DBB. The volume density of MGCs (Va) is defined as its volume (Vb) per unit volume of graft materials (Vc): Va = Vb/Vc. To evaluate the degradation of BioCaP granules, the volume of BioCaP before implantation (time 0, as control) was evaluated by the same histological method. Six chemically fixed and plastic-embedded samples (0.58 g of BioCaP granules per sample) were specifically reserved for this purpose.

## Statistical Analysis

All data are presented as mean ± standard deviation (SD). Data were compared using one way analysis of variance (ANOVA), and Bonferroni's correction was used for *post-hoc* comparison. The significance level was set at $p < 0.05$.

# RESULTS

## *In-vitro* Characterization

BMP2.BioCaP grafts with random shape and 0.25–1.00 mm size were successfully synthesized. BMP2-int.BioCaP showed a homogeneous rough surface (**Figures 2A–C**). BMP2-sur.BioCaP showed the crystalline surface (**Figures 2D–F**). SEM images indicate that the biomimetic technique of BMP2 incorporation in BioCaP to develop BMP2.BioCaP graft did not affect the surface morphology (**Figures 2A,F**). The internal protein incorporation technique ensured the homogenous distribution of protein (green color) in the outer and inner part of the BioCaP (**Figure 2G**). In surface protein incorporated BioCaP, the protein was localized only on the periphery of the graft (**Figure 2H**). ELISA results indicated that BMP2-sur.BioCaP loaded 2 times higher dose of BMP2 (19.28 μg vs. 9.95 μg) compared to BMP2-int.BioCaP graft (**Table 2**).

## Micro-CT Analysis

**Figure 3** shows the micro-CT images of bone defects after 4 weeks of surgery. An almost empty defect was observed in the no graft group. The homogeneous distribution of graft materials was observed in all other groups (**Figure 3**). **Figure 4** shows the micro-CT images of bone defects after 8 weeks of surgery. The newly formed bone was observed in the periphery of the no graft group. In the autologous bone graft group, newly formed bone was observed in the center and periphery with some empty area. This empty area might be the result of faster degradation properties of autologous bone graft. In the synthetic bone graft groups, the faded white color indicates the newly formed bone and the sharp white color indicates the remaining graft materials (**Figure 4**). In DBB and BioCaP group, the defect area was mainly covered by graft materials and with a meager amount of newly formed bone. BMP2-sur.BioCaP and BMP2-int.BioCaP group showed a comparatively bigger area of newly formed bone.

## Histological Analysis

**Figures 5A–F** represents the McNeal's tetrachrome, basic fuchsine, and toluidine blue stained histological images of tissue sections from bone defects at week 4. Histological images showed an empty defect in no graft group (**Figure 5A**). The newly formed bone surrounding the autologous graft was observed in the autologous bone graft group (**Figure 5B**). The newly formed bone was hardly observed in the DBB and BioCaP group (**Figures 5C,D**). Homogeneous distribution of newly formed bone surrounding the graft and in space between graft materials was observed in BMP2-sur.BioCaP and BMP2-int.BioCaP group. **Figures 5A1–F1** represents the histological images of tissue sections from bone defects at week 8. Histological images from 8 weeks showed a higher amount of newly formed bone in all the groups compared to images from 4 weeks of the respective group (**Figures 5A1–F1**). This result indicates the active bone regeneration process during bone defect healing. Newly formed bone was spotted only in the periphery of the defect in no graft group (**Figure 5A1**). The autologous bone graft group mainly showed newly formed bone with almost no remaining graft materials (**Figure 5B1**). Big areas of empty spaces were noticed in the autologous bone graft group, possibly due to the faster degradation nature of the autologous bone graft. The newly formed bone surrounding the graft material was also observed in the DBB and BioCaP group (**Figures 5C1,D1**). However, the area covered by newly formed bone in DBB or BioCaP group was less compared to BMP2.BioCaP or autologous group. This indicates the lack of osteoinductive properties in DBB or BioCaP grafts. A robust amount of new bone was formed surrounding the graft materials and in spaces between the graft materials in BMP2-sur.BioCaP and BMP2-int.BioCaP groups (**Figures 5E1,F1**). The results of histology images are per the results of micro-CT images (**Figures 3–5**).

## Active Bone Regeneration and Bone Remodeling in BMP2.BioCaP Graft Groups

**Figure 6** represents the higher magnification histological images of bone defects at week 4. No graft group was mainly covered with fibrous tissues at week 4. Robust osteogenesis around the graft and in space between the grafts was observed in the autologous bone graft group. DBB and BioCaP group showed sporadic thin layers of newly formed bone around the graft materials and in space between the grafts. Both the BMP2.BioCaP graft groups showed robust bone regeneration throughout the defect compared to the DBB or BioCaP group. **Figure 7** represents the higher magnification histological images of bone defects at week 8. Newly formed bone was hardly observed in the no graft group. The autologous graft group showed big areas

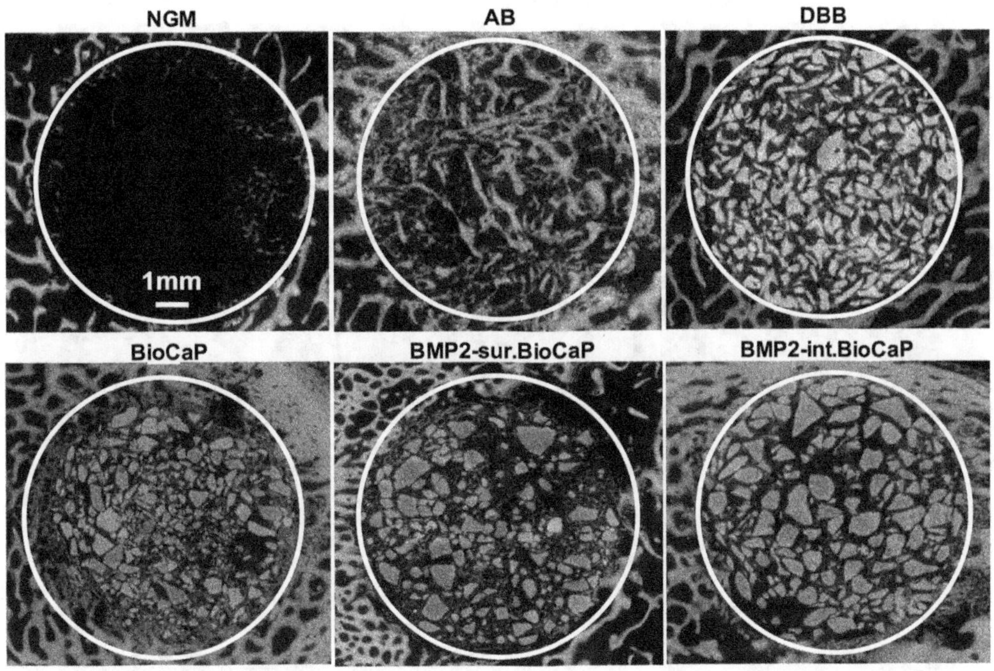


**FIGURE 3** | Micro-CT images showing newly formed bone and grafted biomaterials in the defect site after 4 weeks of grafting.

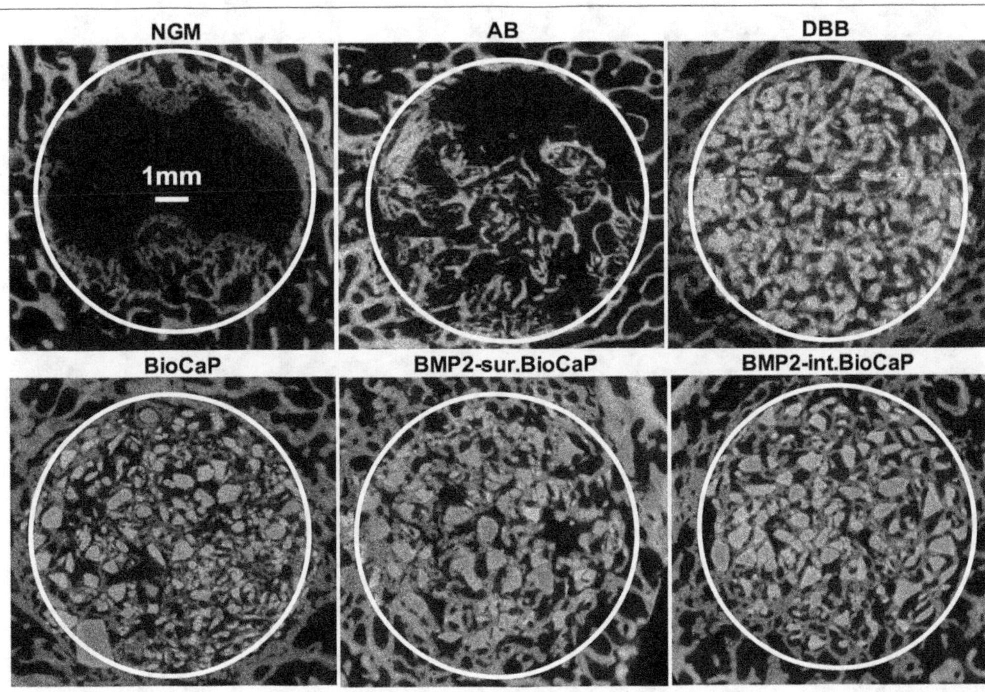


**FIGURE 4** | Micro-CT images showing newly formed bone and grafted biomaterials in the defect site after 8 weeks of grafting.

of newly formed bone but no graft material was left. BMP2-sur.BioCaP and BMP2-int.BioCaP groups showed phenomenal bone regeneration compared to DBB or BioCaP group. All the groups with higher bone regeneration showed the woven bone. BMP2.BioCaP group showed the higher area with trabecular bone appearance, indicating active bone remodeling of woven bone in these groups. In both time points (week 4 and 8), it was difficult to recognize coating around the BMP2.BioCaP, indicating complete degradation of coating possibly by the effect of biological fluid or/and multinucleated giant cells.

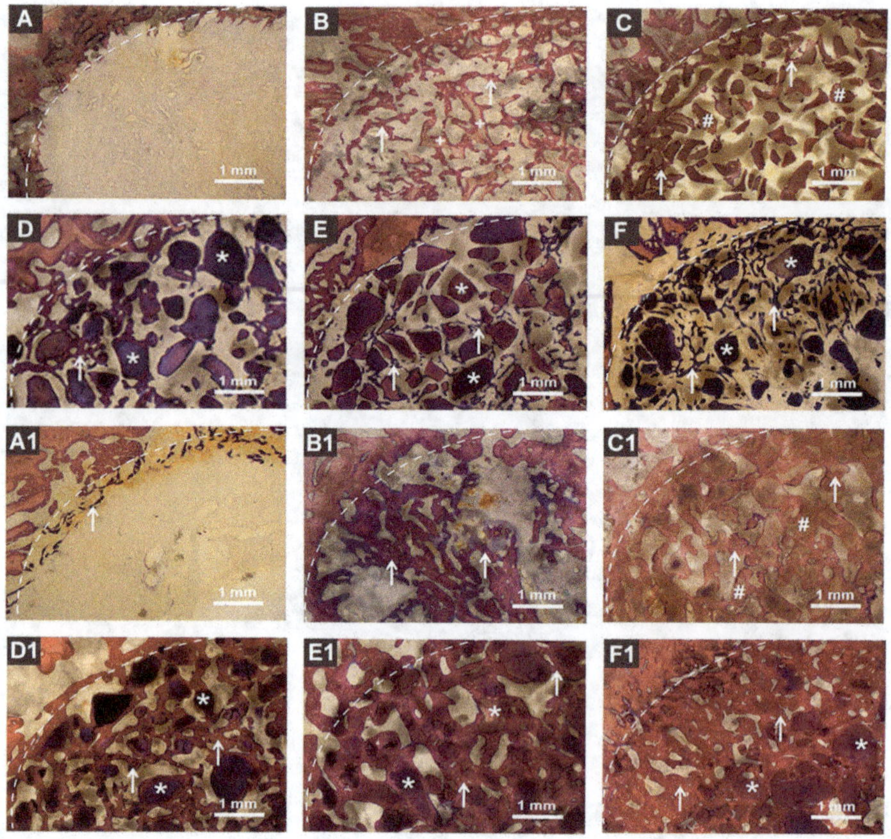


**FIGURE 5 |** Histological images in showing newly formed bone and remaining bone grafts. **(A)** no graft, **(B)** autologous bone, **(C)** DBB, **(D)** BioCaP, **(E)** BMP2-sur.BioCaP, and **(F)** BMP2-int.BioCaP after 4 weeks of grafting. **(A1)** no graft, **(B1)** autologous bone, **(C1)** DBB, **(D1)** BioCaP, **(E1)** BMP2-sur.BioCaP-group, and **(F1)** BMP2-int.BioCaP after 8 weeks of grafting. White dot line: demarcation between native bone and newly formed bone; white stars: remaining graft materials; +: remaining autologous bone; #: remaining DBB.

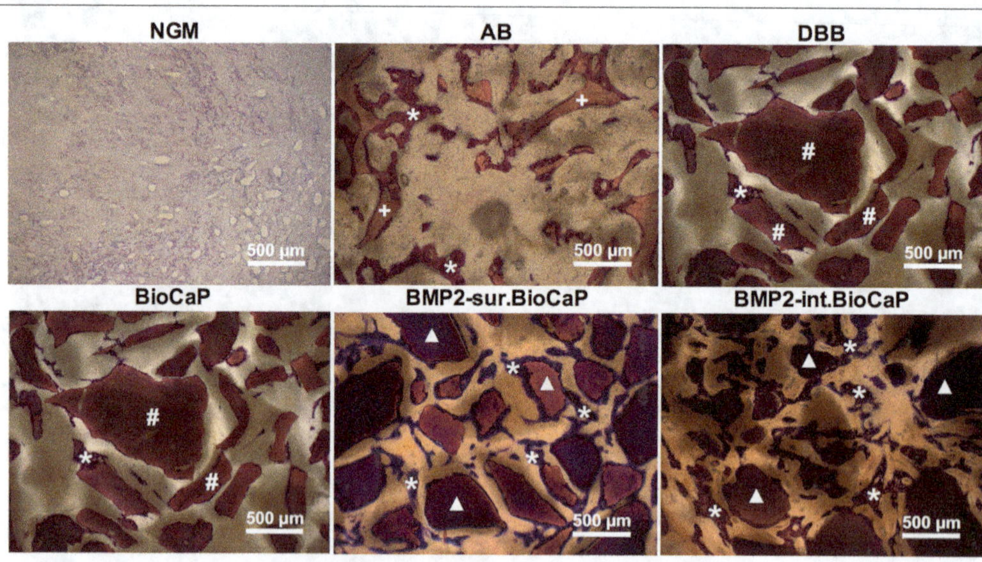


**FIGURE 6 |** Histological images in higher magnification showing newly formed bone and grafted biomaterials in the defect site after 4 weeks of grafting. White stars: remaining graft materials; +: remaining autologous bone; #: remaining DBB.

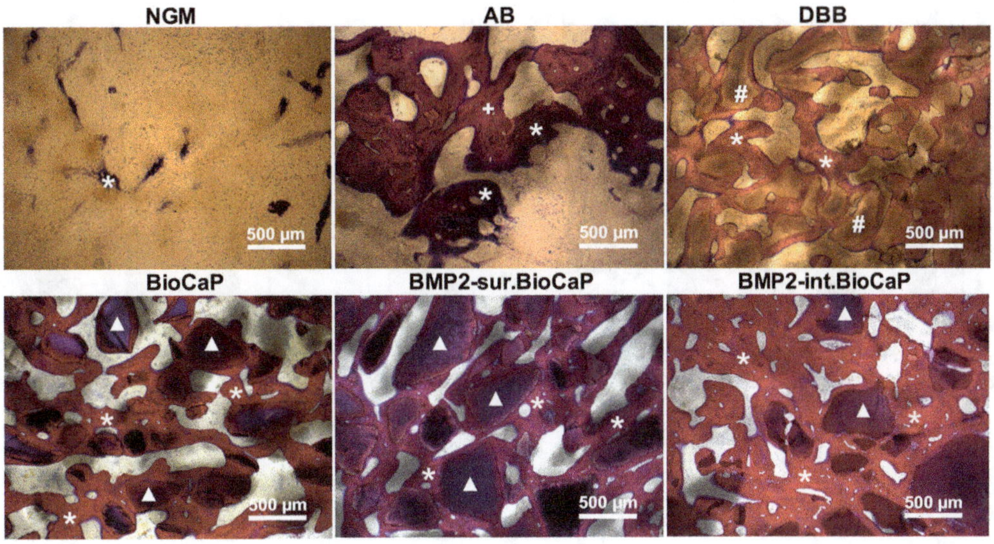


**FIGURE 7 |** Histological images in higher magnification showing newly formed bone and grafted biomaterials in the defect site after 8 weeks of grafting. White stars: newly formed bone; +: remaining autologous bone; #: remaining DBB.

Further high-resolution magnification of histological images indicated active bone regeneration and bone remolding activities at week 4 and 8. Representative histological images of BMP2.BioCaP grafts showed the presence of abundant cells, mainly mononuclear immune cells in the space between the graft materials (**Supplementary Figure 1**). At week 8, the number of mononuclear immune cells was reduced drastically. Chondrocytes and hypertrophic chondrocytes-like cells were observed in the newly formed bone area indicating the active endochondral ossification. Lining osteoblasts were observed on the surface of the newly formed bone. Moreover, osteocytes in lacunae and osteoids were observed inside the newly formed bone at week 8. Similarly, active multinucleated cells on the surface of newly formed bone indicate the active bone remodeling process during bone defect healing (**Supplementary Figure 2**). Bone marrow-like structures and blood vessel-like structures were observed in the space between the graft materials. Osteoclast-resorbed and bio-actively-degraded irregular edges were observed in the DBB, BioCaP, or BMP2.BioCaP grafts.

## Quantitative Micro-CT and Histomorphometric Analysis

Quantitative micro-CT analysis was performed to analyze bone volume/total volume in the site of the defects at week 4 and 8 (**Figure 8A**). BMP2-int.BioCaP group at week 8 showed higher bone volume/total volume compared to DBB and BioCaP grafts. Bone volume/total volume in BMP2-sur.BioCaP and BMP2-int.BioCaP groups was to a similar extent to that of autologous bone graft group. Histomorphometric analysis was performed to quantify the volume density of newly formed bone, bone marrow-like structure, blood vessel-like structure, multinucleated giant cells, and graft material degradation % in the different materials grafted bone defects. Except in the no graft group, all other groups showed a higher volume density of newly formed bone at week 8 compared to the respective group at week 4 (**Figure 8B**). This result revealed that bone formation significantly increased with the implantation duration. The autologous bone group showed a significantly higher volume density of newly formed bone compared to DBB or BioCaP group at week 4 and 8. BMP2-sur.BioCaP and BMP2-int.BioCaP group showed 3.3-, and 3.7-fold higher volume density of newly formed bone respectively at week 4 compared to the DBB group. BMP2-sur.BioCaP and BMP2-int.BioCaP group had a similar degree volume density of newly formed bone with the autologous bone graft group at week 4 and 8. BMP2-int.BioCaP but not BMP2-sur.BioCaP enhanced bone regeneration compared to the BioCaP group at week 8, indicating the better osteoinductive properties of BMP2-int.BioCaP grafts. The results of quantitative micro-CT analysis on newly formed bone were in accordance with the results from the histomorphometric analysis (**Figures 8A,B**).

There was no bone marrow-like structure in the no graft group at week 4 and 8. In all other groups, the quantitative evaluation revealed a robust increase in the volume density of bone marrow-like structures at week 8 compared to the respective group at week 4. There was no difference in the volume density of bone marrow-like structures among the groups at week 4 (**Figure 8C**). The autologous graft group showed the highest volume density of bone marrow-like structures at week 8. BioCaP, BMP2-sur.BioCaP, or BMP2-int.BioCaP group showed a higher volume density of bone marrow-like structures compared to the DBB group at week 8. BioCaP and BMP2.BioCaP groups showed an almost similar degree of the volume density of bone marrow-like structures to the autologous group at week 8 (**Figure 8C**).

There was no significant difference in the volume density of newly formed blood vessel-like structures among the groups at week 4 or 8 (**Supplementary Figure 3A**). Multinucleated giant cells were hardly visualized in the no graft or autologous group at week 4 and 8. In the remaining four groups, the volume density of multinucleated giant cells significantly was reduced at week 8 compared to the respective group at week 4 (**Figure 8D**).

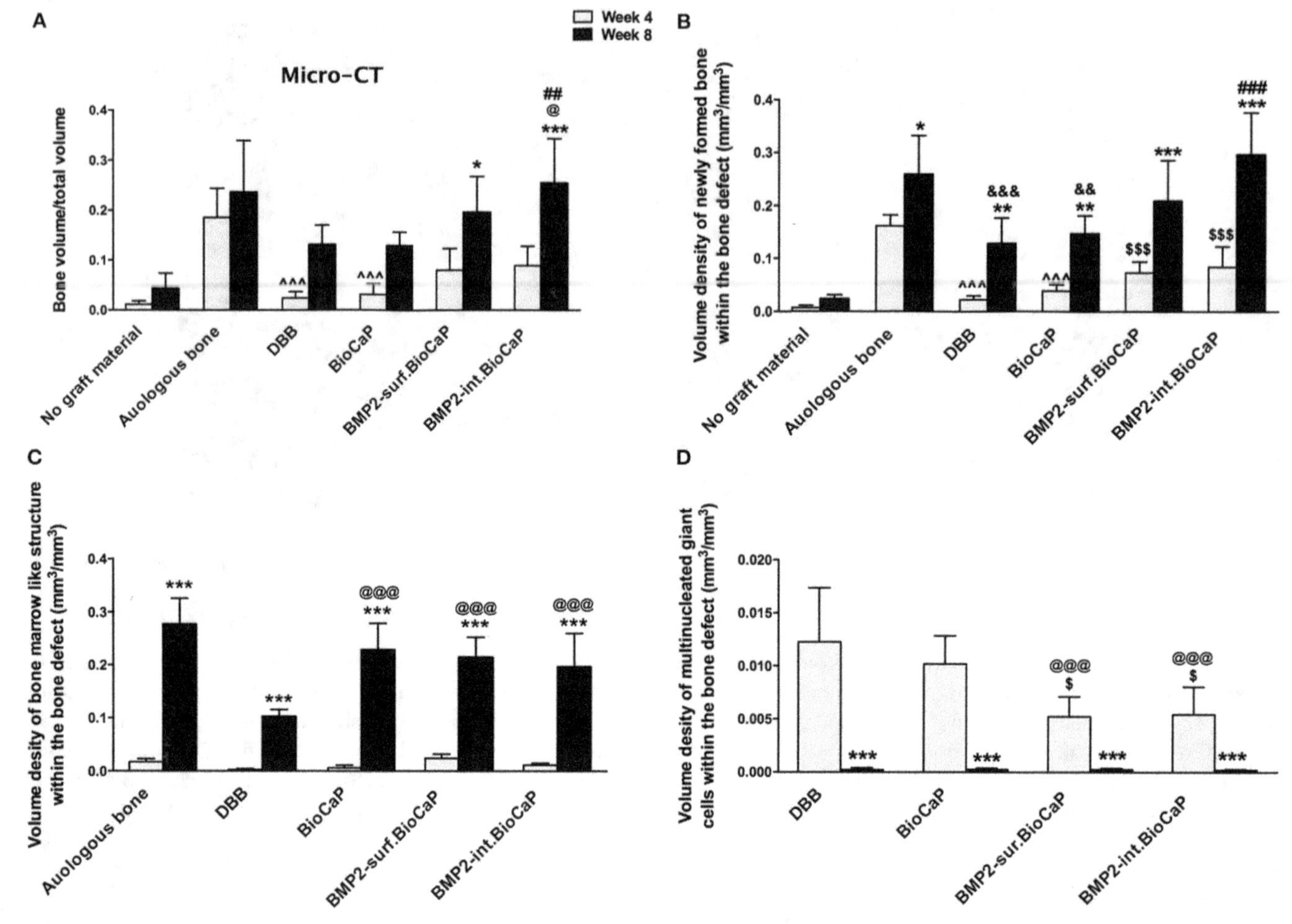


**FIGURE 8 | (A)** Bone volume/Total volume of newly formed bone analyzed from micro-CT data. Volume density of: **(B)** newly formed bone, **(C)** bone marrow-like structures, and **(D)** multinucleated giant cells analyzed form histological images. Data are presented as mean ± SD ($n$ = 6). Significant difference compared to respective week 4-group, $^{*}p < 0.05$, $^{**}p < 0.01$, and $^{***}p < 0.001$; compared to BioCaP week 4-group, $^{\$}p < 0.05$ and $^{\$\$\$}p < 0.001$; compared to DBB week 8-group or week 4-group, $^{@}p < 0.05$, $^{@@@}p < 0.001$; compared to BioCaP week 8-group, $^{\#\#}p < 0.01$, $^{\#\#\#}p < 0.001$; compared to autologous bone week 4-group, $^{\wedge\wedge\wedge}p < 0.001$; compared to autologous bone week 8-group, $^{\&\&}p < 0.01$, $^{\&\&\&}p < 0.001$.

BMP2-sur.BioCaP or BMP2-int.BioCaP group showed a less volume density of multinucleated giant cells compared to DBB or BioCaP group at week 4, indicating less immunogenicity of BMP2.BioCaP grafts. In the autologous group, there was excessive degradation of graft materials at week 4 and almost no graft material was left at week 8. Among the other groups, there was no difference in the graft materials degradation % at week 4 and week 8 (**Supplementary Figure 3B**). The results of this study indicate the osteoconductive, robust osteoinductive, less immunogenic, and phenomenal bone regenerative potential of BMP2-sur.BioCaP and BMP2-int.BioCaP grafts. BMP2-int.BioCaP graft showed better bone defect healing potential than BMP2-sur.BioCaP.

## DISCUSSION

Bone grafts are the second most implanted grafts due to the increase in the cases of bone defects mainly caused by trauma, old-age, and disease-related bone damages. Due to limited sources and other shortcomings of the autografts, allografts, or xenografts, the tissue-engineered biomaterials are being developed as an optional source of the bone grafts for clinical use. Advances in biomaterials had led to the development of osteogenic/angiogenic growth factors loaded tissue-engineered bone grafts. However, osteogenic bioactivity, biosafety, and local/systemic adverse effects are still key issues of synthetic bone grafts that need to be addressed. In this study, we tested the bone defect healing potential of biomimetically fabricated BMP2.BioCaP grafts (BMP2-sur.BioCaP and BMP2-int.BioCaP) in sheep humerus and femoral bone defects.

BMP2-sur.BioCaP and BMP2-int.BioCaP grafts doped ~1000 and 500-fold less BMP2, respectively than used in clinics for bone regeneration (Block and Achong, 2006; Liu et al., 2017). Both Bone grafts showed robustly higher bone defect-healing potential compared to clinically used DBB grafts. The bone defect healing potential of BMP2.BioCaP grafts was as effective as that of the autologous bone graft. Although, BMP2-int.BioCaP graft doped half the amount of BMP2 compared to BMP2-sur.BioCaP graft, the bone defect healing potential of BMP2-int.BioCaP was even robust. Different ways of BMP2 doping did not affect the surface morphology and degradation properties of the graft materials. The BMP2.BioCaP grafts showed less immunogenicity compared to BioCaP or DBB bone grafts. Bone defect sites were healed well without any significant wound complication, signs of inflammation, or adverse host tissue reactions. Our findings indicate the possibility of clinical application of biomimetically fabricated BMP2.BioCaP grafts.

Bone graft biomaterials directly interact with the precursor cells and affect cellular activity and differentiation (Gao et al., 2017). Similarly, the graft material-mediated immunogenicity modulates immune cells' function regulating inflammation in bone defect milieu (Chen Z. T. et al., 2016). Chemical remnants in grafts used for material synthesis can induce graft-related immunogenicity. Biomimetically synthesized biomaterials minimize the immunogenicity and graft material-related local/systemic adverse effects (Greenwald et al., 2001; Fernandez-Yague et al., 2015; Sun et al., 2019; Green et al., 2020). In this study, BMP2.BioCaP grafts were synthesized biomimetically as we reported previously (Liu et al., 2014, 2017; Wang et al., 2017, 2019). BMP2.BioCaP grafts showed less immunogenicity compared to DBB or BioCaP grafts as indicated by the fewer numbers of multinucleated giant immune cells around in BMP2.BioCaP grafts. Foreign body multinucleated giant cells resorb the graft materials and also remodel newly formed bone (Milde et al., 2015; Barbeck et al., 2017). Higher immunogenicity of graft materials triggered the formation of multinucleated cells and inflammatory cascade (Barbeck et al., 2017). In this study, the volume density of multinucleated giant cells was significantly higher in the DBB or BioCaP group compared to BMP2.BioCaP groups at week 4. This result is in accordance with the result from the previous study of ectopic and *in-situ* implantation of BMP2.BioCaP grafts (Liu et al., 2014, 2017). Since, there was no significant difference in the graft materials degradation among the DBB, BioCaP, or BMP2.BioCaP groups, the higher volume density of multinucleated giant cells in DBB or BioCaP might be associated with a higher degree of inflammation.

BMP2.BioCaP grafts give slow and sustained release of low dose BMP2 in the defect area and this release is mainly cellular activity-dependent (Liu et al., 2017). The robust bone regenerative and less immunogenic properties of BMP2.BioCaP grafts might be the effect of this BMP2 release phenomenon. Moreover, slow and sustained release of low dose BMP2 in the defect area might be responsible for the well-healed bone defects without any significant wound complication, signs of inflammation, or adverse host tissue reactions.

Active bone regeneration and bone remodeling are essential for the graft-mediated effective bone defect healing. Recruitment of osteogenic/endothelial precursor cells and immune cells to the graft material is inevitable for bone regeneration and remodeling process (Shi et al., 2016). BMP2.BioCaP graft group showed higher numbers of progenitor cells and immune cells at week 4. The density of immune cells and progenitor cells around the graft materials and newly formed bone was drastically reduced during week 8 of bone defect healing compared to week 4. This indicates the importance of early recruited progenitor cells and immune cells on bone defect healing. During bone defect healing, precursor cells undergo chondrogenic differentiation forming the cartilaginous soft callus that subsequently transfers to the mineralized-bone matrix via endochondral ossification (Nilsson Hall et al., 2020). In this study, we observed chondrocytes and hypertrophic chondrocyte-like structures in or nearby the newly formed bone. This result indicates the endogenous bone regenerative potential of BMP2.BioCaP grafts via endochondral ossification. A prominent number of osteoblast-like lining cells and multinucleated osteoclast-like cells on the surface of the newly formed bone in the BMP2.BioCaP grafts group indicate active bone remodeling. Moreover, A similar extent of the volume density of newly formed bone, bone marrow-like structure, and blood vessel-like structures in BMP2.BioCaP graft groups compared to that in autologous graft group suggests a highly active bone regenerative and bone remodeling potential of BMP2.BioCaP grafts during bone defect healing.

In this study, we analyzed the bone defect healing potential of BMP2.BioCaP grafts in a large animal model. Furthermore, we compared the bone defect healing potential of BMP2.BioCaP graft with the gold standard autologous bone graft and clinically used DBB bone graft. The bone defect healing potential of BMP2.BioCaP grafts was robustly superior compared to BioCaP or DBB graft, and as effective as that of autologous bone graft. Week 4 is the initial stage of new bone formation in the defects of the large animal model as shown by presence of precursor cells and a small amount of newly formed bone in BMP2.BioCaP and autologous bone graft groups. At week 8, the newly formed in mainly woven bone, which requires to undergo the major remodeling for 6–12 months to convert into real load-bearing bone (Hettwer et al., 2019). The use of femoral bone defect in 4 years old adult sheep model allowed us to investigate the biocompatibility, degradation, and bone regenerative potential of the BMP2.BioCaP grafts (Nuss et al., 2006). However, the bone volume, osteoid volume, and mineral apposition rate of 9–10 years old sheep resembles those of 60–70 years humans (Turner, 2001). Therefore, the preclinical study, using segmental bone defect in old age sheep analyzing the major bone remodeling for 6–12 months (Reichert et al., 2009; Hettwer et al., 2019), is further required to understand the bone defect healing potential of BMP2.BioCaP grafts. Early mechanical stimulation is necessary for timely bone defect healing (Tufekci et al., 2018). The current study lacks the role of mechanical stimulation in BMP2.BioCaP-mediated bone defect healing in sheep. The limitation of BMP2.BioCaP graft is the small size of each graft granule (0.25–1.0 mm) that is not suitable to graft in extra-large bone defect and load-bearing site such as segmental bone defects. It is difficult to custom design BMP2.BioCaP granules-based bone graft with a specific shape and certain mechanical strength. However, the biomimetic coating of BMP2.BioCaP on the surface of CaP-based 3D-printed scaffolds could osteogenically functionalize the large size bone grafts designed for critical size bone defects (Lin et al., 2020).

## CONCLUSIONS

Biomimetically fabricated BMP2.BioCaP grafts reduce the clinical dose BMP2. BMP2.BioCaP grafts showed biocompatibility and robust bone regenerative potential in the ectopic model and in *in-situ* bone defects of small and large animals. Our results warrant the pre-clinical studies in critical size segmental bone defect of large animals to access the bone defect healing potential of BMP2.BioCaP grafts.

## ETHICS STATEMENT

The animal study was reviewed and approved by the Ethical Committee of School of Stomatology, Zhejiang University.

## AUTHOR CONTRIBUTIONS

TL, WF, JP, and YL: study concept, design, and data interpretation. YL and TL: data acquisition and analysis. TL and WF: experiment and manuscript writing. GW: BMP2.BioCaP preparation and manuscript editing. All authors read and approved the submitted version.

grant (2008-015), KNAW grant (08CDP043, 09CDP036, and 11CDP011), and High-Level University Construction Talents of Guangzhou Medical University of China (B185006003014 and B195002003017).

## ACKNOWLEDGMENTS

We thank Daniel Wismeijer for his scientific input on the design of this project.

## SUPPLEMENTARY MATERIAL

**Supplementary Figure 1 |** Histological images showing active bone regeneration process during 4 and 8 weeks of grafting in the BMP2-sur.BioCaP group. White star: newly formed bone; white triangle: remaining graft; black arrow: mononuclear immune cells; yellow arrow: chondrocytes and hypertrophic chondrocytes-like cells; green arrow: osteoblast lining cells.

**Supplementary Figure 2 |** Histological images showing active multinucleated giant cells, bone marrow-like, and blood vessel-like structures. White star: newly formed bone; white triangle: remaining graft; black arrow: active osteoclasts; yellow arrow: chondrocytes and hypertrophic chondrocytes-like cells; green arrow: osteoblast lining cells; pink arrow: resorbed graft material by active osteoclasts; M: bone marrow-like structure; V: blood vessel-like structure.

**Supplementary Figure 3 |** Quantitative analysis of volume density of blood vessels like structure **(A)**, and graft material degradation (%) **(B)**. Data are presented as mean ± SD ($n = 6$).

## REFERENCES

Barbeck, M., Booms, P., Unger, R., Hoffmann, V., Sader, R., Kirkpatrick, C. J., et al. (2017). Multinucleated giant cells in the implant bed of bone substitutes are foreign body giant cells-New insights into the material-mediated healing process. *J. Biomed. Mater. Res. Part A* 105, 1105–1111. doi: 10.1002/jbm.a.36006

Block, M. S., and Achong, R. (2006). Bone morphogenetic protein for sinus augmentation. *Atlas Oral Maxillofac. Surg. Clin. North Am.* 14, 99–105. doi: 10.1016/j.cxom.2005.11.002

Chen, R., Wang, J., and Liu, C. S. (2016). Biomaterials act as enhancers of growth factors in bone regeneration. *Adv. Funct. Mater.* 26, 8810–8823. doi: 10.1002/adfm.201603197

Chen, Z. T., Klein, T., Murray, R. Z., Crawford, R., Chang, J., Wu, C. T., et al. (2016). Osteoimmunomodulation for the development of advanced bone biomaterials. *Materials Today* 19, 304–321. doi: 10.1016/j.mattod.2015.11.004

Chim, S., Tickner, J., Chow, S., Kuek, V., Guo, B., Zhang, G., et al. (2013). Angiogenic factors in bone local environment. *Cytokine Growth Factor Rev.* 24, 297–310. doi: 10.1016/j.cytogfr.2013.03.008

Cruz-Orive, L. M., and Weibel, E. R. (1990). Recent stereological methods for cell biology: a brief survey. *Am. J. Physiol.* 258, 148–156. doi: 10.1152/ajplung.1990.258.4.L148

Fernandez-Yague, M. A., Abbah, S. A., Mcnamara, L., Zeugolis, D. I., Pandit, A., and Biggs, M. J. (2015). Biomimetic approaches in bone tissue engineering: integrating biological and physicomechanical strategies. *Adv. Drug Deliv. Rev.* 84, 1–29. doi: 10.1016/j.addr.2014.09.005

Ferreira, J. R., Padilla, R., Urkasemsin, G., Yoon, K., Goeckner, K., Hu, W. S., et al. (2013). Titanium-enriched hydroxyapatite-gelatin scaffolds with osteogenically differentiated progenitor cell aggregates for calvaria bone regeneration. *Tissue Eng. Part A* 19, 1803–1816. doi: 10.1089/ten.tea.2012.0520

Gao, C., Peng, S., Feng, P., and Shuai, C. (2017). Bone biomaterials and interactions with stem cells. *Bone Res* 5:17059. doi: 10.1038/boneres.2017.59

Green, D. W., Stamboulis, A., and Ben-Nissan, B. (2020). Specifiable biomimetic microsponges for timed release of crystal entrapped biomolecules useful in bone repair. *J. Mater. Chem. B* 8, 7143–7148. doi: 10.1039/D0TB01491E

Greenwald, A. S., Boden, S. D., Goldberg, V. M., Khan, Y., Laurencin, C. T., Rosier, R. N., et al. (2001). Bone-graft substitutes: facts, fictions, and applications. *J. Bone Joint Surg. Am.* 83, 98–103. doi: 10.2106/00004623-200100022-00007

Gundersen, H. J., and Jensen, E. B. (1987). The efficiency of systematic sampling in stereology and its prediction. *J. Microsc.* 147, 229–263. doi: 10.1111/j.1365-2818.1987.tb02837.x

Halloran, D., Durbano, H. W., and Nohe, A. (2020). Bone morphogenetic protein-2 in development and bone homeostasis. *J. Dev. Biol* 8:19. doi: 10.3390/jdb8030019

Haugen, H. J., Lyngstadaas, S. P., Rossi, F., and Perale, G. (2019). Bone grafts: which is the ideal biomaterial? *J. Clin. Periodontol.* 46, 92–102. doi: 10.1111/jcpe.13058

Hettwer, W., Horstmann, P. F., Bischoff, S., Gullmar, D., Reichenbach, J. R., Poh, P. S. P., et al. (2019). Establishment and effects of allograft and synthetic bone graft substitute treatment of a critical size metaphyseal bone defect model in the sheep femur. *APMIS* 127, 53–63. doi: 10.1111/apm.12918

Ho-Shui-Ling, A., Bolander, J., Rustom, L. E., Johnson, A. W., Luyten, F. P., and Picart, C. (2018). Bone regeneration strategies: engineered scaffolds, bioactive molecules and stem cells current stage and future perspectives. *Biomaterials* 180, 143–162. doi: 10.1016/j.biomaterials.2018.07.017

Huang, R. L., Kobayashi, E., Liu, K., and Li, Q. (2016). Bone graft prefabrication following the *in vivo* bioreactor principle. *EBioMedicine* 12, 43–54. doi: 10.1016/j.ebiom.2016.09.016

Ingavle, G. C., Gionet-Gonzales, M., Vorwald, C. E., Bohannon, L. K., Clark, K., Galuppo, L. D., et al. (2019). Injectable mineralized microsphere-loaded composite hydrogels for bone repair in a sheep bone defect model. *Biomaterials* 197, 119–128. doi: 10.1016/j.biomaterials.2019.01.005

James, A. W., Lachaud, G., Shen, J., Asatrian, G., Nguyen, V., Zhang, X., et al. (2016). A review of the clinical side effects of bone morphogenetic protein-2. *Tissue Eng. Part B Rev.* 22, 284–297. doi: 10.1089/ten.teb.2015.0357

Jones, A. C., Arns, C. H., Hutmacher, D. W., Milthorpe, B. K., Sheppard, A. P., and Knackstedt, M. A. (2009). The correlation of pore morphology, interconnectivity and physical properties of 3D ceramic scaffolds with bone ingrowth. *Biomaterials* 30, 1440–1451. doi: 10.1016/j.biomaterials.2008.10.056

Jung, R. E., Glauser, R., Scharer, P., Hammerle, C. H., Sailer, H. F., and Weber, F. E. (2003). Effect of rhBMP-2 on guided bone regeneration in humans. *Clin. Oral Implants Res.* 14, 556–568. doi: 10.1034/j.1600-0501.2003.00921.x

Kobayashi, H., Turner, A. S., Seim, H. B. III, Kawamoto, T., and Bauer, T. W. (2010). Evaluation of a silica-containing bone graft substitute in a vertebral defect model. *J. Biomed. Mater. Res. A* 92, 596–603. doi: 10.1002/jbm.a.32397

Kumar, B. P., Venkatesh, V., Kumar, K. A., Yadav, B. Y., and Mohan, S. R. (2016). Mandibular reconstruction: overview. *J. Maxillofac. Oral Surg.* 15, 425–441. doi: 10.1007/s12663-015-0766-5

Lin, X., Chen, J., Liao, Y., Pathak, J. L., Li, H., and Liu, Y. (2020). Biomimetic calcium phosphate coating as a drug delivery vehicle for bone tissue engineering: a mini-review. *Coatings* 10:1118. doi: 10.3390/coatings10111118

Liu, T., Wu, G., Zheng, Y., Wismeijer, D., Everts, V., and Liu, Y. (2014). Cell-mediated BMP-2 release from a novel dual-drug delivery system promotes bone formation. *Clin. Oral Implants Res.* 25, 1412–1421. doi: 10.1111/clr.12283

Liu, T., Zheng, Y., Wu, G., Wismeijer, D., Pathak, J. L., and Liu, Y. (2017). BMP2-coprecipitated calcium phosphate granules enhance osteoinductivity of deproteinized bovine bone, and bone formation during critical-sized bone defect healing. *Sci. Rep.* 7:41800. doi: 10.1038/srep41800

Liu, Y., De Groot, K., and Hunziker, E. B. (2005). BMP-2 liberated from biomimetic implant coatings induces and sustains direct ossification in an ectopic rat model. *Bone* 36, 745–757. doi: 10.1016/j.bone.2005.02.005

Mcgovern, J. A., Griffin, M., and Hutmacher, D. W. (2018). Animal models for bone tissue engineering and modelling disease. *Dis. Model. Mech.* 11:dmm033084. doi: 10.1242/dmm.033084

Milde, R., Ritter, J., Tennent, G. A., Loesch, A., Martinez, F. O., Gordon, S., et al. (2015). Multinucleated giant cells are specialized for complement-mediated phagocytosis and large target destruction. *Cell Rep.* 13, 1937–1948. doi: 10.1016/j.celrep.2015.10.065

Mulder, L., Koolstra, J. H., and Van Eijden, T. M. (2006). Accuracy of MicroCT in the quantitative determination of the degree and distribution of mineralization in developing bone. *Acta Radiol.* 47, 882–883. doi: 10.1080/02841850600854944

Nilsson Hall, G., Mendes, L. F., Gklava, C., Geris, L., Luyten, F. P., and Papantoniou, I. (2020). Developmentally engineered callus organoid bioassemblies exhibit predictive *in vivo* long bone healing. *Adv. Sci.* 7:1902295. doi: 10.1002/advs.201902295

Nkenke, E., Weisbach, V., Winckler, E., Kessler, P., Schultze-Mosgau, S., Wiltfang, J., et al. (2004). Morbidity of harvesting of bone grafts from the iliac crest for preprosthetic augmentation procedures: a prospective study. *Int. J. Oral Maxillofac. Surg.* 33, 157–163. doi: 10.1054/ijom.2003.0465

Nuss, K. M., Auer, J. A., Boos, A., and Von Rechenberg, B. (2006). An animal model in sheep for biocompatibility testing of biomaterials in cancellous bones. *BMC Musculoskelet. Disord.* 7:67. doi: 10.1186/1471-2474-7-67

Oortgiesen, D. A., Walboomers, X. F., Bronckers, A. L., Meijer, G. J., and Jansen, J. A. (2014). Periodontal regeneration using an injectable bone cement combined with BMP-2 or FGF-2. *J. Tissue Eng. Regen. Med.* 8, 202–209. doi: 10.1002/term.1514

Pearce, A. I., Richards, R. G., Milz, S., Schneider, E., and Pearce, S. G. (2007). Animal models for implant biomaterial research in bone: a review. *Eur. Cell. Mater* 13, 1–10. doi: 10.22203/eCM.v013a01

Rao, S. M., Ugale, G. M., and Warad, S. B. (2013). Bone morphogenetic proteins: periodontal regeneration. *N. Am. J. Med. Sci.* 5, 161–168. doi: 10.4103/1947-2714.109175

Reichert, J. C., Cipitria, A., Epari, D. R., Saifzadeh, S., Krishnakanth, P., Berner, A., et al. (2012). A tissue engineering solution for segmental defect regeneration in load-bearing long bones. *Sci. Transl. Med.* 4:141ra193. doi: 10.1126/scitranslmed.3003720

Reichert, J. C., Saifzadeh, S., Wullschleger, M. E., Epari, D. R., Schutz, M. A., Duda, G. N., et al. (2009). The challenge of establishing preclinical models for segmental bone defect research. *Biomaterials* 30, 2149–2163. doi: 10.1016/j.biomaterials.2008.12.050

Samavedi, S., Whittington, A. R., and Goldstein, A. S. (2013). Calcium phosphate ceramics in bone tissue engineering: a review of properties and their influence on cell behavior. *Acta Biomater.* 9, 8037–8045. doi: 10.1016/j.actbio.2013.06.014

Schulten, E. A., Prins, H. J., Overman, J. R., Helder, M. N., Ten Bruggenkate, C. M., and Klein-Nulend, J. (2013). A novel approach revealing the effect of a collagenous membrane on osteoconduction in maxillary sinus floor elevation with beta-tricalcium phosphate. *Eur. Cell. Mater.* 25, 215–228. doi: 10.22203/eCM.v025a16

Selvig, K. A., Sorensen, R. G., Wozney, J. M., and Wikesjo, U. M. (2002). Bone repair following recombinant human bone morphogenetic protein-2 stimulated periodontal regeneration. *J. Periodontol.* 73, 1020–1029. doi: 10.1902/jop.2002.73.9.1020

Shi, J., Sun, J., Zhang, W., Liang, H., Shi, Q., Li, X., et al. (2016). Demineralized bone matrix scaffolds modified by CBD-SDF-1alpha promote bone regeneration via recruiting endogenous stem cells. *ACS Appl. Mater. Interfaces* 8, 27511–27522. doi: 10.1021/acsami.6b08685

Sun, X., Liu, C., Shi, Y., Li, C., Sun, L., Hou, L., et al. (2019). The assessment of xenogeneic bone immunotoxicity and risk management study. *Biomed. Eng. Online* 18:108. doi: 10.1186/s12938-019-0729-z

Transperancy Market Research Report (2020). Bone Graft Substitutes Market. (Albany, NY:Transparency Market Research).

Tufekci, P., Tavakoli, A., Dlaska, C., Neumann, M., Shanker, M., Saifzadeh, S., et al. (2018). Early mechanical stimulation only permits timely bone healing in sheep. *J. Orthop. Res.* 36, 1790–1796. doi: 10.1002/jor.23812

Turner, A. S. (2001). Animal models of osteoporosis–necessity and limitations. *Eur. Cell. Mater.* 1, 66–81. doi: 10.22203/eCM.v001a08

Van Der Stok, J., Van Lieshout, E. M. M., El-Massoudi, Y., Van Kralingen, G. H., and Patka, P. (2011). Bone substitutes in the Netherlands - a systematic literature review. *Acta Biomater.* 7, 739–750. doi: 10.1016/j.actbio.2010.07.035

Wang, D., Liu, Y., Liu, Y., Yan, L., Zaat, S. A. J., Wismeijer, D., et al. (2019). A dual functional bone-defect-filling material with sequential antibacterial and osteoinductive properties for infected bone defect repair. *J. Biomed. Mater. Res. A* 107, 2360–2370. doi: 10.1002/jbm.a.36744

Wang, D., Tabassum, A., Wu, G., Deng, L., Wismeijer, D., and Liu, Y. (2017). Bone regeneration in critical-sized bone defect enhanced by introducing osteoinductivity to biphasic calcium phosphate granules. *Clin. Oral Implants Res.* 28, 251–260. doi: 10.1111/clr.12791

Wang, J., Zheng, Y., Zhao, J., Liu, T., Gao, L., Gu, Z., et al. (2012). Low-dose rhBMP2/7 heterodimer to reconstruct peri-implant bone defects: a micro-CT evaluation. *J. Clin. Periodontol.* 39, 98–105. doi: 10.1111/j.1600-051X.2011.01807.x

Wei, L. F., Teng, F., Deng, L. Q., Liu, G. F., Luan, M. Y., Jiang, J., et al. (2019). Periodontal regeneration using bone morphogenetic protein 2 incorporated biomimetic calcium phosphate in conjunction with barrier membrane: a pre-clinical study in dogs. *J. Clin. Periodontol.* 46, 1254–1263. doi: 10.1111/jcpe.13195

Weigand, A., Beier, J. P., Schmid, R., Knorr, T., Kilian, D., Gotzl, R., et al. (2017). Bone tissue engineering under xenogeneic-free conditions in a large animal model as a basis for early clinical applicability. *Tissue Eng. Part A* 23, 208–222. doi: 10.1089/ten.tea.2016.0176

Wu, G., Hunziker, E., Zheng, Y., Wismeijer, D., and Liu, Y. (2011). Functionalization of deproteinized bovine bone with a coating-incorporated depot of BMP-2 renders the material efficiently osteoinductive and suppresses foreign-body reactivity. *Bone* 49, 1323–1330. doi: 10.1016/j.bone.2011.09.046

Zhang, L., Yang, G., Johnson, B. N., and Jia, X. (2019). Three-dimensional (3D) printed scaffold and material selection for bone repair. *Acta Biomater.* 84, 16–33. doi: 10.1016/j.actbio.2018.11.039

Zhang, M., Sara, J. D., Wang, F. L., Liu, L. P., Su, L. X., Zhe, J., et al. (2015). Increased plasma BMP-2 levels are associated with atherosclerosis burden and coronary calcification in type 2 diabetic patients. *Cardiovasc. Diabetol.* 14:64. doi: 10.1186/s12933-015-0214-3

5

# Multifaceted Functions and Novel Insight into the Regulatory Role of RNA N⁶-Methyladenosine Modification in Musculoskeletal Disorders

*Wenchao Zhang[1,2], Lile He[2,3], Zhongyue Liu[1,2], Xiaolei Ren[1,2], Lin Qi[1,2], Lu Wan[1,2], Wanchun Wang[1,2], Chao Tu[1,2*] and Zhihong Li[1,2*]*

*[1] Department of Orthopedics, The Second Xiangya Hospital, Central South University, Changsha, China, [2] Hunan Key Laboratory of Tumor Models and Individualized Medicine, The Second Xiangya Hospital, Central South University, Changsha, China, [3] Department of Cardiovascular Surgery, The Second Xiangya Hospital, Central South University, Changsha, China*

***Correspondence:**
*Chao Tu*
*tuchao@csu.edu.cn*
*Zhihong Li*
*lizhihong@csu.edu.cn*

RNA modifications have emerged as key regulators of transcript expression in diverse physiological and pathological processes. As one of the most prevalent types of RNA modifications, $N^6$-methyladenosine ($m^6A$) has become the highlight in modulation of various diseases through interfering RNA splicing, translation, nuclear export, and decay. In many cases, the detailed functions of $m^6A$ in cellular processes and diseases remain unclear. Notably, recent studies have determined the relationship between $m^6A$ modification and musculoskeletal disorders containing osteosarcoma, osteoarthritis, rheumatoid arthritis, osteoporosis, etc. Herein, this review comprehensively summarizes the recent advances of $m^6A$ modification in pathogenesis and progression of musculoskeletal diseases. Specifically, the underlying molecular mechanisms, detection technologies, regulatory functions, clinical implications, and future perspectives of $m^6A$ in musculoskeletal disorders are discussed, with the aim to provide a novel insight into their association.

**Keywords: RNA $N^6$-methyladenosine, METTL3, FTO, musculoskeletal disorders, epigenetics**

## INTRODUCTION

Currently, a growing number of studies have shed light on a new hereditary manner, the epigenetics, which refers to changes in phenotype without DNA or RNA sequences alteration (Harvey et al., 2018). Several epigenetics manners have been identified, comprising the histone modification, DNA and RNA methylation, and noncoding RNA (ncRNA) modification. Of note, there have been more than 100 modifications demonstrated within RNAs over the past few years, including the $N^1$-methyladenosine ($m^1A$), $m^6A$, 5-methylcytosine ($m^5C$), 7-methylguanosine ($m^7G$), $m^1G$, $m^2G$, $m^6G$, etc. Among them, the $m^6A$ has received considerable attention because of its high abundance. It relates to a dynamic and reversible RNA modification that participate in a wide range of biological and pathological processes, such as the cancer progression (Lan et al., 2019) and inflammation (Zong et al., 2019). Specifically, it can manipulate the RNA splicing, export, translation, and degradation through methylation and demethylation mediated by multiple enzymes (Cao et al., 2016).

Musculoskeletal disorders are a set of prevalent diseases characterized by dysfunction of bone and skeletal muscle, including, but not limited to, osteosarcoma (OS), osteoarthritis (OA), rheumatoid arthritis (RA), osteoporosis (OP), etc. (Madan and Grime, 2015). Several epigenetics manners have been investigated in this field (Tu et al., 2019; van Wijnen and Westendorf, 2019). Among them, the alteration of $m^6A$ modification has been associated with the initiation and progression of musculoskeletal diseases.

In this review, we broadly summarize the functional repertoire of $m^6A$ in various musculoskeletal disorders, aiming to expand our understanding and discuss the putative perspective for adopting $m^6A$ as a novel biomarker and therapeutic target in musculoskeletal diseases.

## RNA M$^6$A MODIFICATION

As aforementioned, $m^6A$ modification is a dynamic and reversible epigenetic change (Zhang et al., 2020), which affects the stability and function of RNAs, thereby modulating the pathogenesis and progression of diseases (Qin et al., 2020; Wang et al., 2020; Zhu et al., 2020). $M^6A$ modification has been identified in more than 7,000 human genes, and it preferentially occurred at the site of stop codons and long internal exons within the RRACH sequence (R = G or A; H = A, C, or U) (Dominissini et al., 2012). Based on current evidences, $m^6A$ modification is able to interfere in RNA processing, splicing, export, degradation, and translation through the "writers," "erasers," and "readers" proteins (Chen et al., 2019). The detailed graphical description of the RNA $m^6A$ mechanism is presented in **Figure 1**.

Writers refer to the RNA methyltransferases, including methyltransferase-like 3 (METTL3), methyltransferase-like 14 (METTL14), methyltransferase-like 16 (METTL16), Wilms tumor 1-associated protein (WTAP), RNA-binding motif 15, etc. They are in charge of installing $m^6A$ to the RNA strand. In particular, METTL3 and METTL14 are the most studied key regulators in this process. They contain an S-adenosylmethionine–binding motif and are capable of adding methyl to the adenosine. Meanwhile, these two proteins can form a heterodimer core complex to modulate the cellular $m^6A$ deposition (Liu et al., 2014), in which they adopted a class I methyltransferase fold and interacted with each other through hydrogen bonding. Additionally, biochemical analysis revealed that METTL3 principally acted as the catalytic core, whereas METTL14 mainly functioned as an RNA-binding platform (Wang et al., 2016). Besides, the cofactor WTAP itself shows no methyltransferase activity, whereas it could interplay with the core complex to mediate its localization in nuclear spots (Ping et al., 2014). Furthermore, it has been reported that WTAP protein homeostasis in turn relied on the METTL3 protein levels (Sorci et al., 2018). Therefore, these writers cooperate to exert their function of $m^6A$ methylation within the specific RNA sites.

In contrast to the "writers," the "erasers" are demethylases that function in methyl removal, canonically involving the fat mass and obesity-associated protein (FTO) and alkB homolog 5 (ALKBH5). FTO can oxidize $m^6A$ to generate the N(6)-hydroxymethyladenosine and N(6)-formyladenosine that have a half-life time less than 3 h (Fu et al., 2013). Generally, FTO erase methyl in either the selective or nonselective way. In the selective way, FTO recognizes and binds to the specific $m^6A$-containing motif in cells (Li et al., 2019a). Because the association between FTO and RNA is weak, the additional cellular factors can corporately work with FTO to recognize and choose the target sites (Li et al., 2019a). In addition, the $m^6A$ itself can act as a "conformational marker" and interfere with the interaction between $m^6A$ and FTO via altering conformational outcomes in RNAs, which is the nonselective way of FTO-mediated demethylation (Zou et al., 2016). ALKBH5 is a 2-oxoglutarate and ferrous iron–dependent nucleic acid oxygenase that induces the demethylation of multiple RNAs. It was illuminated that ALKBH5 could occupy a similar region as L1 loop of the FTO protein that was associated with the single-strand RNA selectivity (Aik et al., 2014). Taken together, FTO and ALKBH5 are both the core regulators of $m^6A$ demethylation.

Readers are a group of proteins that discern the $m^6A$ modification and determine the functions of RNA transcripts. YTH domain (YTHD) family members (consisting of YTHDF1, YTHDF2, YTHDF3, YTHDC1, and YTHDC2) constitute a large class of $m^6A$ readers. They are located in nucleus or cytoplasm (specifically, YTHDF1 and YTHDF2 are located both in cytoplasm and nucleus, whereas YTHDF3 is only found in the cytoplasm) (Reichel et al., 2019), and characterized by containing the YT521B homology (YTH) domain that possesses an exquisite pocket with two conserved tryptophan residues (W377 and W428) for specific recognition of the methyl group (Xu et al., 2014). YTHDF1 is shown to promote translation of mRNA and enhance protein synthesis through impacting on the translation machinery, ensuring the sufficient protein generation is marked by $m^6A$ (Wang et al., 2015). Conversely, YTHDF2 mediates the degradation of its target $m^6A$ transcripts via reducing their stability (Li et al., 2018). Additionally, YTHDF3 participates in either promoting the protein synthesis in synergy with YTHDF1 or facilitating RNA degradation via interaction with YTHDF2. Thus, these three YTHDF proteins read the $m^6A$ modification in a cooperative way (Ni et al., 2019). Moreover, the nuclear YTHDC1 is associated with the RNA splicing (Kasowitz et al., 2018) and the export of $m^6A$ modified RNAs from nucleus to cytoplasm (Roundtree et al., 2017), whereas YTHDC2 engages in the elongation-promoting effect of $m^6A$ methylated RNA coding region (Mao et al., 2019). In addition to the YTHD family, the family of heterogeneous nuclear ribonucleoproteins (HNRNPs) is another set of $m^6A$ readers, which binds to pre-mRNA to interfere its stability and splicing (Geuens et al., 2016). HNRNPA2B1 has been well-accepted as a nuclear reader of $m^6A$, binding to the RGm$^6$AC containing sites on RNA to affect the alternative splicing and the processing of miRNAs (Alarcón et al., 2015). As to HNRNPC, because the $m^6A$ residues within RNA strand can destabilize the RNA duplexes (Kierzek and Kierzek, 2003), the structure of RNA may be altered when it is $m^6A$ modified. Given this, the $m^6A$ has been proposed to make the UUUUU tract within RNA to become more unfolded and

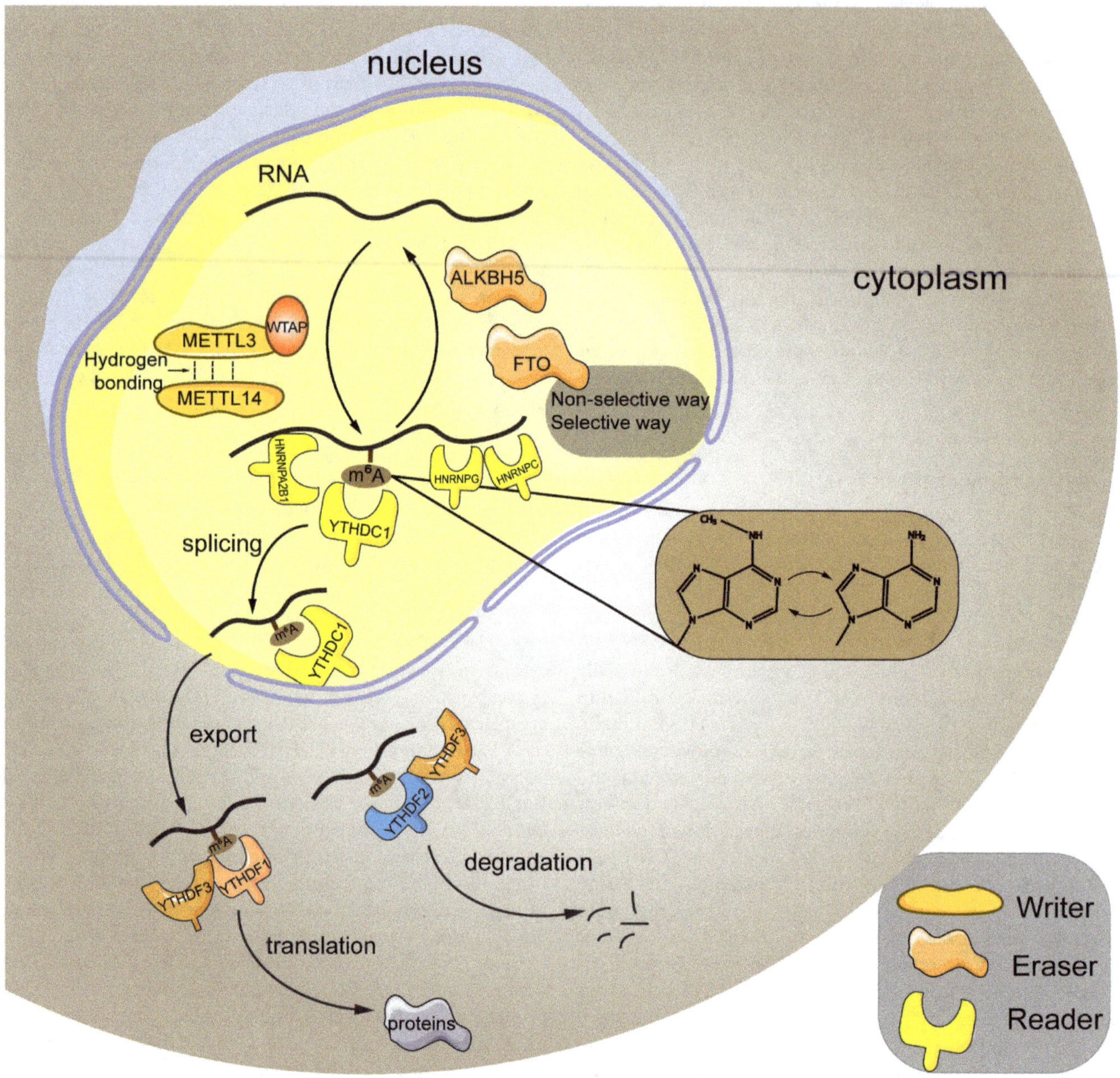


**FIGURE 1 |** Mechanism of m$^6$A RNA modification. M$^6$A modification is a reversible process mediated by its regulatory proteins, including the writers (MELTT3, METTL14, WTAP, etc.), erasers (FTO, ALKBH5, etc.), and readers (YTHDF1, YTHDF2, YTHDF3, etc.). METTL3, methyltransferase-like 3; METTL14, methyltransferase-like 14; WTAP, Wilms tumor 1-associated protein; FTO, fat mass and obesity-associated protein; ALKBH5, alkB homolog 5; YTHDF1, YTH domain family; member 1; HNRNPA2B1, heterogeneous nuclear ribonucleoprotein A2B1; HNRNPC, heterogeneous nuclear ribonucleoprotein C; HNRNPG, heterogeneous nuclear ribonucleoprotein G.

accessible to HNRNPC (Liu et al., 2015), which is termed as the "m$^6$A switch." Moreover, HNRNPG also recognizes the m$^6$A through "m$^6$A switch." HNRNPG has a low-complexity region that can discern a specific motif exposed by m$^6$A-mediated RNA structural change (Liu et al., 2017), subsequently modulating the cotranscriptional pre-mRNA splicing (Zhou et al., 2019). Furthermore, the insulin-like growth factor 2 mRNA-binding proteins (IGF2BPs) can target the mRNA transcripts in an m$^6$A-dependent way through recognizing their GG(m$^6$A)C sequences, subsequently stabilizing the targeted RNAs under both the normal and stress conditions (Huang et al., 2018).

## ADVANCES IN TECHNOLOGIES FOR M$^6$A DETECTION

Currently, a massive number of technologies have been developed for m$^6$A detection based on the immunohistochemistry or hybridization properties (Ovcharenko and Rentmeister, 2018). According to their detection performance, these technologies can be classified into the semiquantitative, quantitative, and precise location detection methods (Zhu et al., 2019; **Table 1**).

## Semiquantitative Methods

Semiquantitative detection strategies, including the dot blot, methyl sensitivity of MazF RNA endonucleases, and immune-Northern blot, are used to determine the presence of $m^6A$ modification rather than the amount. Among them, dot blot is applied to detect the global change of $m^6A$ by using antibodies that specifically bind to the $m^6A$ site. It is relatively simple and fast but not quantitative (Zhu et al., 2019), with low sensitivity when the $m^6A$ RNA fragment is small in the samples (Nagarajan et al., 2019). A modified dot blot method has been adopted to increase the sensitivity through adding an immunoprecipitation step to enrich the $m^6A$ RNA before detection (Nagarajan et al., 2019). Further, *Escherichia coli* MazF is a sequence-specific endoribonuclease, which cleave the 5′-ACA-3′ sequence but not the 5′-($m^6A$)CA-3′ sequence within RNA strand, whereby it is an $m^6A$-sensitive RNA cleavage enzyme. Based on this technology, a new high-throughput detection method for $m^6A$ has been established by researchers (Imanishi et al., 2017). Immuno-Northern blot is another way for semiquantitative detection of various types of RNA modifications. In this way, RNAs are separated and transferred onto a nylon membrane, followed by immunoblotting for measurement (Mishima et al., 2015).

## Quantitative Methods

Unlike semiquantitative methods, the quantitative methods, including photo-crosslinks–based quantitative proteomics, electrochemical immunosensor method, and support vector machine–based method, can be utilized to determine the amount of $m^6A$ RNA. Arguello et al. (2017) have proposed that the photo-crosslinkers, a widely used method to stabilize the protein–RNA interaction, could combine with quantitative proteomics to detect $m^6A$ RNA. Meanwhile, a diazirine containing RNA probes has been recently synthesized to improve its efficiency (Arguello et al., 2017). Moreover, in the electrochemical immunosensor method (Yin et al., 2017), an anti-$m^6A$ antibody has been applied to recognize and capture the $m^6A$-5′-triphosphate. Silver nanoparticles and amine-PEG3-biotin functionalized $SiO_2$ nanospheres (Ag@$SiO_2$) were used to amplify the signal, and phos-tag-biotin was employed as a bridge to connect the $m^6ATP$ and Ag@$SiO_2$. This approach is convenient, low-cost, and of high

**TABLE 1** | Technologies for $m^6A$ detection.

| Classification | Detection method | Mechanism | Advantages | Disadvantages | References |
|---|---|---|---|---|---|
| Semiquantitative | Dot blot | Using antibodies that specifically bind to the $m^6A$ | Simplicity, speediness | Not quantitative, sensitivity is low when the $m^6A$ RNA fragment is small | Nagarajan et al., 2019; Zhu et al., 2019 |
| | Methyl sensitivity of MazF RNA endonucleases | MazF selectively cleave the 5′-ACA-3′ but not the 5′-($m^6A$)CA-3′ sequence | Simple analyses of both $m^6A$ demethylase and methyltransferase activity | Not quantitative, only able to cleave the 5′-ACA-3′ site in single-stranded RNA | Imanishi et al., 2017 |
| | Immuno-Northern blot | Immunoblotting using antibodies against modified nucleosides | High specificity, sensitivity, and potential quantitative capability | Not quantitative | Mishima et al., 2015 |
| Quantitative | Photo-crosslinks based quantitative proteomics | Stabilizing protein–RNA interaction and detecting via synthetic probes | Quantitative, high efficiency | Requirement of the synthesis of the probe | Arguello et al., 2017 |
| | Electrochemical immunosensor method | Antibody–antigen interaction | Simplicity, low-cost, high specificity and sensitivity | N/A | Yin et al., 2017 |
| | Support vector machine–based method | Computational prediction based on existent high-throughout data | Simplicity, saving the experiment cost | Relying on the existent experimental data | Chen W. et al., 2016 |
| Gene specific location detection | MeRIP-Seq | Combination of the ChIP-Seq and RNA-Seq | High-throughput | Poor reproducibility | Meyer et al., 2012; McIntyre et al., 2020 |
| | $m^6A$-LAIC-seq | Sequencing intact full-length RNA in both $m^6A$-positive and -negative fractions post-RIP | Detecting $m^6A$ in differential RNA isoform, determining the $m^6A$ levels in each gene | Cannot stoichiometrically analyze the methylation of a single modified nucleotide | Molinie et al., 2016 |
| Nucleotide-specific location detection | HRM | Detecting the alteration of nucleic acid duplex melting properties | High-throughput, high-resolution | Relying on the previous knowledge of the modified nucleoside position at a particular RNA site | Golovina et al., 2014 |
| | SCARLET | RNAs are cleaved, radiolabeled, digested, and analyzed by TLC | High-resolution | N/A | Liu et al., 2013 |
| | miCLIP | Inducing specific mutational signatures to $m^6A$ antibody | High-resolution | N/A | Linder et al., 2015 |

*HRM, high-resolution melting; $m^6A$-LAIC-seq, $m^6A$ level and isoform-characterization sequencing; MeRIP-Seq, methylated RNA immunoprecipitation next generation sequencing; miCLIP, $m^6A$ individual nucleotide resolution cross linking and immunoprecipitation; N/A, not available; SCARLET, site-specific cleavage and radioactive labeling followed by ligation-assisted extraction and thin-layer chromatography.*

specificity and sensitivity. Besides, the support vector machine-based method is a computational way to predict the m$^6$A site within RNA strand based on the existent high-throughput experiment data (Chen W. et al., 2016).

### M$^6$A Location Detection Methods

To figure out the specific location of m$^6$A within RNAs, several detection methods have been further developed by researchers (Ovcharenko and Rentmeister, 2018). Generally, these techniques can be divided into two sorts, namely, the gene-specific and the nucleoside-specific detection method. The former one comprises methylated RNA immunoprecipitation next-generation sequencing (MeRIP-Seq), m$^6$A level and isoform-characterization sequencing (m$^6$A-LAIC-seq), etc. While the latter contains high-resolution melting (HRM) analysis, site-specific cleavage, and radioactive labeling followed by ligation-assisted extraction and thin-layer chromatography (SCARLET), m$^6$A individual nucleotide resolution cross-linking and immunoprecipitation (miCLIP), etc.

MeRIP-Seq combines the ChIP-Seq and RNA-Seq (Meyer et al., 2012), in which the anti-m$^6$A antibody is incubated with the RNA fragments, and the precipitated fragments then are sequenced. Hence, it can determine the origin of m$^6$A at a gene level. However, a more recent study reported that this method was of poor reproducibility because it was easily influenced by the noise (McIntyre et al., 2020). On the basis of MeRIP-seq, m$^6$A-LAIC-seq (Molinie et al., 2016) is further developed to detect the dynamic range and isoform complexity of m$^6$A content in a single gene, in which the intact full-length RNAs in both m$^6$A-positive and m$^6$A-negative fractions post-RIP are sequenced, and thus the differential isoform usages in each transcripts are detectable.

HRM (Golovina et al., 2014) is a high-throughput method for m$^6$A detection at a specific site within the RNA strand. This method works by detecting the alteration of nucleic acid duplex melting properties caused by m$^6$A modification. For instance, it has been observed that the melting temperature of RNA–DNA duplex was reduced by the presence of m$^6$A modification (Golovina et al., 2014). SCARLET (Liu et al., 2013) is a method that enables detection of m$^6$A status at any site in mRNA/long ncRNA (lncRNA), in which the m$^6$A-containing candidate sites are cleaved, radiolabeled, and site-specific ligated, followed by complete nuclease digestion. The digested m$^6$A residue is then measured by thin-layer chromatography (TLC). Moreover, MiCLIP can be used to determine the m$^6$A site at a nucleotide-specific level (Linder et al., 2015). M$^6$A antibodies bind to the m$^6$A sites within RNA strands, and the m$^6$A residues are then located by inducing specific mutational signatures after ultraviolet light–induced antibody-RNA cross-linking and reverse transcription.

## RNA M$^6$A METHYLATION IN MUSCULOSKELETAL BIOLOGY

Musculoskeletal system mainly consists of skeleton and skeletal muscle, which directly participates in the motor function of human body. Diverse transcriptional factors have been reported to involve in the genesis and maintenance of musculoskeletal system. M$^6$A modification is a widely discovered and annotated epigenetic manner that takes part in the biology of musculoskeletal system. Herein, we discuss the mechanism and regulatory function of m$^6$A in this process (**Figure 2**).

### M$^6$A in Bone Remodeling

Bone is a connective tissue functioning in mechanical support, mineral homeostasis, hematopoiesis, etc., which maintains its metabolic balance principally through bone remodeling, a dynamic process involved in the formation of bone matrix through osteoblasts and removal of bone mass via osteoclasts (Hadjidakis and Androulakis, 2006). Osteoblast is derived from the bone marrow mesenchymal stem cells (BMSCs) under the impact of numerous regulators, which can produce matrix to form the bone tissue. With the development of bone matrix, some osteoblasts finally reorganized and embedded into the matrix as osteocytes (Blair et al., 2017). Accordingly, osteocytes play a vital role in monitoring the bone quality and sensing the mechanotransduction, as well as secreting regulatory factors associated with bone anabolism (Tresguerres et al., 2020). By contrast, osteoclasts are multinuclear cells derived from myeloid precursors, which function in degradation and resorption of bone through secreting proteolytic enzymes and acid (Charles and Aliprantis, 2014). The osteoblasts and osteoclasts couple with each other to maintain the dynamic homeostasis of bones (Weivoda et al., 2016). Any impairment of the homeostasis under pathological condition may contribute to the bone disorder.

As an indispensable part of epigenetic regulation, m$^6$A modification is suggested as a crucial regulator participating in either the osteogenic or osteoclastogenic processes of bone. For instance, the expression of m$^6$A methyltransferases (METTL3 and METTL14) was found significantly elevated in BMSCs undergoing osteogenic induction. Accordingly, knockdown of METTL3 reduced the mRNA level of genes related to BMSC proliferation and differentiation such as the Vegfa-164 and Vegfa-188 (Tian et al., 2019). Apart from this, MYD88 gene, a vital upstream regulator of nuclear factor κB (NF-κB) signaling, was methylated by METTL3, followed by activation of NF-κB and repression of osteogenic progression. Meanwhile, the METTL3-mediated osteogenic differentiation tendency could be reversed by demethylase ALKBH5 (Yu et al., 2020). Moreover, silencing METTL3 decreased the osteogenic markers, Smad signaling, and mineralized nodules in preosteoblast MC3T3-E1 cells, indicating the reduction of osteoblast differentiation (Zhang Y. et al., 2019). Hence, the METTL3-mediated m$^6$A methylation significantly contributes to the maintenance of osteogenesis. Conversely, METTL3-mediated m$^6$A methylation was also reported to facilitate the osteoclast differentiation. METTL3 level was elevated during osteoclastogenesis, and METTL3 depletion suppressed the differentiation and bone-resorbing ability of osteoclasts. Mechanistically, Atp6v0d2 mRNA, the principal regulator of osteoclast precursor cells fusion (Kim et al., 2009) was stabilized

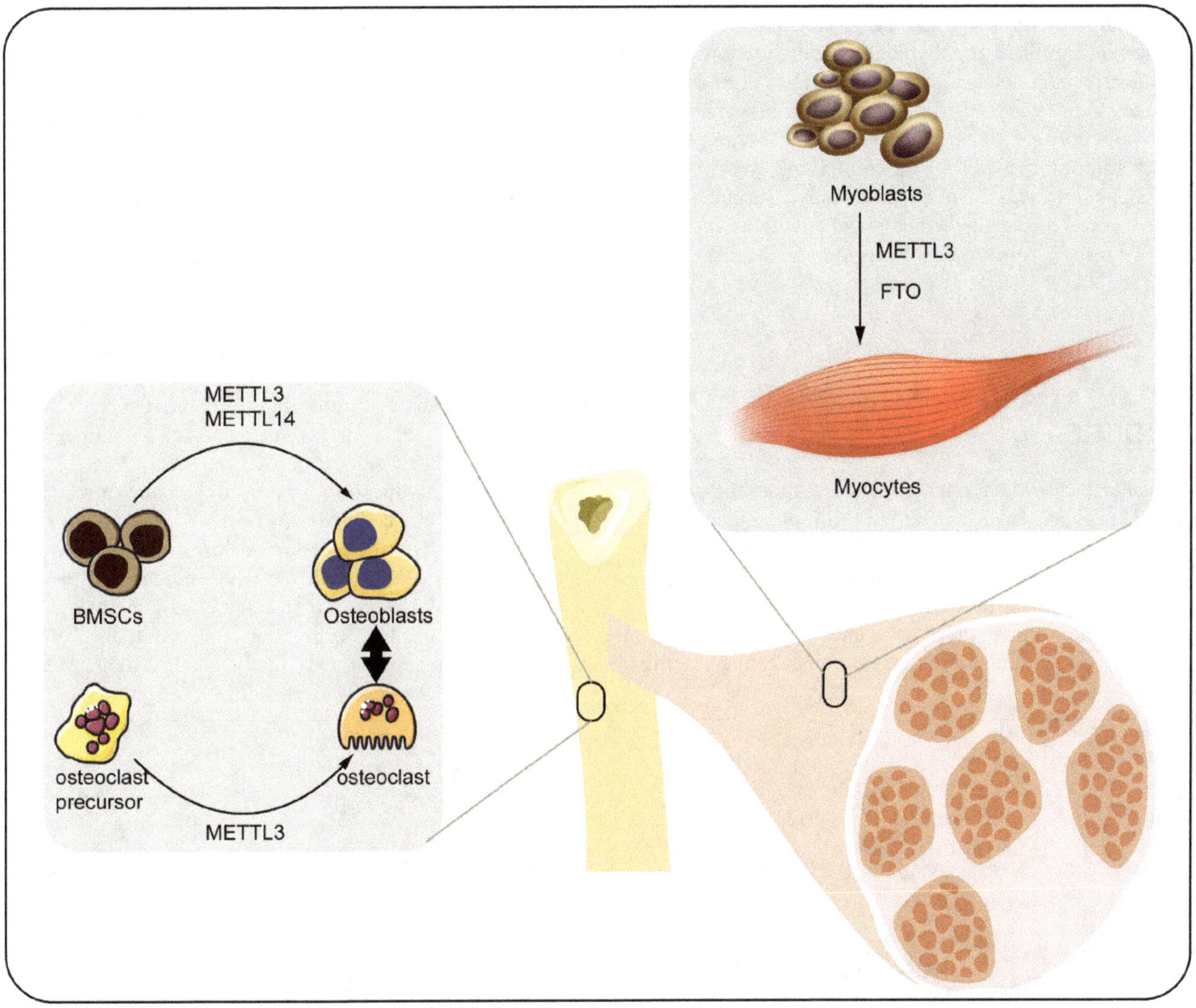


**FIGURE 2 |** Roles of m$^6$A modification in musculoskeletal biology. M$^6$A regulatory proteins participate in differentiation of BMSCs, osteoclast precursors, and myoblasts. METTL3, methyltransferase-like 3; METTL14, methyltransferase-like 14; FTO, fat mass and obesity-associated protein; BMSCs, bone marrow mesenchymal stem cells.

by the m$^6$A-binding protein YTHDF2 when the METTL3 was abolished (Li et al., 2020).

Taken together, the present studies have implicated the function of METTL3-mediated m$^6$A in either the osteogenic or the osteoclastogenic differentiation of bone remodeling.

## M$^6$A in Skeletal Muscle Regulation

Skeletal muscle comprises almost 40% of the total body weight, which functions in both the mechanical and metabolic processes of the body such as force generation and heat production (Frontera and Ochala, 2015). Retaining skeletal muscle mass is crucial for its physiological function, which is principally determined by the size and amount of muscle fibers. Skeletal muscle fibers are generated from myoblasts via myoblasts fusion, a process named as myogenesis (Sampath et al., 2018). Epigenetic modifications involving the histone modification (Machado et al., 2017), ncRNA (Liu M. et al., 2019), DNA methylation (Miyata et al., 2015), etc. have been unraveled to play a part in this process. Among them, m$^6$A was proposed as a concernful regulator.

In the previous analyses, m$^6$A modification can modulate the activity of skeletal muscle via modifying the muscle mass and interfering with the myoblasts differentiation: (1) modifying the muscle mass. For instance, upregulation of FTO gene expression was closely associated with skeletal muscle mass increase in overweight individuals (Doaei et al., 2019). Moreover, maternal high-fat intake could even disturb the m$^6$A modification and FTO gene expression in skeletal muscle of its offspring (Li et al., 2016). Wu et al. (2017) have confirmed that activation of AMPK decreases the lipid accumulation in skeletal muscle cells through inversely regulating FTO expression and FTO-mediated demethylation. (2) Interfering with the myoblasts differentiation. It has been elucidated that FTO downregulation inhibited the myoblasts differentiation of mice through affecting the activity of mTOR-PGC-1α-mitochondria axis, which suppressed the mitochondria biogenesis and energy production of skeletal muscle cells (Wang et al., 2017). In addition, myoblast differentiation was regulated by METTL3-promoted MyoD. Specifically, suppression of METTL3 downregulated the activation of MyoD by modifying the sites within 5' untranslated region of MyoD mRNA (Kudou et al., 2017).

## ROLES OF M$^6$A IN MUSCULOSKELETAL DISORDERS

Musculoskeletal disorders refer to abnormalities of skeleton or skeletal muscle, emerging as the tumor, inflammation, trauma, etc., which may lead to disability and paralysis. Although previous work has shed light on the roles of m$^6$A in musculoskeletal disorders, the details of m$^6$A function and its involvement in the pathogenesis and progression remain unclear. Here, we summarize the current evidences concerning the pleiotropic functions of m$^6$A in musculoskeletal diseases, as presented in **Figure 3** and **Table 2**.

### M$^6$A in OS

OS is the most common primary malignant bone tumor that mainly occurs in teenagers and adolescents with an annual incidence of 3.1 case per million (Gianferante et al., 2017). Although considerable advancement has been achieved in the past decades, the comprehensive mechanism network of OS has not yet been fully investigated. Currently, the standardized therapy for OS is limb salvage surgery or amputation combined with multiregimen-based chemotherapy. However, the survival rate of patients is unsatisfactory because of potential chemoresistance, lung metastasis, or tumor relapses. Recently, increasing studies have explored new therapeutic strategies for OS such as the molecular target therapy (Corre et al., 2020).

Epigenetic modification has been globally investigated in OS (Nebbioso et al., 2018). Almost all types of epigenetics, ranging from DNA methylation to histone modification, have been suggested to involve in the development and progression of OS (Cui et al., 2011). For instance, DNA methylation could downregulate miR-449c expression and eventually contributed to the tumorigenesis of OS (Li Q. et al., 2017). Meanwhile,

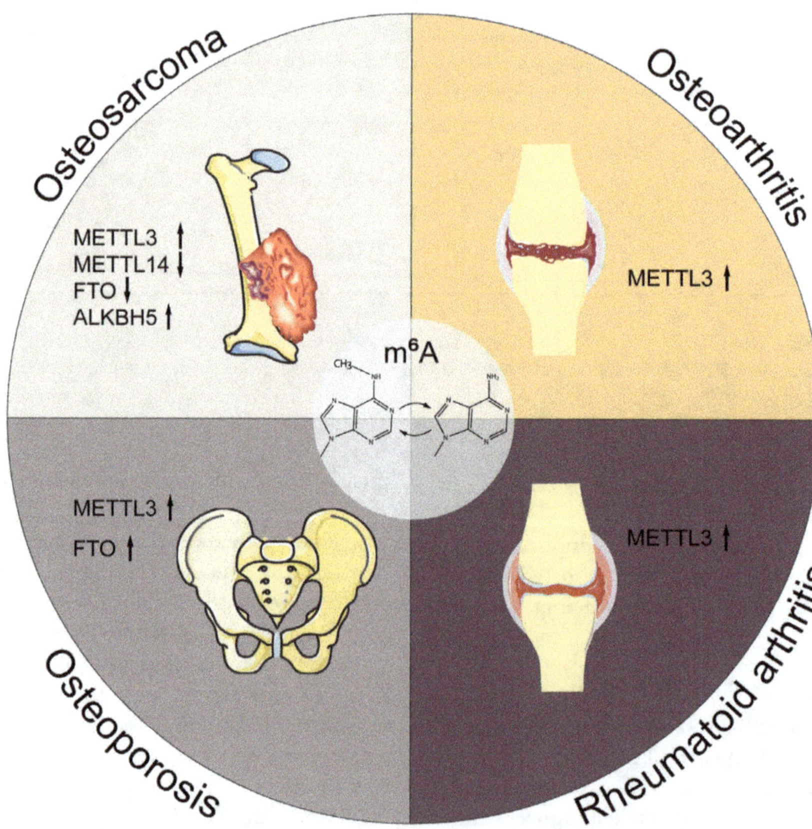


**FIGURE 3** | M$^6$A in musculoskeletal disorders. M$^6$A is associated with the progression of multiple musculoskeletal diseases, including osteosarcoma, osteoarthritis, rheumatoid arthritis, and osteoporosis. METTL3, methyltransferase-like 3; METTL14, methyltransferase-like 14; FTO, fat mass and obesity-associated protein; ALKBH5, alkB homolog 5; YTHDF1, YTH domain family, member 1.

**TABLE 2** | The role of m$^6$A in musculoskeletal disorders.

| Diseases | M$^6$A component | Samples and condition | Function | Regulation | Target | Role in disease | References |
|---|---|---|---|---|---|---|---|
| OS | METTL14, METTL3, FTO, ALKBH5 | MG63/ DXR (doxorubicin treatment) | Oncogene | ↓:METTL14/FTO; ↑:METTL3/ALKBH5 | Wnt signaling | Emergence and maintaining of OSCs, promoting drug resistance | Wang Y. et al., 2019 |
| | ALKBH5 | 70 pairs of OS and normal tissues Osteoblast cell line and OS cell lines | Oncogene | ↑ | PVT1 | Promoting OS cell proliferation | Chen et al., 2020 |
| | METTL3 | HOS, SAOS-2, U2OS, and MG63 cells | Oncogene | ↑ | ATAD2 | Enhancing OS cell growth and metastasis | Zhou et al., 2020 |
| | METTL3 | 28 pairs of OS cancerous and paracancerous tissues; hFOB1.19 and OS cell lines | Oncogene | ↑ | DRG1 | Promoting OS progression | Ling et al., 2020 |
| | METTL3 | 40 paired of OS tissues and adjacent tissues Osteoblast cells and OS cell lines | Oncogene | ↑ | LEF1 | Promoting OS progression | Miao et al., 2019 |
| OA | METTL3 | ATDC5 cells | promotor | ↑ | NF-κB signaling | Promoting inflammatory response, collagen synthesis and degradation, and cell apoptosis in chondrocytes | Liu Q. et al., 2019 |
| RA | METTL3 | 47 RA patients and 30 health controls; THP-1 cell | promotor | ↑ | NF-κB signaling | Promoting RA disease activity | Wang J. et al., 2019 |
| OP | METTL3 | METTL3 knock-out and knock-in mice; primary MSCs | Suppressor | ↓ | PTH/Pth1r signaling | Impairing bone formation | Wu et al., 2018 |
| | METTL3 | Female OP patients and control subjects; METTL3$^{+/-}$ mice | Suppressor | ↓ | miR320/ RUNX2 | Promoting OP development | Yan et al., 2020 |
| | FTO | 44 female/male individuals with/without OP Young and aged C57BL/6J mice | promotor | ↑ | Pparg | Promoting the shift of osteoporotic BMSC fate to adipocyte | Shen et al., 2018 |
| | FTO | FTO$^{flx/flx}$ (FTO$^{f/f}$) mice | Suppressor | ↑ | ER stress pathway | Protecting osteoblasts from genotoxic damage Maintaining bone mass | Zhang Q. et al., 2019 |

*↑, Upregulation; ↓, Downregulation; ALKBH5, alkB homolog 5, ATAD2, ATPase family AAA domain containing 2; DRG1, GTP-binding protein 1; ER, endoplasmic reticulum; FTO, fat mass and obesity-associated protein; LEF1, lymphoid enhancer binding factor 1; METTL3, methyltransferase-like 3; METTL14, methyltransferase-like 14; NF-κB, nuclear factor κB; OA, osteoarthritis; OP, osteoporosis; OS, osteosarcoma; Pparg, peroxisome proliferator-activated receptor γ; PTH/Pth1r, parathyroid hormone /parathyroid hormone receptor-1; PVT1, plasmacytoma variant translocation 1; RA, rheumatoid arthritis; RUNX2, runt-related transcription factor 2.*

histone methyltransferase has been discovered to regulate the chemosensitivity in OS (Jiang et al., 2018; He et al., 2019). Additionally, potential roles of multiple ncRNAs also have been validated in OS, such as the circRNA (Tu et al., 2020) and lncRNA (Ren et al., 2020; Xu et al., 2020). Li X. et al. (2017) reported that HOX transcript antisense intergenic RNA (HOTAIR) could enhance the development of OS via DNA methylation of CDKN2A gene. Notably, there have been some indications that m$^6$A modification exerts pivotal functions in OS.

An integrative study performed by Wang J. et al. (2019) analyzing the transcriptome-wide m$^6$A methylome enriched by chemotherapy in OS stem cells (OSCs) has revealed that several m$^6$A-related enzymes (METTL3, METTL14, FTO, ALKBH5) were altered in OS cells compared with noncancerous counterparts. The aberrantly expressed genes were associated with pluripotency regulation of the OSCs (Wang J. et al., 2019). Further, it has been shown that lncRNA plasmacytoma variant translocation 1 (PVT1) transcript was upregulated because of m$^6$A methylation decrease mediated by ALKBH5, which reduced the binding of reader protein YTHDF2 in PVT1, subsequently lessening the degradation of PVT1 and promoting tumorigenesis of OS (Chen et al., 2020). METTL3 was found localizing in both cytoplasm and nucleus of OS cells, which is also on the map of OS modulation. Downregulation of METTL3 was reported to suppress the expression of ATPase family AAA domain containing 2 (ATAD2), in conjunction with inhibition of OS cell growth and metastasis (Zhou et al., 2020). In addition, knockdown of METTL3 has been demonstrated to be associated with decreased m$^6$A methylation of GTP-binding protein (DRG) 1. Concomitant with the decreased m$^6$A methylation, the stability and expression level of DRG1 were reduced (Ling et al., 2020), resulting in suppression of the OS development, migration, and colony formation. Meanwhile, silence of METTL3 decreased the m$^6$A methylation and expression of lymphoid enhancer binding factor 1 (LEF1), followed by the advent of Wnt/β-catenin signaling pathway deactivation. Consequently, aberration of Wnt/β-catenin pathway contributed to the development of OS (Miao et al., 2019).

Collectively, based on the current evidences, the m$^6$A writers, mainly the METTL3, are found extensively involved in the tumorigenesis, progression, and migration of OS via methylating their target genes. However, the current recognition is still restricted because of the limited number and depth of studies.

## M$^6$A in OA

OA is the most prevalent chronic joint disease that mainly occurs in aging and obesity population. The prevalence of OA is still in continuous growth, and it is estimated that the proportion of OA in population 45 years or older will increase from 26.6 to 29.5% by 2032 (Hunter and Bierma-Zeinstra, 2019). Symptoms of OA typically include stiffness, pain, and movement restriction with a high risk of disability, which can bring substantial socioeconomic burden (Hunter et al., 2014). The pathogenesis of OA principally involves in degradation of cartilage matrix, which consists of collagen type II, minor collagen types IX and XI, and gel-like negatively charged proteoglycans (Kannu et al., 2009). Likewise, many inflammation-related molecules have been suggested to engage in this process such as the growth factors [transforming growth factor β, fibroblast growth factor 2 (FGF-2), and FGF-18], Wnt, β-catenin, HIF-2α, etc. (Xia et al., 2014). Targeting the inflammation pathways is regarded as a promising way for OA therapy. Particularly, epigenetic regulation has been reported to be in connection with the inflammatory factors and response (Shen et al., 2017). As an indispensable way of epigenetic regulation, $m^6A$ has also been partially studied in OA.

It was expounded that METTL3 regulated OA process via enhancing inflammatory response and extracellular matrix (ECM) synthesis (Liu Q. et al., 2019). Mechanistically, silencing METTL3 inhibited the inflammatory cytokines level and nuclear factor κB signaling in OA cells, thereby deactivating the progression of OA. Meanwhile, suppression of METTL3 boosted the degradation of chondrocytes ECM through downregulating the matrix metalloprotease-13 and collagenase type X, consequently promoting the development of OA (Liu M. et al., 2019). In addition, the association between OA and FTO has also been explored in some genome-wide association studies in which they clarified that FTO-mediated overweight increased the susceptibility of OA (Zeggini et al., 2012; Panoutsopoulou et al., 2014). However, another study performed by Dai et al. (2018) showed that the FTO polymorphism (rs8044769) was not linked to OA in the Chinese Han population, and their association may be mediated by other genes. Therefore, the correlation between FTO and OA remains elusive and requires further exploration.

## M⁶A in RA

With a symptom of pain, swelling, and stiffness, RA is a common chronic inflammatory disease that primarily attacks the synovial joint (Littlejohn and Monrad, 2018). RA can bring substantial burden to both the individuals and socioeconomics because of its high morbidity and mortality (Hu et al., 2018). Besides, RA is in close linkage with the occurrence of cardiovascular diseases (Blum and Adawi, 2019). Autoimmune-mediated inflammation is a well-known cause of RA (Derksen et al., 2017), in which both the genetic regulation (Scott et al., 2010) and epigenetic regulation (Doody et al., 2017) are proposed to play indispensable roles.

The relationship between $m^6A$ modification and RA has been partially unraveled in several studies. A large-scale genome-wide association study identifying the $m^6A$-associated SNPs ($m^6A$-SNPs) that affected the progression of RA has been conducted. Thirty-seven RA-related $m^6A$-SNPs were discovered, and 27 of them were verified to affect expression of 24 local genes in different RA cells or tissues, which indicated the potential roles of $m^6A$-SNPs in RA (Mo et al., 2018b). Moreover, METTL3 was validated to significantly suppress the inflammatory response of macrophages in RA. Specifically, METTL3 inhibited the generation of IL-6 and TNF-α in macrophages via restraining the phosphorylation of NF-κB. Therefore, METTL3 may serve as a potential biomarker for diagnosis of RA (Wang J. et al., 2019). However, because of the limitation of current studies, we can only hypothesize that $m^6A$ can decelerate the progression of RA via regulating the inflammatory response of immune cells; studies are still needed to provide more evidences.

## M⁶A in OP

Characterizing by depletion of bone mass and impairment of bone structure, OP is mostly a condition of postmenopausal women and aging, which may lead to disastrous fracture in some cases (Armas and Recker, 2012; Boyanov et al., 2014).

Several researches have enhanced our recognition of the roles of $m^6A$ modification in OP. A genome-wide identification study was indicative of the potential roles of $m^6A$-SNPs in bone mineral density. The results revealed that 138, 125, and 993 $m^6A$-SNPs were in linkage to femoral neck density disorders, lumbar spine density disorders, and heel density disorders, respectively (Mo et al., 2018a). Currently, it becomes obvious that factors associated with regulation of BMSCs differentiation are closely associated with OP. The imbalance between BMSC-derived osteoblasts and adipocytes was deemed underlying progression of OP (Chen Q. et al., 2016). It has been demonstrated that METTL3-mediated $m^6A$ methylation affected the function of BMSCs through several pathways. In the first place, knockdown of $m^6A$ methyltransferase METTL3 in mice induced pathological features related to the occurrence of OP via decreasing parathyroid hormone (PTH)/parathyroid hormone receptor-1 (Pth1r) signaling axis, interfering the PTH-induced osteogenic response of BMSCs (Wu et al., 2018). Moreover, downregulation of METTL3 in BMSCs inhibited the methylation of runt-related transcription factor 2 (RUNX2) and precursor (pre-) miR320 (Yan et al., 2020). RUNX2 is an essential regulator of osteoblast progenitor proliferation and osteogenic differentiation, which can enhance the bone mineralization, and multiple factors were reported to participate in the osteogenic process via targeting RUNX2 (Hou et al., 2019; Komori, 2019).

Conversely, the FTO, represented as the RNA demethylase, was reported to promote the shift of osteoporotic BMSC fate to adipocyte and impede the bone formation through a growth differentiation factor 11 (GDF11)-FTO-peroxisome proliferator-activated receptor γ (Pparg) axis, whereby high FTO expression indicated high risk of OP (Shen et al., 2018). Meanwhile, the expression of FTO could be repressed by overexpression of miR-149-3p, followed by a higher potential of BMSCs to differentiate into adipocytes (Li et al., 2019b). In addition, of SNPs in multitude utilizing the association analyses, it was shown that a FTO such as rs1421085, rs1558902 and rs1121980 were associated with bone mineral density and risk of fracture (Guo et al., 2011; Tran et al., 2014). Interestingly, although FTO inhibited the BMSCs from differentiating into osteoblasts, it could exert a protective role in differentiated osteoblasts.

Osteoblasts with FTO suppression were prone to develop cell death, which was illustrated to be caused by the interruption of DNA repair pathway. Specifically, FTO was able to stabilize the endoplasmic reticulum stress pathway components, such as Hsp70, protecting osteoblasts from genotoxic damage (Zhang Q. et al., 2019).

Taken together, m$^6$A modification is involved in the occurrence and development of OP via (1) METTL3-mediated differentiation of BMSCs to osteocyte, (2) FTO-mediated differentiation of BMSCs to adipocyte, and (3) FTO-mediated protection of osteoblasts from genotoxic damage. Herein, we assume that m$^6$A may play a dual role in OP, by which it can either promote or decelerate the progression of OP via different modifications.

## CLINICAL UTILIZATIONS OF M$^6$A IN MUSCULOSKELETAL DISORDERS

RNA target therapy has become a hotspot and shown convincing prospects in treatment of many diseases with high specificity and efficacy (Crooke et al., 2018). The broad involvement of m$^6$A in musculoskeletal disorders, as outlined previously, has driven extensive research efforts at m$^6$A-based therapy. The functions of the m$^6$A regulatory proteins including FTO, METTL3, ALKBH5, etc. have been determined in OS, OA, RA, and OP as mentioned previously. As a result, the possibility is then opened for developing inhibitors or promoters of them to control the diseases.

Some natural products have been discovered showing significant activity in FTO inhibition. The natural product rhein is the first identified small-molecule inhibitor of human FTO demethylase, which competitively binds to the FTO active site and inhibit the demethylation *in vitro* (Chen et al., 2012). Additionally, by using the structure-based hierarchical virtual screening, researchers have found that entacapone directly bound to FTO and subsided its activity (Peng et al., 2019). And the natural compound radicicol also has been recognized as a potent FTO inhibitor, which suppressed the FTO demethylation activity in a dose-dependent manner (Wang et al., 2018). Besides, the meclofenamic acid (MA), a nonsteroidal anti-inflammatory drug, was identified as a specific inhibitor of FTO. Mechanically, MA competed with FTO for the binding sites within the m$^6$A modified RNA, reducing activity of FTO-mediated demethylation (Huang et al., 2015). Further, FTO may interfere the reaction of human body to other drugs. For instance, it has been elucidated that the rs7195994 variant at the FTO gene locus hereditarily impacted the TNF inhibitor response in RA patients, and the customized treatment based on the FTO genetic stratification of patients could improve the efficacy (Massey et al., 2018).

Similarly, because METTL3 up-regulation in OS, OA, and RA contributes to the progression of diseases, METTL3 may also be targeted for treatment. Although METTL3 inhibitor is not available so far, it provides us with a novel direction. The fact that several drug screening technologies for RNA-modifying enzymes such as the self-assembled monolayer desorption/ionization have been developed illustrates a promising future for METTL3-based drugs (Buker et al., 2020). Recently, the first series of small molecule inhibitors of METTL3 have been identified via high-throughput docking into the SAM binding site and protein X-ray crystallography, in which seven compounds belonging to N-substituted amide of ribofuranuronic acid analogs of adenosine or adenosine mimics with a six-member ring were uncovered to be the effective METTL3 inhibitors (Bedi et al., 2020).

In summary, m$^6$A-modifying proteins can serve as potential targets for drugs with which the FTO and METTL3 inhibitor may have great prospect in the treatment of musculoskeletal disorders.

## DISCUSSION

Epigenetics has been widely illuminated in multiple diseases over the past decades, and researchers are consistently seeking for new remedy from this field (Prachayasittikul et al., 2017). Currently, a diverse set of RNA modifications has been identified and annotated. Of note, m$^6$A is the most abundant among them (Linder et al., 2015). Even though the recent advances have highlighted the crucial role of m$^6$A in a multitude of diseases, only a small percentage of them focus on the musculoskeletal disorders. In this review, we have discussed the molecular mechanisms, detection technologies, regulatory functions, and clinical implications of m$^6$A in musculoskeletal diseases. As we summarized previously, m$^6$A modification is of great potential in disease prediction and drug development, yet the current studies are insufficient.

The first issue is how to choose and optimize the laboratory used technology for m$^6$A detection in clinical practice. Although a diverse set of methods have been continually developed in experiment to detect the m$^6$A modification or analyze the m$^6$A residue locations within RNA site over the past decades, the use in clinic has not been investigated yet. Here, we envision that we can associate the disease progression with the m$^6$A presence patterns that may be presented as the presence of m$^6$A, the proportion of m$^6$A, or the specific site of m$^6$A. With the appropriate detection method, doctors will be able to figure out the situation of musculoskeletal diseases through the m$^6$A examination results.

Furthermore, it has remained a significant challenge to dissect the mechanism of m$^6$A in musculoskeletal disorders because limited studies have been performed toward it, especially for OA and RA. Meanwhile, the current studies of m$^6$A in musculoskeletal disorders focus only on the "writers" and "erasers," whereas clues toward the "readers" are scarce. As a matter of fact, roles of the "readers" have been investigated in other diseases. For instance, high YTHDF1 expression was a significant predictor of malignant tumor behaviors and poor prognosis in colorectal cancer (Nishizawa et al., 2018). IGF2BPs was demonstrated to participate in suppression of glycolysis and stemness properties of breast cancer cells via a FGF13-AS1/IGF2BPs/Myc feedback loop (Ma et al., 2019). Thus, the "readers" may also engage in the pathophysiological processes of musculoskeletal disorders.

Besides, $m^6A$-based drugs remain poorly understood. Only a limited number of FTO and METTL3 inhibitors have been identified, yet their efficacy and safety are inconclusive. Notably, there are currently no $m^6A$-based drugs developed for musculoskeletal disorders. Therefore, to address these limitations, we still have a long way to go.

## CONCLUSION

As the most abundant RNA modification in eukaryotic cells, it is beyond doubt that $m^6A$ is a central node of the regulatory network of diseases. The illustration of $m^6A$ function has revealed its great importance in both the biological and pathological processes of bone and skeletal muscle. $M^6A$ modification has been partially studied in musculoskeletal disorders, including OS, OA, RA, OP, etc. Regarding its pivotal role in regulating the progression and development of diseases, $m^6A$ modification is of great potential to serve as the diagnostic biomarker or therapeutic target in musculoskeletal diseases, although more evidences are still warranted for validation in the future. Furthermore, a growing number of technologies have been developed for the $m^6A$ detection, and it has become evident that $m^6A$ is detectable and usable in disease prediction. Even with all of the effort over the recent years to figure out the detection methods for $m^6A$, it should be noted that there is no clear indication for selecting the most suitable detection method for clinical application. Simplified $m^6A$ detection methods with high specificity/sensitivity and low costing, such as dot blot, immuno-Northern blot, and electrochemical immunosensor method, may be the promising methods to be utilized.

## AUTHOR CONTRIBUTIONS

WZ and CT conceived and designed the work. WZ, LH, and ZLiu contributed to material preparation and performed data collection and analysis. WZ wrote the first draft of the manuscript. XR, LQ, LW, and WW wrote sections of the manuscript. All authors commented on previous versions of the manuscript. CT revised the manuscript. ZLi contributed to manuscript drafting, critical revision, and final approval of the version to be published. All authors read and approved the final manuscript.

## REFERENCES


Aik, W., Scotti, J. S., Choi, H., Gong, L., Demetriades, M., Schofield, C. J., et al. (2014). Structure of human RNA $N^6$-methyladenine demethylase ALKBH5 provides insights into its mechanisms of nucleic acid recognition and demethylation. *Nucleic Acids Res.* 42, 4741–4754. doi: 10.1093/nar/gku085

Alarcón, C. R., Goodarzi, H., Lee, H., Liu, X., Tavazoie, S., and Tavazoie, S. F. (2015). HNRNPA2B1 is a mediator of m(6)A-dependent nuclear RNA processing events. *Cell* 162, 1299–1308. doi: 10.1016/j.cell.2015.08.011

Arguello, A. E., DeLiberto, A. N., and Kleiner, R. E. (2017). RNA Chemical Proteomics Reveals the N(6)-Methyladenosine (m(6)A)-Regulated Protein-RNA Interactome. *J. Am. Chem. Soc.* 139, 17249–17252. doi: 10.1021/jacs.7b09213

Armas, L. A., and Recker, R. R. (2012). Pathophysiology of osteoporosis: new mechanistic insights. *Endocrinol. Metab. Clin. North Am.* 41, 475–486. doi: 10.1016/j.ecl.2012.04.006

Bedi, R. K., Huang, D., Eberle, S. A., Wiedmer, L., Śledź, P., and Caflisch, A. (2020). Small-molecule inhibitors of METTL3, the major human epitranscriptomic writer. *ChemMedChem* 15, 744–748. doi: 10.1002/cmdc.202000011

Blair, H. C., Larrouture, Q. C., Li, Y., Lin, H., Beer-Stoltz, D., Liu, L., et al. (2017). Osteoblast differentiation and bone matrix formation *in vivo* and *in vitro*. *Tissue Eng. Part B Rev.* 23, 268–280. doi: 10.1089/ten.TEB.2016.0454

Blum, A., and Adawi, M. (2019). Rheumatoid arthritis (RA) and cardiovascular disease. *Autoimmun. Rev.* 18, 679–690. doi: 10.1016/j.autrev.2019.05.005

Boyanov, M., Shinkov, A., Psachoulia, E., Intorcia, M., and Petkova, R. (2014). Increased bone mineral density (Bmd) in postmenopausal women with osteoporosis (Op) receiving two denosumab injections in routine clinical practice in bulgaria. *Value Health* 17:A389. doi: 10.1016/j.jval.2014.08.2662

Buker, S. M., Gurard-Levin, Z. A., Wheeler, B. D., Scholle, M. D., Case, A. W., Hirsch, J. L., et al. (2020). A mass spectrometric assay of METTL3/METTL14 methyltransferase activity. *SLAS Discov.* 25, 361–371. doi: 10.1177/2472555219878408

Cao, G., Li, H. B., Yin, Z., and Flavell, R. A. (2016). Recent advances in dynamic m6A RNA modification. *Open Biol.* 6:160003. doi: 10.1098/rsob.160003

Charles, J. F., and Aliprantis, A. O. (2014). Osteoclasts: more than 'bone eaters'. *Trends Mol. Med.* 20, 449–459. doi: 10.1016/j.molmed.2014.06.001

Chen, B., Ye, F., Yu, L., Jia, G., Huang, X., Zhang, X., et al. (2012). Development of cell-active N6-methyladenosine RNA demethylase FTO inhibitor. *J. Am. Chem. Soc.* 134, 17963–17971. doi: 10.1021/ja3064149

Chen, Q., Shou, P., Zheng, C., Jiang, M., Cao, G., Yang, Q., et al. (2016). Fate decision of mesenchymal stem cells: Adipocytes or osteoblasts? *Cell Death Differ.* 23, 1128–1139. doi: 10.1038/cdd.2015.168

Chen, S., Zhou, L., and Wang, Y. (2020). ALKBH5-mediated m(6)A demethylation of lncRNA PVT1 plays an oncogenic role in osteosarcoma. *Cancer Cell Int.* 20:34. doi: 10.1186/s12935-020-1105-6

Chen, W., Feng, P., Ding, H., and Lin, H. (2016). Identifying N (6)-methyladenosine sites in the Arabidopsis thaliana transcriptome. *Mol. Genet. Genomics* 291, 2225–2229. doi: 10.1007/s00438-016-1243-7

Chen, X. Y., Zhang, J., and Zhu, J. S. (2019). The role of m(6)A RNA methylation in human cancer. *Mol. Cancer* 18:103. doi: 10.1186/s12943-019-1033-z

Corre, I., Verrecchia, F., Crenn, V., Redini, F., and Trichet, V. (2020). The osteosarcoma microenvironment: a complex but targetable ecosystem. *Cells* 9:976. doi: 10.3390/cells9040976

Crooke, S. T., Witztum, J. L., Bennett, C. F., and Baker, B. F. (2018). RNA-Targeted Therapeutics. *Cell Metab.* 27, 714–739. doi: 10.1016/j.cmet.2018.03.004

Cui, J., Wang, W., Li, Z., Zhang, Z., Wu, B., and Zeng, L. (2011). Epigenetic changes in osteosarcoma. *Bull. Cancer* 98, E62–E68. doi: 10.1684/bdc.2011.1400

Dai, J., Ying, P., Shi, D., Hou, H., Sun, Y., Xu, Z., et al. (2018). FTO variant is not associated with osteoarthritis in the Chinese Han population: replication study for a genome-wide association study identified risk loci. *J. Orthop. Surg. Res.* 13:65. doi: 10.1186/s13018-018-0769-2

Derksen, V., Huizinga, T. W. J., and van der Woude, D. (2017). The role of autoantibodies in the pathophysiology of rheumatoid arthritis. *Semin. Immunopathol.* 39, 437–446. doi: 10.1007/s00281-017-0627-z

Doaei, S., Kalantari, N., Mohammadi, N. K., Izadi, P., Gholamalizadeh, M., Eini-Zinab, H., et al. (2019). Up-regulation of FTO gene expression was associated with increase in skeletal muscle mass in overweight male adolescents. *Arch. Med. Sci.* 15, 1133–1137. doi: 10.5114/aoms.2019.87239

Dominissini, D., Moshitch-Moshkovitz, S., Schwartz, S., Salmon-Divon, M., Ungar, L., Osenberg, S., et al. (2012). Topology of the human and mouse m6A RNA methylomes revealed by m6A-seq. *Nature* 485, 201–206. doi: 10.1038/nature11112

Doody, K. M., Bottini, N., and Firestein, G. S. (2017). Epigenetic alterations in rheumatoid arthritis fibroblast-like synoviocytes. *Epigenomics* 9, 479–492. doi: 10.2217/epi-2016-0151

Frontera, W. R., and Ochala, J. (2015). Skeletal muscle: a brief review of structure and function. *Calcif. Tissue Int.* 96, 183–195. doi: 10.1007/s00223-014-9915-y

Fu, Y., Jia, G., Pang, X., Wang, R. N., Wang, X., Li, C. J., et al. (2013). FTO-mediated formation of N6-hydroxymethyladenosine and N6-formyladenosine in mammalian RNA. *Nat. Commun.* 4:1798. doi: 10.1038/ncomms2822

Geuens, T., Bouhy, D., and Timmerman, V. (2016). The hnRNP family: insights into their role in health and disease. *Hum. Genet.* 135, 851–867. doi: 10.1007/s00439-016-1683-5

Gianferante, D. M., Mirabello, L., and Savage, S. A. (2017). Germline and somatic genetics of osteosarcoma - connecting aetiology, biology and therapy. *Nat. Rev. Endocrinol.* 13, 480–491. doi: 10.1038/nrendo.2017.16

Golovina, A. Y., Dzama, M. M., Petriukov, K. S., Zatsepin, T. S., Sergiev, P. V., Bogdanov, A. A., et al. (2014). Method for site-specific detection of m6A nucleoside presence in RNA based on high-resolution melting (HRM) analysis. *Nucleic Acids Res.* 42:e27. doi: 10.1093/nar/gkt1160

Guo, Y., Liu, H., Yang, T. L., Li, S. M., Li, S. K., Tian, Q., et al. (2011). The fat mass and obesity associated gene, FTO, is also associated with osteoporosis phenotypes. *PLoS One* 6:e27312. doi: 10.1371/journal.pone.0027312

Hadjidakis, D. J., and Androulakis, I. I. (2006). Bone remodeling. *Ann. N. Y. Acad. Sci.* 1092, 385–396. doi: 10.1196/annals.1365.035

Harvey, Z. H., Chen, Y., and Jarosz, D. F. (2018). Protein-based inheritance: epigenetics beyond the chromosome. *Mol. Cell* 69, 195–202. doi: 10.1016/j.molcel.2017.10.030

He, C., Liu, C., Wang, L., Sun, Y., Jiang, Y., and Hao, Y. (2019). Histone methyltransferase NSD2 regulates apoptosis and chemosensitivity in osteosarcoma. *Cell Death Dis.* 10:65. doi: 10.1038/s41419-019-1347-1

Hou, Z., Wang, Z., Tao, Y., Bai, J., Yu, B., Shen, J., et al. (2019). KLF2 regulates osteoblast differentiation by targeting of Runx2. *Lab. Invest.* 99, 271–280. doi: 10.1038/s41374-018-0149-x

Hu, H., Luan, L., Yang, K., and Li, S. C. (2018). Burden of rheumatoid arthritis from a societal perspective: a prevalence-based study on cost of this illness for patients in China. *Int. J. Rheum. Dis.* 21, 1572–1580. doi: 10.1111/1756-185x.13028

Huang, H., Weng, H., Sun, W., Qin, X., Shi, H., Wu, H., et al. (2018). Recognition of RNA N(6)-methyladenosine by IGF2BP proteins enhances mRNA stability and translation. *Nat. Cell Biol.* 20, 285–295. doi: 10.1038/s41556-018-0045-z

Huang, Y., Yan, J., Li, Q., Li, J., Gong, S., Zhou, H., et al. (2015). Meclofenamic acid selectively inhibits FTO demethylation of m6A over ALKBH5. *Nucleic Acids Res.* 43, 373–384. doi: 10.1093/nar/gku1276

Hunter, D. J., and Bierma-Zeinstra, S. (2019). Osteoarthritis. *Lancet* 393, 1745–1759. doi: 10.1016/s0140-6736(19)30417-9

Hunter, D. J., Schofield, D., and Callander, E. (2014). The individual and socioeconomic impact of osteoarthritis. *Nat. Rev. Rheumatol.* 10, 437–441. doi: 10.1038/nrrheum.2014.44

Imanishi, M., Tsuji, S., Suda, A., and Futaki, S. (2017). Detection of N(6)-methyladenosine based on the methyl-sensitivity of MazF RNA endonuclease. *Chem. Commun.* 53, 12930–12933. doi: 10.1039/c7cc07699a

Jiang, C., He, C., Wu, Z., Li, F., and Xiao, J. (2018). Histone methyltransferase SETD2 regulates osteosarcoma cell growth and chemosensitivity by suppressing Wnt/β-catenin signaling. *Biochem. Biophys. Res. Commun.* 502, 382–388. doi: 10.1016/j.bbrc.2018.05.176

Kannu, P., Bateman, J. F., Belluoccio, D., Fosang, A. J., and Savarirayan, R. (2009). Employing molecular genetics of chondrodysplasias to inform the study of osteoarthritis. *Arthritis Rheum.* 60, 325–334. doi: 10.1002/art.24251

Kasowitz, S. D., Ma, J., Anderson, S. J., Leu, N. A., Xu, Y., Gregory, B. D., et al. (2018). Nuclear m6A reader YTHDC1 regulates alternative polyadenylation and splicing during mouse oocyte development. *PLoS Genet.* 14:e1007412. doi: 10.1371/journal.pgen.1007412

Kierzek, E., and Kierzek, R. (2003). The thermodynamic stability of RNA duplexes and hairpins containing N6-alkyladenosines and 2-methylthio-N6-alkyladenosines. *Nucleic Acids Res.* 31, 4472–4480. doi: 10.1093/nar/gkg633

Kim, T., Ha, H. I., Kim, N., Yi, O., Lee, S. H., and Choi, Y. (2009). Adrm1 interacts with Atp6v0d2 and regulates osteoclast differentiation. *Biochem. Biophys. Res. Commun.* 390, 585–590. doi: 10.1016/j.bbrc.2009.10.010

Komori, T. (2019). Regulation of proliferation, differentiation and functions of osteoblasts by Runx2. *Int. J. Mol. Sci.* 20:1694. doi: 10.3390/ijms20071694

Kudou, K., Komatsu, T., Nogami, J., Maehara, K., Harada, A., Saeki, H., et al. (2017). The requirement of Mettl3-promoted MyoD mRNA maintenance in proliferative myoblasts for skeletal muscle differentiation. *Open Biol.* 7:170119. doi: 10.1098/rsob.170119

Lan, Q., Liu, P. Y., Haase, J., Bell, J. L., Hüttelmaier, S., and Liu, T. (2019). The critical role of RNA m(6)A methylation in cancer. *Cancer Res.* 79, 1285–1292. doi: 10.1158/0008-5472.Can-18-2965

Li, D., Cai, L., Meng, R., Feng, Z., and Xu, Q. (2020). METTL3 modulates osteoclast differentiation and function by controlling RNA stability and nuclear Export. *Int. J. Mol. Sci.* 21:1660. doi: 10.3390/ijms21051660

Li, M., Zhao, X., Wang, W., Shi, H., Pan, Q., Lu, Z., et al. (2018). Ythdf2-mediated m(6)A mRNA clearance modulates neural development in mice. *Genome Biol.* 19:69. doi: 10.1186/s13059-018-1436-y

Li, Q., Li, H., Zhao, X., Wang, B., Zhang, L., Zhang, C., et al. (2017). DNA methylation mediated downregulation of miR-449c controls osteosarcoma cell cycle progression by directly targeting oncogene c-Myc. *Int. J. Biol. Sci.* 13, 1038–1050. doi: 10.7150/ijbs.19476

Li, X., Lu, H., Fan, G., He, M., Sun, Y., Xu, K., et al. (2017). A novel interplay between HOTAIR and DNA methylation in osteosarcoma cells indicates a new therapeutic strategy. *J. Cancer Res. Clin. Oncol.* 143, 2189–2200. doi: 10.1007/s00432-017-2478-3

Li, X., Yang, J., Zhu, Y., Liu, Y., Shi, X., and Yang, G. (2016). Mouse maternal high-fat intake dynamically programmed mRNA m$^6$a modifications in adipose and skeletal muscle tissues in offspring. *Int. J. Mol. Sci.* 17:1336. doi: 10.3390/ijms17081336

Li, Y., Wu, K., Quan, W., Yu, L., Chen, S., Cheng, C., et al. (2019a). The dynamics of FTO binding and demethylation from the m(6)A motifs. *RNA Biol.* 16, 1179–1189. doi: 10.1080/15476286.2019.1621120

Li, Y., Yang, F., Gao, M., Gong, R., Jin, M., Liu, T., et al. (2019b). miR-149-3p regulates the switch between adipogenic and osteogenic differentiation of BMSCs by targeting FTO. *Mol. Ther. Nucleic Acids* 17, 590–600. doi: 10.1016/j.omtn.2019.06.023

Linder, B., Grozhik, A. V., Olarerin-George, A. O., Meydan, C., Mason, C. E., and Jaffrey, S. R. (2015). Single-nucleotide-resolution mapping of m6A and m6Am throughout the transcriptome. *Nat. Methods* 12, 767–772. doi: 10.1038/nmeth.3453

Ling, Z., Chen, L., and Zhao, J. (2020). m6A-dependent up-regulation of DRG1 by METTL3 and ELAVL1 promotes growth, migration, and colony formation in osteosarcoma. *Biosci. Rep.* 40:BSR20200282. doi: 10.1042/bsr20200282

Littlejohn, E. A., and Monrad, S. U. (2018). Early diagnosis and treatment of rheumatoid arthritis. *Prim. Care* 45, 237–255. doi: 10.1016/j.pop.2018.02.010

Liu, J., Yue, Y., Han, D., Wang, X., Fu, Y., Zhang, L., et al. (2014). A METTL3-METTL14 complex mediates mammalian nuclear RNA N6-adenosine methylation. *Nat. Chem. Biol.* 10, 93–95. doi: 10.1038/nchembio.1432

Liu, M., Li, B., Peng, W., Ma, Y., Huang, Y., Lan, X., et al. (2019). LncRNA-MEG3 promotes bovine myoblast differentiation by sponging miR-135. *J. Cell. Physiol.* 234, 18361–18370. doi: 10.1002/jcp.28469

Liu, N., Dai, Q., Zheng, G., He, C., Parisien, M., and Pan, T. (2015). N(6)-methyladenosine-dependent RNA structural switches regulate RNA-protein interactions. *Nature* 518, 560–564. doi: 10.1038/nature14234

Liu, N., Parisien, M., Dai, Q., Zheng, G., He, C., and Pan, T. (2013). Probing N6-methyladenosine RNA modification status at single nucleotide resolution in mRNA and long noncoding RNA. *RNA* 19, 1848–1856. doi: 10.1261/rna.041178.113

Liu, N., Zhou, K. I., Parisien, M., Dai, Q., Diatchenko, L., and Pan, T. (2017). N6-methyladenosine alters RNA structure to regulate binding of a low-complexity protein. *Nucleic Acids Res.* 45, 6051–6063. doi: 10.1093/nar/gkx141

Liu, Q., Li, M., Jiang, L., Jiang, R., and Fu, B. (2019). METTL3 promotes experimental osteoarthritis development by regulating inflammatory response and apoptosis in chondrocyte. *Biochem. Biophys. Res. Commun.* 516, 22–27. doi: 10.1016/j.bbrc.2019.05.168

Ma, F., Liu, X., Zhou, S., Li, W., Liu, C., Chadwick, M., et al. (2019). Long non-coding RNA FGF13-AS1 inhibits glycolysis and stemness properties of breast cancer cells through FGF13-AS1/IGF2BPs/Myc feedback loop. *Cancer Lett.* 450, 63–75. doi: 10.1016/j.canlet.2019.02.008

Machado, L., Esteves de Lima, J., Fabre, O., Proux, C., Legendre, R., Szegedi, A., et al. (2017). *In situ* fixation redefines quiescence and early activation of skeletal muscle stem cells. *Cell Rep.* 21, 1982–1993. doi: 10.1016/j.celrep.2017.10.080

Madan, I., and Grime, P. R. (2015). The management of musculoskeletal disorders in the workplace. *Best Pract. Res. Clin. Rheumatol.* 29, 345–355. doi: 10.1016/j.berh.2015.03.002

Mao, Y., Dong, L., Liu, X. M., Guo, J., Ma, H., Shen, B., et al. (2019). m(6)A in mRNA coding regions promotes translation via the RNA helicase-containing YTHDC2. *Nat. Commun.* 10:5332. doi: 10.1038/s41467-019-13317-9

Massey, J., Plant, D., Hyrich, K., Morgan, A. W., Wilson, A. G., Spiliopoulou, A., et al. (2018). Genome-wide association study of response to tumour necrosis factor inhibitor therapy in rheumatoid arthritis. *Pharmacogenomics J.* 18, 657–664. doi: 10.1038/s41397-018-0040-6

McIntyre, A. B. R., Gokhale, N. S., Cerchietti, L., Jaffrey, S. R., Horner, S. M., and Mason, C. E. (2020). Limits in the detection of m(6)A changes using MeRIP/m(6)A-seq. *Sci. Rep.* 10:6590. doi: 10.1038/s41598-020-63355-3

Meyer, K. D., Saletore, Y., Zumbo, P., Elemento, O., Mason, C. E., and Jaffrey, S. R. (2012). Comprehensive analysis of mRNA methylation reveals enrichment in 3', UTRs and near stop codons. *Cell* 149, 1635–1646. doi: 10.1016/j.cell.2012.05.003

Miao, W., Chen, J., Jia, L., Ma, J., and Song, D. (2019). The m6A methyltransferase METTL3 promotes osteosarcoma progression by regulating the m6A level of LEF1. *Biochem. Biophys. Res. Commun.* 516, 719–725. doi: 10.1016/j.bbrc.2019.06.128

Mishima, E., Jinno, D., Akiyama, Y., Itoh, K., Nankumo, S., Shima, H., et al. (2015). Immuno-northern blotting: detection of RNA modifications by using antibodies against modified nucleosides. *PLoS One* 10:e0143756. doi: 10.1371/journal.pone.0143756

Miyata, K., Miyata, T., Nakabayashi, K., Okamura, K., Naito, M., Kawai, T., et al. (2015). DNA methylation analysis of human myoblasts during *in vitro* myogenic differentiation: de novo methylation of promoters of muscle-related genes and its involvement in transcriptional down-regulation. *Hum. Mol. Genet.* 24, 410–423. doi: 10.1093/hmg/ddu457

Mo, X. B., Zhang, Y. H., and Lei, S. F. (2018a). Genome-wide identification of m(6)A-associated SNPs as potential functional variants for bone mineral density. *Osteoporos Int.* 29, 2029–2039. doi: 10.1007/s00198-018-4573-y

Mo, X. B., Zhang, Y. H., and Lei, S. F. (2018b). Genome-Wide Identification of N(6)-Methyladenosine (m(6)A) SNPs associated with rheumatoid arthritis. *Front. Genet.* 9:299. doi: 10.3389/fgene.2018.00299

Molinie, B., Wang, J., Lim, K. S., Hillebrand, R., Lu, Z. X., Van Wittenberghe, N., et al. (2016). m(6)A-LAIC-seq reveals the census and complexity of the m(6)A epitranscriptome. *Nat. Methods* 13, 692–698. doi: 10.1038/nmeth.3898

Nagarajan, A., Janostiak, R., and Wajapeyee, N. (2019). Dot Blot Analysis for Measuring Global N(6)-Methyladenosine Modification of RNA. *Methods Mol. Biol.* 1870, 263–271. doi: 10.1007/978-1-4939-8808-2_20

Nebbioso, A., Tambaro, F. P., Dell'Aversana, C., and Altucci, L. (2018). Cancer epigenetics: moving forward. *PLoS Genet.* 14:e1007362. doi: 10.1371/journal.pgen.1007362

Ni, W., Yao, S., Zhou, Y., Liu, Y., Huang, P., Zhou, A., et al. (2019). Long noncoding RNA GAS5 inhibits progression of colorectal cancer by interacting with and triggering YAP phosphorylation and degradation and is negatively regulated by the m(6)A reader YTHDF3. *Mol. Cancer* 18:143. doi: 10.1186/s12943-019-1079-y

Nishizawa, Y., Konno, M., Asai, A., Koseki, J., Kawamoto, K., Miyoshi, N., et al. (2018). Oncogene c-Myc promotes epitranscriptome m(6)A reader YTHDF1 expression in colorectal cancer. *Oncotarget* 9, 7476–7486. doi: 10.18632/oncotarget.23554

Ovcharenko, A., and Rentmeister, A. (2018). Emerging approaches for detection of methylation sites in RNA. *Open Biol.* 8:180121. doi: 10.1098/rsob.180121

Panoutsopoulou, K., Metrustry, S., Doherty, S. A., Laslett, L. L., Maciewicz, R. A., Hart, D. J., et al. (2014). The effect of FTO variation on increased osteoarthritis risk is mediated through body mass index: a Mendelian randomisation study. *Ann. Rheum. Dis.* 73, 2082–2086. doi: 10.1136/annrheumdis-2013-203772

Peng, S., Xiao, W., Ju, D., Sun, B., Hou, N., Liu, Q., et al. (2019). Identification of entacapone as a chemical inhibitor of FTO mediating metabolic regulation through FOXO1. *Sci. Transl. Med.* 11:eaau7116. doi: 10.1126/scitranslmed.aau7116

Ping, X. L., Sun, B. F., Wang, L., Xiao, W., Yang, X., Wang, W. J., et al. (2014). Mammalian WTAP is a regulatory subunit of the RNA N6-methyladenosine methyltransferase. *Cell Res.* 24, 177–189. doi: 10.1038/cr.2014.3

Prachayasittikul, V., Prathipati, P., Pratiwi, R., Phanus-Umporn, C., Malik, A. A., Schaduangrat, N., et al. (2017). Exploring the epigenetic drug discovery landscape. *Expert Opin. Drug Discov.* 12, 345–362. doi: 10.1080/17460441.2017.1295954

Qin, L., Min, S., Shu, L., Pan, H., Zhong, J., Guo, J., et al. (2020). Genetic analysis of N6-methyladenosine modification genes in Parkinson's disease. *Neurobiol. Aging.* 93, 143.e9–143.e13. doi: 10.1016/j.neurobiolaging.2020.03.018

Reichel, M., Köster, T., and Staiger, D. (2019). Marking RNA: m6A writers, readers, and functions in Arabidopsis. *J. Mol. Cell Biol.* 11, 899–910. doi: 10.1093/jmcb/mjz085

Ren, X., He, J., Qi, L., Li, S., Zhang, C., Duan, Z., et al. (2020). Prognostic and clinicopathologic significance of long non-coding RNA opa-interacting protein 5-antisense RNA 1 in multiple human cancers. *Artif. Cells Nanomed. Biotechnol.* 48, 353–361. doi: 10.1080/21691401.2019.1709854

Roundtree, I. A., Luo, G. Z., Zhang, Z., Wang, X., Zhou, T., Cui, Y., et al. (2017). YTHDC1 mediates nuclear export of N(6)-methyladenosine methylated mRNAs. *eLife* 6:e31311. doi: 10.7554/eLife.31311

Sampath, S. C., Sampath, S. C., and Millay, D. P. (2018). Myoblast fusion confusion: the resolution begins. *Skelet. Muscle* 8:3. doi: 10.1186/s13395-017-0149-3

Scott, D. L., Wolfe, F., and Huizinga, T. W. (2010). Rheumatoid arthritis. *Lancet* 376, 1094–1108. doi: 10.1016/s0140-6736(10)60826-4

Shen, G. S., Zhou, H. B., Zhang, H., Chen, B., Liu, Z. P., Yuan, Y., et al. (2018). The GDF11-FTO-PPARγ axis controls the shift of osteoporotic MSC fate to adipocyte and inhibits bone formation during osteoporosis. *Biochim. Biophys. Acta Mol. Basis Dis.* 1864, 3644–3654. doi: 10.1016/j.bbadis.2018.09.015

Shen, J., Abu-Amer, Y., O'Keefe, R. J., and McAlinden, A. (2017). Inflammation and epigenetic regulation in osteoarthritis. *Connect Tissue Res.* 58, 49–63. doi: 10.1080/03008207.2016.1208655

Sorci, M., Ianniello, Z., Cruciani, S., Larivera, S., Ginistrelli, L. C., Capuano, E., et al. (2018). METTL3 regulates WTAP protein homeostasis. *Cell Death Dis.* 9:796. doi: 10.1038/s41419-018-0843-z

Tian, C., Huang, Y., Li, Q., Feng, Z., and Xu, Q. (2019). Mettl3 regulates osteogenic differentiation and alternative splicing of vegfa in bone marrow mesenchymal stem cells. *Int. J. Mol. Sci.* 20:551. doi: 10.3390/ijms20030551

Tran, B., Nguyen, N. D., Center, J. R., Eisman, J. A., and Nguyen, T. V. (2014). Association between fat-mass-and-obesity-associated (FTO) gene and hip fracture susceptibility. *Clin. Endocrinol.* 81, 210–217. doi: 10.1111/cen.12335

Tresguerres, F. G. F., Torres, J., López-Quiles, J., Hernández, G., Vega, J. A., and Tresguerres, I. F. (2020). The osteocyte: a multifunctional cell within the bone. *Ann. Anat.* 227:151422. doi: 10.1016/j.aanat.2019.151422

Tu, C., He, J., Chen, R., and Li, Z. (2019). The emerging role of exosomal non-coding RNAs in musculoskeletal diseases. *Curr. Pharm. Des.* 25, 4523–4535. doi: 10.2174/1381612825666191113104946

Tu, C., He, J., Qi, L., Ren, X., Zhang, C., Duan, Z., et al. (2020). Emerging landscape of circular RNAs as biomarkers and pivotal regulators in osteosarcoma. *J. Cell. Physiol.* doi: 10.1002/jcp.29754 [Epub ahead of print].

van Wijnen, A. J., and Westendorf, J. J. (2019). Epigenetics as a new frontier in orthopedic regenerative medicine and oncology. *J. Orthop. Res.* 37, 1465–1474. doi: 10.1002/jor.24305

Wang, J., Yan, S., Lu, H., Wang, S., and Xu, D. (2019). METTL3 attenuates LPS-induced inflammatory response in macrophages via NF-κB signaling pathway. *Mediators Inflamm.* 2019:3120391. doi: 10.1155/2019/3120391

Wang, R., Han, Z., Liu, B., Zhou, B., Wang, N., Jiang, Q., et al. (2018). Identification of natural compound radicicol as a Potent FTO inhibitor. *Mol. Pharm.* 15, 4092–4098. doi: 10.1021/acs.molpharmaceut.8b00522

Wang, T., Kong, S., Tao, M., and Ju, S. (2020). The potential role of RNA N6-methyladenosine in Cancer progression. *Mol. Cancer* 19:88. doi: 10.1186/s12943-020-01204-7

Wang, X., Feng, J., Xue, Y., Guan, Z., Zhang, D., Liu, Z., et al. (2016). Structural basis of N(6)-adenosine methylation by the METTL3-METTL14 complex. *Nature* 534, 575–578. doi: 10.1038/nature18298

Wang, X., Huang, N., Yang, M., Wei, D., Tai, H., Han, X., et al. (2017). FTO is required for myogenesis by positively regulating mTOR-PGC-1α pathway-mediated mitochondria biogenesis. *Cell Death Dis.* 8:e2702. doi: 10.1038/cddis.2017.122

Wang, X., Zhao, B. S., Roundtree, I. A., Lu, Z., Han, D., Ma, H., et al. (2015). N(6)-methyladenosine modulates messenger RNA translation efficiency. *Cell* 161, 1388–1399. doi: 10.1016/j.cell.2015.05.014

Wang, Y., Zeng, L., Liang, C., Zan, R., Ji, W., Zhang, Z., et al. (2019). Integrated analysis of transcriptome-wide m(6)A methylome of osteosarcoma stem cells enriched by chemotherapy. *Epigenomics* 11, 1693–1715. doi: 10.2217/epi-2019-0262

Weivoda, M. M., Ruan, M., Pederson, L., Hachfeld, C., Davey, R. A., Zajac, J. D., et al. (2016). Osteoclast TGF-β Receptor Signaling Induces Wnt1 Secretion and Couples Bone Resorption to Bone Formation. *J. Bone Miner. Res.* 31, 76–85. doi: 10.1002/jbmr.2586

Wu, W., Feng, J., Jiang, D., Zhou, X., Jiang, Q., Cai, M., et al. (2017). AMPK regulates lipid accumulation in skeletal muscle cells through FTO-dependent demethylation of N(6)-methyladenosine. *Sci. Rep.* 7:41606. doi: 10.1038/srep41606

Wu, Y., Xie, L., Wang, M., Xiong, Q., Guo, Y., Liang, Y., et al. (2018). Mettl3-mediated m(6)A RNA methylation regulates the fate of bone marrow mesenchymal stem cells and osteoporosis. *Nat. Commun.* 9:4772. doi: 10.1038/s41467-018-06898-4

Xia, B., Di, C., Zhang, J., Hu, S., Jin, H., and Tong, P. (2014). Osteoarthritis pathogenesis: a review of molecular mechanisms. *Calcif. Tissue Int.* 95, 495–505. doi: 10.1007/s00223-014-9917-9

Xu, C., Wang, X., Liu, K., Roundtree, I. A., Tempel, W., Li, Y., et al. (2014). Structural basis for selective binding of m6A RNA by the YTHDC1 YTH domain. *Nat. Chem. Biol.* 10, 927–929. doi: 10.1038/nchembio.1654

Xu, S., Gong, Y., Yin, Y., Xing, H., and Zhang, N. (2020). The multiple function of long noncoding RNAs in osteosarcoma progression, drug resistance and prognosis. *Biomed. Pharmacother.* 127:110141. doi: 10.1016/j.biopha.2020.110141

Yan, G., Yuan, Y., He, M., Gong, R., Lei, H., Zhou, H., et al. (2020). m(6)A methylation of precursor-miR-320/RUNX2 controls osteogenic potential of bone marrow-derived mesenchymal stem cells. *Mol. Ther. Nucleic Acids* 19, 421–436. doi: 10.1016/j.omtn.2019.12.001

Yin, H., Wang, H., Jiang, W., Zhou, Y., and Ai, S. (2017). Electrochemical immunosensor for N6-methyladenosine detection in human cell lines based on biotin-streptavidin system and silver-SiO(2) signal amplification. *Biosens. Bioelectron.* 90, 494–500. doi: 10.1016/j.bios.2016.10.066

Yu, J., Shen, L., Liu, Y., Ming, H., Zhu, X., Chu, M., et al. (2020). The m6A methyltransferase METTL3 cooperates with demethylase ALKBH5 to regulate osteogenic differentiation through NF-κB signaling. *Mol. Cell. Biochem.* 463, 203–210. doi: 10.1007/s11010-019-03641-5

Zeggini, E., Panoutsopoulou, K., Southam, L., Rayner, N. W., Day-Williams, A. G., Lopes, M. C., et al. (2012). Identification of new susceptibility loci for osteoarthritis (arcOGEN): a genome-wide association study. *Lancet* 380, 815–823. doi: 10.1016/s0140-6736(12)60681-3

Zhang, H., Shi, X., Huang, T., Zhao, X., Chen, W., Gu, N., et al. (2020). Dynamic landscape and evolution of m6A methylation in human. *Nucleic Acids Res.* 19:88. doi: 10.1093/nar/gkaa347

Zhang, Q., Riddle, R. C., Yang, Q., Rosen, C. R., Guttridge, D. C., Dirckx, N., et al. (2019). The RNA demethylase FTO is required for maintenance of bone mass and functions to protect osteoblasts from genotoxic damage. *Proc. Natl. Acad. Sci. U.S.A.* 116, 17980–17989. doi: 10.1073/pnas.1905489116

Zhang, Y., Gu, X., Li, D., Cai, L., and Xu, Q. (2019). METTL3 regulates osteoblast differentiation and inflammatory response via Smad Signaling and MAPK Signaling. *Int. J. Mol. Sci.* 21:199. doi: 10.3390/ijms21010199

Zhou, K. I., Shi, H., Lyu, R., Wylder, A. C., Matuszek, Ż., Pan, J. N., et al. (2019). Regulation of Co-transcriptional Pre-mRNA Splicing by m(6)A through the Low-Complexity Protein hnRNPG. *Mol. Cell* 76, 70–81.e9. doi: 10.1016/j.molcel.2019.07.005

Zhou, L., Yang, C., Zhang, N., Zhang, X., Zhao, T., and Yu, J. (2020). Silencing METTL3 inhibits the proliferation and invasion of osteosarcoma by regulating ATAD2. *Biomed. Pharmacother.* 125:109964. doi: 10.1016/j.biopha.2020.109964

Zhu, W., Wang, J. Z., Xu, Z., Cao, M., Hu, Q., Pan, C., et al. (2019). Detection of N6-methyladenosine modification residues (Review). *Int. J. Mol. Med.* 43, 2267–2278. doi: 10.3892/ijmm.2019.4169

Zhu, Z. M., Huo, F. C., and Pei, D. S. (2020). Function and evolution of RNA N6-methyladenosine modification. *Int. J. Biol. Sci.* 16, 1929–1940. doi: 10.7150/ijbs.45231

Zong, X., Zhao, J., Wang, H., Lu, Z., Wang, F., Du, H., et al. (2019). Mettl3 deficiency sustains long-chain fatty acid absorption through suppressing Traf6-dependent inflammation response. *J. Immunol.* 202, 567–578. doi: 10.4049/jimmunol.1801151

Zou, S., Toh, J. D., Wong, K. H., Gao, Y. G., Hong, W., and Woon, E. C. (2016). N(6)-Methyladenosine: a conformational marker that regulates the substrate specificity of human demethylases FTO and ALKBH5. *Sci. Rep.* 6:25677. doi: 10.1038/srep25677

6

# BMSC-Derived Exosomal miR-29a Promotes Angiogenesis and Osteogenesis

*Guo-dong Lu[1†], Peng Cheng[2†], Ting Liu[3*] and Zhong Wang[1*]*

*[1] Department of Cardiology, The First Affiliated Hospital of Shihezi University Medical College, Shihezi, China, [2] Division of Geriatric Endocrinology, The First Affiliated Hospital, Nanjing Medical University, Nanjing, China, [3] Department of Endocrinology, Changsha Central Hospital, Changsha, China*

***Correspondence:**
*Ting Liu*
*2649547299@qq.com*
*Zhong Wang*
*wangzhong2014@163.com*

*† These authors have contributed equally to this work*

Angiogenesis and osteogenesis are tightly coupled during bone modeling and remodeling processes. Here we reported that bone marrow mesenchymal stem cell (BMSC)-derived exosomal miR-29a promotes angiogenesis and osteogenesis *in vitro* and *in vivo*. BMSC-derived exosomes (BMSCs-Exos) can be taken up by human umbilical vein endothelial cells (HUVECs) and promote the proliferation, migration, and tube formation of HUVECs. MiRNA-29a level was high in BMSCs-Exos and can be transported into HUVECs to regulate angiogenesis. VASH1 was identified as a direct target of miR-29a, mediating the effects of BMSC-derived exosomal miR-29a on angiogenesis. More interestingly, miR29a-loaded exosomes from engineered BMSCs (miR-29a-loaded BMSCs-Exos) showed a robust ability of promoting angiogenesis and osteogenesis *in vivo*. Taken together, these findings suggest that BMSC-derived exosomal miR-29a regulates angiogenesis and osteogenesis, and miR-29a-loaded BMSCs-Exos may serve as a potential therapeutic target for osteoporosis.

**Keywords: BMSCs-exosomes, miRNA-29a, angiogenesis, osteogenesis, osteoporosis**

## INTRODUCTION

Bone undergoes sustained modeling and remodeling processes throughout life to ensure the integrity and structure of the skeleton (Wu et al., 2010). Angiogenesis is tightly coupled with bone formation and regeneration for proper bone homeostasis (Hui et al., 2014; Kusumbe et al., 2014; Yang et al., 2017). Recently, extracellular vesicles (EVs), such as exosomes and microvesicles, have been attracting a strong research interest for use as natural drug delivery systems (Chen et al., 2018; Tang and Wang, 2020). Mesenchymal stem cell (MSC)-derived exosomes have been reported to be involved in multiple physiology and pathology activities including osteogenesis, bone regeneration, osteoarthritis, cardiomyoblast hypoxia–reperfusion, cognitive impairment, inflammation, stroke, sepsis, and tumorigenesis (Zheng et al., 2018; Huang et al., 2020; Jin et al., 2020; Nakano et al., 2020; Tan et al., 2020; Venkat et al., 2020; Xu et al., 2020; Zou et al., 2020). Jia et al. (2020) report that exosomes secreted by young MSCs promote osteogenesis and bone formation in older rats. Liu et al. (2020) find that MSC-derived exosomes promote bone fracture healing by transferring miR-126. Zuo et al. (2019) report that bone marrow MSC (BMSC)-derived exosomes alleviate radiation-induced bone loss by activating Wnt/β-catenin signaling. However, the effects of BMSC-derived exosomes (BMSCs-Exos), especially the key microRNAs within the BMSCs-Exos, on angiogenesis and osteogenesis are not well studied.

MicroRNAs are a class of small non-coding RNAs of 19–22 nucleotides and involved in almost all cellular processes as a negative mediator of mRNA translational efficiency (Li et al., 2015). MicroRNAs post-transcriptionally decrease targeted gene expression through binding the sequence in the 3′ untranslated region (UTR) of the target mRNAs (Li et al., 2015). Recently, miRNAs were reported to be secreted and delivered into distal or local tissue and cells through circulation within exosomes (Hu et al., 2018; Vilaca-Faria et al., 2019; Song et al., 2020; Sun et al., 2020). Exosomes are EVs, with sizes arranged from 30 to 150 nm, released from multiple cell types. The functions of containing and transporting of bioactive protein, mRNAs, and miRNAs to other cells make exosomes a research hotspot of intracellular communications (Li and Tang, 2020). Recent studies report that exosomes from MSCs (Gong et al., 2017), smooth muscle cells (Zheng et al., 2017), tumor cells (Zhang et al., 2016), leukemia cells, and macrophages (Li M. et al., 2019) mediate angiogenesis. MSC-derived exosomes containing miR-30b, miR-30c, and miR-424 promote angiogenesis through targeting DLL4 (Ghosh et al., 2010; Bridge et al., 2012; Gong et al., 2017). Exosomal miR-301 derived from MSCs inhibits myocardial autophagy to protect myocardial infarction (Li Y. et al., 2019). MiR-155 within exosomes from smooth muscle cells induces endothelial injury and promotes atherosclerosis (Zheng et al., 2017). In gastric carcinoma, cell-derived microvesicles delivered miR-29a/c to suppress angiogenesis (Zhang et al., 2016). Li M. et al. (2019) report that macrophage-derived exosomes suppress the inflammation and promote the proliferation and migration of endothelial cells during wound healing. Li's group reported that human induced pluripotent stem cell-derived exosomes promote bone defect repair through enhancing angiogenesis and osteogenesis in ovariectomy-induced osteoporotic rat model (Qi et al., 2016). However, the exact molecular mechanisms responsible for the effects of BMSCs-Exos on angiogenesis and osteogenesis remain elusive.

In this study, we reported that BMSCs-Exos can be transported into endothelial cells and promote the proliferation, migration, and tube formation of endothelial cells. MiRNA-29a level was high in BMSCs-Exos and promoted angiogenesis. VASH1 was identified as a direct target of miR-29a, mediating the effects of BMSC-derived exosomal miR-29a on angiogenesis. Moreover, miR-29a-loaded BMSCs-Exos showed a strong ability to promote angiogenesis and osteogenesis *in vivo*.

## MATERIALS AND METHODS

### Animals and Treatment

Three-month-old male C57BL/6J mice were injected with miR-29a-loaded BMSCs-Exo, BMSCs-Exo, or phosphate-buffered saline (PBS) control *via* the tail vein (100 μg exosomes dissolved with 100 μl PBS or an equal volume of PBS) twice per week for 2 months. Then, the femurs were collected for analysis of angiogenesis and osteogenesis by immunostaining and micro-CT analysis. Animal care and experimental protocol were approved by the Animal Care and Use Committees of the Laboratory Animal Research Center at Shihezi University First Affiliated Hospital. The animals were maintained in a pathogen-free facility of the Laboratory Animal Research Center at Shihezi University First Affiliated Hospital, with free access to food and water prior to the initiation of experiments.

### BMSC-Derived Exosome Isolation and Characterization

We isolated BMSC exosomes based on the protocols described previously (Ying et al., 2017). Briefly, we dissected femora from C57BL/6J mice. Then, we crushed and digested the femurs with collagenase II at 37°C for 15 min to make a single-cell suspension. The BMSCs were FACS-sorted using (Sca-$1^+CD29^+CD45^-CD11b^-$) strategy and cultured in exosome-free medium for 72 h. We collected the medium of BMSCs and centrifuged such to remove dead cells or debris. The collected medium was subjected to ultracentrifugation at 100,000 *g* for 4-6 h at 4°C after filtration with a 0.22-μm filter. The exosome-containing pellet was washed and resuspended with PBS. We characterized the exosomes by detecting the expression of exosome-specific markers syntenin 1 and TSG101 by western blot, concentration by NanoSight analysis (Particle Metrix), and size distribution and morphology by transmission electron microscopy imaging (Hitachi H7500 TEM). For the *in vitro* experiments, exosomes (2 μg of exosomes per $1 \times 10^5$ recipient cells) were added to the culture medium for 12 h, and then tube formation was measured.

### Tube Formation Assay

Fifty microliters of Matrigel (BD Biosciences) was plated in 96-well culture plates and then incubated at 37°C. Human umbilical vein endothelial cells (HUVECs) were cultured on Matrigel with different exosomes or other treatments. After incubation at 37°C for 4 h, tube formation was visualized under microscopy and analyzed by measuring the cumulative tube lengths.

### MTS Assay

The tetrazolium-dye-based MTS assay was used to evaluate cell growth rate as described previously (Zheng et al., 2017). In brief, $1 \times 10^4$ cells per well were seeded in triplicate into 96-well plates for 24 h. Then, the cells were treated with different treatments according to design. After treatment, the cells were washed twice with PBS and treated with 2 mg/ml Hank's buffer and incubated for 1 h. Then, the dark blue crystal should be seen under light microscopy. The crystals were dissolved in dimethyl sulfoxide, and the absorbance was measured with a Thermo Fluoroscan Ascent spectrometer at 570 nm.

### Wound-Healing Assay

A total of $5 \times 10^5$ HUVECs were seeded in six-well plates. Scratch wounds were created using 100-ml sterile pipette tips when the cells grew to 95% confluence. The plates were washed twice with PBS to remove the suspended cells. Images were captured in three defined fields at 0 and 48 h, respectively.

### Immunoblotting

We performed western blotting analysis as previously described (Li et al., 2016b; Li C. et al., 2017). Exosome lysates were separated by SDS-PAGE blotted on polyvinylidene fluoride membranes (Millipore). The membranes were incubated with primary antibodies against syntenin 1(PA5-28826), TSG101 (ab125011), and VASH1 (EPR17420). All the primary antibodies were incubated at 4°C overnight, and specific proteins were visualized by enhanced chemiluminescence (ECL Kit; Amersham Biosciences).

## qRT-PCR Analysis

The total RNAs were extracted by Trizol (Thermo Fisher Scientific). Qiagen miRNeasy Mini Kit was used to extract exosomal miRNAs. cDNA was prepared using the SuperScript First-Strand Synthesis System (Invitrogen) for qRT-PCR analysis by SYBR GreenMaster Mix (Qiagen). 2-CT method was used to calculate the relative expression after normalization with GAPDH and U6 (Li et al., 2016a).

## Luciferase Activity Assay

Luciferase activity assays were conducted as reported previously (Yang et al., 2017). We constructed the wild-type and mutated VASH1 3′ UTR luciferase reporter plasmids with the potential binding site of miR-29a-3p and co-transfected them with miR-29a-3p mimics or miR-NC into HEK293 cells, respectively. Renilla luciferase reporter plasmids were used as internal control. The luciferase activities were measured by a Dual-Glo Luciferase Assay Kit (Promega).

## Quantification and Statistical Analysis

All data are presented as mean ± SEM. For comparisons between two groups, a two-tailed Student's *t*-test was used. Comparisons between multiple groups were made using ANOVA, followed by Bonferroni post-test. All experiments were repeated at least three times, and representative experiments are shown. $p < 0.05$ was considered statistically significant.

# RESULTS

## BMSC-Derived Exosomes Promoted Angiogenesis

To obtain BMSCs-Exos, BMSCs were isolated from C57BL/6J mice by fluorescence-activated sorting ($Sca\text{-}1^{+}CD29^{+}CD45^{-}CD11b^{-}$) and then cultured with exosome-free medium for 72 h. The BMSCs-Exos were isolated by ultracentrifugation after the removal of dead cells and debris from the conditional medium. The exosomes were round-shaped vesicles with a bilayer membrane structure, as observed by electron microscopy (**Figure 1A**). The concentration of exosomes was around 1 to 2 × $10^{10}$ particles/ml, and the diameter predominantly ranged from 30 to 150 nm (**Figure 1B**). The exosome-specific protein markers (syntenin 1 and TSG 101) were highly expressed in these exosomes as evidenced by Western blotting analysis (**Figure 1C**).

Next, we tested the effects of BMSCs-Exos on angiogenesis. BMSCs-Exos and PBS control were added to the culture medium of HUVECs, respectively, for tube-like structure formation assay. The cumulative tube length was significantly longer in HUVECs treated with BMSCs-Exos compared to those treated with PBS control (**Figures 1D,E**). Furthermore, the proliferation and migration of BMSCs-Exos-treated HUVECs were dramatically increased compared to the PBS-treated control (**Figures 1F,G**). These data indicated that BMSCs-Exos promoted the proliferation and migration of endothelial cells and thus enhanced angiogenesis.

## BMSC-Derived Exosomal miR-29a Transported Into Endothelial Cells

Exosomes contain and transport bioactive proteins, mRNAs, and microRNAs into distal and nearby cells. Next, we measured the angiogenesis-related miRNA (miR-19b, miR-21, miR-27, miR-29a, miR-125b, miR-126b, and miR-214) expression in BMSCs-Exos. A qPCR analysis revealed that miR-29a-3p, but not miR-29a-5p, was the most highly expressed microRNA among the detected miRNAs within BMSCs-Exos (**Figure 2A**). Thus, we chose miR-29a-3p to study. Our previous study found that exosomal miR-29a could be taken up by adipocytes, myocytes, and hepatocytes and then regulate insulin resistance (Liu T. et al., 2019). In this study, we tested whether exosomal miR-29a could be transferred into endothelial cells to affect angiogenesis. First, we tested whether BMSCs-Exos can be transferred into endothelial cells. The BMSCs-Exos were labeled with the fluorescent dye PKH26 and then added into the culture medium of HUVECs. The red fluorescence staining showed that HUVECs exhibited an efficient uptake of BMSCs-Exos (**Figure 2B**). Furthermore, after culturing with BMSCs-Exos, the miR-29a level in these recipient HUVECs was significantly higher than those cultured with PBS control (**Figure 2C**).

## BMSCs-Exosomal miR-29a Promoted Angiogenesis

Next, we tested whether BMSCs-Exosomal miR-29a could regulate angiogenesis. First, miR-29a mimic was transfected into HUVECs to measure the effects of miR-29a on angiogenesis. MiR-29a level was dramatically increased in HUVECs transfected with miR-29a mimic compared to the control mimic group, indicating successful and effective transfection (**Figure 3A**). A tube-like structure formation assay showed that the cumulative tube length was significantly longer in miR-29a mimic-transfected HUVECs, in contrast to the control group (**Figures 3B,C**). As expected, HUVECs with the overexpression of miR-29a showed an enhanced ability of proliferation and migration in contrast to the control group (**Figures 3D,E**). Furthermore, BMSCs-Exos with miR-29a deficiency obtained from BMSCs with transfection of antagomir-29a were added into the culture medium of HUVECs. Consistently, BMSCs-Exos dramatically promoted tube-like structure formation, proliferation, and migration of HUVECs compared to those treated with the PBS control. However, the effects of BMSCs-Exos on angiogenesis were blunted with miR-29a deficiency in BMSCs-Exos (**Figures 3F–J**). These data indicated that miR-29a within exosomes played a key role in promoting angiogenesis by BMSCs-Exos.

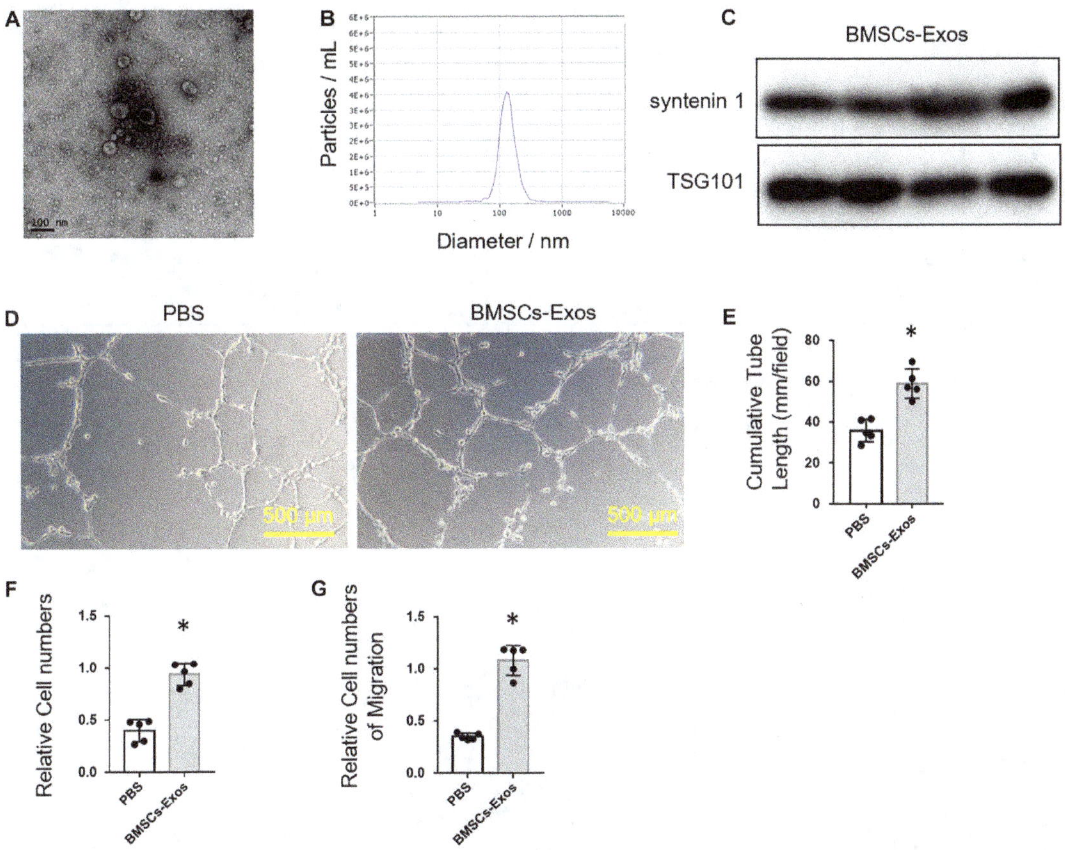


**FIGURE 1** | Bone marrow mesenchymal stem cell (BMSC)-derived exosomes promoted angiogenesis. **(A)** Representative picture of BMSC-derived exosomes collected by ultracentrifugation. Scale bar: 100 nm. **(B)** Size distribution profile of BMSC-derived exosomes. **(C)** Western blot analysis of exosome-specific markers, syntenin 1 and TSG101. Representative images of tube formation **(D)** and quantitative data of cumulative tube length **(E)** of human umbilical vein endothelial cell (HUVEC) cultured with phosphate-buffered saline control or BMSCs-Exos. Scale bars, 500 μm. **(F)** MTS assay was used to detect the proliferation of HUVECs. **(G)** Wound-healing assay was used to detect the migration of HUVECs; $N = 5$. Data are presented as mean ± SEM. $^*P < 0.05$ as determined by Student's *t*-test.

## BMSCs-Exosomal miR-29a Regulated Angiogenesis *via* VASH1

miRNAs bind to the amino acid coding sequence or 3′ UTRs of target genes to regulate gene expression. Target Scan was used to identify the targets of miR-29a. Among the predicted genes, we chose VASH1 for further study (**Figure 4A** and **Supplementary Table S1**). The reason that we chose VASH1 to study is that, among these target genes of miR-29a, VASH1 is a robust negative regulator of angiogenesis. Thus, we speculate that miR-29a might promote angiogenesis through post-transcriptional inhibition of VASH1. We have also listed the target genes that associated with osteogenesis and angiogenesis in **Supplementary Table S1**. The mRNA and protein levels of VASH1 were measured in HUVECs treated with miR-29a mimic or control by qPCR and western blotting analysis. miR-29a mimics downregulated VASH1 protein level but not mRNA level, indicating the post-transcriptional regulation of miR-29a on VASH1 gene (**Figures 4B,C**). A sequence analysis revealed that the binding site of miR-29a in the 3′UTR of VASH1 was from position 2244 to 2250 (**Figure 4A**). The direct binding of miR-29a on the seed region of VASH1 3′UTR was confirmed by luciferase reporter assay. Luciferase reporter constructs with wild-type 3′UTR of VASH1 (pGL3-VASH1$^{WT-3'UTR}$) was generated and transfected into HEK293 cells with co-transfection of miR-29a mimics. The analysis of luciferase enzyme activity showed that miR-29a mimics significantly suppressed the luciferase activity of VASH1 3′UTR reporter gene. However, the mutation of two nucleotides in the putative binding sites in 3′UTR of VASH1 completely abolished these effects (**Figure 4D**). Furthermore, whether VASH1 mediates the effects of miR-29a on angiogenesis was tested. HUVECs transfected with miR-29a mimics were replenished with rVASH1, and a tube-like structure formation assay was conducted. Interestingly, the effect of miR-29a mimics on tube formation was blunted with the replenishment of rVASH1 (**Figures 4E,F**). These data indicated that VASH1, as a direct target, mediated the regulation of miR-29a on angiogenesis.

## BMSCs-miR-29a Exosomes Promoted Angiogenesis and Osteogenesis *in vivo*

These above *in vitro* lead us to test the effects of BMSCs-Exos and miR-29a-loaded BMSCs-Exos on angiogenesis and

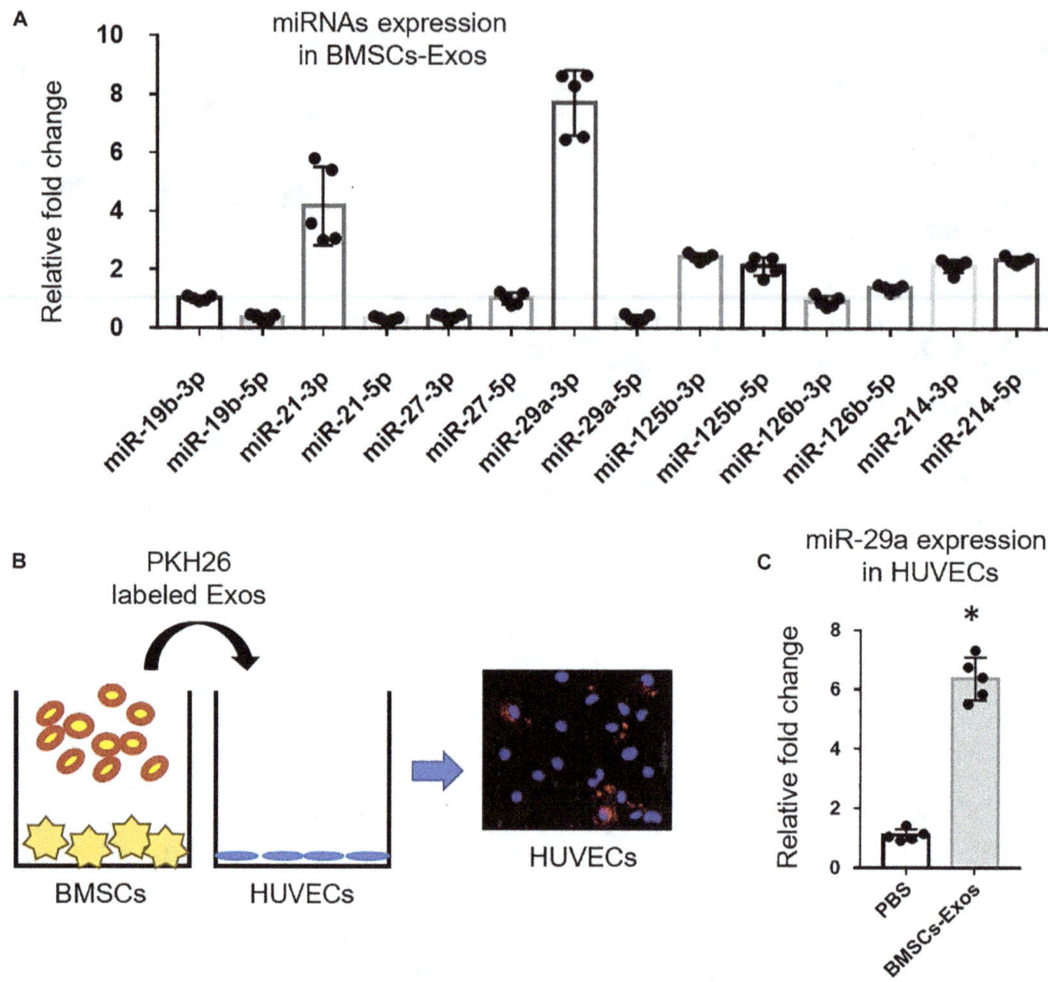


**FIGURE 2 |** miR-29a was increased in bone marrow mesenchymal stem cells (BMSCs)-Exo and transported into endothelial cells. **(A)** qPCR analysis of angiogenesis-related miRNA expression in BMSCs. **(B)** Exos from BMSCs were labeled with PKH26 and then added to human umbilical vein endothelial cell (HUVEC) cultures. **(C)** After treatment of BMSCs-Exos for 24 h, the levels of miR-29a in HUVECs were measured by qPCR analysis. Data are presented as mean ± SEM; $N = 5$ per group. $^{*}p < 0.05$, Student's *t*-test.

osteogenesis *in vivo*. First, we isolated BMSCs-Exos from an age-related osteoporotic mouse model to measure the miR-29a level within exosomes. We found that the miR-29a level was dramatically decreased in aged BMSCs-Exo compared to young BMSCs-Exo, implying that the decreased level of miR-29a in aged exosome might contribute to age-related bone loss (**Figures 5A,B**). Next, BMSCs transfected with miR-29a mimics were subjected to collect the miR-29a-loaded BMSCs-Exos. The 3-month-old mice were treated with miR-29a-loaded BMSCs-Exos, BMSCs-Exos, or PBS control for 2 months. An immunostaining analysis revealed that the number of CD31-positive endothelial cells increased in mice treated with BMSCs-Exos compared to the PBS-treated control. More interestingly, mice with treatment of miR-29a-loaded BMSCs-Exos showed a greater number of endothelial cells than BMSCs-Exo-treated mice (**Figures 5C,D**) as angiogenesis is tightly coupled with osteogenesis. Next, we measured the effects of miR-29a-loaded BMSCs-Exos on osteogenesis. As expected, mice treated with miR-29a-loaded BMSCs-Exos have a greater number of osteocalcin-positive osteoblasts in bone surface compared with BMSCs-Exos- or PBS-treated mice (**Figures 5E,F**).

## miR-29a-Loaded BMSCs-Exos Increased Trabecular Bone Mass

Next, we tested the function of miR-29a-loaded BMSCs-Exos on bone mass. The 3-month-old mice were treated with miR-29a-loaded BMSCs-Exos, BMSCs-Exos, or PBS control for 2 months. A micro-CT analysis revealed that mice with treatment of BMSCs-Exos showed increased bone mineral density (BMD), trabecular bone volume (BV/TV), trabecular bone number (Tb.N), and lower trabecular separation (Tb. Sp) in contrast to the PBS-treated control. Moreover, the miR-29a-loaded BMSCs-Exos-treated mice showed additive elevation in BMD, BV/TV, and Tb.N when compared to BMSCs-Exos-treated mice (**Figures 6A–F**). We have also measured the effects of miR-29a-loaded BMSCs-Exos on cortical

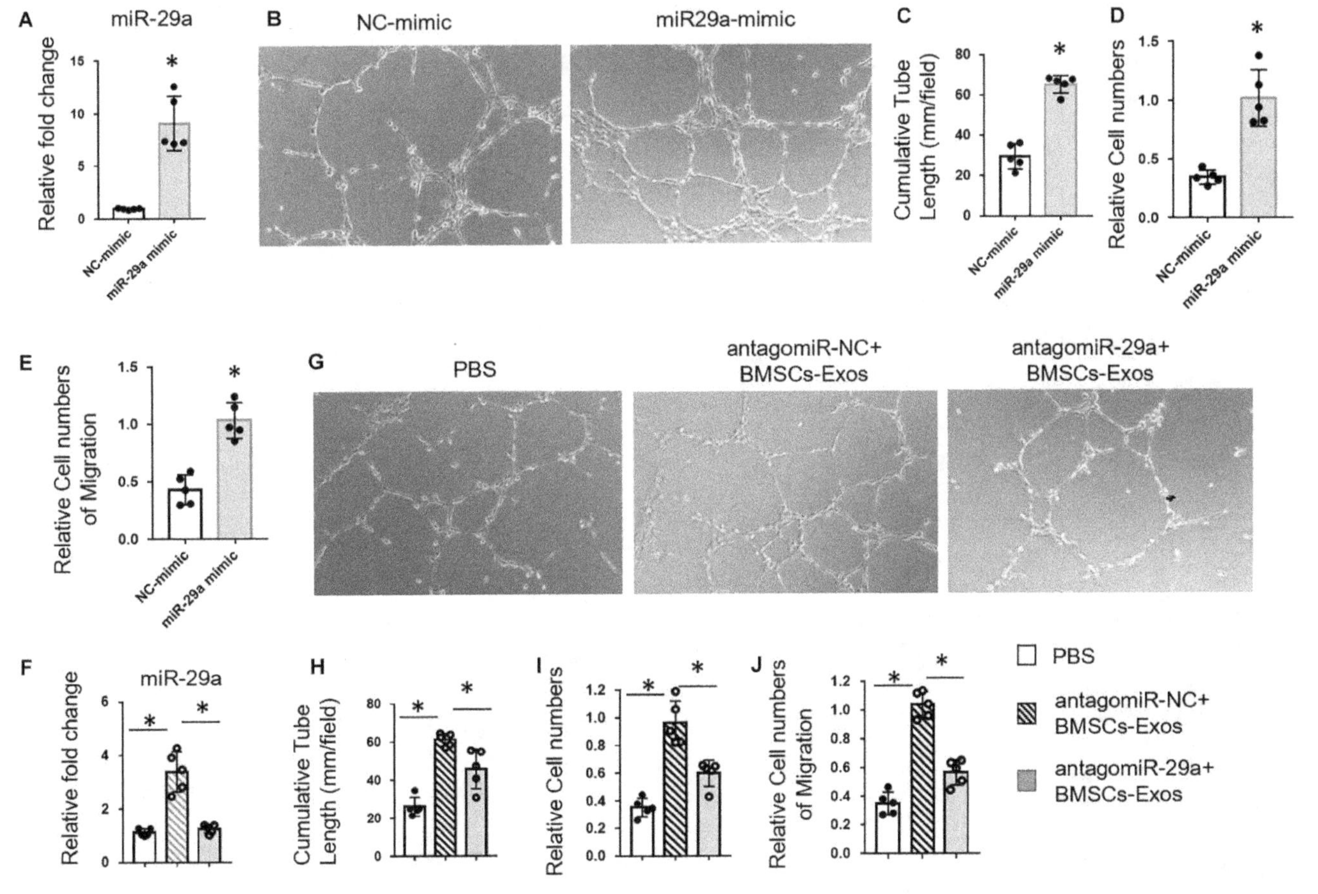


**FIGURE 3** | Bone marrow mesenchymal stem cells (BMSCs)-exosomal miR-29a promoted angiogenesis. **(A)** qPCR analysis of miR-29a expression in human umbilical vein endothelial cells (HUVECs) transfected with miR-29a mimic. Representative images of tube formation **(B)** and quantitative data of cumulative tube length **(C)** of HUVECs transfected with miR-29a or control mimics. **(D)** MTS assay was used to detect the proliferation of HUVECs. **(E)** Wound-healing assay was used to detect the migration of HUVECs. **(F)** qPCR analysis of miR-29a expression in exosomes collected from BMSCs with transfection of antagomir-29a. Representative images of tube formation **(G)** and quantitative data of cumulative tube length **(H)** of HUVECs with different treatments as indicated. **(I)** MTS assay was used to detect the proliferation of HUVECs. **(J)** Wound-healing assay was used to detect the migration of HUVECs; $N = 5$. Data are presented as mean ± SEM. $^{*}P < 0.05$, Student's *t*-test for **(A–E)** and ANOVA for **(F–J)**.

bone phenotype. However, we did not observe a significant change in cortical bone thickness in miR-29a-loaded BMSCs-Exos-treated mice compared to BMSCs-Exos- or PBS-treated mice (**Figures 6G,H**). These data indicate that miR-29a-loaded BMSCs-Exos have a robust ability of increasing bone mass in mice.

## DISCUSSION

In this study, we have shown that BMSCs-Exos promote angiogenesis and osteogenesis. BMSCs-Exos can be taken up by endothelial cells and regulate angiogenesis. BMSCs-Exos promoted the tube-like structure formation, proliferation, and migration of HUVECs. We found that the miR-29a level was high in BMSCs-Exos and played key roles in regulating angiogenesis. Downregulation of miR-29a level in BMSCs-Exos showed blunted effects on promoting angiogenesis. Furthermore, we identified that VASH1, as a direct target of miR-29a, mediated the effects of BMSCs-Exos on angiogenesis. miR-29a-loaded BMSCs-Exos have a robust ability of increasing bone mass in mice. More interestingly, we found that miR-29a level was dramatically decreased in aged BMSCs-Exos compared to young BMSCs-Exos, implying that the decreased level of miR-29a in aged exosome might contribute to age-related bone loss, and miR-29a-loaded BMSCs-Exo might be a potential way to treat age-related osteoporosis. It is worthwhile to investigate the effect of miR-29a-loaded BMSCs-Exo in aged mice in a future study.

miR-29a belongs to miR-29 family which has been reported to regulate angiogenesis (Li Z. et al., 2017). miR-29a mimics regulate the angiogenesis of gastric carcinoma cells and downregulate VEGF level (Zhang et al., 2016). Besides the endogenous regulation, miR-29a/c can be secreted into microvesicles and transported into endothelial cells to affect angiogenesis. Zhang et al. (2016) found that upregulation of miR-29a/c level in microvesicles by transfection of miR-29a/c mimics in HEK293 cells suppresses VEGF expression and angiogenesis in gastric carcinoma cells. We found that BMSCs-exosomal miR-29a

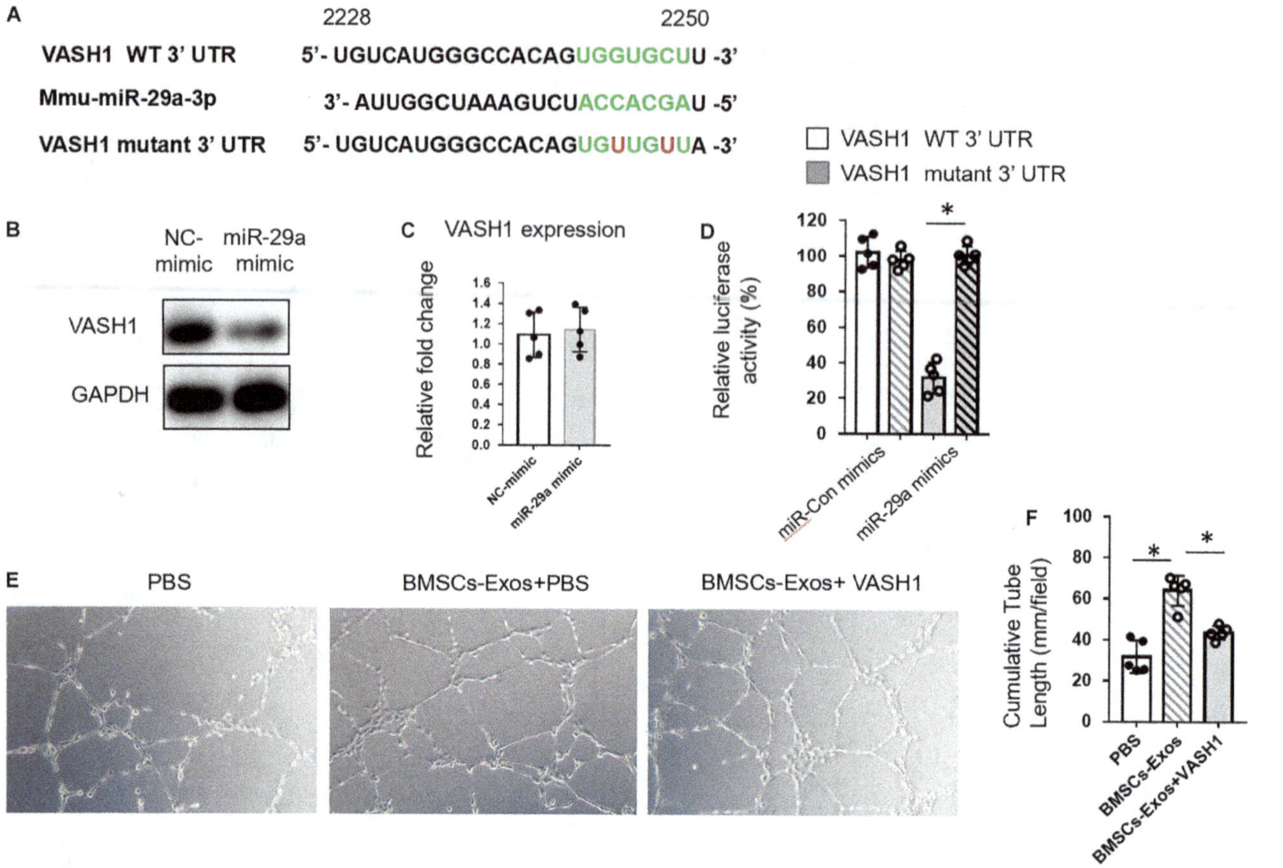


**FIGURE 4 |** BMSCs-exosomal miR-29a regulated angiogenesis *via* VASH1. **(A)** The miR-29a targets were predicted using TargetScan. Western blot analysis **(B)** and qPCR analysis **(C)** of VASH1 in human umbilical vein endothelial cells (HUVECs) transfected with miR-29a or control mimics. **(D)** The impact of miR-29a mimics on WT-VASH1; the mutant-VASH1 luciferase activity in 293T cells is shown. Representative images of tube formation **(E)** and quantitative data of cumulative tube length **(F)** of HUVECs with different treatments as indicated; $N = 5$. Data are presented as mean ± SEM. $^*P < 0.05$ as determined by Student's *t*-test for **(C)** and ANOVA for **(D,F)**.

promoted angiogenesis. Although we found that miR-29a within BMSCs-Exos plays a vital role in regulating angiogenesis, we cannot exclude the possibilities that other microRNAs or small molecules within exosomes also contribute to the regulation of BMSCs-Exos on angiogenesis. Zheng et al. (2017) found that miR-155 mediates endothelial injury and atherosclerosis. MSC-derived exosomes promote endothelial cell angiogenesis by transferring miR-125a (Gong et al., 2017). Thus, screening other potential components in BMSCs-Exos regulating angiogenesis is worthy of future study.

Other than MSCs, other cell types, such as smooth muscle cells, adipose tissue macrophages, and tumor cells, also secret exosomes to mediate angiogenesis. Exosomal miR-155 from smooth muscle cells has been reported to induce endothelial injury and promote atherosclerosis (Zheng et al., 2017). Ovarian cancer cell-derived PKR1-positive exosomes promote migration and tube formation of HUVECs *in vitro* (Zhang et al., 2020). Adipocytes can secret exosomes to regulate angiogenesis in diabetic mice (Wang et al., 2018). The reason we chose BMSCs to study is that as functionally and numerically dominant in bone marrow, BMSCs show robust abilities of regulating angiogenesis and osteogenesis (Li et al., 2013, 2016a, 2018; Li C. et al., 2017). The effects of BMSCs-Exos and the key components within exosome on angiogenesis and osteogenesis in mice are not well studied. Thus, in this study, we tested the function of BMSCs-Exos on angiogenesis and osteogenesis.

Type H vessel has been reported to be coupled with osteogenesis in recent years. In this study, we found that miR-29a within BMSCs-Exos promoted angiogenesis. However, among the predicted target genes of miR-29a, there is no gene reported to be involved in the signaling or pathway associated with type H vessel formation. Thus, we did not test the effects of BMSC-derived exosomal miR-29a on type H vessel formation, whereas there is a possibility that miR-29a might regulate type H vessel formation through undefined signaling or pathway. It is worthwhile to test this hypothesis in a future study.

In our study, we observed increased bone mass in mice with the treatment of miR-29a-loaded BMSCs-Exos. In this study, we focus on the effects of miR-29a-loaded BMSCs-Exos on angiogenesis. We speculate that the increased angiogenesis may contribute to the increased bone mass in response

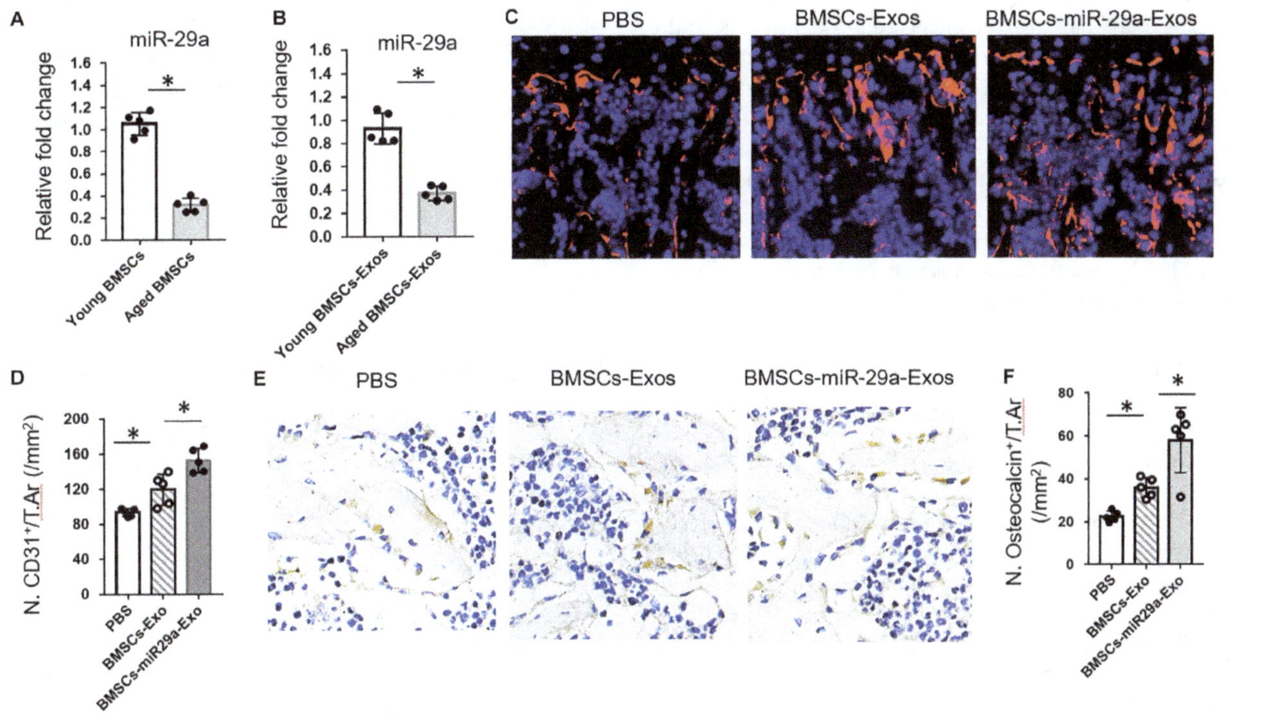


**FIGURE 5 |** Bone marrow mesenchymal stem cells (BMSCs)-miR-29a exosomes promoted angiogenesis and osteogenesis. **(A,B)** qPCR analysis of miRNA-29a-3p expression in young (3 months) and aged (18 months) BMSCs and of exosomes isolated from young and aged BMSCs. The 3-month-old mice were injected with BMSCs-Exos, BMSCs-miR29a-Exos, or phosphate-buffered saline for 2 months. **(C)** Representative images of CD31 (red) immunostaining. Nuclei, 4′,6-diamidino-2-phenylindole (blue). **(D)** Quantitative analysis of $CD31^{+}$ endothelial cells in distal femora. **(E)** Representative images of osteocalcin immunostaining. **(F)** Quantitative analysis of $osteocalcin^{+}$ osteoblasts in distal femora ($N$ = 5 mice in each group). Data are mean ± SD. $^{*}P < 0.05$ as determined by ANOVA.

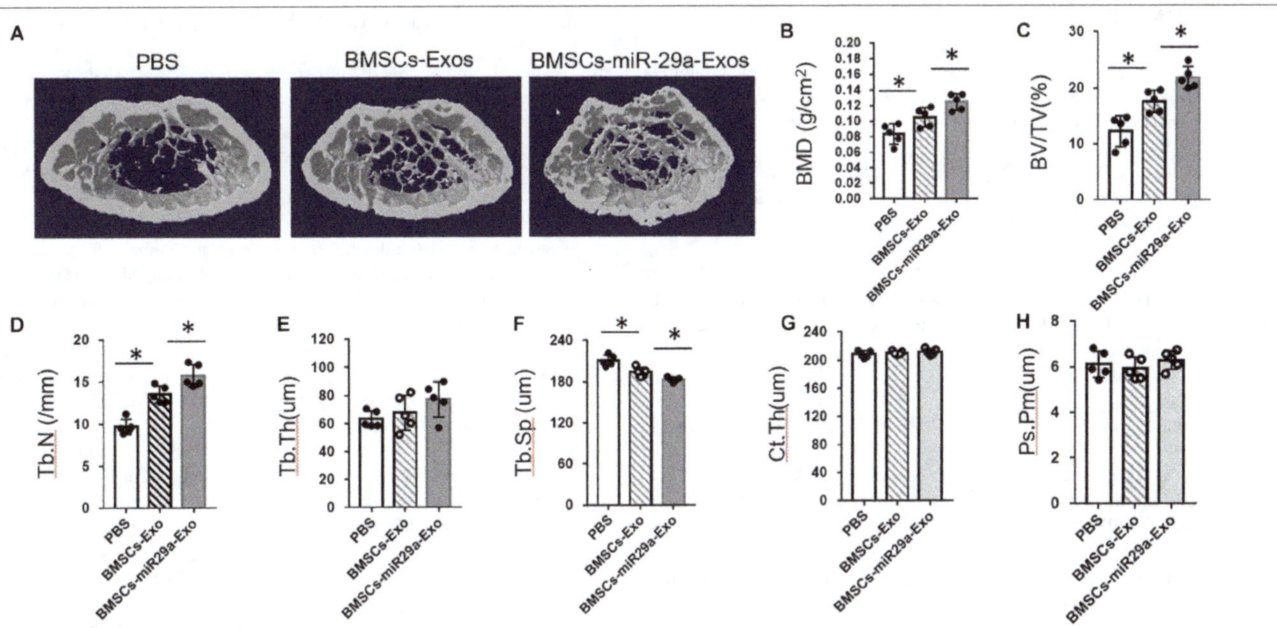


**FIGURE 6 |** miR-29a-loaded bone marrow mesenchymal stem cells (BMSCs)-exosomes increased trabecular bone mass. The 3-month-old female mice were injected with BMSCs-Exos, BMSCs-miR29a-Exos, or phosphate-buffered saline for 2 months. Representative micro-CT images **(A)** and quantitative micro-CT analysis **(B–H)** of bone mineral density, trabecular bone volume (BV/TV), trabecular bone number (Tb.N), trabecular thickness (Tb. Th), trabecular separation (Tb. Sp), cortical thickness (Ct. Th), and periosteal perimeter (Ps. Pm) in femurs ($N$ = 5 mice in each group). Data are mean ± SD (ANOVA). $^{*}P < 0.05$ as determined by ANOVA.

to miR-29a-loaded BMSCs-Exos. However, miR-29a-loaded BMSCs-Exos may have direct effects on osteogenesis and/or osteoclastogenesis. Recent studies reported that microRNA-29a can repress osteoclastogenesis to counteract glucocorticoid-induced bone loss (Wu et al., 2019). Lian et al. (2019) found that miR-29a regulates PCAF-mediated RANKL and CXCL12 to repress osteoclast formation. MiR-29a has also been reported to regulate osteoblast differentiation of BMSCs in a high-fat environment through modulating Frizzled 4 (Liu F. et al., 2019). Thus, miR-29a-loaded BMSCs-Exos may have multiple effects on angiogenesis, osteogenesis, and osteoclastogenesis.

We did not observe a significant increase in cortical bone from mice treated with miR-29a-loaded BMSCs-Exos in contrast to those from PBS-treated mice. This may be because of the way and period of administration of exosomes. Previous studies reported that majority of exosomes accumulated in the liver and lung through tail vein injection as measured by fluorescence molecular tomography imaging system. Xie's group reported that BMSC-specific aptamer conjugated exosomes have a high efficiency of bone tissue accumulation (Luo et al., 2019). Whereas they did not show the effects of BMSC-specific aptamer conjugated exosomes' effect on cortical bone, the effects of bone tissue-targeted delivery of exosomes with a prolonged treatment time on cortical bone are an attractive topic for future study.

In this study, we found that miR29a-loaded BMSCs-Exos promote angiogenesis and osteogenesis. BMSCs-Exos promote the proliferation, migration, and tube formation of HUVECs. MiRNA-29a level was high in BMSCs-Exos and can be transported into HUVECs to regulate angiogenesis in a VASH1-dependent way. More interestingly, miR29a-loaded BMSCs-Exos have a robust ability of promoting angiogenesis and osteogenesis in mice. Thus, these findings suggest that BMSC-derived exosomal miR-29a regulates angiogenesis and osteogenesis, and miR-29a-loaded BMSCs-Exos may serve as a potential therapeutic target for osteoporosis.

## ETHICS STATEMENT

Animal care and experimental protocol were approved by the Animal Care and Use Committees of the Laboratory Animal Research Center at Shihezi University First Affiliated Hospital.

## AUTHOR CONTRIBUTIONS

ZW and TL designed the experiments, supervised the experiments, analyzed results, and wrote the manuscript. GL and PC carried out most of the experiments. All authors contributed to the article and approved the submitted version.

## REFERENCES


Bridge, G., Monteiro, R., Henderson, S., Emuss, V., Lagos, D., Georgopoulou, D., et al. (2012). The microRNA-30 family targets DLL4 to modulate endothelial cell behavior during angiogenesis. *Blood* 120, 5063–5072. doi: 10.1182/blood-2012-04-423004

Chen, C. Y., Rao, S. S., Ren, L., Hu, X. K., Tan, Y. J., Hu, Y., et al. (2018). Exosomal DMBT1 from human urine-derived stem cells facilitates diabetic wound repair by promoting angiogenesis. *Theranostics* 8, 1607–1623. doi: 10.7150/thno.22958

Ghosh, G., Subramanian, I. V., Adhikari, N., Zhang, X., Joshi, H. P., Basi, D., et al. (2010). Hypoxia-induced microRNA-424 expression in human endothelial cells regulates HIF-α isoforms and promotes angiogenesis. *J. Clin. Invest.* 120, 4141–4154. doi: 10.1172/jci42980

Gong, M., Yu, B., Wang, J., Wang, Y., Liu, M., Paul, C., et al. (2017). Mesenchymal stem cells release exosomes that transfer miRNAs to endothelial cells and promote angiogenesis. *Oncotarget* 8, 45200–45212. doi: 10.18632/oncotarget.16778

Hu, Y., Rao, S. S., Wang, Z. X., Cao, J., Tan, Y. J., Luo, J., et al. (2018). Exosomes from human umbilical cord blood accelerate cutaneous wound healing through miR-21-3p-mediated promotion of angiogenesis and fibroblast function. *Theranostics* 8, 169–184. doi: 10.7150/thno.21234

Huang, C. C., Kang, M., Lu, Y., Shirazia, S., Diaza, J. I., Cooper, L. F., et al. (2020). Functionally engineered extracellular vesicles improve bone regeneration. *Acta Biomater.* 109, 182–194. doi: 10.1016/j.actbio.2020.04.017

Hui, X., Zhuang, C., Long, W., Xia, Z., Hu, Y., Xian, L., et al. (2014). PDGF-BB secreted by preosteoclasts induces angiogenesis during coupling with osteogenesis. *Nat. Med.* 20, 1270–1278. doi: 10.1038/nm.3668

Jia, Y., Qiu, S., Xu, J., Kang, Q., and Chai, Y. (2020). Exosomes secreted by young mesenchymal stem cells promote new bone formation during distraction osteogenesis in older rats. *Calcif. Tissue Int.* 106, 509–517. doi: 10.1007/s00223-019-00656-4

Jin, Z., Ren, J., and Qi, S. (2020). Exosomal miR-9-5p secreted by bone marrow-derived mesenchymal stem cells alleviates osteoarthritis by inhibiting syndecan-1. *Cell Tissue Res.* 381, 99–114. doi: 10.1007/s00441-020-03193-x

Kusumbe, A. P., Ramasamy, S. K., and Adams, R. H. (2014). Coupling of angiogenesis and osteogenesis by a specific vessel subtype in bone. *Nature* 507, 323–328. doi: 10.1038/nature13145

Li, C., Chai, Y., Wang, L., Gao, B., Chen, H., Gao, P., et al. (2017). Programmed cell senescence in skeleton during late puberty. *Nat. Commun.* 8:1312.

Li, C., Wang, W., Xie, L., Luo, X., Cao, X., and Wan, M. (2016a). Lipoprotein receptor-related protein 6 is required for parathyroid hormone-induced Sost suppression. *Ann. N. Y. Acad. Sci.* 1364, 62–73. doi: 10.1111/nyas.12750

Li, C., Xing, Q., Yu, B., Xie, H., Wang, W., Shi, C., et al. (2013). Disruption of LRP6 in osteoblasts blunts the bone anabolic activity of PTH. *J. Bone Miner. Res.* 28, 2094–2108. doi: 10.1002/jbmr.1962

Li, C., Zhen, G., Chai, Y., Xie, L., Crane, J. L., Farber, E., et al. (2016b). RhoA determines lineage fate of mesenchymal stem cells by modulating CTGF-VEGF complex in extracellular matrix. *Nat. Commun.* 7:11455.

Li, C. J., Cheng, P., Liang, M. K., Chen, Y. S., Lu, Q., Wang, J. Y., et al. (2015). MicroRNA-188 regulates age-related switch between osteoblast and adipocyte differentiation. *J. Clin. Invest.* 125, 1509–1522. doi: 10.1172/jci77716

Li, C. J., Xiao, Y., Yang, M., Su, T., Sun, X., Guo, Q., et al. (2018). Long noncoding RNA Bmncr regulates mesenchymal stem cell fate during skeletal aging. *J. Clin. Invest.* 128, 5251–5266. doi: 10.1172/jci99044

Li, M., Wang, T., Tian, H., Wei, G., Zhao, L., and Shi, Y. (2019). Macrophage-derived exosomes accelerate wound healing through their anti-inflammation effects in a diabetic rat model. *Artif. Cells Nanomed. Biotechnol.* 47, 3793–3803. doi: 10.1080/21691401.2019.1669617

Li, X., and Tang, M. (2020). Exosomes released from M2 macrophages transfer miR-221-3p contributed to EOC progression through targeting CDKN1B. *Cancer Med.* 9, 5976–5988. doi: 10.1002/cam4.3252

Li, Y., Yang, R., Guo, B., Zhang, H., Zhang, H., Liu, S., et al. (2019). Exosomal miR-301 derived from mesenchymal stem cells protects myocardial infarction by inhibiting myocardial autophagy. *Biochem. Biophys. Res. Commun.* 514, 323–328. doi: 10.1016/j.bbrc.2019.04.138

Li, Z., Jiang, R., Yue, Q., and Peng, H. (2017). MicroRNA-29 regulates myocardial microvascular endothelial cells proliferation and migration in association with IGF1 in type 2 diabetes. *Biochem. Biophys. Res. Commun.* 487, 15–21. doi: 10.1016/j.bbrc.2017.03.055

Lian, W. S., Ko, J. Y., Chen, Y. S., Ke, H.-J., Hsieh, C.-K., Kuo, C.-W., et al. (2019). MicroRNA-29a represses osteoclast formation and protects against osteoporosis by regulating PCAF-mediated RANKL and CXCL12. *Cell Death Dis.* 10:705.

Liu, F., Wang, Z. F., Liu, F. F., Xu, J. Z., Liu, Q., and Lan, J. (2019). [MicroRNA-29a-3p regulates osteoblast differentiation and peri-implant osseointegration in a rat model of hyperlipidemia by modulating Frizzled 4 expression]. *Hua Xi Kou Qiang Yi Xue Za Zhi* 37, 200–207.

Liu, T., Sun, Y. C., Cheng, P., and Shao, H. G. (2019). Adipose tissue macrophage-derived exosomal miR-29a regulates obesity-associated insulin resistance. *Biochem. Biophys. Res. Commun.* 515, 352–358. doi: 10.1016/j.bbrc.2019.05.113

Liu, W., Li, L., Rong, Y., Qian, D., Chen, J., Zhou, Z., et al. (2020). Hypoxic mesenchymal stem cell-derived exosomes promote bone fracture healing by the transfer of miR-126. *Acta Biomater.* 103, 196–212. doi: 10.1016/j.actbio.2019.12.020

Luo, Z. W., Li, F. X., Liu, Y. W., Rao, S. S., Yin, H., Huang, J., et al. (2019). Aptamer-functionalized exosomes from bone marrow stromal cells target bone to promote bone regeneration. *Nanoscale* 11, 20884–20892. doi: 10.1039/c9nr02791b

Nakano, M., Kubota, K., Kobayashi, E., Chikenji, T. S., Saito, Y., Konari, N., et al. (2020). Bone marrow-derived mesenchymal stem cells improve cognitive impairment in an Alzheimer's disease model by increasing the expression of microRNA-146a in hippocampus. *Sci. Rep.* 10:10772.

Qi, X., Zhang, J., Yuan, H., Xu, Z., Li, Q., Niu, X., et al. (2016). Exosomes secreted by human-induced pluripotent stem cell-derived mesenchymal stem cells repair critical-sized bone defects through enhanced angiogenesis and osteogenesis in osteoporotic rats. *Int. J. Biol. Sci.* 12, 836–849. doi: 10.7150/ijbs.14809

Song, W., Chen, Y., Zhu, G., Xie, H., Yang, Z., and Li, L. (2020). Exosome-mediated miR-9-5p promotes proliferation and migration of renal cancer cells both in vitro and in vivo by targeting SOCS4. *Biochem. Biophys. Res. Commun.* 529, 1216–1224. doi: 10.1016/j.bbrc.2020.06.114

Sun, W., Zhao, P., Zhou, Y., Xing, C., Zhao, L., Li, Z., et al. (2020). Ultrasound targeted microbubble destruction assisted exosomal delivery of miR-21 protects the heart from chemotherapy associated cardiotoxicity. *Biochem. Biophys. Res. Commun.* 532, 60–67. doi: 10.1016/j.bbrc.2020.05.044

Tan, S. H. S., Wong, J. R. Y., Sim, S. J. Y., Tjio, C. K. E., Wong, K. L., Chew, J. R. J., et al. (2020). Mesenchymal stem cell exosomes in bone regenerative strategies-a systematic review of preclinical studies. *Mater. Today Bio* 7:100067. doi: 10.1016/j.mtbio.2020.100067

Tang, T. T., and Wang, B. (2020). Extracellular vesicle-encapsulated IL-10 as novel nanotherapeutics against ischemic AKI. *Sci. Adv.* 6:eaaz0748. doi: 10.1126/sciadv.aaz0748

Venkat, P., Zacharek, A., Landschoot-Ward, J., Wang, F., Culmone, L., Chen, Z., et al. (2020). Exosomes derived from bone marrow mesenchymal stem cells harvested from type two diabetes rats promotes neurorestorative effects after stroke in type two diabetes rats. *Exp. Neurol.* 334:113456. doi: 10.1016/j.expneurol.2020.113456

Vilaca-Faria, H., Salgado, A. J., and Teixeira, F. G. (2019). Mesenchymal stem cells-derived exosomes: a new possible therapeutic strategy for Parkinson's disease? *Cells* 8:118. doi: 10.3390/cells8020118

Wang, F., Chen, F. F., Shang, Y. Y., Li, Y., Wang, Z. H., Han, L., et al. (2018). Insulin resistance adipocyte-derived exosomes aggravate atherosclerosis by increasing vasa vasorum angiogenesis in diabetic ApoE(-/-) mice. *Int. J. Cardiol.* 265, 181–187. doi: 10.1016/j.ijcard.2018.04.028

Wu, R. W., Lian, W. S., Chen, Y. S., Kuo, C. W., Ke, H. C., Hsieh, C. K., et al. (2019). MicroRNA-29a counteracts glucocorticoid induction of bone loss through repressing TNFSF13b modulation of osteoclastogenesis. *Int. J. Mol. Sci.* 20:5141. doi: 10.3390/ijms20205141

Wu, X., Pang, L., Lei, W., Lu, W., Li, J., Li, Z., et al. (2010). Inhibition of Sca-1-positive skeletal stem cell recruitment by alendronate blunts the anabolic effects of parathyroid hormone on bone remodeling. *Cell Stem Cell* 7, 571–580. doi: 10.1016/j.stem.2010.09.012

Xu, Y., Liu, N., Wei, Y., Zhou, D., Lin, R., Wang, X., et al. (2020). Anticancer effects of miR-124 delivered by BM-MSC derived exosomes on cell proliferation, epithelial mesenchymal transition, and chemotherapy sensitivity of pancreatic cancer cells. *Aging (Albany NY)* 12, 19660–19676. doi: 10.18632/aging.103997

Yang, M., Li, C. J., Sun, X., Guo, Q., Xiao, Y., Su, T., et al. (2017). MiR-497 approximately 195 cluster regulates angiogenesis during coupling with osteogenesis by maintaining endothelial Notch and HIF-1alpha activity. *Nat. Commun.* 8:16003.

Ying, W., Riopel, M., Bandyopadhyay, G., Dong, Y., Birmingham, A., Seo, J. B., et al. (2017). Adipose tissue macrophage-derived exosomal miRNAs can modulate in vivo and in vitro insulin sensitivity. *Cell* 171, 372–384.e12.

Zhang, H., Bai, M., Deng, T., Liu, R., Wang, X., Qu, Y., et al. (2016). Cell-derived microvesicles mediate the delivery of miR-29a/c to suppress angiogenesis in gastric carcinoma. *Cancer Lett.* 375, 331–339. doi: 10.1016/j.canlet.2016.03.026

Zhang, X., Sheng, Y., Li, B., Wang, Q., Liu, X., and Han, J. (2020). Ovarian cancer derived PKR1 positive exosomes promote angiogenesis by promoting migration and tube formation in vitro. *Cell Biochem. Funct.* doi: 10.1002/cbf.3583 [Epub ahead of print].

Zheng, B., Yin, W. N., Suzuki, T., Zhang, X. H., Zhang, Y., Song, L. L., et al. (2017). Exosome-mediated miR-155 transfer from smooth muscle cells to endothelial cells induces endothelial injury and promotes atherosclerosis. *Mol. Ther.* 25, 1279–1294. doi: 10.1016/j.ymthe.2017.03.031

Zheng, G., Huang, R., Qiu, G., Ge, M., Wang, J., Shu, Q., et al. (2018). Mesenchymal stromal cell-derived extracellular vesicles: regenerative and immunomodulatory effects and potential applications in sepsis. *Cell Tissue Res.* 374, 1–15. doi: 10.1007/s00441-018-2871-5

Zou, L., Ma, X., Wu, B., Chen, Y., Xie, D., and Peng, C. (2020). Protective effect of bone marrow mesenchymal stem cell-derived exosomes on cardiomyoblast hypoxia-reperfusion injury through the miR-149/let-7c/Faslg axis. *Free Radic. Res.* 15, 1–19. doi: 10.1080/10715762.2020.1837793

Zuo, R., Liu, M., Wang, Y., Li, J., Wang, W., Wu, J., et al. (2019). BM-MSC-derived exosomes alleviate radiation-induced bone loss by restoring the function of recipient BM-MSCs and activating Wnt/beta-catenin signaling. *Stem Cell Res. Ther.* 10:30.

7

# Functions and Clinical Significance of Super-Enhancers in Bone-Related Diseases

*Jian Qu[1,2†], Zhanbo Ouyang[1,2†], Wenqiang Wu[3], Guohua Li[1,2], Jiaojiao Wang[1,2], Qiong Lu[1,2*] and Zhihong Li[2,4*]*

[1] Department of Pharmacy, The Second Xiangya Hospital, Central South University, Changsha, China, [2] Hunan Key Laboratory of Tumor Models and Individualized Medicine, The Second Xiangya Hospital, Central South University, Changsha, China, [3] Mathematical Engineering Academy of Chinese Medicine, Guangzhou University of Chinese Medicine, Guangzhou, China, [4] Department of Orthopedics, The Second Xiangya Hospital, Central South University, Changsha, China

***Correspondence:**
Qiong Lu
christy_luq@csu.edu.cn
Zhihong Li
lizhihong@csu.edu.cn

† These authors have contributed equally to this work

Super-enhancers (SEs) are a large cluster of *cis*-regulatory DNA elements that contain many binding motifs, which master transcription factors and cofactors bind to with high density. SEs usually regulate the expression of genes that can control the cell identity and fate, and SEs can be used to explain the patterns of the expression of cell-specific genes. Hence, it shows great potential for application in the treatment of diseases like cancer. At present, the clinical treatments for osteosarcoma, Ewing sarcoma, and other bone-related diseases remain challenging. The poor prognosis and difficult treatment of these diseases imposes heavy economic burden on patients and society. In recent years, research on SEs with respect to bone-related diseases has attracted increasing attention. In this paper, we first review the identification and functional mechanisms of SEs. Then, we integrate the findings of the emerging studies on SEs in bone-related diseases. Finally, we summarize recent strategies for targeting SEs for the treatment of bone-related diseases. This review aims to provide comprehensive insights into the roles of SEs in bone-related diseases.

**Keywords: super-enhancers, bone-related diseases, osteosarcoma, Ewing sarcoma, multiple myeloma**

## INTRODUCTION

Since the Human Genome Project was launched in 1990, our understanding of the regulatory mechanism of genes has evolved drastically. Nowadays, many scientists believe that gene transcription is controlled by types of regulatory elements known as enhancers and super-enhancers (SEs). Bulger and Groudine, 2011 proposed that enhancers are functionally defined as non-coding elements that can activate gene transcription through long-range *cis* chromatin interactions. Initially, enhancers only meant the typical enhancers (TEs). However, Hnisz et al. (2013) proposed the concept of SEs in 2013. They put forward that although TEs and SEs are similar with respect to carrying the same components such as transcription factors (TFs), cofactors, mediator complex, and RNA polymerase II (pol II) complex, SEs harbors these factors on an average 10-fold higher density than do TEs (Hnisz et al., 2013; Whyte et al., 2013; Thandapani, 2019). The difference between the function and structure of TEs and SEs are shown in **Figure 1**. SEs are a large cluster of *cis*-regulatory DNA elements densely bound by transcription factors and cofactors and play critical roles in defining cell fate and

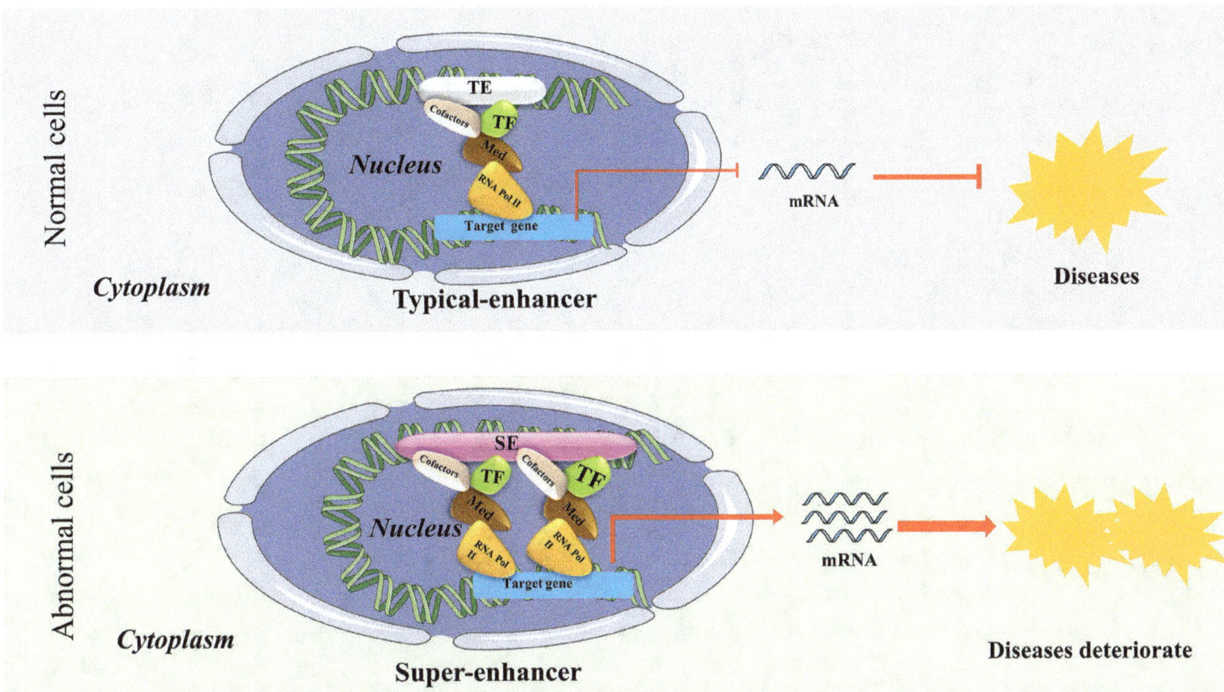


**FIGURE 1 |** The structure and possible functional mechanism of super-enhancers (SEs) vs. typical enhancers (TEs). SEs are a large cluster of *cis*-regulatory DNA elements densely bound by transcription factors and cofactors. SEs are often found near genes that have cell type-specific functions and genes closely associated with the progress of bone-related diseases. It usually causes diseases or accelerates the progress of diseases by regulating the expression of disease-specific genes.

identity (Hnisz et al., 2013). Histone marks such as H3K27ac, H3K4me1, and the transcription cofactor p300 are often used to define SEs (Riggi et al., 2014; Kennedy et al., 2015; Niederriter et al., 2015). Ever since their discovery, SEs have been the focus of increasing research to investigate their roles in cancers and inflammatory diseases like osteoarthritis. For example, previous research indicated that SEs frequently drive high-level expression of prominent oncogenes in cancer cells (Hnisz et al., 2013; Chipumuro et al., 2014; Kwiatkowski et al., 2014). Other groups found that SEs play a critical role in autoimmune diseases like juvenile idiopathic arthritis (Peeters et al., 2015). Shin (2018) proposed that SEs can be used as biomarkers to develop novel disease diagnostic tools and establish new directions in clinical therapeutic strategies. Hence, SEs can be considered novel targets in diseases, and targeting SEs should be a promising therapeutic strategy.

The clinical treatment of bone-related diseases such as osteosarcoma, Ewing sarcoma, osteoporosis, cartilage dysplasia, chordoma, rheumatoid arthritis, osteoarthritis, and multiple myeloma continue to remain challenging. Although the incidence of these bone-related diseases is relatively lower than cancers like lung cancer, the poor prognosis and difficult treatment imposes a heavy burden on patients and caregivers. To address this complex problem, researchers have aimed to develop high-efficiency, novel therapies based on targeting SEs to treat bone-related diseases. In recent years, the functional mechanism of SEs in these bone-related diseases has attracted increasing attention. Thus, this review will mainly focus on integrating the findings of the emerging studies on SEs (shown in **Table 1**) in bone-related diseases and summarizing the strategies of targeting SEs as a clinical treatment for bone-related diseases. We believe it can provide new insights and angles for future studies and optimum treatment strategies using SEs in bone-related diseases.

## THE IDENTIFICATION OF SEs

Diseases-related cells acquire SEs through various mechanisms, including (i)mutations and genomic alterations like deletions, duplications, translocations, insertions, inversions (Mansour et al., 2014; Oldridge et al., 2015; Zhang et al., 2019); (ii) single-nucleotide polymorphisms (SNPs) (Zhu et al., 2018); (iii) chromosomal rearrangements (Affer et al., 2014; Gröschel et al., 2014; Demchenko et al., 2016); and (iv) 3D genome structural changes (Furlong and Levine, 2018). Once the SEs originated through the above mechanisms, resulting in the dysregulation of nearby SEs-target genes, which ultimately accelerates the deterioration of diseases.

With rapid developments in genetic research, many refractory diseases with complex disease mechanisms have been well studied. However, despite researchers having identified some effective treatments, osteosarcoma, Ewing sarcoma, and other bone-related diseases remain difficult to treat. The poor prognosis and difficulty in treatment impose heavy economic burden on patients and society. Although many studies have proposed

**TABLE 1** | Summary of the researches about the SEs in bone-related diseases.

| Diseases* | Cell/tissue* | SEs-targeted genes | Methods | Findings | References |
|---|---|---|---|---|---|
| OS | OS cell lines (U2OS/SJSA-1) | *MYC*, *STAT3* | ChIP-Seq of H3K27ac | THZ2 can inhibit the progression of osteosarcoma by targeting SE-associated genes like *MYC*, *STAT3* | Zhang et al., 2020 |
| OS | OS cell lines (143B and SJSA1), primary OS cells (ZOS and ZOSM), and OS tissue | *LIF* | ChIP-Seq of H3K27ac | SEs function as an activator of NOTCH1 pathway through regulating LIF/STAT3 pathway in promoting the progression of osteosarcoma | Lu et al., 2020 |
| ES | ES cell lines (A673/SKNMC) | *BCL11B*, *GLG1* | Analysis of ChIP-Seq data of H3K27ac | SEs-targeted genes *BCL11B* and *GLG1* are novel biomarkers for the diagnosis of Ewing sarcoma | Baldauf et al., 2018 |
| ES | ES cell lines (A673/SKNMC) | *MEIS1* | ChIP-Seq of H3K27ac | SEs-associated gene *MEIS1* promotes transcriptional dysregulation in Ewing sarcoma in co-operation with EWS-FLI1 | Lin et al., 2018 |
| ES | ES cell lines (TC32/TC71) | *CCND1* | ChIP-Seq of H3K27ac | SEs-associated gene *CCND1* promotes the progression of Ewing sarcoma | Kennedy et al., 2015 |
| ES | ES cell lines-A673 cells treated with JQ1 | *EWS-FLI1* | ChIP of BRD4 and analysis of ChIP-Seq data of H3K27ac | SE-inhibitors like JQ1 can repress the progression of Ewing sarcoma through impacting *EWS-FLI1*' expression | Jacques et al., 2016 |
| Chordoma | Chordoma cell lines and chordoma tissue | *TBXT* | ChIP-Seq of H3K27ac | The dysregulation of *TBXT* regulated by SEs is the main cause for the tumorigenesis of chordoma | Sharifnia et al., 2019 |
| MM | Primary cells isolated from MM tissue and Myeloma cell lines | *IRF4*, *FLI1* | ChIP-Seq of H3K27ac | *IRF4* and *FLI1* showed significant overlap with SEs. They can promote the progress of MM | Jin et al., 2018 |
| MM | MM1.S MM cells | *MYC* | ChIP-Seq of H3K27ac, BRD4, MED1 | SE-inhibitors treatment like JQ1 results in preferential loss of BRD4 in *MYC*-SE, which can repress the progress of MM | Loven et al., 2013 |
| OP | GM12878 cells/osteoblast | *RANKL* | Analysis of ChIP-Seq data of H3K27ac from ENCODE | The dysregulated expression of the SE-associated gene *RANKL* is critical for the progress of osteoporosis | Zhu et al., 2018 |
| CD | Rat chondrosarcoma cells | *SOX9*, *SOX6*, *SOX5* | ChIP-Seq 0f H3K27ac | The dysregulation of the SE- associated genes may cause cartilage dysplasia | Liu and Lefebvre, 2015 |
| RA | CD4 + T cell | *BACH2* | ChIP-Seq of P300 protein | SEs-associated gene *BACH2* which is critical for the progress of RA | Vahedi et al., 2015 |
| OS | Chondrocyte cell (sw1353 and chondrocytes isolated from OA tissue) | *HMGB1* | ChIP of BRD4 and analysis of ChIP-Seq data of H3K27ac | SEs may mediate the BRD4 regulating role in the expression of *HMGB1* | Jiang et al., 2017 |

**OS cell, osteosarcoma cell; ES cell, Ewing sarcoma cell; OP cell, osteoporosis cell; CD cell, cartilage dysplasia cell; chordoma, RA cell, rheumatoid arthritis cell; OA cell, osteoarthritis cell; and MM cell, multiple myeloma cell.*

different treatment options for bone-related diseases, the effects of these treatments are not satisfactory. Therefore, significant research is on-going in an attempt to discover satisfactory treatment methods for these diseases.

Loven et al. (2013) and Whyte et al. (2013) first identified SEs in mouse embryonic stem cells and human cells. Since then, several publications have cited the SEs and identified its applications in different diseases (Chapuy et al., 2013; Loven et al., 2013; Whyte et al., 2013; Brown et al., 2014; Vaharautio and Taipale, 2014). Besides, an SE database—dbSUPER—in the mouse and human genome has been established by Khan and Zhang (2016). It is the first integrated and interactive database of SEs and serves as a reference for further studies related to transcriptional control of cell identity and disease. Pott and Lieb (2015) summarized the characteristics of SEs based on these publications: (i) SEs are enriched for motifs related to cell type-specific master transcription factors, and are often found near genes that have cell type-specific functions, including known master regulators; (ii) SEs are enriched for trait-associated variants; (iii) SEs overlap with previously defined large-scale regulatory domains and (iv) SEs in cancer cells are enriched in the vicinity of oncogenes. Summarizing from previous studies, abnormal SEs in disease states may form because of focal amplification, genomic regulatory elements rearrangements (Affer et al., 2014; Walker et al., 2014), and small insertions and deletions.

In recent years, research on SEs in diseases has become an important focus of clinical and basic research. As for the functional mechanism of the SEs (shown in **Figure 1**), Sengupta and George (2017) concluded that transcription factor (TF) binding to enhancers results in recruitment of the mediator complex. This, in turn, facilitates enhancer interaction with the basal transcription machinery and RNA polymerase II (Pol II) at the promoter regions in a gene-specific manner, a process mediated by "looping" of the loaded enhancer to the cognate promoter (Hnisz et al., 2016; Sur and Taipale, 2016). Thus, SEs can influence disease progression by initiating downstream transcription of the affected genes (Sengupta and George, 2017).

## SEs IN BONE-RELATED DISEASES

### SEs in Osteosarcoma

Osteosarcoma (OS) is the most common primary sarcoma occurring in children and adolescents. Metastasis and recurrence of osteosarcoma are the main influencing factors for the poor survival rate. The overall 5-year survival rate for patients with non-metastatic osteosarcoma is approximately 60–70%, while that for patients with metastatic and recurrent osteosarcoma is significantly reduced (Kempf-Bielack et al., 2005; Luetke et al., 2014; Kwiatkowski et al., 2014). Researchers have found that SEs play a critical role in the progression of osteosarcoma by promoting its growth and metastasis.

Chen et al. (2018) found a significant increase in *MYC* expression in metastatic osteosarcoma samples, suggesting that *MYC* may be an important therapeutic target for osteosarcoma treatment. They further tested the recently developed small-molecule SE-inhibitors of osteosarcoma and found that the SE-inhibitors were effective in inhibiting the proliferation, migration, and invasion of osteosarcoma cells. This is likely due to the inhibition of a large population of SEs containing the *MYC* target gene by THZ1 [a SE-inhibitor that also functions as a CDK7 (cyclin-dependent kinase) inhibitor] treatment. They also reported that the chosen sensitivity of some SE genes are more sensitive to THZ1 treatment than others, indicating that *MYC* binding strength, SE size and intensity, basic gene expression levels, and the activity of transcription factors and cofactors may lead to differential responses of the SEs gene to THZ1 treatment. Chen et al. (2018) have experimentally demonstrated that SE-inhibitors are promising small-molecule drugs for patients with osteosarcoma by targeting the MYC signaling pathway in osteosarcoma.

Zhang et al. (2020) found THZ2 can target SE-associated oncogenes in osteosarcoma. Using ChIP-Seq, they found that SEs are associated with oncogenic genes in osteosarcoma cells. They further reported several SE-associated genes to be sensitive to THZ2 treatment. Finally, they proved their hypothesis that THZ2 can inhibit the progression of osteosarcoma by targeting SE-associated genes such as *MYC*, *STAT3*, and *HMOX1*. These findings indicate that THZ2 has the potential to become a promising targeting drug for osteosarcoma treatment.

Morrow et al. (2018) suggested that enhancer elements can confer metastatic ability to osteosarcoma cells. They found that metastatic osteosarcoma and non-metastatic osteosarcoma have different enhancer activities for metastatic genes, and proposed a new concept of Metastatic Variant Enhancer Loci (Met-VELs). Comparing the activity of the gene with Met-VELs with the activity of SE-associated genes, they proved the existence of different Met-VELs in related metastasis genes, which lead to differences in metastatic ability between metastatic and non-metastatic osteosarcoma. Further, genes with Met-VELs were reportedly more related to osteosarcoma metastasis, while those with SE-associated genes were more related to the tumorigenesis and survival of osteosarcoma.

Lee et al. (2015) found the following phenomenon in the study of the treatment mechanism of JQ1—a bromodomain and extra terminal domain (BET) protein inhibitor—in human osteosarcoma: although the inhibition of bromodomain-containing protein 4 (BRD4) by JQ1 could inhibit the growth of osteosarcoma cells *in vitro*. They showed that the level of c-MYC protein in the cells treated with JQ1 remained unchanged. Meanwhile, some studies showed that JQ1 treatment significantly decreased the expression of *RUNX2* gene, which can be regulated by SEs with the region enriched for H3K27Ac (Encode Project Consortium, 2004; Loven et al., 2013; Whyte et al., 2013). Thus, Lee et al. (2015) suggested that the downstream target gene of JQ1 in osteosarcoma is *RUNX2* but not *MYC*, and they proved it through experiments such as ChIP-seq assay.

By profiling the epigenetic characteristics and SEs landscape of the osteosarcoma and some clinical specimens, Lu et al. (2020) found the SE-mediated regulator LIF can promote osteosarcoma stemness gene expression. Mechanistically, they found SEs function as an activator of the NOTCH1 pathway through regulating the LIF/STAT3 pathway in promoting the progression of osteosarcoma. They believe that their findings will provide new insights for the treatments of osteosarcoma. The possible functional mechanism of SEs in osteosarcoma is shown in **Figure 2**.

## SEs in Ewing Sarcoma

Ewing sarcoma is the second most common and devastating primary malignant tumor, and mainly occurs in children and adolescents. Despite advances in treatment over the past few decades, patient survival remains unsatisfactory. Thus, there is an urgent need for more effective treatments based on the molecular basis of cancer (Riggi and Stamenkovic, 2007; Mackintosh et al., 2010; Stoll et al., 2013). Several studies have shown that SEs play a critical role in the tumorigenesis, proliferation, and metastasis of Ewing sarcoma (Kennedy et al., 2015; Jacques et al., 2016; Baldauf et al., 2018; Lin et al., 2018).

Recent studies have indicated that the disease-associated fusion protein EWS-FLI1 activates or inhibits enhancer elements in Ewing sarcoma through different chromatin remodeling patterns (Riggi et al., 2014; Tomazou et al., 2015). Baldauf et al. (2018) found out that the EWSR1-ETS-targeted genes—*BCL11B* and *GLG1*—are driven by SEs through immunohistochemistry analysis. They found that both *BCL11B* and *GLG1* are more specific than *CD99* for Ewing sarcoma, suggesting that *BCL11B* and *GLG1* can be used as novel biomarkers for the diagnosis of Ewing sarcoma. Therefore, the discovery of *BCL11B* and *GLG1* may significantly reduce the number of misdiagnosed patients, thereby improving the care of patients with Ewing sarcoma.

Lin et al. (2018) used epigenetic genomics analysis to characterize transcriptional disorders in Ewing sarcoma. By focusing on SEs and its associated transcriptional regulatory mechanisms, they demonstrated that SE-associated transcripts are significantly enriched in the *EWS-FLI1* target gene, which contributes to aberrant transcription in Ewing sarcoma and mediates the specific sensitivity of Ewing sarcoma to transcriptional repression. Through comprehensive analysis, the authors identified *MEIS1* as a SE-driven oncogene that synergizes with *EWS-FLI1* in transcriptional regulation and plays a key role in pro-survival in Ewing sarcoma. Besides, they identified that the SE-related gene *APCCD1*, a downstream target of *MEIS1* and *EWS-FLI1*, was also a novel tumor-promoting factor for Ewing sarcoma.

The main known carcinogenic event in Ewing sarcoma is somatic chromosomal translocation that occurs most commonly between chromosomes 11 and 22 and results in a fusion between the 5′ region of the *EWS* gene and the 3′ region of the ETS family gene *FLI1* (Delattre et al., 1992). Kennedy et al. (2015) suggested that while direct targeting of aberrant transcription factors remains a pharmacological challenge, identifying the dependence of *EWS/FLI1* expression will provide new therapeutic avenues. They used SE analysis, near-genome shRNA assay, and small-molecule screening to identify cyclin D1 and CDK to characterize the selective dependence of Ewing sarcoma. They found that SEs regulate cyclin D1 and promote its expression in Ewing sarcoma. Moreover, Ewing sarcoma cells require CDK4 and cyclin D1 to survive and do not rely on adherent growth. Pharmacological inhibition through CDK4 with selective CDK4/6 inhibitors results in cytostasis and cell death of Ewing sarcoma cell lines *in vitro* as well as growth retardation in the Ewing sarcoma xenograft model *in vivo*. These results showed the dependence of Ewing sarcoma on CDK4 and cyclin D1; hence, CDK4/6 inhibitors can be explored further for the treatment of patients with Ewing sarcoma.

Jacques et al. (2016) focused on the *EWS-FLI1* gene, the most popular target of Ewing sarcoma, and inspired by related research, hypothesized that the expression of *EWS-FLI1* gene may be regulated by the SEs and activated by BET bromodomain activity. Based on this, they proposed that JQ1 can directly target the *EWS-FLI1* gene, releasing BRD4 from the *EWS-FLI1* promoter, thereby resulting in down-regulation of *EWS-FLI1* gene expression and inhibiting the progression and metastasis of Ewing sarcoma (Jacques et al., 2016). They proved that JQ1 can down-regulate the expression of *EWS-FLI1*, as well as inhibit the downstream gene expression of *EWS-FLI1* through a series of cell proliferation, qRT-PCR, western blotting, and CHIP analysis experiments. Hence, it was proposed as a good therapeutic drug for Ewing sarcoma. The possible functional mechanism of SEs in Ewing sarcoma is shown in **Figure 2**.

## SEs in Chordoma

Chordoma is a major bone tumor that originates from the residual spinal cord tissue and occurs in the skull base, spine, and tibia (Salisbury, 1993; McMaster et al., 2001). Chordoma usually presents as a slow-growing but locally aggressive malignant tumor. There is still a recurrence tendency after surgery and radiotherapy. Given the inadequate understanding of the disease mechanism of chordoma, patients with advanced disease usually show poor prognosis because of the lack of effective therapies (Barry et al., 2011; Stacchiotti and Sommer, 2015).

Sharifnia et al. (2019) identified a SE-associated oncogenic TF named TBXT (developmental transcription factor T) with high expression in chordoma using comprehensive methods such as CRISPR-Cas9 screening, RNA-seq, and RT-qPCR. They found that CDK inhibitors can inhibit the proliferation of chordoma cells. They further demonstrated that TBXT is a SE-associated TF in chordoma. Similar to other diseases, SEs are associated with genes (*TBXT* in chordoma) that are critical for disease identity and maintenance. The dysregulation of *TBXT* regulated by SEs is the main feature of the regulatory environment in chordoma cells (Sharifnia et al., 2019). The possible functional mechanism of SEs in chordoma is shown in **Figure 2**.

## SEs in Multiple Myeloma

Multiple myeloma (MM) is a malignant tumor that originates from antibody-secreting plasma cells and is driven by many genetic and epigenetic changes (Landgren et al., 2009; Weiss et al., 2009; Kuehl and Bergsagel, 2012). Research efforts have revealed the involvement of SEs-associated genes such as *IRF4* (Jin et al., 2018) and *MYC* (Loven et al., 2013; Affer et al., 2014). Studies showed that these SEs-associated genes are critical for the tumorigenesis and development of MM.

Amorim et al. (2016) proposed that bromodomain binds to the acetylated lysine residue on the histone tail, allowing the

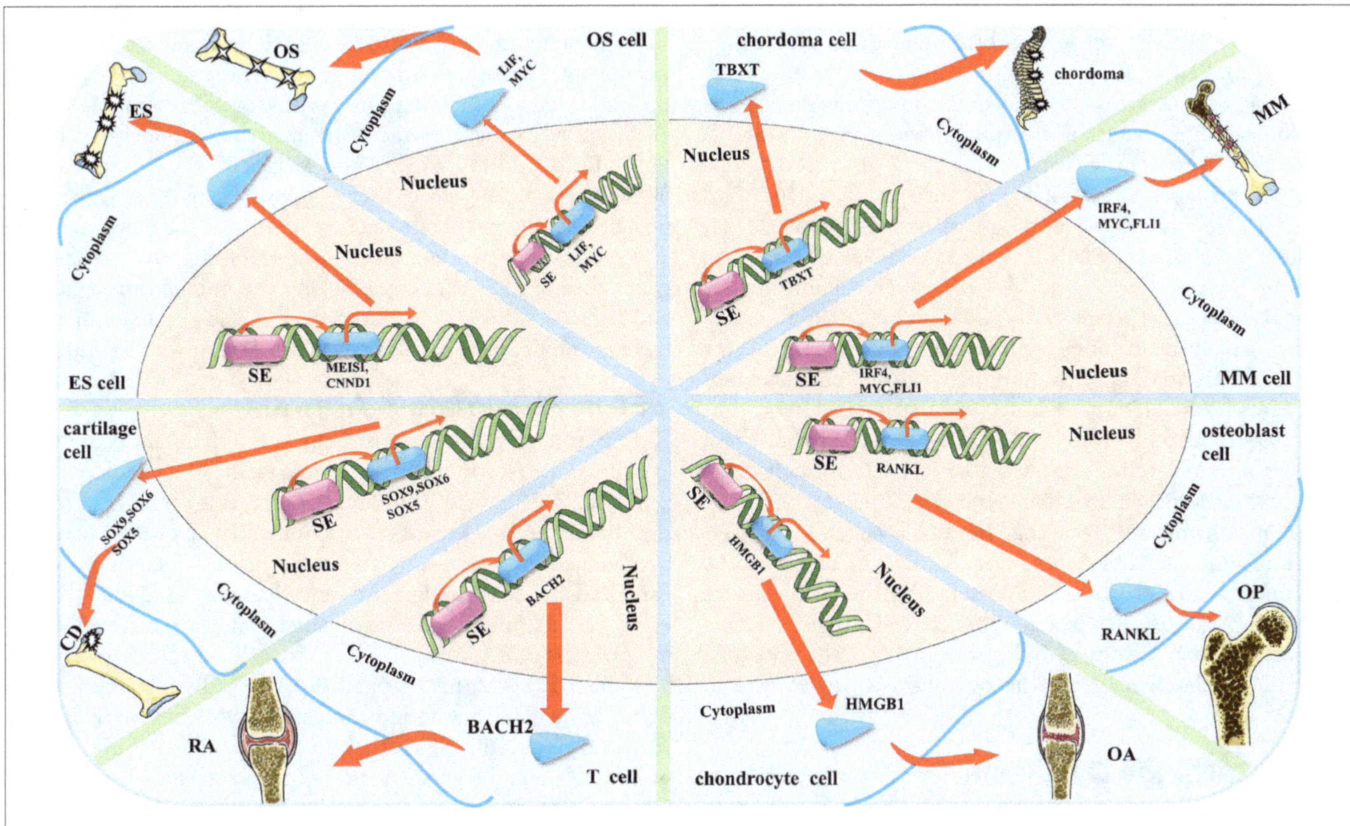


**FIGURE 2 |** The possible mechanism of super enhancers (SEs) in the eight main bone-related diseases discussed in this review. SE accelerates the progress of the four bone-related diseases by activating or up-regulating the expression of bone-related disease-specific genes that are near the related SEs (OS, osteosarcoma; ES, Ewing sarcoma; OP, osteoporosis; CD, cartilage dysplasia; RA, rheumatoid arthritis; OA, osteoarthritis; and MM, multiple myeloma).

extension complex that binds to the terminal portion of the protein to enter the promoter region of the gene, triggering gene transcription. Fulciniti et al. (2018) discovered that non-overlapping control of the promoter and SE-dependent transcriptomes in MM contributed to the growth and proliferation of MM. They also discovered the relationship between the transcription factor E2F and the transcriptional coactivator BRD4 in MM. They demonstrated the existence of two different regulatory pathways and showed that they can synergistically promote the growth and proliferation of MM. The discovered transcriptional regulatory mechanisms provide a theoretical basis for the development of new treatments for MM and other malignancies.

Affer et al. (2014) proposed that the *MYC* locus in MM has a loose rearrangement of enhancers and SEs that causes dysregulation of *MYC*. They proposed that rearrangement like this reposition of *MYC* nearby the genes related to SEs accelerates the progress of MM (Affer et al., 2014).

Although MM is well characterized in terms of genome and transcription, the abnormal regulatory network of the gene that supports this disease is still not well understood. Jin et al. (2018) described the regulatory elements and TF footprint in primary MM cells by RNA-seq and ChIP-seq assay. They established a SE-related TF-based regulatory network and identified several novel TFs critical for the biology of MM based on the newly established regulatory network. Their study indicated that *IRF4* and *FLI1* showed significant overlap with 92% of all SEs in MM cells and could promote the growth and proliferation of MM. These findings will provide potential therapeutic targets and new solutions for the treatment of MM.

Chromatin regulatory factors have become attractive targets for cancer therapy, but the mechanisms involved in inhibiting the gene-specific effects of tumor cells caused by these common regulatory factors are not well understood yet. Loven et al. (2013) investigated the mechanisms involved in the selective inhibition of *MYC* oncogenes in MM caused by inhibition of transcriptional coactivator BRD4. They found that treatment of MM tumor cells with the BET domain inhibitor, JQ1, resulted in preferential loss of BRD4 in *MYC*-SEs and subsequent transcriptional extension defects, which preferentially affected SE-associated genes such as *MYC*. This also consequently inhibited the progression of MM. The possible functional mechanism of SEs in MM is shown in **Figure 2**.

## SEs in Osteoporosis

Osteoporosis is a metabolic disease caused by reduced bone formation and/or increased bone resorption, which results in decreased bone mass and increased bone fragility. It is characterized by reduced bone mineral density (BMD) and low bone mass. Osteoporosis has become a global health concern.

Zhu et al. (2018) found a SE-associated gene—*RANKL*—was critical for the progress of osteoporosis, by analyzing the ChIP-seq Data from ENCODE.

Some significant genome-wide association studies (GWAS) have shown that single nucleotide polymorphisms (SNPs) near *RANKL* are associated with osteoporosis on chromosome 13q14.11 (Zhang et al., 2014; Kuosmanen et al., 2016). Zhu et al. (2018) identified five BMD-associated SNPs (rs9533094, rs9533090, rs9594738, rs8001611, and rs9533095) that may be related to osteoporosis in the SEs region via bioinformatics data analysis and experimental validation. *RANKL* is a key regulator involved in bone remodeling and is critical for osteoclast differentiation, activation, survival, and enhancement of bone resorption (Lacey et al., 1998; Hsu et al., 1999; Jimi et al., 1999; Sobacchi et al., 2007). They proposed that these five SNPs up-regulate the expression of *RANKL* through long-range chromosomal interaction with SEs, thereby affecting bone metabolism and resulting in an imbalance between bone resorption and bone formation, leading to osteoporosis. These findings are critical to understanding the pathogenesis of osteoporosis. Research about *RANKL* will provide a new approach to the treatment of osteoporosis. The possible functional mechanism of SEs in osteoporosis are shown in **Figure 2**.

## SEs in Cartilage Dysplasia

During the development of vertebrate embryo, chondrocytes build hundreds of vital cartilage anlagen that provide morphological and skeletal support. Their unique elongation property can rapidly drive body growth (Liu and Lefebvre, 2015). Cartilage dysplasia (CD) can seriously affect people's bone formation and growth (Warman et al., 2011). If cartilage dysplasia occurs in childhood, it will lead to lifelong defects like dwarfism or may even be fatal. Therefore, it is necessary to clarify the mechanisms related to cartilage development. Ohba et al. (2015) reported that *SOX9*-related SEs up-regulate the expression of *SOX9* gene which can promote cartilage formation. Liu and Lefebvre (2015) showed that three SOX proteins (SOX9, SOX6, and SOX5) play critical roles in chondrocyte development through SEs.

Using ChIP-seq, Ohba et al. (2015) discovered that the upstream region of key cartilage-related genes such as *SOX9* binds to a large number of enhancers and is rich in H3K27ac protein (characteristic of SEs). They found that the expression of the SEs-related genes (key cartilage-associated genes such as *SOX9*) is significantly higher than those associated with TEs. With reference to the above findings, Symon and Harley (2017) speculated that *SOX9*-related SEs up-regulate the expression of *SOX9* gene that can promote cartilage formation.

Liu and Lefebvre (2015) studied the target genes and functional modes of three SOX proteins (SOX9, SOX6, and SOX5) on chondrocytes using GWAS. They used rat chondrosarcoma (RCS) cell lines as a reliable model for chondrocytes and found that SOX6 and SOX9 bind thousands of genomic loci that are often close to each other. Although SOX proteins bind to a small number of TEs, they bind multiple sites on almost all SEs in RCS cells. These SEs are primarily associated with cartilage-specific genes. The three SOX proteins work together to activate these SEs. It is required for *in vivo* expression of their associated genes. These genes encode key regulatory factors including these three SOX proteins, as well as all essential cartilage extracellular matrix components. Chst11, Fgfr3, Runx2, and Runx3 are new targets for the three identified SOX proteins. Therefore, they proposed that these three SOX proteins closely cooperate with each other in the whole genome and effectively activate a large number of chondrocyte-specific genes through SEs, thereby realizing the unique differentiation and regulation process of chondrocytes. The possible functional mechanism of SEs in cartilage dysplasia are shown in **Figure 2**.

## SEs in Rheumatoid Arthritis

Rheumatoid arthritis (RA) is a chronic inflammatory synovitis systemic disease of unknown etiology. It is characterized by multiple, symmetric, and invasive arthritis of the joints of the hands and feet, often accompanied by extra-articular involvement and serum positivity for rheumatoid factor, which can lead to joint deformity and loss of function. Vahedi et al. (2015) found a SEs-associated gene *BACH2* critical for the progress of RA.

Vahedi et al. (2015) mapped the T-cell SEs through a series of experiments. They found that many cytokines and cytokine receptor genes with SEs structure are essential for the process of RA. *BACH2*, the gene encoding the key negative regulator of effector differentiation, is the most prominent T-cell SE. This reveals a network by which SE-related genes essential for T cell biology are inhibited by *BACH2*. Immune-mediated diseases (including RA) typically occur when disease-related SNPs are highly enriched in T-cell SEs rather than TEs. Treatment of T cells with the JAK inhibitor tofacitinib disproportionately alters the expression of RA risk genes with SEs structure. Based on these findings, the depiction of SEs can accurately identify key regulatory nodes in T cells that can be preferentially regulated by pharmacological interventions. It may provide new targets for the treatment of RA or other diseases. The possible functional mechanism of SEs in RA are shown in **Figure 2**.

## SEs in Osteoarthritis

Osteoarthritis is a common age-related degenerative disease that causes severe joint pain and physical dysfunction and is one of the important causes of disability in the elderly population (Xing et al., 2016). Despite its high incidence, the disease mechanism is poorly understood. Therefore, clarifying its etiology and pathogenesis can provide new drug targets for the clinical treatment of the disease. Jiang et al. (2017) found that SE inhibitor JQ1 can inhibit the progression of osteoarthritis by regulating the expression of *HMGB1*.

A growing number of studies have reported an important role for BRD4 in the pathology of inflammatory diseases which suggest its enormous potential as a drug target. Jiang et al. (2017) found that the BRD4 inhibitor, JQ1, inhibits the progression of osteoarthritis through dual effects on HMGB1 and NF-κB signaling pathways, proving that BRD4 may be a new target for the treatment of osteoarthritis. They found that BRD4 is enriched in the upstream non-promoter region of *HMGB1* by using the ChIP assay. In addition, treatment with JQ1 induced BRD4 release from the non-promoter and binding sites of *HMGB1*. They also found abundant enrichment of H3K27ac in the *HMGB1* promoter and upstream non-promoter region. Therefore, they speculated that the SEs may mediate the regulatory role of BRD4 in the expression of HMGB1. However, they could only prove that BRD4 may be a new target for the treatment of osteoarthritis, as the mechanism of SEs on BRD4 and HMGB1 was not investigated in their study. The possible functional mechanism of SEs in osteoarthritis are shown in **Figure 2**.

## TARGETING SEs FOR BONE-RELATED DISEASE THERAPY

Notably, as SEs harbor TFs binding sites with high density, a small change in the number of binding TFs can cause significant changes in associated gene transcription. Thus, disruption of the SEs structure and function should be the focus of disease therapy. Besides, as bone-related diseases prefer hijacking SEs to drive their aberrant transcription program which promotes disease processes like growth and metastasis, SEs have been exploited as a drug target with great potential for clinical treatment of bone-related diseases. Therefore, many researchers proposed that SEs can be considered as therapeutic targets. Accordingly, several types of small molecule inhibitors have been developed for the clinical treatment of bone-related diseases (shown in **Table 2**). Thus far, BET inhibitors and CDK inhibitors are the most widely used small molecule inhibitors (Jia et al., 2019). To a certain extent, drugs that target key components of SEs, such as BRD4 and CDK7, provide a novel strategy for better treatment of bone-related diseases.

### BET Inhibitors Targeting SEs

The BET family proteins including BRD2, BRD3, BRD4, and BRDT play a key role in chromatin remodeling and transcriptional regulation. JQ1, the first BET inhibitor applied to target BET bromodomain was discovered by Filippakopoulos et al. (2010). Recently, many studies have shown that JQ1 has anti-proliferative activity against many cancers, and it exhibits anti-proliferative activity mainly via inhibiting c-MYC expression and up-regulating p21 expression (Delmore et al., 2011; Dang, 2012). Jia et al. (2019) concluded that JQ1 treatment displaces BRD4 preferably from histone proteins and disrupts SEs. Partly, the mechanism by which BET inhibitors like JQ1 inhibit bone-related disease progression is through repressing the SE-associated genes that are critical for bone-related diseases. As mentioned above, JQ1 treatment on MM cells decreased BRD4 binding at SEs and subsequently repressed the SE-associated genes of MM (Loven et al., 2013). It is also reported that JQ1 can inhibit the growth and disease process of osteosarcoma by repressing the SEs containing oncogenes by limiting *MYC* expression (Chen et al., 2018). However, others found that JQ1 treatment inhibits the growth and disease process of osteosarcoma by targeting *RUNX2* instead of *MYC* through influencing SEs (Lee et al., 2015). Another study initiated by

**TABLE 2** | Inhibitor which targeting SEs in bone-related diseases.

| Diseases | Inhibitor | Target of the inhibitor | Effect on SEs-driven transcription | Effects of SEs inhibition on diseases | References |
|---|---|---|---|---|---|
| Multiple myeloma | JQ1 | BRD4 | Decrease of BRD4 binding at SEs and downregulation of SEs associated genes | Repression of the progression of multiple myeloma | Loven et al., 2013 |
| Osteosarcoma | JQ1 | BRD4 | Restraining of the expression of *MYC* | Inhibition of the growth and proliferation of osteosarcoma | Chen et al., 2018 |
| Osteosarcoma | JQ1 | BRD4 | Restraining of the expression of *RUNX2* | Inhibition of the growth and proliferation of osteosarcoma | Lee et al., 2015 |
| Osteosarcoma | THZ1 | CDK7 | Downregulation of SEs associated genes | Suppressing the proliferation, migration of osteosarcoma | Chen et al., 2018 |
| Chordoma | THZ1 | CDK7 | Downregulation of SEs associated genes *TBXT* | Suppressing the proliferation of chordoma | Sharifnia et al., 2019 |
| Osteosarcoma | THZ2 | CDK7 | Downregulation of SEs associated genes *LIF*, *STAT3*, *NOTCH1* | Impeding the proliferation and metastasis of osteosarcoma | Zhang et al., 2020 |
| Ewing sarcoma | LEE011 | CDK4/6 | Downregulation of SEs associated genes | Impairing the progression of Ewing sarcoma | Kennedy et al., 2015 |
| Osteoarthritis | JQ1 | BRD4 | Downregulation of SEs associated gene *HMGB1* | Inhibiting the progression of osteoarthritis | Jiang et al., 2017 |

Jacques et al. proposed that the use of JQ1 can repress the expression of *EWS-FLI1* by disrupting the *EWS-FLI1*-associated SEs and subsequently control the disease process in Ewing sarcoma (Jacques et al., 2016). Besides, Jiang et al. (2017) showed that JQ1 treatment-induced BRD4 release from the non-promoter and binding sites of *HMGB1*. They also hypothesized that it can inhibit the progression of osteoarthritis. In conclusion, SEs are sensitive to bromodomain inhibition. BET inhibitors have great therapeutic potential in bone-related diseases.

Up to now, researchers have initialed clinical trials about BET inhibitors applied in treatment for bone-related diseases. NCT03068351, one clinical trial, found that BET inhibitor RO6870810 may apply for combination therapy for MM. Another clinical trial, NCT02157636, demonstrated that BET inhibitor CPI-0610 can inhibit the progress of MM. But there aren't clinical trials related to the above SEs-inhibitors initiated. In addition, there aren't study articles about these two BET-inhibitors, with completed or registered clinical trials carried out, repress the progression of bone-related diseases through SEs reported. So, it's necessary to verify the clinical treatment effect of the above potential SEs-inhibitors of bone-related diseases through clinical trials.

### CDK Inhibitors Targeting SEs

RNA Pol II, the central enzyme functioning in protein-coding gene transcription, initiation, and elongation, is particularly regulated by CDK7—one of the CDKs (Larochelle et al., 2012). CDK7 can phosphorylate the carboxyl-terminal domain of RPB1 (CTD) of RNA Pol II (RNAPIICTD), thereby regulating transcriptional initiation and pause release, as well as elongation (Palancade and Bensaude, 2003; Glover-Cutter et al., 2009; Larochelle et al., 2012). An increasing number of CDK7 inhibitors have been developed including THZ1 and THZ2. THZ1 is an advanced CDK7 inhibitor that has been reported to have the ability to target the general transcriptional elements and disrupt SEs (Kwiatkowski et al., 2014). Consistent with this, other similar findings of CDK7 inhibitor and SEs have been reported in bone-related cancers. For instance, THZ1 can suppress the proliferation, migration, and invasion of osteosarcoma cells by inhibiting the expression of important SE-containing oncogenic genes (Chen et al., 2018). Sharifnia et al. (2019) found that CDK inhibitors like THZ1 can substantially suppress the growth of chordoma by inhibiting the SEs which is critical for the expression of the important oncogene gene *TBXT* for chordoma. However, Li et al. (2017) reported that the translational significance and clinical application of THZ1 are limited by its short half-life. Compared with THZ1, THZ2 is a newly developed CDK7 inhibitor with a fivefold increase of half-life. Zhang et al. (2020) found that THZ2 can impede the proliferation and metastasis of osteosarcoma via targeting SE-associated oncogenes. Overall, CDK7 inhibition is another promising target treatment therapy for bone-related diseases. Besides CDK7 inhibitors, researchers also suggested that CDK4/6 inhibitors like LEE011 can target SEs. Kennedy et al. (2015) reported that LEE011 can impair the progression of Ewing sarcoma by inhibiting the expression of CDK4/6. In conclusion, SEs are sensitive to CDK inhibition. CDK inhibitors like THZ1, THZ2, and LEE011 also have great therapeutic potential for bone-related diseases.

To date, some clinical trials have been carried out to test the treatment effect of CDK inhibitors on bone-related diseases. For example, NCT01096342, a clinical trial carried out by Kumar et al. (2015) showed that CDK inhibitor-dinaciclib (SCH 727965) can repress the progression of MM. Based on this trial, they reported an article that demonstrates the activity of dinaciclib in relapsed MM (Kumar et al., 2015). But this article didn't demonstrate that dinaciclib can repress the progression of relapsed MM through influencing SEs in MM. Unfortunately, there aren't completed or registered clinical trials related to the above SEs-inhibitors initiated. Thus, it's necessary to verify the clinical treatment effect of the above potential CDK-inhibitors of bone-related diseases through clinical trials.

### Developing New Downstream Target Genes of SEs for Bone-Related Diseases

Super-enhancers inhibitors mainly repress the progression of bone-related diseases by disrupting the SEs associated with bone-related diseases and subsequently influencing the critical oncogenes that are targeted by SEs. There are no studies yet to indicate whether SE inhibitors can be used for the potential treatment of bone-related diseases like osteoporosis, cartilage dysplasia, and RA. In the future, besides carrying out studies using the above two kinds of SEs inhibitors as a treatment approach for bone-related diseases, we should focus more on developing new downstream target genes of SEs for the diagnosis and treatment of bone-related diseases. This approach may ensure sufficient and varied treatment strategies for bone-related diseases.

## SUMMARY AND PERSPECTIVE

The rapid development of bioinformatics technology has driven the study of the genetic mechanism of diseases, which has helped researchers and clinicians to better understand the underlying mechanisms of several disease conditions. Furthermore, some intractable diseases have become less difficult to treat. However, the pathogenic mechanisms of many other complex diseases remain unclear, such as osteosarcoma, Ewing sarcoma, and other bone-related diseases with poor prognosis. Multiple studies have reported novel insights of which many include SEs-associated genes such as *MYC* (Loven et al., 2013; Zhang et al., 2020) LIF, (Lu et al., 2020), and *EWS-FLI1* (Jacques et al., 2016), and SEs-inhibitors with therapeutic effects such as JQ1 (Loven et al., 2013; Lee et al., 2015; Jiang et al., 2017; Chen et al., 2018), THZ1 (Chen et al., 2018; Sharifnia et al., 2019), and THZ2 (Zhang et al., 2020) on diseases like osteosarcoma, Ewing sarcoma, MM, chordoma, and osteoarthritis. However, for osteoporosis, cartilage dysplasia, and RA, only a few therapeutic drugs have been reported that can efficiently target SEs or SEs-associated genes. Besides, there are rarely completed or registered clinical trials that investigate the clinical treatment effect of the potential SEs-inhibitors initiated. Therefore, future research should focus more on the SEs-associated mechanism of the above bone-related diseases and it is so urgent to initiate more clinical trials that testify the potential clinical application of the above-mentioned SEs-inhibitors.

In summary, the above studies on SEs in bone-related diseases focused on the identification of disease-specific SEs and their target genes, followed by verification of the effects of the screened target gene through related *in vitro* and *in vivo* experiments. The specific stepwise method is as follows: first, identifying the bone cancer-related SEs and verifying the most related SEs by techniques such as ChIP-seq. Second, screening target genes associated with the SEs through bioinformatics analysis for building therapies for bone cancer. Finally, testing the potential and accuracy of target genes via *in vitro* and *in vivo* experiments. We believe that the findings from SEs studies will be helpful for the treatment for difficult-to-treat bone-related diseases in the future. However, to a certain degree, as the SEs-related studies most involve in cancer field, the SEs-related studies in skeleton field are rare. So, we can explore the role of SEs in skeleton field in future studies.

The discovery of SEs is a scientific and clinical breakthrough. Many studies have proven that the abnormal expression of SEs is closely related to the disease process. Therefore, research on SEs has gained immense clinical importance. By studying the expression of SEs in diseases, clarifying the pathogenesis of diseases, and finding accurate and efficient target genes, new treatment options can be developed. Thus, it is necessary to study the functions of SEs in bone-related diseases. Recent years have witnessed rapid advancements in technologies like ChIP with high-throughput sequencing (Schmidt et al., 2009) and CRISPR genome editing tool (Burgess, 2013), which offer novel insights into the function and biophysical formation of SEs, as well as the regulatory mechanisms of the targeted gene. With the accumulation of related research, the role of SEs in bone-related diseases is becoming more and more clear. However, as shown above, many studies are on the phenomenon level, and the mechanism researches such as how SEs are regulated and the detailed molecular mechanism of how SEs regulate its target genes are still insufficient. Therefore, the research on the deep and detailed mechanism needs to be strengthened in the future. Besides, the potential of the clinical application of SEs inhibitors in bone-related diseases needs to be further explored. Therefore, future studies of SEs should focus on how to better utilize SEs in the targeted therapy of bone-related diseases in clinical.

## AUTHOR CONTRIBUTIONS

QL and ZL conceived of this review. ZO and JQ drafted the manuscript. WW and ZO designed the figures. GL and JW designed the tables. JQ revised the manuscript. All authors were involved in the critical revision of the manuscript and approved the final version.

## REFERENCES


Affer, M., Chesi, M., Chen, W. G., Keats, J. J., Demchenko, Y. N., Roschke, A. V., et al. (2014). Promiscuous MYC locus rearrangements hijack enhancers but mostly super-enhancers to dysregulate MYC expression in multiple myeloma. *Leukemia* 28, 1725–1735. doi: 10.1038/leu.2014.70

Amorim, S., Stathis, A., Gleeson, M., Iyengar, S., Magarotto, V., Leleu, X., et al. (2016). Bromodomain inhibitor OTX015 in patients with lymphoma or multiple myeloma: a dose-escalation, open-label, pharmacokinetic, phase 1 study. *Lancet Haematol.* 3, e196–e204. doi: 10.1016/S2352-3026(16)00021-1

Baldauf, M. C., Orth, M. F., Dallmayer, M., Marchetto, A., Gerke, J. S., Rubio, R. A., et al. (2018). Robust diagnosis of Ewing sarcoma by immunohistochemical detection of super-enhancer-driven EWSR1-ETS targets. *Oncotarget* 9, 1587–1601. doi: 10.18632/oncotarget.20098

Barry, J. J., Jian, B. J., Sughrue, M. E., Kane, A. J., Mills, S. A., Tihan, T., et al. (2011). The next step: innovative molecular targeted therapies for treatment of intracranial chordoma patients. *Neurosurgery* 68, 231–241. doi: 10.1227/NEU.0b013e3181fd2ac5

Brown, J. D., Lin, C. Y., Duan, Q., Griffin, G., Federation, A., Paranal, R. M., et al. (2014). NF-kappaB directs dynamic super enhancer formation in inflammation and atherogenesis. *Mol. Cell* 56, 219–231. doi: 10.1016/j.molcel.2014.08.024

Bulger, M., and Groudine, M. (2011). Functional and mechanistic diversity of distal transcription enhancers. *Cell* 144, 327–339. doi: 10.1016/j.cell.2011.01.024

Burgess, D. J. (2013). Technology: a CRISPR genome-editing tool. *Nat. Rev. Genet.* 14:80. doi: 10.1038/nrg3409

Chapuy, B., McKeown, M. R., Lin, C. Y., Monti, S., Roemer, M. G., Qi, J., et al. (2013). Discovery and characterization of super-enhancer-associated dependencies in diffuse large B cell lymphoma. *Cancer Cell* 24, 777–790. doi: 10.1016/j.ccr.2013.11.003

Chen, D., Zhao, Z., Huang, Z., Chen, D., Zhu, X., Wang, Y., et al. (2018). Super enhancer inhibitors suppress MYC driven transcriptional amplification and tumor progression in osteosarcoma. *Bone Res.* 6:11. doi: 10.1038/s41413-018-0009-8

Chipumuro, E., Marco, E., Christensen, C. L., Kwiatkowski, N., Zhang, T., Hatheway, C. M., et al. (2014). CDK7 inhibition suppresses super-enhancer-linked oncogenic transcription in MYCN-driven cancer. *Cell* 159, 1126–1139. doi: 10.1016/j.cell.2014.10.024

Dang, C. V. (2012). MYC on the path to cancer. *Cell* 149, 22–35. doi: 10.1016/j.cell.2012.03.003

Delattre, O., Zucman, J., Plougastel, B., Desmaze, C., Melot, T., Peter, M., et al. (1992). Gene fusion with an ETS DNA-binding domain caused by chromosome translocation in human tumours. *Nature* 359, 162–165. doi: 10.1038/359162a0

Delmore, J. E., Issa, G. C., Lemieux, M. E., Rahl, P. B., Shi, J., Jacobs, H. M., et al. (2011). BET bromodomain inhibition as a therapeutic strategy to target c-Myc. *Cell* 146, 904–917. doi: 10.1016/j.cell.2011.08.017

Demchenko, Y., Roschke, A., Chen, W. D., Asmann, Y., Bergsagel, P. L., and Kuehl, W. M. (2016). Frequent occurrence of large duplications at reciprocal genomic rearrangement breakpoints in multiple myeloma and other tumors. *Nucleic Acids Res.* 44, 8189–8198. doi: 10.1093/nar/gkw527

Encode Project Consortium (2004). The ENCODE (ENCyclopedia Of DNA Elements) Project. *Science* 306, 636–640. doi: 10.1126/science.1105136

Filippakopoulos, P., Qi, J., Picaud, S., Shen, Y., Smith, W. B., Fedorov, O., et al. (2010). Selective inhibition of BET bromodomains. *Nature* 468, 1067–1073. doi: 10.1038/nature09504

Fulciniti, M., Lin, C. Y., Samur, M. K., Lopez, M. A., Singh, I., Lawlor, M. A., et al. (2018). Non-overlapping control of transcriptome by promoter- and super-enhancer-associated dependencies in multiple myeloma. *Cell. Rep.* 25, 3693–3705. doi: 10.1016/j.celrep.2018.12.016

Furlong, E., and Levine, M. (2018). Developmental enhancers and chromosome topology. *Science* 361, 1341–1345. doi: 10.1126/science.aau0320

Glover-Cutter, K., Larochelle, S., Erickson, B., Zhang, C., Shokat, K., Fisher, R. P., et al. (2009). TFIIH-associated Cdk7 kinase functions in phosphorylation of C-terminal domain Ser7 residues, promoter-proximal pausing, and termination by RNA polymerase II. *Mol. Cell Biol.* 29, 5455–5464.doi: 10.1128/MCB.00637-09

Gröschel, S., Sanders, M. A., Hoogenboezem, R., de Wit, E., Bouwman, B., Erpelinck, C., et al. (2014). A single oncogenic enhancer rearrangement causes concomitant EVI1 and GATA2 deregulation in leukemia. *Cell* 157, 369–381. doi: 10.1016/j.cell.2014.02.019

Hnisz, D., Abraham, B. J., Lee, T. I., Lau, A., Saint-André, V., Sigova, A. A., et al. (2013). Super-enhancers in the control of cell identity and disease. *Cell* 155, 934–947. doi: 10.1016/j.cell.2013.09.053

Hnisz, D., Day, D. S., and Young, R. A. (2016). Insulated neighborhoods: structural and functional units of mammalian gene control. *Cell* 167, 1188–1200. doi: 10.1016/j.cell.2016.10.024

Hsu, H., Lacey, D. L., Dunstan, C. R., Solovyev, I., Colombero, A., Timms, E., et al. (1999). Tumor necrosis factor receptor family member RANK mediates osteoclast differentiation and activation induced by osteoprotegerin ligand. *Proc. Natl. Acad. Sci. U.S.A.* 96, 3540–3545. doi: 10.1073/pnas.96.7.3540

Jacques, C., Lamoureux, F., Baud'Huin, M., Calleja, L. R., Quillard, T., Amiaud, J., et al. (2016). Targeting the epigenetic readers in Ewing Sarcoma inhibits the oncogenic transcription factor EWS/Fli1. *Oncotarget* 7, 24125–24140. doi: 10.18632/oncotarget.8214

Jia, Y., Chng, W. J., and Zhou, J. (2019). Super-enhancers: critical roles and therapeutic targets in hematologic malignancies. *J. Hematol. Oncol.* 12:77. doi: 10.1186/s13045-019-0757-y

Jiang, Y., Zhu, L., Zhang, T., Lu, H., Wang, C., Xue, B., et al. (2017). BRD4 has dual effects on the HMGB1 and NF-kappa B signalling pathways and is a potential therapeutic target for osteoarthritis. *Biochim. Biophys. Acta Mol. Basis Dis.* 1863, 3001–3015. doi: 10.1016/j.bbadis.2017.08.009

Jimi, E., Akiyama, S., Tsurukai, T., Okahashi, N., Kobayashi, K., Udagawa, N., et al. (1999). Osteoclast differentiation factor acts as a multifunctional regulator in murine osteoclast differentiation and function. *J. Immunol.* 163, 434–442.

Jin, Y., Chen, K., De Paepe, A., Hellqvist, E., Krstic, A. D., Metang, L., et al. (2018). Active enhancer and chromatin accessibility landscapes chart the regulatory network of primary multiple myeloma. *Blood* 131, 2138–2150. doi: 10.1182/blood-2017-09-808063

Kempf-Bielack, B., Bielack, S. S., Jurgens, H., Branscheid, D., Berdel, W. E., Exner, G. U., et al. (2005). Osteosarcoma relapse after combined modality therapy: an analysis of unselected patients in the cooperative osteosarcoma study group (COSS). *J. Clin. Oncol.* 23, 559–568. doi: 10.1200/JCO.2005.04.063

Kennedy, A. L., Vallurupalli, M., Chen, L., Crompton, B., Cowley, G., Vazquez, F., et al. (2015). Functional, chemical genomic, and super-enhancer screening identify sensitivity to cyclin D1/CDK4 pathway inhibition in Ewing sarcoma. *Oncotarget* 6, 30178–30193. doi: 10.18632/oncotarget.4903

Khan, A., and Zhang, X. (2016). dbSUPER: a database of super-enhancers in mouse and human genome. *Nucleic Acids Res.* 44, D164–D171. doi: 10.1093/nar/gkv1002

Kuehl, W. M., and Bergsagel, P. L. (2012). Molecular pathogenesis of multiple myeloma and its premalignant precursor. *J. Clin. Invest.* 122, 3456–3463. doi: 10.1172/JCI61188

Kumar, S. K., LaPlant, B., Chng, W. J., Zonder, J., Callander, N., Fonseca, R., et al. (2015). Dinaciclib, a novel CDK inhibitor, demonstrates encouraging single-agent activity in patients with relapsed multiple myeloma. *Blood* 125, 443–448. doi: 10.1182/blood-2014-05-573741

Kuosmanen, S. M., Viitala, S., Laitinen, T., Perakyla, M., Polonen, P., Kansanen, E., et al. (2016). The Effects of Sequence Variation on Genome-wide NRF2 Binding–New Target Genes and Regulatory SNPs. *Nucleic Acids Res.* 44, 1760–1775. doi: 10.1093/nar/gkw052

Kwiatkowski, N., Zhang, T., Rahl, P. B., Abraham, B. J., Reddy, J., Ficarro, S. B., et al. (2014). Targeting transcription regulation in cancer with a covalent CDK7 inhibitor. *Nature* 511, 616–620. doi: 10.1038/nature13393

Lacey, D. L., Timms, E., Tan, H. L., Kelley, M. J., Dunstan, C. R., Burgess, T., et al. (1998). Osteoprotegerin ligand is a cytokine that regulates osteoclast differentiation and activation. *Cell* 93, 165–176. doi: 10.1016/s0092-8674(00)81569-x

Landgren, O., Kyle, R. A., Pfeiffer, R. M., Katzmann, J. A., Caporaso, N. E., Hayes, R. B., et al. (2009). Monoclonal gammopathy of undetermined significance (MGUS) consistently precedes multiple myeloma: a prospective study. *Blood* 113, 5412–5417. doi: 10.1182/blood-2008-12-194241

Larochelle, S., Amat, R., Glover-Cutter, K., Sanso, M., Zhang, C., Allen, J. J., et al. (2012). Cyclin-dependent kinase control of the initiation-to-elongation switch of RNA polymerase II. *Nat. Struct. Mol. Biol.* 19, 1108–1115. doi: 10.1038/nsmb.2399

Lee, D. H., Qi, J., Bradner, J. E., Said, J. W., Doan, N. B., Forscher, C., et al. (2015). Synergistic effect of JQ1 and rapamycin for treatment of human osteosarcoma. *Int. J. Cancer* 136, 2055–2064. doi: 10.1002/ijc.29269

Li, B., Ni, C. T., Fan, Y., Madden, S. F., Klinger, R., O'Connor, A. E., et al. (2017). Therapeutic rationale to target highly expressed CDK7 conferring poor outcomes in triple-negative breast cancer. *Cancer Res.* 77, 3834–3845. doi: 10.1158/0008-5472.CAN-16-2546

Lin, L., Huang, M., Shi, X., Mayakonda, A., Hu, K., Jiang, Y. Y., et al. (2018). Super-enhancer-associated MEIS1 promotes transcriptional dysregulation in Ewing sarcoma in co-operation with EWS-FLI1. *Nucleic Acids Res.* 47, 1255–1267. doi: 10.1093/nar/gky1207

Liu, C., and Lefebvre, V. (2015). The transcription factors SOX9 and SOX5/SOX6 cooperate genome-wide through super-enhancers to drive chondrogenesis. *Nucleic Acids Res.* 43, 8183–8203. doi: 10.1093/nar/gkv688

Loven, J., Hoke, H. A., Lin, C. Y., Lau, A., Orlando, D. A., Vakoc, C. R., et al. (2013). Selective inhibition of tumor oncogenes by disruption of super-enhancers. *Cell* 153, 320–334. doi: 10.1016/j.cell.2013.03.036

Lu, B., He, Y., He, J., Wang, L., Liu, Z., Yang, J., et al. (2020). Epigenetic profiling identifies LIF as a super-enhancer-controlled regulator of stem cell-like properties in osteosarcoma. *Mol. Cancer Res.* 18, 57–67. doi: 10.1158/1541-7786.MCR-19-0470

Luetke, A., Meyers, P. A., Lewis, I., and Juergens, H. (2014). Osteosarcoma treatment - where do we stand? A state of the art review. *Cancer Treat. Rev.* 40, 523–532. doi: 10.1016/j.ctrv.2013.11.006

Mackintosh, C., Madoz-Gurpide, J., Ordonez, J. L., Osuna, D., and Herrero-Martin, D. (2010). The molecular pathogenesis of Ewing sarcoma. *Cancer Biol. Ther.* 9, 655–667. doi: 10.4161/cbt.9.9.11511

Mansour, M. R., Abraham, B. J., Anders, L., Berezovskaya, A., Gutierrez, A., Durbin, A. D., et al. (2014). Oncogene regulation. An oncogenic super-enhancer formed through somatic mutation of a noncoding intergenic element. *Science* 346, 1373–1377. doi: 10.1126/science.1259037

McMaster, M. L., Goldstein, A. M., Bromley, C. M., Ishibe, N., and Parry, D. M. (2001). Chordoma: incidence and survival patterns in the United States, 1973-1995. *Cancer Causes Control* 12, 1–11.

Morrow, J. J., Bayles, I., Funnell, A. P. W., Miller, T. E., Saiakhova, A., Lizardo, M. M., et al. (2018). Positively selected enhancer elements endow osteosarcoma cells with metastatic competence. *Nat. Med.* 24:176. doi: 10.1038/nm.4475

Niederriter, A., Varshney, A., Parker, S., and Martin, D. (2015). Super enhancers in cancers, complex disease, and developmental disorders. *Genes* 6, 1183–1200. doi: 10.3390/genes6041183

Ohba, S., He, X., Hojo, H., and McMahon, A. P. (2015). Distinct transcriptional programs underlie Sox9 regulation of the mammalian chondrocyte. *Cell Rep.* 12, 229–243. doi: 10.1016/j.celrep.2015.06.013

Oldridge, D. A., Wood, A. C., Weichert-Leahey, N., Crimmins, I., Sussman, R., Winter, C., et al. (2015). Genetic predisposition to neuroblastoma mediated by a LMO1 super-enhancer polymorphism. *Nature* 528, 418–421. doi: 10.1038/nature15540

Palancade, B., and Bensaude, O. (2003). Investigating RNA polymerase II carboxyl-terminal domain (CTD) phosphorylation. *Eur. J. Biochem.* 270, 3859–3870. doi: 10.1046/j.1432-1033.2003.03794.x

Peeters, J. G., Vervoort, S. J., Tan, S. C., Mijnheer, G., de Roock, S., Vastert, S. J., et al. (2015). Inhibition of super-enhancer activity in autoinflammatory site-derived T cells reduces disease-associated gene expression. *Cell. Rep.* 12, 1986–1996. doi: 10.1016/j.celrep.2015.08.046

Pott, S., and Lieb, J. D. (2015). What are super-enhancers? *Nat. Genet.* 47, 8–12. doi: 10.1038/ng.3167

Riggi, N., Knoechel, B., Gillespie, S. M., Rheinbay, E., Boulay, G., Suva, M. L., et al. (2014). EWS-FLI1 utilizes divergent chromatin remodeling mechanisms to directly activate or repress enhancer elements in Ewing sarcoma. *Cancer Cell* 26, 668–681. doi: 10.1016/j.ccell.2014.10.004

Riggi, N., and Stamenkovic, I. (2007). The biology of Ewing sarcoma. *Cancer Lett.* 254, 1–10. doi: 10.1016/j.canlet.2006.12.009

Salisbury, J. R. (1993). The pathology of the human notochord. *J. Pathol.* 171, 253–255. doi: 10.1002/path.1711710404

Schmidt, D., Wilson, M. D., Spyrou, C., Brown, G. D., Hadfield, J., and Odom, D. T. (2009). ChIP-seq: using high-throughput sequencing to discover protein-DNA interactions. *Methods* 48, 240–248. doi: 10.1016/j.ymeth.2009.03.001

Sengupta, S., and George, R. E. (2017). Super-enhancer-driven transcriptional dependencies in cancer. *Trends Cancer* 3, 269–281. doi: 10.1016/j.trecan.2017.03.006

Sharifnia, T., Wawer, M. J., Chen, T., Huang, Q. Y., Weir, B. A., Sizemore, A., et al. (2019). Small-molecule targeting of brachyury transcription factor addiction in chordoma. *Nat. Med.* 25, 292–300. doi: 10.1038/s41591-018-0312-3

Shin, H. Y. (2018). Targeting super-enhancers for disease treatment and diagnosis. *Mol. Cells* 41, 506–514. doi: 10.14348/molcells.2018.2297

Sobacchi, C., Frattini, A., Guerrini, M. M., Abinun, M., Pangrazio, A., Susani, L., et al. (2007). Osteoclast-poor human osteopetrosis due to mutations in the gene encoding RANKL. *Nat. Genet.* 39, 960–962. doi: 10.1038/ng2076

Stacchiotti, S., and Sommer, J. (2015). Building a global consensus approach to chordoma: a position paper from the medical and patient community. *Lancet Oncol.* 16, e71–e83. doi: 10.1016/S1470-2045(14)71190-8

Stoll, G., Surdez, D., Tirode, F., Laud, K., Barillot, E., Zinovyev, A., et al. (2013). Systems biology of Ewing sarcoma: a network model of EWS-FLI1 effect on proliferation and apoptosis. *Nucleic Acids Res.* 41, 8853–8871. doi: 10.1093/nar/gkt678

Sur, I., and Taipale, J. (2016). The role of enhancers in cancer. *Nat. Rev. Cancer* 16, 483–493. doi: 10.1038/nrc.2016.62

Symon, A., and Harley, V. (2017). SOX9: A genomic view of tissue specific expression and action. *Int. J. Biochem. Cell Biol.* 87, 18–22. doi: 10.1016/j.biocel.2017.03.005

Thandapani, P. (2019). Super-enhancers in cancer. *Pharmacol. Ther.* 199, 129–138. doi: 10.1016/j.pharmthera.2019.02.014

Tomazou, E. M., Sheffield, N. C., Schmidl, C., Schuster, M., Schoenegger, A., Datlinger, P., et al. (2015). Epigenome mapping reveals distinct modes of gene regulation and widespread enhancer reprogramming by the oncogenic fusion protein EWS-FLI1. *Cell Rep.* 10, 1082–1095. doi: 10.1016/j.celrep.2015.01.042

Vaharautio, A., and Taipale, J. (2014). Cancer. Cancer by super-enhancer. *Science* 346, 1291–1292. doi: 10.1126/science.aaa3247

Vahedi, G., Kanno, Y., Furumoto, Y., Jiang, K., Parker, S., Erdos, M. R., et al. (2015). Super-enhancers delineate disease-associated regulatory nodes in T cells. *Nature* 520:558. doi: 10.1038/nature14154

Walker, B. A., Wardell, C. P., Brioli, A., Boyle, E., Kaiser, M. F., Begum, D. B., et al. (2014). Translocations at 8q24 juxtapose MYC with genes that harbor superenhancers resulting in overexpression and poor prognosis in myeloma patients. *Blood Cancer J.* 4:e191. doi: 10.1038/bcj.2014.13

Warman, M. L., Cormier-Daire, V., Hall, C., Krakow, D., Lachman, R., LeMerrer, M., et al. (2011). Nosology and classification of genetic skeletal disorders: 2010 revision. *Am. J. Med. Genet. A* 155A, 943–968. doi: 10.1002/ajmg.a.33909

Weiss, B. M., Abadie, J., Verma, P., Howard, R. S., and Kuehl, W. M. (2009). A monoclonal gammopathy precedes multiple myeloma in most patients. *Blood* 113, 5418–5422. doi: 10.1182/blood-2008-12-195008

Whyte, W. A., Orlando, D. A., Hnisz, D., Abraham, B. J., Lin, C. Y., Kagey, M. H., et al. (2013). Master transcription factors and mediator establish super-enhancers at key cell identity genes. *Cell* 153, 307–319. doi: 10.1016/j.cell.2013.03.035

Xing, D., Xu, Y., Liu, Q., Ke, Y., Wang, B., Li, Z., et al. (2016). Osteoarthritis and all-cause mortality in worldwide populations: grading the evidence from a meta-analysis. *Sci. Rep.* 6:24393. doi: 10.1038/srep24393

Zhang, J., Liu, W., Zou, C., Zhao, Z., Lai, Y., Shi, Z., et al. (2020). Targeting super-enhancer-associated oncogenes in osteosarcoma with THZ2, a covalent CDK7 inhibitor. *Clin Cancer Res.* 26, 2681–2692. doi: 10.1158/1078-0432.CCR-19-1418

Zhang, L., Choi, H. J., Estrada, K., Leo, P. J., Li, J., Pei, Y. F., et al. (2014). Multistage genome-wide association meta-analyses identified two new loci for bone mineral density. *Hum. Mol. Genet.* 23, 1923–1933. doi: 10.1093/hmg/ddt575

Zhang, X., Wang, Y., Chiang, H. C., Hsieh, Y. P., Lu, C., Park, B. H., et al. (2019). BRCA1 mutations attenuate super-enhancer function and chromatin looping in haploinsufficient human breast epithelial cells. *Breast Cancer Res.* 21:51. doi: 10.1186/s13058-019-1132-1

Zhu, D. L., Chen, X. F., Hu, W. X., Dong, S. S., Lu, B. J., Rong, Y., et al. (2018). Multiple functional variants at 13q14 risk locus for osteoporosis regulate RANKL expression through long-range super-enhancer. *J. Bone Miner. Res.* 33, 1335–1346. doi: 10.1002/jbmr.3419

8

# Medium-Intensity Treadmill Exercise Exerts Beneficial Effects on Bone Modeling Through Bone Marrow Mesenchymal Stromal Cells

*Lingli Zhang[1], Yu Yuan[1], Wei Wu[1], Zhongguang Sun[1], Le Lei[1], Jing Fan[2], Bo Gao[2]* and Jun Zou[1]**

[1] *School of Kinesiology, Shanghai University of Sport, Shanghai, China,* [2] *Institute of Orthopedic Surgery, Xijing Hospital, Fourth Military Medical University, Xi'an, China*

***Correspondence:***
*Bo Gao*
*gaobofmmu@hotmail.com*
*Jun Zou*
*junzou@sus.edu.cn*

As a type of multipotential cells, bone marrow mesenchymal stromal cells (BMMSCs) can differentiate into chondrocytes, osteoblasts, and adipocytes under different loading condition or specific microenvironment. Previous studies have shown that BMMSCs and their lineage-differentiated progeny (for example, osteoblasts), and osteocytes are mechanosensitive in bone. The appropriate physical activity and exercise could help attenuate bone loss, effectively stimulate bone formation, increase bone mineral density (BMD), prevent the progression of osteoporosis, and reduce the risk of bone fractures. Bone morphogenetic protein (BMP) is originally discovered as a protein with heterotopic bone-inducing activity in the bone matrix that exerts a critical role in multiple stages of bone metabolism. In the present study, the medium-intensity treadmill exercise enhanced bone formation and increased *osteocalcin (OCN)* and *osteopontin (OPN)* mRNA expression as well as activation of the BMP-Smad signaling pathway *in vivo*. In order to investigate the effect of a BMP-Smad signaling pathway, we injected mice with activated enzyme inhibitors (LDN-193189HCL) and subjected the mice to treadmill exercise intervention. LDN-193189HCL attenuated the BMD and bone mass mediated by medium-intensity exercise and BMP-Smad signaling pathway.

**Keywords: treadmill exercise, bone morphogenetic protein, BMP-Smad signaling pathway, bone marrow mesenchymal stromal cell, bone formation, enzyme inhibitor**

## INTRODUCTION

Bone is critical for the sports system. The existence and structure of bone depends completely on the formation, quantity, and activity of bone cells that are regulated by several factors, such as mechanical and chemical stimuli, receptor and signal transduction, transcription and translation, heredity, nutrition, and endocrines (Rodan, 1998). Exercise or mechanical stimulation is one of the main factors affecting bone mass; it does not completely inhibit the loss of bone mineral content with increasing age and menopause and has a positive effect on several circulational index of bone metabolism (Smith et al., 2014). The appropriate physical activity and exercise could help attenuate bone loss, effectively stimulate bone formation, increase bone mineral density (BMD), prevent the progression of osteoporosis, and reduce the risk of bone fractures (Smith and Gilligan, 1991). The exercise can also reduce the risk of falls and increase the bone strength, flexibility, balance, and reaction time (Smith and Gilligan, 1991). Thus, exercise is known to improve bone health based on two aspects primarily by increasing the growth period of peak bone mass (PBM) in children and adolescents and maintaining or slowing down the aging (especially emphasizes the premenopausal women) with respect to bone absorption rate (Sumida et al., 2014; Winther et al., 2014; Tucker et al., 2015). Long-time high-intensity exercise or physical activity were bad for bone healthy, such as soldiers and marathon runners.

Recent studies have greatly expanded the knowledge of mechanoresponse of mesenchymal stem cells and their roles on the maintenance of bone homeostasis (Potier et al., 2010). Many studies in the mechanosensibility of bone marrow mesenchymal stromal cells (BMMSCs) have indicated central roles of BMMSCs in locomotion induced bone mass increase (Casazza et al., 2012; Shin et al., 2013; Monika et al., 2015). As a type of multipotential cells, BMMSCs can differentiate into chondrocytes, osteoblasts, and adipocytes under different loading condition (Zhang et al., 2016) or specific microenvironment. Previous studies have shown that BMMSCs and their lineage-differentiated progeny (for example, osteoblasts), and osteocytes are mechanosensitive in bone (Wang et al., 2020). And it is suggested that constant loading in an appropriate intensity is able to switch the differentiation direction of BMMSCs from adipogenesis to osteoblastogenesis (Casazza et al., 2012; Monika et al., 2015). Besides, the increase of BMMSC proliferation induced by fluid shear stress also contributes to the number of total bone cell population (Riddle et al., 2005). Accordingly, a direct connection between locomotion and enhancement of bone quality is built in light of the mechanical ability of BMMSCs. It is still unclear how these ubiquious signals arising from mechanical stimulation are perceived by BMMSCs and then how the cells respond to them. The key regulatory signals are generated during exercise and that these factors are first and foremost mechanical in nature.

The differentiation of BMMSCs toward an osteogenic lineage relies on various of signaling pathways including: Bone morphogenetic protein (BMP), IGF, NOTCH, Hedgehog and Wnt signaling (James, 2013). BMP is originally discovered as a protein with heterotopic bone-inducing activity in the bone matrix. BMPs are multi-functional growth factors that belong to the transforming growth factor beta (TGF-β) superfamily (Di et al., 2003). The signaling transduction by BMPs occurs specifically via both canonical Smad-dependent pathways (TGF-β/BMP ligands, receptors and Smads) and non-canonical Smad-independent signaling pathway (MAPK pathway) (Chen et al., 2012). Mechanical load can stimulate the activation of osteoblasts. Effective osteogenesis differentiation is highly dependent on the growth factor signals and mechanical load. It is still unclear how exercise type, intensity, duration, and frequency affect bone mass and strength. Hitherto, exercise and mechanical load promoted the expression of BMP-related target genes in osteoblasts and improved the morphological structure and mechanical properties of bone.

In order to investigate the effect of a BMP-Smad signaling pathway, we injected mice with activated enzyme inhibitors (LDN-193189HCL) and subjected the mice to treadmill exercise intervention. BMD, bone mass, the content of osteoblasts and osteoclasts, and the index of serum and urine were tested. In this study, we aimed to investigate the influence of exercise on bone metabolism in mice with or without the inhibition of BMP-Smad signaling pathway.

## MATERIALS AND METHODS

### Treatment of Animals

Twelve 2-month-old C57BL/6 male mice were randomly divided into two groups with six mice in each group: control group (Control), and exercise group (Exercise) in part one experiment. Exercise group was assigned treadmill running for 5 weeks, 6 days per week. The exercise program was adapted from previous studies (Mehl et al., 2005; Ferreira et al., 2007). Briefly, the mice were trained on a treadmill (**Figure 1A**). The speed of exercise group was equivalent to 85% maximal oxygen uptake ($VO_{2max}$).

Seventy-two 7-week-old C57BL/6 male mice were divided into four groups in accordance with weight and BMD of mice with 18 mice in each group: control group (C), exercise group (E), LDN group (LDN+C), and exercise with LDN group (LDN+E) in part two experiment. Mice in the exercise group and exercise with LDN group were assigned treadmill running exercise at intensities for 6 weeks, 6 days per week (**Figure 2A**).

All mice were maintained at five mice per cage, and provided food and water *ad libitum*. All mice were housed in an environment maintained on a 12-h light–dark cycle at 22 ± 2°C. All the mice were anesthetized with ether inhalation the animals were euthanized by cervical vertebra dislocation.

### LDN-193189HCL Injection

Mice in the LDN groups were injected with LDN (LDN-193189HCL, Selleckchem) on Wednesday from the third to sixth week by intraperitoneal injection (Yu et al., 2008a; Lee et al., 2011; Katagiri and Tsukamoto, 2013). LDN (3 mg/kg body weight) was mixed with DMSO and slowly added this DMSO liquor into physiological saline. LDN powder was completely dissolved using water bath ultrasonic and dissolved by 0.22 μm filter. Each mouse was weighed before injecting and the doses of LDN were adjusted.

### Calcein Injection

A 20.0 mg calcein was mixed with 5 ml 4% $NaHCO_3$ (PH: 8.0–8.5) and 5 ml stroke-physiological saline solution. Mouse bones were labeled with subcutaneously injected calcein (5 μl/g) at day 1 and 8 before the mice were killed at day 9.

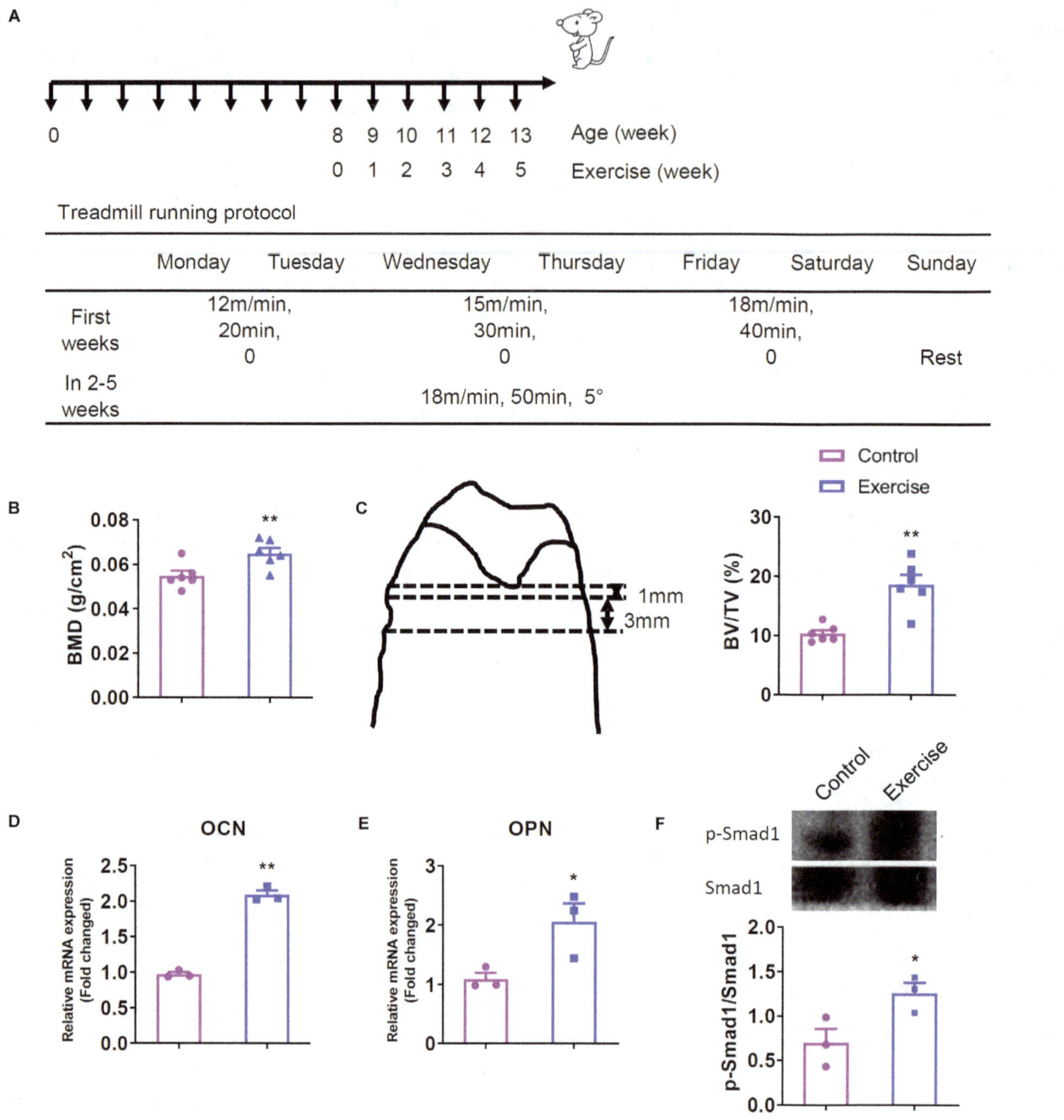


**FIGURE 1** | Exercise increased bone mineral density (BMD) and trabecular bone volume (BV/TV) of the femurs and activated bone morphogenetic protein signaling (BMPS) pathway. Mice were exercised for 5 weeks and then killed. The femurs of these mice were used for BMD and bone mass determination, and tibias were used for evaluating the mRNA expression and protein activation. **(A)** Treadmill running protocol. **(B)** BMD values of mice ($n = 6$). **(C)** The area of bone histomorphometry was used for calculating the bone mass and BV/TV values of mice ($n = 6$). **(D)** *OCN* mRNA expression of mice ($n = 3$). **(E)** *OPN* mRNA expression of mice ($n = 3$). **(F)** Activation of Smad1 proteins in mice ($n = 3$). $^*P < 0.05$, $^{**}P < 0.01$ as compared to the control group.

## BMMSCs Cultures and ALP Staining

The femurs of mice were used for BMMSCs extraction and culture. The bone marrow cells were washed out with α-MEM (HyClone, United States). After being centrifuged at 1000 rpm for 10 min, the pellets were resuspended in α-MEM supplemented with 10% fetal bovine serum (FBS) (Gibco, United States), and 1% penicillin-streptomycin (Invitrogen, United States). The cells were seeded at a density of $5 \times 10^6$ cells/well in 12-well plates. Alkaline phosphatase (ALP) staining was performed 7 days after seeding (Sigma-Aldrich ALP stain kit, United States), and images were captured using a microscope (Nikon Eclipse 90i and Nikon Elements AR 3

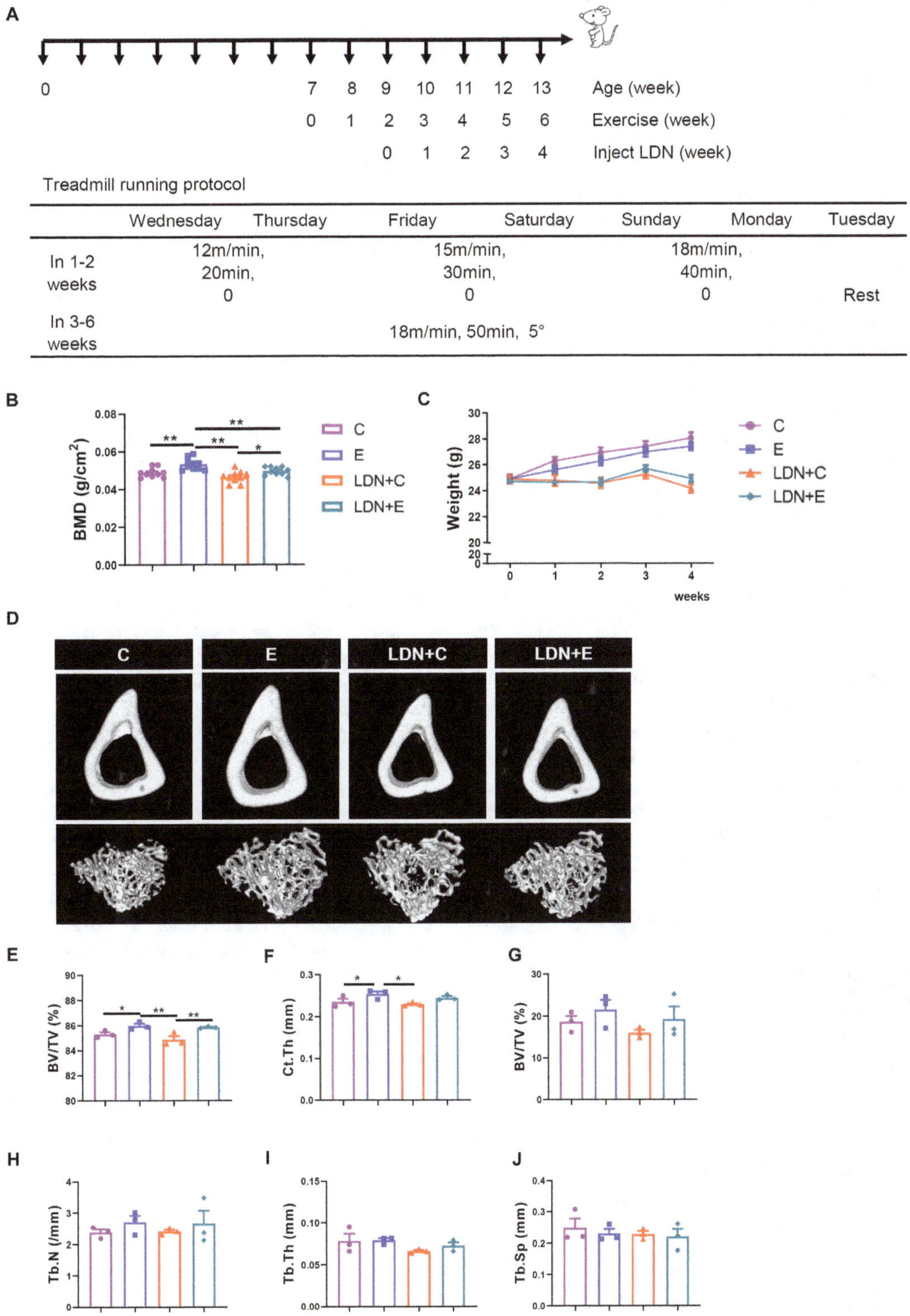


**FIGURE 2 |** Effects of exercise and LDN injection on mouse body weight and bone mineral density (BMD) of the femurs. Exercise increased cortical bone volume (BV/TV), and cortical thickness (Ct.Th) of tibia. Mice were exercised for 6 weeks in the presence or absence of LDN and then killed. The femurs of these mice were used for BMD determination. Body weights of mice in the four groups were recorded every week during the exercise. **(A)** Treadmill running protocol. **(B)** BMD values of mice ($n$ = 10). **(C)** Average body weight was shown ($n$ = 18). **(D)** Representative μCT images showed two-dimensional cortical and trabecular architecture in mouse tibia ($n$ = 3). **(E)** Cortical bone volume per tissue volume (BV/TV). **(F)** Cortical thickness (Ct.Th). **(G)** Trabecular bone volume per tissue volume (BV/TV). **(H)** Trabecular number (Tb.N). **(I)** Trabecular thickness (Tb.Th). **(J)** Trabecular separation (Tb.Sp). $^*P < 0.05$, $^{**}P < 0.01$.

software, Japan). Colony-forming units (CFUs) were calculated from those images.

## BMD Measurement of Total Femurs

The left femurs were used for BMD. Special attention was paid to avoiding damage of the bone cortex when removing the skin, muscles, and connective tissues. Before testing, the specimens were observed under a microscope to make sure all specimens were intact. The dual energy X-ray absorptiometry method was used for measurement of BMD (Osteocore3 Digital 2D, France) of the total left femurs.

## Bone Histomorphometry

The right femurs were isolated, fixed in 4% paraformaldehyde (PFA) after washing with PBS, and then dehydrated in 70% ethanol. The specimens were dehydrated sequentially in ascending concentrations of ethanol (95%, 100%) and xylene, and then embedded in methyl methacrylate. The femurs were cut at 4-μm thickness using a microtome (Leica RM2265, Germany), transferred onto gelatin-coated slides, and dried overnight in an oven at 60°C. After the slices were stained using Masson's method, the digitizing morphometric system (Osteomeasure High Resolution Color Subsystem) was used to measure the bone histomorphometric parameters. In the present study, the region of cancellous bone measured was 1–4 mm distal to the lower margin of the growth plate in the proximal femur (**Figure 1C**). The measured parameters for cancellous bone included bone volume (BV), the total tissue volume (TV), bone surface (BS), single-labeled surfaces (sLS), double-labeled surfaces (dLS) and so on. These data were used to calculate the percent cancellous mineral apposition rate (MAR), bone formation rate/bone volume (BFR/BV), bone formation rate/total tissue volume (BFR/TV), bone formation rate/bone surface (BFR/BS), bone volume (BV/TV), trabecular number (Tb.N), trabecular thickness (Tb.Th), and trabecular separation (Tb.Sp).

## μCT for BMD and Bone Histomorphometry

The right tibias were observed under a microscope to ensure all specimens were intact. After fixation with 4% PFA and dehydrated in 70% ethanol, the specimens were scanned by a μCT scanner (Skyscan 1174; Bruker, Kontich, Belgium) with acquisition settings of: 40 kVp, 555 uA, filter AL 0.5 mm, and 9 micron isotropic resolution. Bone microarchitecture parameters of cortical bone and trabecular bone were measured using the built-in software as follows: bone volume (BV/TV), cortical thickness (Ct.Th), Tb.N, Tb.Th, and Tb.Sp.

## Methods for Bone Biomechanics Measurement

The three-point bending method was performed for biomechanics analysis (Reger RGM-2020, China) immediately after BMD measurement. Then, a vernier caliper was used for measurement of femoral short axis, and minor axis in the central part of the direction of Tb.Th. When testing, the proximal and distal ends of the femur were fixed on the machine pedestal, with a 12-mm span and specimens in horizontal position. The probe moved continuously down at a speed of 1 mm/min for bending test with no preload. Data including maximum load, yield stress, and elastic modulus were automatically calculated by a computer program.

## Real-Time PCR

The total RNA was isolated from the left tibias of mice using TRIzol (Sigma, United States) and reverse-transcription (Revert Aid first strand cDNA Synthesis Kit, Cat.#:K1622, Thermo Scientific, United States) was conducted using 1 μg of total RNA with oligo-dT primers at 42°C for 1 h. All PCRs were performed using 2 μg of respective cDNA with SYBR Green qPCR Master Mix (Roche, Switzerland). *Osteocalcin (OCN)* mRNA, *osteopontin (OPN)* mRNA, *Osterix (OSX)* mRNA, *runt related transcription factor 2 (Runx2)* mRNA, *msh homeobox-2 (MSX2)* mRNA, *distal-less homeobox 5 (DLX5)* mRNA, and *GAPDH* mRNA were measured by quantitative testing. Quantification of mRNA was performed using Step One Plus$^{TM}$ Sequencing Detection System (Life Technologies, United States). The mouse primers used in this study are presented in **Table 1**.

## Western Blot Assay

The total proteins were extracted from other tibias with RIPA Lysis Buffer (Biyuntian, China) containing a protease inhibitor cocktail (Roche, Switzerland). Proteins were separated by 10% SDS-PAGE with 80 to 120 V, and then transferred onto a 0.45 μm PVDF membrane (Millipore, United States) with 300 mA for 2 h. The blotting membranes were blocked with 5% skim milk powder in 1 × TBS-Tween (TBST) for 1 h. After washing with 1 × TBST three times for 10 min once, the blotting membranes incubated with phospho-Smad1 (CST, #9553), Smad1 (CST, #9743), phospho-p44/42 MAPK (CST, #5726), p44/42 MAPK (CST, #9102), phospho-p38 MAPK (CST, #9211), p38 MAPK (CST, #9212), and β-Actin (CST, #5057). The molecular weight and gray value of the target strip were analyzed by the Image J system.

**TABLE 1** | RT-PCR primer Sequences.

| mRNA | Primer | Sequences (5′–3′) |
|---|---|---|
| OCN | Forward | AGCAGGAGGGCAATAAGGTAGT |
| | Reverse | ACCGTAGATGCGTTTGTAGGC |
| OPN | Forward | CAGCCTGCACCCAGATCCTA |
| | Reverse | GCGCAAGGAGATTCTGCTTCT |
| OSX | Forward | TGGTACAAGGCAGGCATCCA |
| | Reverse | GGAGCAAAGTCAGATGGGTAAGT |
| Runx2 | Forward | TTTAGGGCGCATTCCTCATC |
| | Reverse | TGTCCTTGTGGATTAAAAGGACTTG |
| MSX2 | Forward | AACACAAGACCAACCGGAAG |
| | Reverse | GCCGTATATGGATGCTGCTT |
| DLX5 | Forward | CACCACCCGTCTCAGGAATC |
| | Reverse | GCTTTGCCATAAGAAGCAGAGG |
| GAPDH | Forward | CCACAGTCCATGCCATCAC |
| | Reverse | CATACCAGGAAATGAGCTTGAC |

## Serum and Urine Biochemical Maker Analysis

Massage technique was used to obtain urine samples, which were stored at −80°C until further analysis. All the mice were anesthetized with ether inhalation; after blood samples were collected, the animals were euthanized by cervical vertebra dislocation. The serum samples were collected from the blood. The levels of serum calcium and phosphorus were measured by colorimetric assays (Total Calcium LiquiColor kit: Stanbio, TX, United States; inorganic phosphorus mensuration reagent kit: Shanghai, China). Urinary deoxypyridinoline (DPD) levels were measured by enzyme-linked immunosorbent assay (DPD EIA kit; METRA, San Diego, CA, United States). Urinary carboxy-terminal collagen cross-linking telopeptide of type I collagen (CTX-I) levels were measured by enzyme-linked immunosorbent assay (RatLaps$^{TM}$ CTX-I EIA kit; Boldon, United Kingdom). Urinary creatinine (UCr) levels were measured by creatinine colorimetric assay using a creatinine mensuration reagent kit (Hubei, China).

## Serum Starvation

The mouse embryo fibroblasts (MEFs) were extracted from embryo of C57BL/6 mice (Anna et al., 2014), 14–16 days pregnant. Embryo washed three times with PBS. After being detached with 0.25% trypsin-EDTA (Gibco, United States) for 30 min, the pellets were resuspended in high-MEM supplemented with 10% FBS (Gibco, United States), and 1% penicillin-streptomycin (Invitrogen, United States) at 37°C in 5%$CO_2$ incubator. The cells were seeded in six-well plates. When cells reached 80–90% confluence, the essential medium was changed to high-MEM supplemented 1% penicillin-streptomycin without FBS for 4 h. After 4 h, four six-well plates were divided into four groups with six wells in each group, then supplemented with 1% penicillin-streptomycin and mice serum in different groups, respectively. After 30 min, the cells were collected and used for measuring the phospho-Smad1, Smad1, and β-Actin. After 1 h, another cells were collected and used for measuring the phospho-p44/42 MAPK, p44/42 MAPK, phospho-p38 MAPK, p38 MAPK, and β-Actin.

## Statistical Analysis

All the data were expressed as mean ± SEM. Two-way analysis of variance (ANOVA) was performed, and statistical differences were calculated using independent sample *T*-test. Values of $P < 0.05$ were considered statistically significant. All statistical analysis was performed by statistical software SPSS 13.0 for Windows (version 13, SPSS, Chicago, IL, United States).

# RESULTS

## Treadmill Exercise Increases BMD, Bone Volume of 2-Month-Old Male Mice and Activates BMP-Smad Signaling Pathway

In the present study, 2-month-old male mice undergo 5-week treadmill exercise were analyzed for BMD and bone histomorphometry. We found that treadmill exercise significantly improved bone mass and quality including BMD and BV/TV compared to control littermates (**Figures 1B,C**), and was efficient to up-regulated the expression of *OCN* and *OPN* (**Figures 1D,E**). Mechanistically, western blot analysis showed that exercise activated the Smad1 protein phosphorylation (**Figure 1F**).

## Treadmill Exercise Increases BMD, Cortical Bone BV/TV and Ct.Th of Tibia, and LDN Injection Shows a Significant Effect on Mouse Body Weight

To further investigate the role of BMP signaling in treadmill exercise-induced bone formation, 7-week-old male mice were performed a 6-week round exercise and injected specific BMP singnaling inhibitor - LDN. The mice ran at the speed of 18 m/min on a 5° slope, which is categorized as medium-intensity exercise. We found that 6 weeks of medium-intensity exercise significantly increased mice BMD. BMD in the E group was significantly higher than that in the C group ($P < 0.01$), and BMD in the LDN+E group was higher than that in the LDN+C group ($P < 0.05$); four times inhibition of BMP signaling decreased the BMD that was significantly lower in the LDN+E group than that in the E group ($P < 0.01$) (**Figure 2B**). Mouse body weight was measured every week during exercise and inhibition of BMP signaling (**Table 2** and **Figure 2C**). Inhibition of BMP signaling decreased the mouse body weight; however, the exercise did not show a significant effect on mouse body weight during Inhibition of BMP signaling for 3 weeks. These results suggested that medium-intensity exercise increased the BMD in mice, whereas LDN attenuated the BMD.

Next, exercise was found to increase the cortical bone BV/TV and Ct.Th of tibia (**Figure 2D**): cortical bone BV/TV in the E group was higher than that in the C group ($P < 0.05$), cortical bone BV/TV in the LDN+E group was significantly higher than that in the LDN+C group ($P < 0.01$) (**Figure 2E**); whereas, the Ct.Th in the E group was higher than that in the C group ($P < 0.05$) (**Figure 2F**). Inhibition of BMP signaling alone did not have any effect on the bone mass of tibia (**Figures 2G–J**). The data of three-point bending experiment including maximum load, yield stress, and elastic modulus were no difference between groups (**Supplementary Figures S1A–C**).

## Medium-Intensity Exercise Increases Bone Formation and Inhibits Bone Resorption, and LDN Injection Inhibits the Exercise–Mediated Bone Formation and Promotes Bone Resorption

Mouse bones were labeled with subcutaneously injected calcein (5 μL/g) at days 1 and 8. After the slices were made, the bone volume was examined using bone histomorphometry (**Figure 3A**). We found that exercise increased the bone formation and LDN injection inhibited the exercise-based improvement in the bone formation. In addition, exercise

**TABLE 2 |** Effects of exercise and LDN on mouse body weight.

| Group | N | Weight (g) | | | | |
|---|---|---|---|---|---|---|
| | | 0 | 1 | 2 | 3 | 4 |
| C | 18 | 24.92 ± 1.43 | 26.31 ± 1.33 | 26.94 ± 1.62 | 27.42 ± 1.68 | 28.07 ± 1.73 |
| E | 18 | 24.92 ± 1.13 | 25.61 ± 1.09 | 26.28 ± 1.46 | 27.00 ± 1.55 | 27.41 ± 1.24 |
| LDN+C | 18 | 24.91 ± 1.18 | 24.79 ± 1.68** | 24.58 ± 1.63** | 25.27 ± 1.45** | 24.17 ± 1.39**△△ |
| LDN+E | 18 | 24.72 ± 0.33 | 24.64 ± 0.57△△ | 24.67 ± 0.95△△ | 25.70 ± 0.97△ | 24.93 ± 1.13**△△ |

*$^{**}P < 0.01$ as compared to the C group. $^{\triangle}$ $P < 0.05$, $^{\triangle\triangle}$ $P < 0.01$ as compared to the E group.*

increased the bone formation of femur: BV/TV and Tb.N in the LDN+E group were higher than those in the LDN+C group (**Figures 3B,C**), Tb.Sp in the LDN+E group was lower than that in the LDN+C group (**Figure 3E**), BFR/TV and BFR/BS in the E group were higher than those in the C group (**Figures 3H,I**). Also, we found that LDN injection inhibited the exercise-improved bone formation: BFR/BV, BFR/TV, and BFR/BS were lower in the LDN+E group than the E group ($P < 0.05$) (**Figures 3G,I**). Mice that were exercised for 6 weeks or injected with LDN alone revealed that BV/TV, Tb.N, and BFR/TV in the LDN+C group were lower than those in the E group (**Figures 3B,C,H**), while Tb.Sp in the LDN+C group was higher than that in the E group (**Figure 3E**). Tb.Th and MAR were no statistical differences (**Figures 3D,F**).

After the slices were stained using Masson's method, the femur bones of 6 mice were used for bone histomorphometry analysis (**Figure 3J**). Consequently, exercise could increase the bone formation of femur: BV/TV and Tb.N in the E group were higher than those in the C group (**Figures 3K,L**), while Tb.Sp in the E group was lower than that in the C group (**Figure 3N**). Moreover, BV/TV in the LDN+C group was lower than that in the E group (**Figure 3K**), while Tb.Sp in the LDN+C group was higher than that in the E group (**Figure 3N**) when mice were exercised for 6 weeks or injected with LDN alone. Tb.Th was no statistical difference (**Figure 3M**).

We measured the calcium and phosphorus levels in the serum and found that inhibition of BMP signaling increased these levels. The serum calcium level in the LDN+C group was significantly higher than that in the C group ($P < 0.01$) (**Figure 3O**), while the serum calcium and phosphorus levels were significantly higher in the LDN+E group than that in the E group ($P < 0.01$) (**Figures 3O,P**). The serum calcium level in the LDN+E group was significantly higher than that in the LDN+C group ($P < 0.05$) (**Figure 3O**). Importantly, we found that medium-intensity exercise significantly decreased circulating DPD and CTX-I level, indicating the inhibition effect of bone resorption potency. Moreover, Inhibition of BMP signaling could attenuate the inhibitory effect of medium-intensity exercise, indicating BMP signaling as the key modulator of treadmill exercise-induced bone remoldling. Also, the urinary DPD and CTX-I levels, two *in vivo* bone resorption markers, were measured. Exercise led to a decrease in the urine CTX-I levels, while Inhibition of BMP signaling promoted the bone resorption. DPD/Ucr in the LDN+C group was significantly higher than that in the C group ($P < 0.01$) (**Figure 3Q**); DPD/Ucr and CTX-I levels were higher in the LDN+E group than the E group ($P < 0.05$) (**Figures 3Q,R**).

## Treadmill Exercise Activates Smad1 Protein Phosphorylation, and LDN Injection Inhibits the Expression of Osteoblast-Related Genes in Tibia

The mRNA expression of *OCN* was lower in the LDN+E group than the E group ($P < 0.05$) (**Figure 4A**). The mRNA expression of OSX, Runx2, MSX2, DLX5 were no statistical differences (**Figures 4B–E**). The left tibias were used for the evaluation of protein activation (**Figure 4F**). Western blot analysis with antibodies to p-Smadl and Smadl showed that p-Smadl expression was higher in the E group than in the C group ($P < 0.05$) (**Figure 4G**), indicating that exercise could activate the Smadl protein phosphorylation. Also, Smadl expression was higher in the LDN+E group than the LDN+C group ($P < 0.05$) (**Figure 4H**), suggesting that exercise improves Smadl protein expression. ERK expression was lower in the E group than the C group ($P < 0.05$) (**Figure 4J**). The ERK and P38 protein phosphorylation, P38 expression were no statistical differences (**Figures 4I,K,L**).

## Medium Level of Exercise Increases Osteogenic Differentiation of BMMSCs and Activates Smad1 Protein Phosphorylation, and LDN Injection Inhibits Smad1 Protein Phosphorylation

To further test whether medium level treadmill exercise have impact on BMMSCs, we isolated BMMSCs followed by previously described protocal and analyzed their colony-forming and osteogenic ability. ALP staining showed that medium level treadmill exercise markedly increase osteogenic differentiation potential. What's more, inhibition of BMP signaling significantly attenuated. The ALP-positive CFU was measured, which indicated the number of osteogenic BMMSCs in the bone marrow. The medium level of exercise increased the number of osteogenic BMMSCs (**Figures 5A,B**).

Mouse embryo fibroblasts were extracted from embryo of C57BL/6 mice, 14–16 days pregnant. The essential medium was changed to high-MEM without FBS for 4 h, supplemented with mice serum in different groups, respectively. After 30 min, the cells were used for measuring the protein activity (**Figure 5C**). Exercise activated Smadl protein phosphorylation, whereas LDN injection inhibited the Smadl protein phosphorylation (**Figures 5D,E**). In addition, Inhibition of BMP signaling did

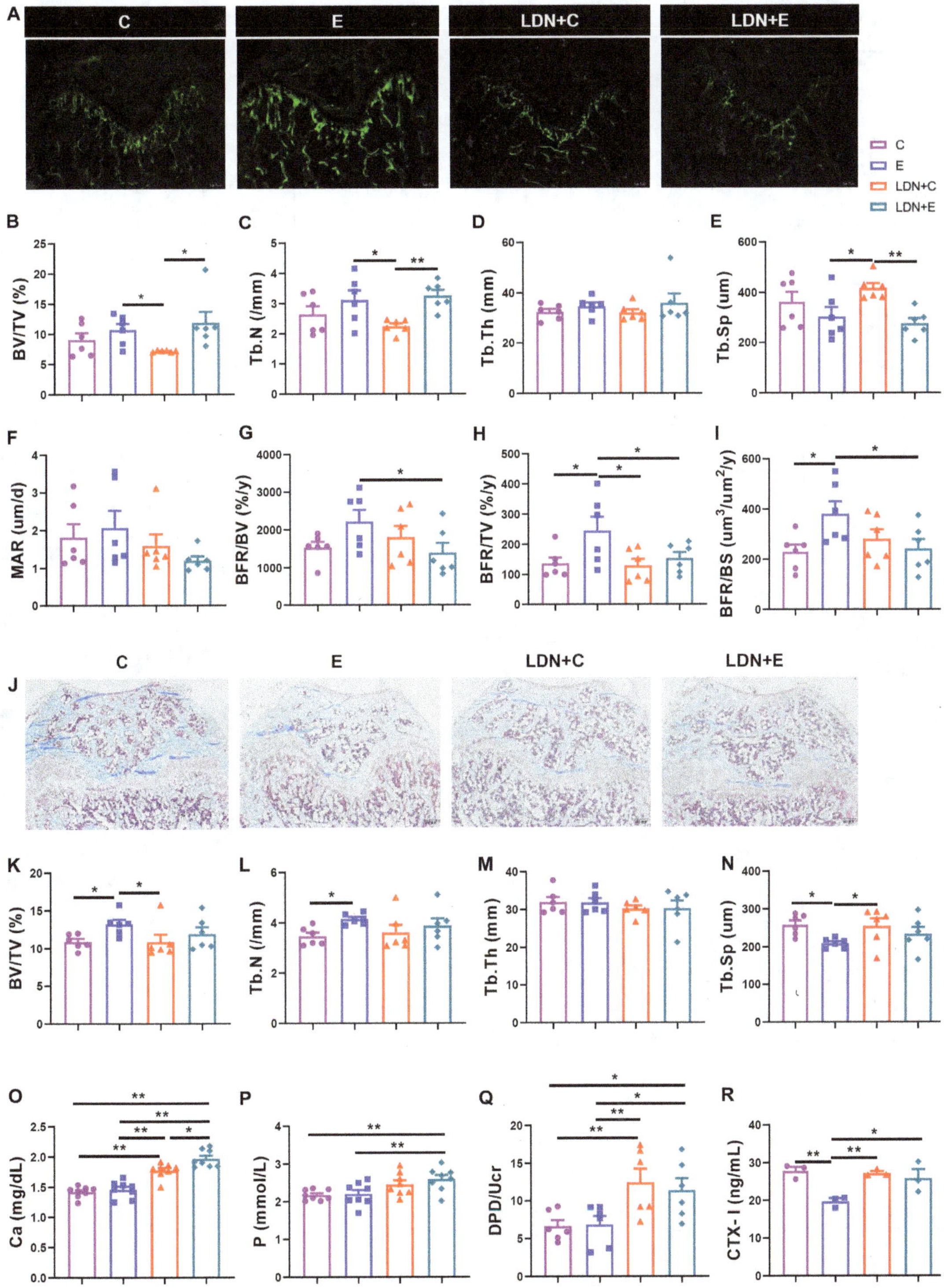


**FIGURE 3 |** Medium-intensity exercise increased bone formation and inhibited bone resorption, and LDN injection inhibited the exercise–mediated bone formation and promoted bone resorption. Mice were exercised for 6 weeks in the presence or absence of LDN and then killed. **(A)** Mouse bones were labeled with subcutaneously injected calcein (5 µl/g) at days 1 and 8 ($n$ = 6). **(B)** Trabecular bone volume (BV/TV). **(C)** Trabecular number (Tb.N). **(D)** Trabecular thickness (Tb.Th). **(E)** Trabecular separation (Tb.Sp). **(F)** Mineral apposition rate (MAR) values of the four groups of mice. **(G)** Bone formation rate/bone volume (BFR/BV) values of the four groups of mice. **(H)** Bone formation rate/total tissue volume (BFR/TV) values of the four groups of mice. **(I)** Bone formation rate/bone surface (BFR/BS) values of the four groups of mice. **(J)** After the slices were stained using Masson's method, the femur bones of six mice were used for bone histomorphometry analysis ($n$ = 6). The photos of the masson staining. **(K)** Trabecular bone volume (BV/TV). **(L)** Trabecular number (Tb.N). **(M)** Trabecular thickness (Tb.Th). **(N)** Trabecular separation (Tb.Sp). **(O)** The serum calcium level ($n$ = 8). **(P)** The serum phosphorus level ($n$ = 8). **(Q)** The urinary deoxypyridinoline (DPD) level ($n$ = 6). **(R)** The urinary carboxy-terminal collagen cross-linking telopeptide of type I collagen (CTX-I) level ($n$ = 3). $^*P < 0.05$, $^{**}P < 0.01$.

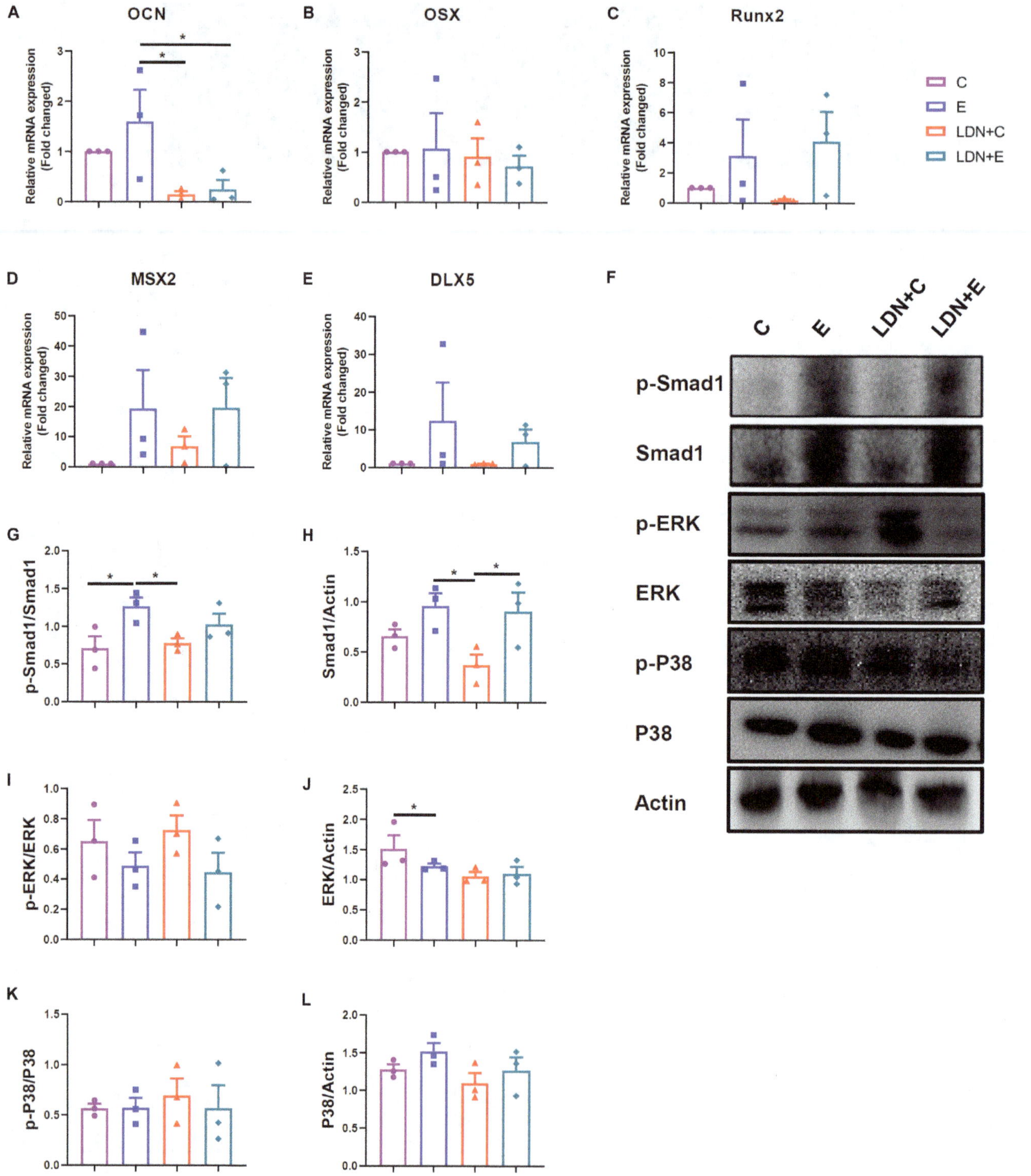


**FIGURE 4 |** Exercise could active Smad1 protein, and LDN injection inhibited the expression of osteoblast-related genes in tibia. Mice were exercised for 6 weeks in the presence or absence of LDN and then killed. The left tibias were used for the evaluation of gene expression and protein activation. **(A)** The mRNA expression of *OCN* ($n = 4$). **(B)** The mRNA expression of *OSX* ($n = 4$). **(C)** The mRNA expression of *Runx2* ($n = 4$). **(D)** The mRNA expression of *MSX2* ($n = 4$). **(E)** The mRNA expression of *DLX5* ($n = 4$). **(F)** Representative images of protein expression by Western blot. **(G,H)** Western blot analysis with antibodies to p-Smad1 and Smad1 ($n = 4$). **(I,J)** Western blot analysis with antibodies to p-ERK and ERK ($n = 4$). **(K,L)** Western blot analysis with antibodies to p-P38 and P38 ($n = 4$). $^{*}P < 0.05$.

not affect the phosphorylation of P38 and ERK proteins (**Figures 5F–I**).

## DISCUSSION

The medium level exercise increased BMD and BV/TV of the femurs of 2-month-old male mice, in addition, increased the expression of osteoblast-related genes (*OCN* and *OPN*), and activated the BMP-Smad signaling pathway *in vivo*. OCN collagen constitutes osteoblast synthesis and secretion and is a specific marker of bone formation (Magni et al., 2016). OPN can stimulate the osteoblast proliferation and calcification, promote the adhesion of osteoclasts and bone matrix, and improve the bone resorption (Zhang et al., 2018). BMP signaling is one of the essential pathways involved in osteogenic differentiation of BMMSCs and regulation of bone formation (Huang et al., 2018). Therefore, we hypothesized that BMP-Smad signaling pathway mediates the treadmill exercise that can regulate BMMSCs to osteoblast differentiation in mice.

Mice were exercised for 6 weeks. Firstly, at the end of 2-week exercise training, the mice body weight of the four groups did not differ significantly. This exercise training was categorized as medium-intensity exercise, and the strength was about 85% $VO_{2max}$ (Droste et al., 2003; Kramer et al., 2006; Petzinger et al., 2013). The results

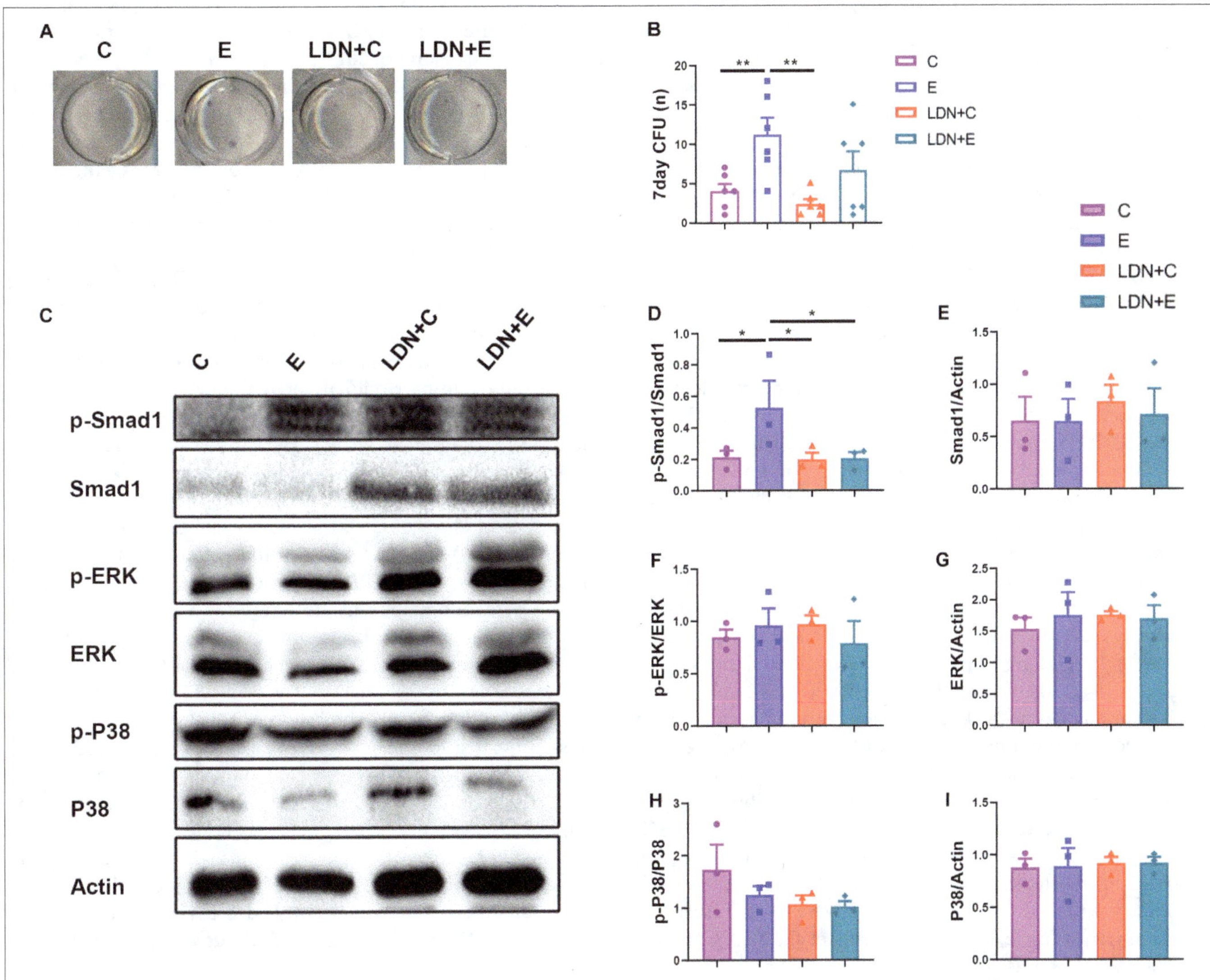


**FIGURE 5 |** Effects of exercise and LDN injection on the number of BMMSCs, and exercise activated Smad1 protein phosphorylation, and LDN injection inhibited Smad1 protein phosphorylation. Mice were exercised for 6 weeks in the presence or absence of LDN and then killed. The bone marrow cells were flushed out, plated, and cultured for 10 days, and then stained for ALP. **(A)** Representative images of colony-forming units (CFU) staining. **(B)** ALP quantitation results ($n = 6$). **(C)** The mouse embryo fibroblasts (MEF) were extracted from embryo of C57BL/6 mice, 14–16 days pregnant. The essential medium was changed to high-MEM without FBS, supplemented with mice serum in different groups, respectively. After 30 min, the cells were used for measuring the protein activity. Representative images of protein expression by Western blot. **(D,E)** Western blot analysis with antibodies to p-Smad1 and Smad1. **(F,G)** Western blot analysis with antibodies to p-ERK and ERK. **(H,I)** Western blot analysis with antibodies to p-P38 and P38. $^*P < 0.05$, $^{**}P < 0.01$.

suggested that the mice can adapt to medium-intensity treadmill exercise for 4 weeks, which is similar to that reported previously (Zhang et al., 2017). In addition, the medium level of exercise could activate Smad1 protein phosphorylation from serum starvation experiment *in vitro*; the experimental results were in agreement with previous studies. However, it did not activate P38 and ERK protein phosphorylation.

Previous studies have shown that resistance exercise stimulates bone formation and only slightly affects bone resorption (Smith et al., 2008, 2014) as exercise renders muscle tension via the mechanical stress pathways and stimulates the bone formation. But running exercise could increase the BMD of growing mice (Huang et al., 2003). After 6 weeks of exercise, the medium level of exercise significantly increased the BMD, the cortical bone volume, and Ct.Th of tibia. Furthermore, bone histomorphometry showed that the medium level of exercise led to an increase in BFR/TV, BFR/BS, trabecular bone volume, and Tb.N, accompanied by a decrease in bone separation. These results are consistent with those from previous studies, which showed that medium-intensity exercise enhanced the bone formation (Ronga et al., 2013; Smith et al., 2014; Iura et al., 2015; Li et al., 2015). There was no significant difference in maximum load, yield stress, and elastic modulus of femurs between groups, which may be due to the stable biomechanical properties of bone. Bone strength mainly includes bone mass and bone quality. Although bone mass determines about 80% of bone biomechanical strength, recent data show that BMD can't completely provide bone biomechanical index (Hasegawa et al., 2001). In addition to bone mass, it is related to the internal structure of bone such as the three-dimensional architecture of bone and the connectivity between trabeculae. Due to the stability of bone biomechanical properties, the effect of external intervention is not significant.

In addition, the ALP-positive CFU, an indication of the number of osteogenic BMMSCs in the bone marrow. Mouse ALP is frequently measured and used as a bone marker in mammalian bone research (Halling et al., 2013). The osteoblasts activity is improved with increased ALP secretion (Shen et al., 2007). Exercise stimulates the ALP production by osteogenic cells in order to increase the mineralization of the newly forming bone (Roussignol et al., 2012; Wang et al., 2018). Supposedly, the increase in bone formation and the number of osteoblasts may be mediated by the increase in the number of osteogenic BMMSCs (Zhang et al., 2017). Osteoclasts constantly resorb old bone, and osteoblasts form osteoid that is converted into mineralized bone. The urinary levels of DPD and CTX-I were bone resorption markers *in vivo* (Woitge et al., 1998; Vesper et al., 2002; Carvalho et al., 2006), and exercise leads to a decrease in the urinary levels of CTX-I. Previous studies have shown that exercise decreases the bone resorption (O'Kane et al., 2006; Kishimoto et al., 2012; Pacheco-Costa et al., 2018). These results indicated that medium level exercise suppressed bone resorption, which contributed to the increase in bone mass.

Bone morphogenetic proteins exert their diverse biological effects through two types of transmembrane receptors: BMP receptor type I (BMPR-I) and type II (BMPR-II) possess intrinsic serine/threonine kinase activity (Heldin et al., 1997). Type I and II BMP receptors are highly homologous transmembrane serine/threonine kinases. Only when two type I and two type II receptors form the heterogeneous dimers in the BMP family, they exhibit a high affinity toward the ligand. An allele-specific RNAi has been established for the mutant type I receptor, ALK2 (Lowery and Rosen, 2012). LDN-193189HCL as a BMP signaling inhibitor have been developed for the specific inhibition of BMP type I receptor-Smad1/5/8 signaling axis (Katagiri and Tsukamoto, 2013; Yu et al., 2017), inhibited the kinase ALK2 (the amino acid sequence of ALK2 login NP001103675) in mice (Lowery and Rosen, 2012). Consecutively, LDN-193189 is a potent derivative of dorsomorphin, the first chemical inhibitor explicitly identified for the receptor-induced phosphorylation of Smad1/5/8s but not the MAP kinase pathway (Yu et al., 2008b; Katagiri and Tsukamoto, 2013).

Inhibition of BMP-Smad signaling reduced the body weight in mice. Thus, LDN injection might potentially lead to weight loss by reducing bone mass. Because LDN-193189 has been shown to reduce the heterotopic bone formation in a transgenic mouse model carrying a mutant *ALK2* gene (Yu et al., 2008a; Katagiri and Tsukamoto, 2013). Furthermore, the pharmacological dose of LDN led to a slight decrease in BMD. The LDN injection further decreased the BFR/BV, BFR/TV, and BFR/BS in combination with the medium level of exercise in young mice. Moreover, the injection also decreased the osteoblast-related *OCN* mRNA expression. Activated Smads regulate the expression of transcriptional factors and transcriptional co-activators vital for osteoblasts differentiations (DLX5, Runx2, and OSX) (Chen et al., 2012). Herein, we have identified the altered expression of the BMP/Smad target gene, *DLX5*, which is an osteoblast-specific and BMP signaling specific transcription factor (Lee et al., 2003), critical for skeletal tissue development (Komori, 2019) and osteoblast differentiation (Tadic et al., 2002). Msx2 is the BMP/Smad target gene (Jovanovic et al., 2018), a homeodomain transcription factor relevant to osteoblast survival, programming (Tong and Lee, 2013), and orthotopic craniofacial bone formation (Jabs et al., 1993). The trend of *MSX2* gene expression was similar to that of *DLX5* and did not differ significantly. In addition, inhibition of BMP signaling increased the serum calcium and phosphorus levels, the bone absorption may be enhanced. The serum calcium and phosphorus levels were critical bone mineral components of the blood (Lin et al., 2012; Orcy et al., 2014). When bone is decomposed or resorbed, it releases calcium, phosphorus, and other minerals in the blood circulation. Injecting LDN could enhance bone resorption, but not significantly decrease the number of osteogenic BMMSCs. Simultaneously, it downregulates the level of Smad1 protein.

Furthermore, we found that the medium level exercise attenuated the decreasing BMD, cortical bone volume, trabecular bone volume, Tb.N, and serum calcium levels caused by LDN injection. Different intensities of exercise training affected the serum calcium levels differentially. The medium level of exercise combined with LDN injection also increased the Smad1 protein expression as compared to LDN injection alone.

## ETHICS STATEMENT

These mice in the study were purchased from the Second Military Medical University Animal Centre (Shanghai SLAC Laboratory Animal Co.) according to the protocols (Approval Number: 2007000563539) authorized by the Ethical Committee of Shanghai University of Sport on the Care and Use of Animal Subjects. We have complied with all relevant ethical regulations for animal testing and research.

## AUTHOR CONTRIBUTIONS

JZ designed this study. LZ, WW, ZS, LL, and JF did the experiments. LZ and YY analyzed the experimental data. LZ and BG were responsible for manuscript writing. JZ revised the manuscript and supervised this entire program. All authors approved the final version of this manuscript.

## REFERENCES


Anna, L., Xuechun, X., James, Y., Huiyi, K., Huijuan, L., Yuji, M., et al. (2014). Pdgf-aa promotes osteogenic differentiation and migration of mesenchymal stem cell by down-regulating pdgfrα and derepressing bmp-smad1/5/8 signaling. *PLoS One* 9:e113785. doi: 10.1371/journal.pone.0113785

Carvalho, D. C., Garlipp, C. R., Bottini, P. V., Afaz, S. H., Moda, M. A., and Cliquet Jr, A. (2006). Effect of treadmill gait on bone markers and bone mineral density of quadriplegic subjects. *Braz. J. Med. Biol. Res.* 39, 1357–1363. doi: 10.1590/s0100-879x2006001000012

Casazza, K., Hanks, L. J., Hidalgo, B., Hu, H. H., and Affuso, O. (2012). Short-term physical activity intervention decreases femoral bone marrow adipose tissue in young children: a pilot study. *Bone* 50, 0–27.

Chen, G., Deng, C., and Li, Y. P. (2012). Tgf-β and bmp signaling in osteoblast differentiation and bone formation. *Int. J. Biol. Sci.* 8, 272–288. doi: 10.7150/ijbs.2929

Di, C., Ming, Z., and Mundy, G. R. (2003). Bone morphogenetic proteins. *Growth Fact.* 22, 233–241.

Droste, S. K., Gesing, A., Ulbricht, S., Müller, M. B., Linthorst, A. C., and Reul, J. M. (2003). Effects of long-term voluntary exercise on the mouse hypothalamic-pituitary-adrenocortical axis. *Endocrinology* 144, 3012–3023. doi: 10.1210/en.2003-0097

Ferreira, J. C., Rolim, N. P., Bartholomeu, J. B., Gobatto, C. A., Kokubun, E., and Brum, P. C. (2007). Maximal lactate steady state in running mice: effect of exercise training. *Clin. Exp. Pharmacol. Physiol.* 34, 760–765. doi: 10.1111/j.1440-1681.2007.04635.x

Halling, L. C., Englund, U. H., Narisawa, S., Millán, J. L., and Magnusson, P. (2013). Isozyme profile and tissue-origin of alkaline phosphatases in mouse serum. *Bone* 53, 399–408. doi: 10.1016/j.bone.2012.12.048

Hasegawa, Y., Schneider, P., and Reiners, C. (2001). Age, sex, and grip strength determine architectural bone parameters assessed by peripheral quantitative computed tomography (pQCT) at the human radius. *J. Biomech.* 34, 497–503. doi: 10.1016/s0021-9290(00)00211-6

Heldin, C. H., Miyazono, K., and Ten, D. P. (1997). Tgf-beta signalling from cell membrane to nucleus through smad proteins. *Nature* 390, 465–471. doi: 10.1038/37284

Huang, H., Dou, L., Song, J., and Luo, J. (2018). Cbfa2t2 is required for bmp-2-induced osteogenic differentiation of mesenchymal stem cells. *Biochem. Biophys. Res. Commun.* 496, 1095–1101. doi: 10.1016/j.bbrc.2018.01.144

Huang, T. H., Lin, S. C., Chang, F. L., Hsieh, S. S., Liu, S. H., and Yang, R. S. (2003). Effects of different exercise modes on mineralization, structure, and biomechanical properties of growing bone. *J. Appl. Physiol.* 95, 300–307. doi: 10.1152/japplphysiol.01076.2002

Iura, A., Mcnerny, E. G., Zhang, Y., Kamiya, N., Tantillo, M., Lynch, M., et al. (2015). Mechanical loading synergistically increases trabecular bone volume and improves mechanical properties in the mouse when bmp signaling is specifically ablated in osteoblasts. *PLoS One* 10:e0141345. doi: 10.1371/journal.pone.0141345

Jabs, E. W., Müller, Ulrich, Li, Xiang, et al. (1993). A mutation in the homeodomain of the human msx2 gene in a family affected with autosomal dominant craniosynostosis. *Cell* 75, 443–450. doi: 10.1016/0092-8674(93)90379-5

James, A. W. (2013). Review of signaling pathways governing msc osteogenic and adipogenic differentiation. *Scientifica* 2013, 1–17. doi: 10.1155/2013/684736

Jovanovic, V., Salti, A., Tilleman, H., Zega, K., Jukic, M., Zou, H., et al. (2018). Bmp/smad pathway promotes neurogenesis of midbrain dopaminergic neuronsin vivoand in human induced pluripotent and neural stem cells. *J. Neuroence* 38, 1540–1517.

Katagiri, T., and Tsukamoto, S. (2013). The unique activity of bone morphogenetic proteins in bone: a critical role of the smad signaling pathway. *Biol. Chem.* 394, 703–714. doi: 10.1515/hsz-2012-0310

Kishimoto, K., Lynch, R. P., Reiger, J., and Yingling, V. R. (2012). Short-term jump activity on bone metabolism in female college-aged nonathletes. *J. Sports Sci. Med.* 11, 31–38.

Komori, T. (2019). Regulation of Proliferation, Differentiation and Functions of Osteoblasts by Runx2. *Int. J. Mol. Sci.* 20:1694. doi: 10.3390/ijms20071694

Kramer, H. F., Witczak, C. A., Fujii, N., Jessen, N., Taylor, E. B., Arnolds, D. E., et al. (2006). Distinct signals regulate as160 phosphorylation in response to insulin, aicar, and contraction in mouse skeletal muscle. *Diabetes* 55, 2067–2076. doi: 10.2337/db06-0150

Lee, M. H., Kim, Y. J., Kim, H. J., Park, H. D., Kang, A. R., and Kyung, H. M. (2003). Bmp-2-induced runx2 expression is mediated by dlx5, and tgf-beta 1 opposes the bmp-2-induced osteoblast differentiation by suppression of dlx5 expression. *J. Biol. Chem.* 278, 34387–34394. doi: 10.1074/jbc.m211386200

Lee, Y. C., Cheng, C. J., Bilen, M. A., Lu, J. F., Satcher, R. L., Yu-Lee, L. Y., et al. (2011). Bmp4 promotes prostate tumor growth in bone through osteogenesis. *Cancer Res.* 71, 5194–5203. doi: 10.1158/0008-5472.can-10-4374

Li, M., Wu, W., Tan, L., Mu, D., Zhu, D., Wang, J., et al. (2015). Low-magnitude mechanical vibration regulates expression of osteogenic proteins in ovariectomized rats. *Biochem. Biophys. Res. Commun.* 465, 344–348. doi: 10.1016/j.bbrc.2015.07.154

Lin, C. F., Huang, T. H., Tu, K. C., Lin, L. L., Tu, Y. H., and Yang, R. S. (2012). Acute effects of plyometric jumping and intermittent running on serum bone markers in young males. *Eur. J. Appl. Physiol.* 112, 1475–1484. doi: 10.1007/s00421-011-2108-8

Lowery, J. W., and Rosen, V. (2012). Allele-specific rna interference in fop silencing the fop gene. *Gene Therapy* 19, 701–702. doi: 10.1038/gt.2011.190

Magni, P., Macchi, C., Sirtori, C. R., and Corsi Romanelli, M. M. (2016). Osteocalcin as a potential risk biomarker for cardiovascular and metabolic diseases. *Clin. Chem. Lab. Med.* 54, 1579–1587.

Mehl, K. A., Davis, J. M., Clements, J. M., Berger, F. G., Pena, M. M., and Carson, J. A. (2005). Decreased intestinal polyp multiplicity is related to exercise mode and gender in apcmin/+ mice. *J. Appl. Physiol.* 98, 2219–2225. doi: 10.1152/japplphysiol.00975.2004

Monika, M., Smieszek, A., Klaudia, C., Katarzyna, B., and Krzysztof, M. (2015). Physical activity increases the total number of bone-marrow-derived mesenchymal stem cells, enhances their osteogenic potential, and inhibits their adipogenic properties. *Stem Cells Int.* 2015, 1–11. doi: 10.1155/2015/379093

O'Kane, J. W., Hutchinson, E., Atley, L. M., and Eyre, D. R. (2006). Sport-related differences in biomarkers of bone resorption and cartilage degradation in endurance athletes. *Osteoarthr. Cartil.* 14, 71–76. doi: 10.1016/j.joca.2005.08.003

Orcy, R., Antunes, M. F., Schiller, T., Seus, T., and Böhlke, M. (2014). Aerobic exercise increases phosphate removal during hemodialysis: a controlled trial. *Hemodial. Int.* 18, 450–458. doi: 10.1111/hdi.12123

Pacheco-Costa, R., Davis, H. M., Atkinson, E. G., Dilley, J. E., Byiringiro, I., Aref, M. W., et al. (2018). Reversal of loss of bone mass in old mice treated with mefloquine. *Bone* 114, 22–31. doi: 10.1016/j.bone.2018.06.002

Petzinger, G. M., Walsh, J. P., Akopian, G., Hogg, E., Abernathy, A., Arevalo, P., et al. (2013). Effects of treadmill exercise on dopaminergic transmission in the 1-methyl-4-phenyl-1,2,3,6-tetrahydropyridine-lesioned mouse model of basal ganglia injury. *J. Neurosci.* 27, 5291–5300. doi: 10.1523/jneurosci.1069-07.2007

Potier, E., Noailly, J., and Ito, K. (2010). Directing bone marrow-derived stromal cell function with mechanics. *J. Biomech.* 43, 807–817. doi: 10.1016/j.jbiomech.2009.11.019

Riddle, R. C., Taylor, A. F., Genetos, D. C., and Donahue, H. J. (2005). Map kinase and calcium signaling mediate fluid flow-induced human mesenchymal stem cell proliferation. *AJP Cell Physiol.* 290, C776–C784.

Rodan, G. A. (1998). Bone homeostasis. *Proc. Natl. Acad. Sci. U S A.* 95, 13361–13362.

Ronga, M., Fagetti, A., Canton, G., Paiusco, E., Surace, M. F., and Cherubino, P. (2013). Clinical applications of growth factors in bone injuries: experience with bmps. *Inj. Int. J. Care Inj.* 44, S34–S39.

Roussignol, X., Currey, C., Duparc, F., and Dujardin, F. (2012). Indications and results for the exogen$^{TM}$ ultrasound system in the management of non-union: a 59-case pilot study. *Orthopaed. Traumatol. Surg. Res.* 98, 206–213. doi: 10.1016/j.otsr.2011.10.011

Shen, C. L., Williams, J. S., Chyu, M. C., Paige, R. L., Stephens, A. L., Chauncey, K. B., et al. (2007). Comparison of the effects of tai chi and resistance training on bone metabolism in the elderly: a feasibility study. *Am. J. Chin. Med.* 35, 369–381. doi: 10.1142/s0192415x07004898

Shin, J. W., Swift, J., Ivanovska, I., Spinler, K. R., Buxboim, A., and Discher, D. E. (2013). Mechanobiology of bone marrow stem cells: from myosin-ii forces to compliance of matrix and nucleus in cell forms and fates. *Differentiation* 86, 77–86. doi: 10.1016/j.diff.2013.05.001

Smith, E. L., and Gilligan, C. (1991). Physical activity effects on bone metabolism. *Calcified Tissue Int.* 49, S50–S54.

Smith, S. M., Abrams, S. A., Davisstreet, J. E., Heer, M., O'Brien, K. O., Wastney, M. E., et al. (2014). Fifty years of human space travel: implications for bone and calcium research. *Annu. Rev. Nutr.* 34, 377–400. doi: 10.1146/annurev-nutr-071813-105440

Smith, S. M., Zwart, S. R., Heer, M., Lee, S. M. C., Baecker, N., Meuche, S., et al. (2008). Wise-2005: supine treadmill exercise within lower body negative pressure and flywheel resistive exercise as a countermeasure to bed rest-induced bone loss in women during 60-day simulated microgravity. *Bone* 42, 572–581. doi: 10.1016/j.bone.2007.11.015

Sumida, S., Iwamoto, J., Uenishi, K., and Otani, T. (2014). One-year changes in bone mineral density and bone turnover markers in premenopausal amateur runners: a prospective study. *Keio J. Med.* 63, 43–51. doi: 10.2302/kjm.2013-0010-oa

Tadic, T., Dodig, M., Erceg, I., Marijanovic, I., Mina, M., Kalajzic, Z., et al. (2002). Overexpression of dlx5 in chicken calvarial cells accelerates osteoblastic differentiation. *J. Bone Miner. Res.* 17, 1008–1014. doi: 10.1359/jbmr.2002.17.6.1008

Tong, M. L., and Lee, E. H. (2013). Transcriptional regulatory cascades in runx2-dependent bone development. *Tissue Engine. Part B Rev.* 19, 254–263. doi: 10.1089/ten.teb.2012.0527

Tucker, L. A., Strong, J. E., Lecheminant, J. D., and Bailey, B. W. (2015). Effect of two jumping programs on hip bone mineral density in premenopausal women: a randomized controlled trial. *Am. J. Health Promot.* 29, 158–164. doi: 10.4278/ajhp.130430-quan-200

Vesper, H. W., Demers, L. M., Eastell, R., Garnero, P., Kleerekoper, M., Robins, S. P., et al. (2002). Assessment and recommendations on factors contributing to preanalytical variability of urinary pyridinoline and deoxypyridinoline. *Clin. Chem.* 48, 220–235. doi: 10.1093/clinchem/48.2.220

Wang, L., You, X., Lotinun, S., Zhang, L., Wu, N., and Zou, W. (2020). Mechanical sensing protein PIEZO1 regulates bone homeostasis via osteoblast-osteoclast crosstalk. *Nat. Commun.* 11:282.

Wang, Y., Newman, M. R., and Benoit, D. S. W. (2018). Development of controlled drug delivery systems for bone fracture-targeted therapeutic delivery: a review. *Eur. J. Pharmaceut. Biopharmaceut.* 127, 223–236. doi: 10.1016/j.ejpb.2018.02.023

Winther, A., Dennison, E., Ahmed, L. A., Furberg, A. S., Grimnes, G., Jorde, R., et al. (2014). The tromsø study: fit futures: a study of norwegian adolescents' lifestyle and bone health. *Arch. Osteopor.* 9:185.

Woitge, H. W., Friedmann, B., Suttner, S., Farahmand, I., Müller, M., Schmidt-Gayk, H., et al. (1998). Changes in bone turnover induced by aerobic and anaerobic exercise in young males. *J. Bone Miner. Res.* 13, 1797–1804. doi: 10.1359/jbmr.1998.13.12.1797

Yu, P. B., Deng, D. Y., Lai, C. S., Hong, C. C., Cuny, G. D., Bouxsein, M. L., et al. (2008a). Bmp type i receptor inhibition reduces heterotopic [corrected] ossification. *Nat. Med.* 14, 1363–1369. doi: 10.1038/nm.1888

Yu, P. B., Hong, C. C., Sachidanandan, C., Babitt, J. L., Deng, D. Y., Hoyng, S. A., et al. (2008b). Dorsomorphin inhibits bmp signals required for embryogenesis and iron metabolism. *Nat. Chem. Biol.* 4, 33–41. doi: 10.1038/nchembio.2007.54

Yu, Y., Lin, Y., Yang, G., and Tian, L. (2017). The interplay between tgf-β/smad and bmp/smad signaling pathways in the epithelial mesenchymal transition of a549 cells induced by silica. *Toxicol. Mech. Methods* 28, 286–292. doi: 10.1080/15376516.2017.1407978

Zhang, J., Cai, L., Tang, L., Zhang, X., Yang, L., Zheng, K., et al. (2018). Highly dispersed lithium doped mesoporous silica nanospheres regulating adhesion, proliferation, morphology, alp activity and osteogenesis related gene expressions of bmscs. *Colloids Surf. B Biointerfaces* 170, 563–571. doi: 10.1016/j.colsurfb.2018.06.038

Zhang, L., Chen, X., Wu, J., Yuan, Y., Guo, J., Biswas, S., et al. (2017). The effects of different intensities of exercise and active vitamin D on mouse bone mass and bone strength. *J. Bone Miner. Metab.* 35, 265–277. doi: 10.1007/s00774-016-0764-9

Zhang, L., Liu, W., Zhao, J., Ma, X., Shen, L., Zhang, Y., et al. (2016). Mechanical stress regulates osteogenic differentiation and rankl/opg ratio in periodontal ligament stem cells by the wnt/β-catenin pathway. *Biochimica Biophysica Acta* 1860:2211–2219. doi: 10.1016/j.bbagen.2016.05.003

# 9

# SLIT2 Overexpression in Periodontitis Intensifies Inflammation and Alveolar Bone Loss, Possibly via the Activation of MAPK Pathway

*Liping Wang[1†], Jing Zheng[1†], Janak L. Pathak[1†], Yunxin Chen[1], Dongliang Liang[1], Luxi Yang[1], Haobo Sun[1], Mei Zhong[1], Lihong Wu[1], Li Li[2], Shuhua Deng[2], Lingyun Zheng[2], Yongyong Yan[1], Dan Hou[1], Lijing Wang[1,2*] and Linhu Ge[1*]*

*[1] Guangzhou Key Laboratory of Basic and Applied Research in Oral Regenerative Medicine, Affiliated Stomatology Hospital of Guangzhou Medical University, Institute of Oral Disease, Guangzhou Medical University, Guangzhou, China, [2] Vascular Biology Research Institute, School of Life Sciences and Biopharmaceutics, Guangdong Pharmaceutical University, Guangzhou, China*

***Correspondence:***
*Lijing Wang*
*2018991265@gzhmu.edu.cn*
*Linhu Ge*
*gelinhu@yeah.net*

*† These authors have contributed equally to this work and share first authorship*

SLIT2, a member of neuronal guidance cues, has been reported to regulate inflammation and cancer progression. Periodontitis is an oral inflammatory disease that degenerates periodontal tissue, alveolar bone and tooth. This study aims to explore the expression pattern of SLIT2 in periodontitis and its role in disease progression and bone loss. Gingival tissue of 20 periodontitis patients and 20 healthy-controls was obtained. Ligature-induced periodontitis (LIP) mice-model was developed in *Slit2-Tg* and wild-type mice. The effect of SLIT2 on inflammation, immune cell infiltration, M1 macrophage polarization, and alveolar bone loss in periodontitis was analyzed extensively. In periodontitis-affected gingival-tissue, SLIT2 expression was 4.4-fold higher compared to healthy-volunteers. LIP enhanced SLIT2 expression in mice periodontitis-affected periodontal tissue (PAPT) and blood circulation of wild-type mice by 4. 6-, and 5.0-fold, respectively. In Slit2-Tg-mice PAPT, SLIT2 expression was 1.8-fold higher compared to wild-type mice. Micro-CT and histomorphometric analysis revealed a 1.3-fold higher cement-enamel-junction to the alveolar-bone-crest (CEJ-ABC) distance and alveolar bone loss in LIP Slit2-Tg-mice compare to LIP wild-type mice. Results from RNA-sequencing, RT-qPCR, and ELISA showed a higher expression of Cxcr2, Il-18, TNF$\alpha$, IL-6, and IL-1$\beta$ in Slit2-Tg-mice PAPT compared to wild-type-mice. Slit2-Tg-mice PAPT showed a higher number of osteoclasts, M1 macrophages, and the upregulation of Robo1 expression. Slit2-Tg-mice PAPT showed upregulation of M1 macrophage marker CD16/32 and osteoclastogenic markers *Acp5*, *Ctsk*, and *Nfatc1*, but osteogenic markers (*Alp, Bglap*) remained unchanged. Immunohistochemistry unveiled the higher vasculature and infiltration of leucocytes and macrophages in Slit2-Tg-mice PAPT. RNA-sequencing, GO-pathway enrichment analysis, and western blot analysis revealed the activation of the MAPK signaling pathway in *Slit2*-Tg mice PAPT. In conclusion,

SLIT2 overexpression in periodontitis intensifies inflammation, immune cells infiltration, M1 macrophage polarization, osteoclastogenesis, and alveolar bone loss, possibly via activation of MAPK signaling, suggesting the role of SLIT2 on exacerbation of periodontitis and alveolar bone loss.

**Keywords: SLIT2, periodontitis, alveolar bone loss, osteoclasts, MAPK signaling**

## INTRODUCTION

SLIT2 protein, a member of neuronal guidance cues, is also expressed in extraneuronal tissues, including kidney, lung, heart, and immune cells (Yuan et al., 1999; Wu et al., 2001; Wong et al., 2002). SLIT2 is aberrantly expressed in various cancers and plays a role in the regulation of cancer cell apoptosis, cancer metastasis, tumor-associated inflammation, and tumor progression (Wang et al., 2003, 2008; Schmid et al., 2007; Avci et al., 2008; Yang et al., 2010; Zhou et al., 2011; Chang et al., 2015; Liu et al., 2018). Moreover, the SLIT2 has been reported to aberrantly regulate the inflammation in different inflammatory diseases and cell types (Zhao et al., 2014; Zhou et al., 2017; Fernando et al., 2018). SLIT2 is a secreted protein that binds to Roundabout (ROBO) receptors, i.e., ROBO1, ROBO2, ROBO3, and ROBO4. Binding of SLIT2 with specific ROBO receptor regulates particular cell functions. SLIT2/ROBO1-axis triggers proinflammatory signaling, and SLIT2/ROBO4-axis alleviates inflammation in endothelial cells during endotoxemia (Zhao et al., 2014). Periodontitis is a 6th most common chronic inflammatory disease worldwide (Kassebaum et al., 2014), affecting periodontal tissue, alveolar bone, and oral health homeostasis (Cochran, 2008; Darveau, 2010; Hajishengallis, 2014; Richards, 2014). Polymicrobial dysbiosis disrupts oral tissue homeostasis, and host immune reaction induces local and systematic inflammation in periodontitis (Darveau, 2010). Based on the existing knowledge about biological functions of SLITs in various pathophysiological conditions, (Zhao et al., 2012) had hypothesized SLIT as an effective immunotherapeutic agent in the treatment of periodontitis. However, the expression pattern of SLIT2 in periodontal tissue during periodontitis and its' role in the pathophysiology of periodontitis is still unknown.

In periodontitis, activated proinflammatory cascade dictates the pathophysiology of the disease. Higher microvessel density (MVD) in periodontitis affected gingival tissue promotes the extravasation of inflammatory immune cells (Aspriello et al., 2009). Recruited immune cells such as macrophages and neutrophils in gingival tissue not only phagocytize the microbes but also release the proinflammatory cytokines. Enhanced macrophage infiltration in gingival tissue is frequently observed in histological images of human or animal periodontitis-affected gingival tissue sections (Yu et al., 2016). M1 macrophage polarization in periodontitis-affected gingival tissue triggers the release of proinflammatory cytokines from the immune cells and amplifies the inflammation (Yu et al., 2016; Zhou et al., 2019). Higher numbers of M1 macrophages in periodontitis-affected gingival tissue positively correlates with clinical features of chronic and aggressive periodontitis (Gonzalez et al., 2015; Yu et al., 2016; Zhou et al., 2019; Zhu et al., 2019). Neutrophil extravasates and infiltrates in periodontitis-affected gingival tissue (Zhang et al., 2020). SLIT2 has been reported to regulate neutrophil chemotaxis during lung inflammation and renal-ischemic perfusion injury (Ye et al., 2010; Chaturvedi and Robinson, 2015). However, the effect of SLIT2 on, the infiltration of leucocytes/macrophages in periodontitis-affected gingival tissue, and regulation of periodontitis-induced inflammatory cascade still need to be investigated.

Periodontitis induces periodontal tissue damage and alveolar bone resorption increasing the risk of tooth loss. Activated inflammatory cascade elevates the level of pro-inflammatory cytokines in periodontal tissue, including IL-6, IL-1β, and TNF-α. Elevated levels of pro-inflammatory cytokines in alveolar bone induce osteoclastogenesis and osteoclastogenic bone resorption (Pan et al., 2019; AlQranei and Chellaiah, 2020; Xu et al., 2020). Activation of MAPK (p38) signaling in various immune cells regulates periodontal disease progression and alveolar bone loss (Li et al., 2012; Xu et al., 2020). SLIT2 contributes to cholestatic fibrosis via activation of MAPK p38 signaling in hepatic stellate cells (Li et al., 2019). However, the effect of SLIT2 on MAPK signaling in periodontal immune cells during periodontitis is still a mystery.

In this study, we aimed to analyze the expression pattern of SLIT2 in periodontitis-affected gingival tissue, and the role of SLIT2 on the pathophysiology of periodontitis. We analyzed SLIT2 expression in the human periodontitis-affected gingival tissue and ligature-induced periodontitis (LIP)-affected mice periodontal tissue. The effect of SLIT2 on the infiltration of immune cells, M1 macrophage polarization, osteoclastogenesis, and alveolar bone loss was extensively analyzed in *Slit2*-Transgenic (Tg) periodontitis mice. Our study elucidated SLIT2 overexpression in human and mice periodontitis-affected tissue. Moreover, SLIT2 overexpression intensifies the infiltration of leucocytes/macrophages, inflammation, M1 macrophage polarization, osteoclastogenesis, alveolar bone loss, and activation of P-P38 signaling in periodontitis.

## MATERIALS AND METHODS

### Collection of Human Gingival Biopsies

Human gingiva, including sulcus/pocket epithelium and underlying connective tissue, were obtained from either healthy controls ($n$ = 20) or patients with periodontitis ($n$ = 20) with alveolar bone loss confirmed by radiography. Patients and healthy controls clinical characteristics and demographics are summarized in **Supplementary Table S1**. Written informed consent was obtained from each patient. Human gingival tissues were used to analyze SLIT2 protein expression by ELISA. The Medical Ethics Committee of the Affiliated Stomatology Hospital of Guangzhou Medical University approved all protocols dealing with patients (approval number: KY2019032).

## Animals

Total of 47 wild-type C57BL/6 and 47 *Slit2* transgenic (*Slit2-Tg*) C57BL/6 mice were used in this study. Wild-type mice were purchased from Guangdong Medical Animal Experiment Center (Guangdong, China). *Slit2-Tg* mice were obtained from Prof. Lijing Wang's lab, Vascular Biology Research Institute, School of Life Sciences and Biopharmaceutics, Guangdong Pharmaceutical University, Guangzhou, China. *Slit2-Tg* mice were generated according to the previously reported protocol (Yang et al., 2010). All the mice used were healthy and immune-normal, euthanized after their experimental periods. All studies were performed in 8-week-old male mice unless otherwise indicated. The Experimental Animal Ethics Committee of Guangzhou Medical University approved all animal care and study protocols (GY2020-004).

## Primary Bone Marrow-Derived Macrophages (BMMs) Culture

Bone marrow-derived macrophages (BMMs) were harvested from the bone marrow of six C57BL/6 mice as described previously (Spiller et al., 2016). BMMs were expanded in T75 culture flasks supplemented with Gibco RPMI 1640 medium (Life Technologies, Carlsbad, CA, United States) and 10% FBS. For the *in vitro* studies cultures were supplemented with 30 ng/ml recombinant mouse macrophage colony-stimulating factor (M-CSF, CB34, Novoprotein, Shanghai, China). Cultures were used for further mRNA and protein expression analysis.

## Development of Periodontitis in Mice

A ligature-induced periodontitis (LIP) model was developed in *Slit2-Tg* and wild-type mice, as described previously (Abe and Hajishengallis, 2013).

## Micro-CT Analysis

Micro-CT scanned the maxilla to evaluate the morphological changes in the alveolar bone. The distance from the mesial buccal cemento-enamel junction to the alveolar bone crest (CEJ-ABC) of the second molar was measured as a reference for bone loss. The level of bone resorption was calculated as described previously (Abe and Hajishengallis, 2013).

## Western Blot Analysis

Periodontitis-affected periodontal tissue (PAPT; 0.5 cm× 0.5 cm × 1.0 cm) surrounding the teeth cut from mice maxilla, including gingiva, periodontal ligament, and a part of alveolar bone, was stored at −80°C for use. Frozen periodontal tissue samples were solubilized in lysis buffer containing 10 mM of Tris–HCl, pH 7.4, 150 mM of NaCl, 1 mM of EDTA, and 1% Triton X-100 at 4°C for 20 min. The tissue lysates were subjected to centrifugation at 15000 × *g* at 4°C for 20 min. The supernatant was collected, and their protein contents were determined using Coomassie Plus Protein Assay Reagent (Pierce, Rockford, IL, United States). Cell lysate protein (50 μg) was separated by sodium dodecyl sulfate-polyacrylamide gel electrophoresis (SDS-PAGE) and transferred to polyvinylidene difluoride (PVDF) membranes. The membranes were then blocked with 5% non-fat dry milk for 1 h and incubated overnight at 4°C with primary antibodies: anti-TRAF6 (1:1000 dilution, ABclonal, Wuhan, China), anti-P38 (1:1000 dilution, ABclonal), anti-P-P38 (1:1000 dilution, Cell Signaling Technology, MA, United States), or anti-TRAP (1:1000 dilution, ABclonal). The membranes were then washed and incubated with HRP-conjugated secondary antibodies (1:5000 dilution, ABclonal) at room temperature. An enhanced chemiluminescence detection system (Thermo Scientific, MA, United States) detected the immunoreactive protein bands. Densitometry data for band intensities results were generated by analyzing the images using ImageJ software. β-actin was used as a reference housekeeping protein.

## Histological Evaluation

After scanning micro-CT images, the collected maxillae were fixed in 4% formaldehyde overnight, followed by decalcification in 10% EDTA, which was exchanged every week for 1 month. The specimens were cut in 3 mm thickness along the long axis of the molars. Next, the samples were dehydrated and embedded in paraffin blocks. Serial sections of 5 μm thickness were cut and mounted on poly-l-lysine-coated slides. Hematoxylin and eosin (H&E) staining was performed separately on consecutive tissue sections. Images were captured using a microscope. The CEJ-ABC distance between the maxillary first and second molars was measured as a net bone loss on tissue sections, using Image J software (Wang et al., 2015).

## Immunohistochemistry

Thick tissue sections (5 μm) were deparaffinized and rehydrated, followed by heat-induced epitope retrieval (Xiao et al., 2017). Methanol containing 3% $H_2O_2$ was used to block the endogenous peroxidase for 20 min. Tissue sections were then blocked with 10% bovine serum albumin (BSA) and incubated for overnight at 4°C with primary antibodies: monoclonal anti-CD34 [EP373Y], (ab81289, Abcam, Cambridge, United Kingdom), anti-CD45 (20103-1-AP, Proteintech, United States), monoclonal anti-F4/80 [BM8], (123110, BioLegend, CA, United States) or isotype controls. After washing with PBS three times, tissue sections were incubated with a corresponding goat anti-rabbit secondary antibody (SolelyBio, Beijing, China) for 30 min at 37°C. Slides were incubated with diaminobenzidine (Cell Signaling Technology, MA, United States) followed by hematoxylin counterstaining. Finally, all stained sections were dehydrated through a series of graded alcohol baths of increasing concentration, cleared in xylene, and mounted with coverslips. Stained tissue sections were visualized under a microscope (Leica, Germany), and images were captured. The visual fields between the first molar and the second molar were photographed. The number of immunostaining-positive cells was counted in the entire area of each image.

## Tartrate-Resistant Acid Phosphatase (TRAP) Staining

Tissue sections were stained using acid phosphatase (TRAP) kit (G1050, Servicebio, Wuhan, China) following the manufacturer's instructions. TRAP stained histological tissue section were examined under microscope, and images of predefined areas were captured. TRAP-positive cells appeared bright red. TRAP-positive osteoclasts, in the alveolar bone tissue section between the first molar and the second molar, were counted.

## Real-Time qPCR

Periodontal tissue removed from mice maxillae (periodontitis-affected and control group) was homogenized in a mortar on liquid nitrogen, and total RNA was isolated using PureLink RNA Mini Kit (12183018A, Thermo Fisher Scientific, United States). RNA samples with 1.8 to 2.0 of the OD260/280 ratio were used for analysis, and total RNA reverse were transcribed using Takara PrimeScriptTM RT Master Mix in T100 Thermal Cycler (Bio-Rad, United States). The transcribed cDNA was used for RT-qPCR using Takara TB-Green Premix Ex Taq in LightCycler RT-PCR system (LC-480 II, Roche, Switzerland). GADPH was used as a reference housekeeping gene. The $2^{-\Delta\Delta Ct}$ method was used to analyze the relative mRNA expression levels. The primers used for RT-qPCR are listed in **Supplementary Table S2**.

## Protein Expression Analysis by ELISA

ELISA analyzed the protein level in human and mice periodontal tissue protein extract, mice serum, conditioned medium of mice BMMs culture, and mice BMMs cell lysates. The procedure of periodontal tissue protein extract has been described in the Western blot analysis section above. For mice serum separation, blood samples were collected from orbital venous plexus, and the serum was separated by 5 min centrifugation at 2,000 rpm. BMMs culture conditioned medium and cell lysates were prepared as follows. On the fifth day of BMMs culture, 100 ng/ml LPS was added. After 48 h of LPS treatment, conditioned medium (CM) was collected, and attached cells in the culture harvested for cell lysate preparation. SLIT2 level in human periodontal tissue lysate was analyzed by human SLIT2 ELISA kit (Cusabio, Wuhan, China) following the manufacturer's instruction. The protein levels of IL-6, IL-1β, and TNF-a in periodontal tissue protein extract and CM were measured by mouse ELISA Standard Kit (RayBiotech, Atlanta, United States). The protein level of CD16/32 in mice periodontal tissue protein extract and the BMMs cell lysate were measured by Mouse ELISA Standard Kit (Cusabio, Wuhan, China). The protein levels of SLIT2 in mice periodontal tissue protein extract and mice serum were measured by mouse SLIT2 ELISA Kit (Cusabio, Wuhan, China) following the manufacturer's instruction.

## Flow Cytometry Analysis

The cell suspension was prepared from mice periodontal tissue, including gingiva, periodontal ligament, and a part of alveolar bone for flow cytometry analysis (Mizraji et al., 2013). Prior to the test, cells were counted and cell viability was evaluated by the Zombie NIR$^{TM}$ Fixable Viability Kit (423105, BioLegend, Beijing, China). Cells were stained with 1 μg of anti-F4/80 (123110, BioLegend, CA, United States) solution, monoclonal anti-CD11b [M1/70], (101206, BioLegend, CA, United States) or anti-rabbit IgG per $1 \times 10^6$ cells for 30 min on ice in the dark. After two times washing with PBS, the cells were resuspended in 300 μl PBS and transferred to flow tubes. Flow cytometric analysis was performed using the FACSAria III Cell Sorter (BD Biosciences, San Jose, CA, United States).

## RNA Sequencing

The wild-type and Slit2-Tg periodontitis mice periodontal tissue samples without enzymatic treatment were used for RNA sequencing. Total RNA was extracted from periodontal tissue using the TRIzol kit (Invitrogen, Carlsbad, CA, United States), according to the manufacturer's protocol. The RNA concentration was determined using Qubit, and RNA amount and purity of each sample was assessed with a NanoDrop spectrophotometer (NanoDrop 2000, Wilmington, DE, United States). RNA was isolated in 40 μl of DEPC water and stored in −80°C. Briefly, RNA-seq libraries were prepared by using the Illumina TruseqTM RNA sample prep Kit and were sequenced using an Illumina HiSeq. Cutadapt was used to obtain paired-end reads (Martin, 2011). The quality of the RNA-samples used for RNA-seq is presented in **Supplementary Table S3**. The reads were aligned with Hisat2 (v 2.1.0) to GRCm38 with default parameters (Kim et al., 2015). Only the data matched to the reference genome were used for subsequent analysis. The mapped reads of each sample were assembled using StringTie (Pertea et al., 2015). Then, the transcriptomes from all samples were merged to reconstruct a comprehensive transcriptome using perl scripts. After the final transcriptome was generated, StringTie (Pertea et al., 2015) and Ballgown (Frazee et al., 2015) was used to estimate the expression levels of all transcripts. Traditional singular enrichment analysis (SEA) (Rodriguez et al., 2016) was used for the enrichment analysis of GO terms and pathways. The enrichment *P*-value calculation was performed with Fisher's exact test. RNA-sequence data are available at **Supplementary Data S1**. All raw RNA-sequencing data can be accessed from NCBI SRA database (SRA accession: PRJNA639904)[1].

## Statistical Analyses

All data are presented as mean ± standard deviation (SD). Statistical analysis was performed using SPSS 19.0 statistical software (SPSS IBM, Armonk, NY, United States). For where appropriate (comparison of two groups only), two-tailed *t*-tests were done. In all cases, data from at least three independent experiments was used, and *P* value of less than 0.05 was considered to indicate a statistically significant difference.

[1]https://www.ncbi.nlm.nih.gov/bioproject/PRJNA639904/

## RESULTS

### Periodontitis Amplifies SLIT2 Expression in Gingival Tissue

First, we examined the SLIT2 expression in human gingival tissues of 20 periodontitis patients and 20 age and gender-matched healthy individuals. The SLIT2 protein level in periodontitis-affected human gingival tissue was 4.4-fold higher compared to healthy gingival tissue (**Figure 1A**). The SLIT2 protein level in the periodontal tissue of *Slit2*-Tg mice was 2.1-fold higher compared to wild-type mice (**Figure 1B**). The SLIT2 protein expression in wild-type mice was upregulated by 4.6-fold compared to healthy periodontal tissue (**Figure 1B**). Similarly, a 3.9-fold higher expression of SLIT2 protein was observed in *Slit2-Tg* mice PAPT compared to healthy periodontal tissue (**Figure 1B**). *Slit2-Tg* mice PAPT showed a 1.8-fold higher expression of SLIT2 protein in comparison to wild-type mice PAPT (**Figure 1B**). Additionally, the serum of wild-type periodontitis mice showed 5.0-fold higher expression of SLIT2 protein compared to wild-type healthy mice (**Figure 1C**). Our results indicate the upregulation of SLIT2 expression in gingival tissue during periodontitis in human and in PAPT of wild-type mice or *Slit2-Tg* mice. Moreover, periodontitis condition upregulates the level of serum SLIT2 in wild-type mice showing the systemic effect of periodontitis.

### Higher Expression of SLIT2 Intensifies Periodontitis and Alveolar Bone Loss

We performed micro-CT scanning to analyze the effect of LIP on alveolar bone loss. Intact periodontal tissue and normal alveolar bone were observed in healthy wild-type and *Slit2*-Tg mice (**Figure 1D**). Loss of periodontal tissue and alveolar bone was observed in LIP wild-type and *Slit2-Tg* mice (**Figure 1D**). The higher CEJ-ABC distance indicates the higher effect of periodontitis on periodontal tissue damage and alveolar bone loss. CEJ-ABC distance in periodontitis wild-type mice was 1.9-fold higher compared to healthy wild-type mice (**Figure 1E**). Similarly, CEJ-ABC distance in periodontitis *Slit2-Tg* mice was 2.3-fold higher compared to healthy *Slit2-Tg* mice (**Figure 1E**). *Slit2-Tg* periodontitis mice showed a 1.3-fold higher CEJ-ABC distance compared to wild-type periodontitis mice (**Figure 1E**). This finding was corroborated by the histological images as well (**Figure 1F**). *Slit2*-Tg mice periodontitis exhibited more bone loss and bone destruction in the alveolar crest height than in wild-type mice periodontitis (**Figures 1D,E**). This effect was further corroborated by the histological images (**Figure 1F**). The histological images showed the infiltration of inflammatory immune cells in gingival epithelial and alveolar bone resorption (**Figure 1F**). Histomorphometric analysis showed 1.3-fold higher periodontitis-induced alveolar bone loss in *Slit2-Tg* mice compared to wild-type mice (**Figure 1G**). Our results indicate that the overexpressed SLIT2 in periodontitis aggravates the consequences of the disease, such as the destruction of periodontal tissue and alveolar bone loss.

### SLIT2 Overexpression Amplifies Osteoclastogenesis and Inflammation in Periodontitis Milieu

Inflammatory cytokines promote osteoclastogenesis, and higher osteoclastogenesis is associated with higher bone loss. In this study, we analyzed the role of the higher SLIT2 expression in periodontitis on osteoclastogenesis. More numbers of TRAP-positive osteoclasts were visualized in the PAPT section of *Slit2-Tg* mice compared to wild type mice (**Figure 2A**). A higher degree of vasculature in gingival tissue aggravates periodontitis. In this study, we performed CD34 immunostaining in PAPT to detect microvasculatures. Higher CD34 expression was observed in PAPT *of Slit2-Tg* mice compared to wild-type mice (**Figure 2B**). Quantitative analysis showed a 1.4-fold higher number of osteoclasts in PAPT in *Slit2-Tg* mice compared to wild-type mice (**Figure 2C**). Quantitative analysis revealed 1.4-fold higher microvessel density (MVD) in PAPT of *Slit2-Tg* mice compared to wild-type mice (**Figure 2D**).

Similarly, we performed immunohistochemical staining for leukocyte specific antigen, CD45, in gingival tissue sections to analyze the effect of SLIT2 overexpression on leucocytes infiltration in PAPT. More numbers of CD45 positive cells were observed in periodontitis-affected gingival tissue of *Slit2-Tg* mice compared to wild-type mice (**Figure 2B**). Quantitative analysis results revealed a 1.2-fold higher number of CD45-positive cells in PAPT of *Slit2-Tg* mice compared to wild-type mice (**Figure 2E**). This indicates that the higher degree of leucocyte infiltration in PAPT of *Slit2-Tg* mice, possibly amplify periodontal inflammation.

RNA sequencing (RNA-seq) of mice PAPT was performed to explore the underlying mechanisms of the regulatory effects of SLIT2 on periodontitis. Among 24 common inflammatory factors, *Cxcr2, Il18,* and *Il1β* were differentially upregulated by more than 2-fold in PAPT of *Slit2-Tg* mice compared to wild-type mice (**Figure 3A (i)**). The heat map corroborated the differential upregulation of *Cxcr2, Il18,* and *Il1β* mRNA in PAPT of *Slit2-Tg* mice compared to wild-type mice (**Figure 3A (ii)**). Highly expressed pro-inflammatory cytokines in periodontal tissue abrogate periodontitis. RT-qPCR results showed 2. 3-, 1. 8-, and 1.6-fold higher expression of *Il6* (**Figure 3B**), *Il1β* (**Figure 3C**), and *Tnf* (**Figure 3D**), respectively, in PAPT of *Slit2-Tg* mice compared to wild-type mice. Protein level expression of IL-6 (**Figure 3E**), IL-1β (**Figure 3F**), and TNF-α (**Figure 3G**) were 8-, 4- and 2.6-fold higher, respectively, in PAPT of *Slit2-Tg* mice compared to wild-type mice. This result indicates that the SLIT2-overexpression intensifies the inflammation in periodontitis.

We further analyzed the differential expression of 32 osteoclastogenesis related genes in PAPT by RAN-seq. The expression of *Fosl2, Il1β, Mapk14, Ncf4,* and *Pik3cb,* was differentially upregulated in PAPT of *Slit2-Tg* mice compared to wild-type mice (**Figures 4A (i),(ii)**). We further analyzed the mRNA expression of the key osteoclastogenesis regulators (*Acp5, Ctsk,* and *Nfatc1*) in PAPT by RT-qPCR. Notably, the expression of *Acp5, Ctsk*, and *Nfatc1* in PAPT of *Slit2-Tg* mice was 18. 4-, 2. 2-, and 1.8-fold higher, respectively, compared to wild-type mice (**Figures 4B–D**). Additionally, the expressions

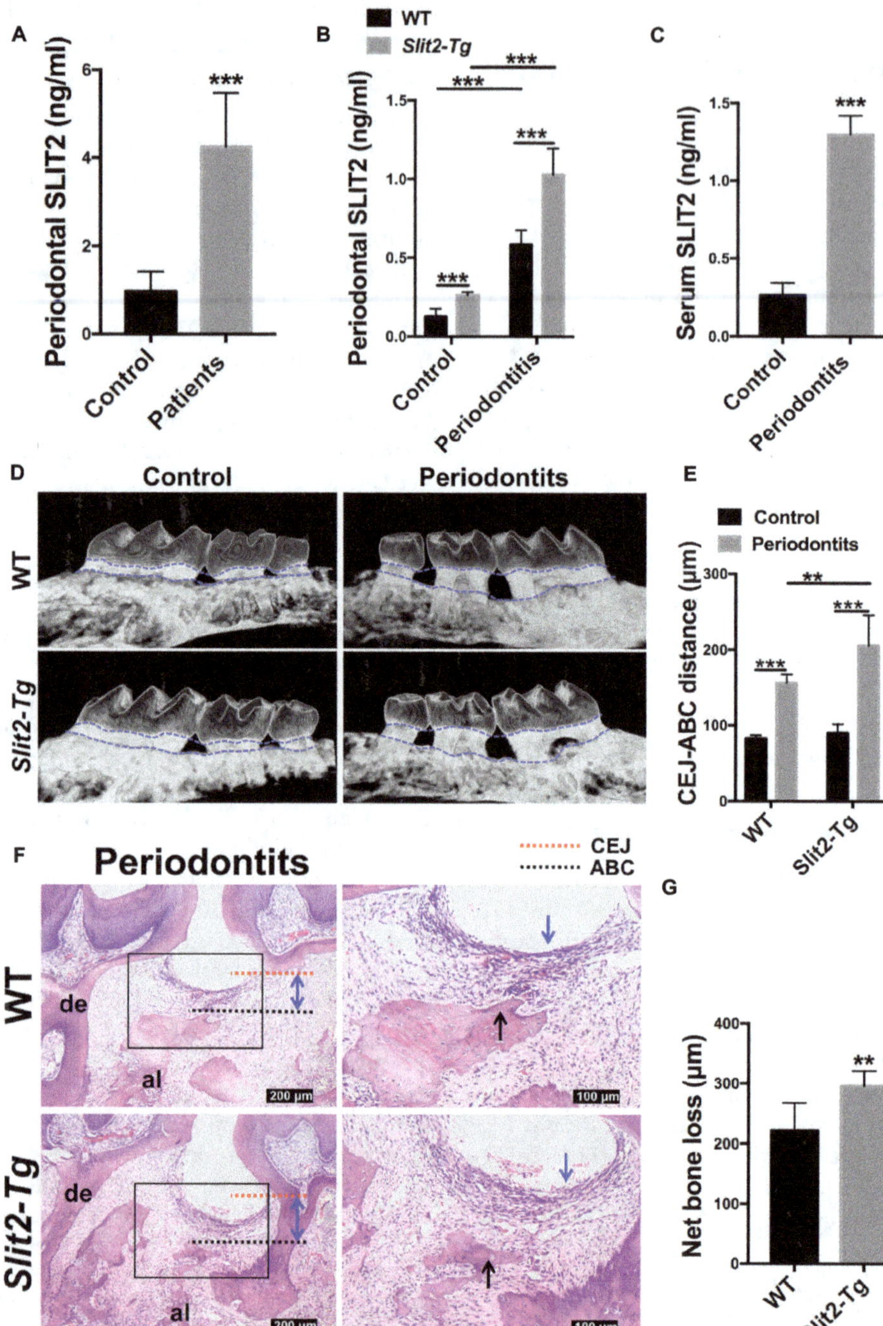


**FIGURE 1 |** Periodontitis-induced SLIT2 aggravates periodontitis and alveolar bone loss. Expression pattern of SLIT2 protein in, **(A)** Gingival tissue of periodontitis patients and healthy individuals ($n$ = 20), and **(B)** periodontal tissue of healthy and periodontitis wild-type or *Slit2-Tg* mice. **(C)** Serum level of SLIT2 protein in wild-type mice ($n$ = 5). **(D)** Micro-CT images of healthy and periodontitis-affected alveolar bone with the intact tooth of wild-type and *Slit2-Tg* mice. **(E)** Quantitative data of CEJ-ABC distance analyzed from micro-CT images. **(F)** H&E stained histological images of PAPT of wild-type and *Slit2-Tg* mice. **(G)** Quantitative data of alveolar bone loss around the periodontitis-affected tooth analyzed from histological images. Data are presented as mean ± SD ($n$ = 6). The significant difference among the groups, *$P < 0.05$, **$P < 0.01$, ***$P < 0.001$. CEJ: cement-enamel junction, ABC: alveolar bone crest, Red dot line: CEJ level, Black dot line: ABC level, al: alveolar bone, de: dentine, blue arrow: inflammatory infiltration of the gingival epithelium, black arrow: alveolar bone resorption, double arrowhead (blue): CEJ-ABC distance, and WT: wild-type.

of the majority of osteoblastogenesis associated genes were not altered in PAPT of *Slit2-Tg* mice compared to wild-type mice. (**Figure 4E** and **Supplementary Figure S1**). These results indicate that the SLIT2 overexpression mainly triggers inflammation-induced osteoclastogenesis but might not affect the osteoblast function during periodontitis.

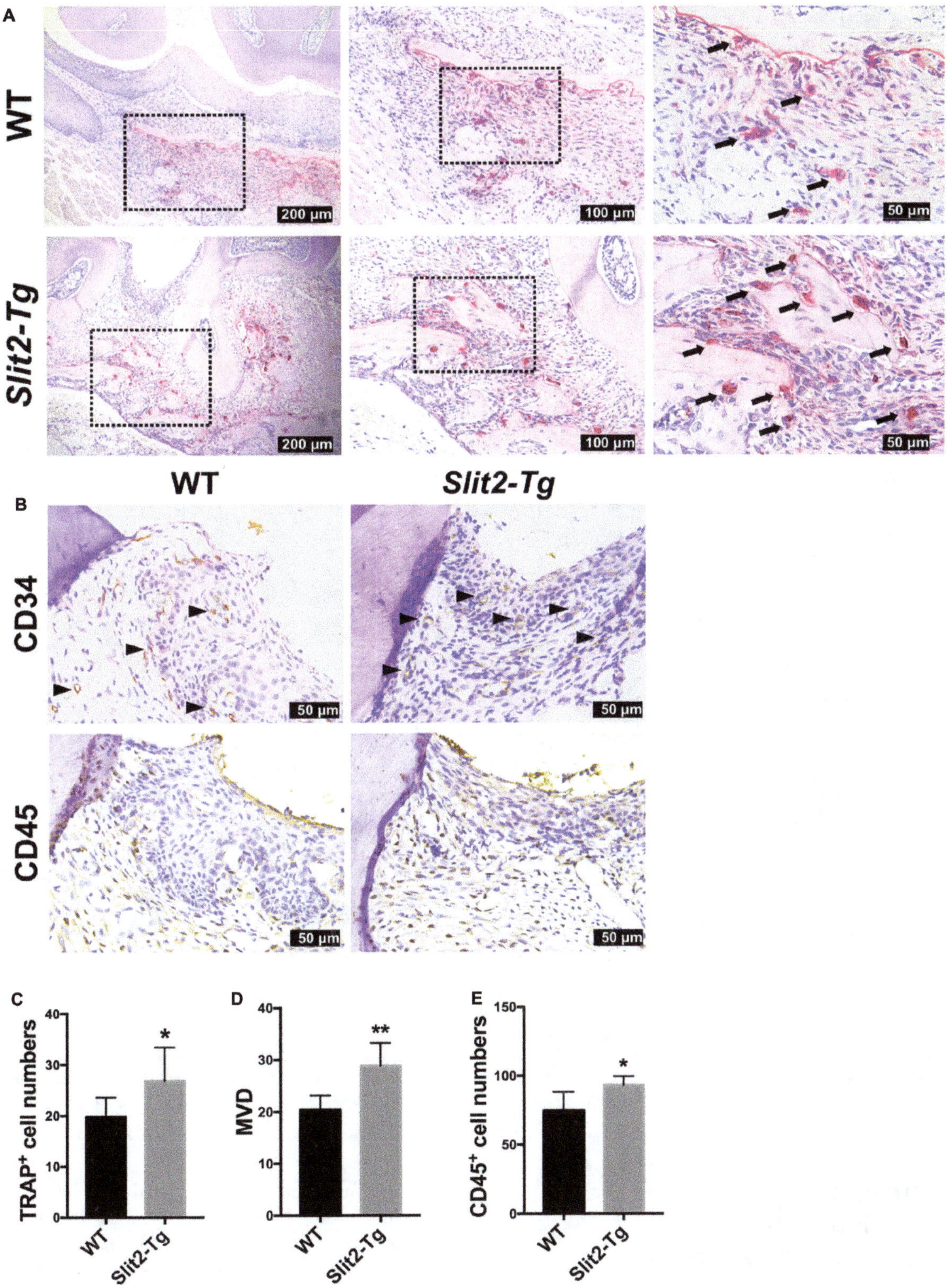


**FIGURE 2** | SLIT2 overexpression augments pathological changes in both periodontal milieu soft and bone tissues during periodontitis. **(A)** Representative histological images of PAPT sections showing TRAP+ osteoclasts. **(B)** Representative CD34 and CD45 immunohistochemistry images of PAPT sections. **(C)** Quantitative analysis of osteoclasts from TRAP-stained histological tissue sections ($n$ = 6). **(D)** Quantification of micro-vessel density from CD34 immunohistochemistry images ($n$ = 5). **(E)** Quantification of CD45 expressing cells from CD45 immunohistochemistry images ($n$ = 6). The significant difference among the groups, $^{*}P < 0.05$, $^{**}P < 0.01$. Black arrow: TRAP+ multinucleated osteoclasts. Black triangle arrowhead: microvessel. WT: wild-type.

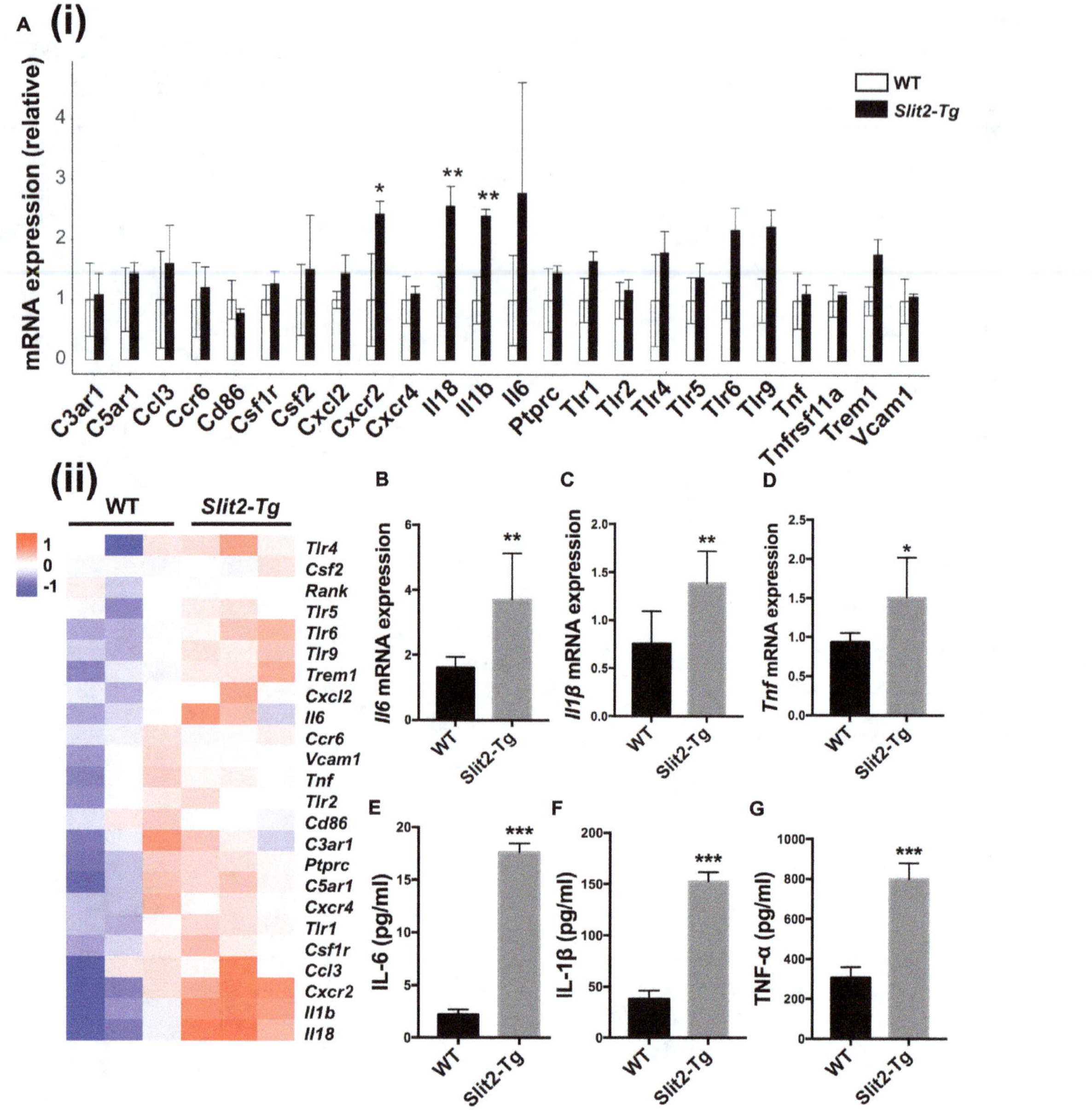


**FIGURE 3 |** SLIT2 overexpression triggers up-regulation of periodontal inflammatory factors. **(A (i))** Relative mRNA expression, and **(A (ii))** Heat map showing the differential expression pattern of inflammatory markers in PAPT analyzed by RNA sequencing ($n$ = 3). Relative mRNA expression of **(B)** *Il6*, **(C)** *Il1β*, and **(D)** *Tnfα* in periodontitis-affected tissue analyzed by RT-qPCR. Protein expression of, **(E)** IL-6, **(F)** IL-1β, and **(G)** TNF-α in periodontitis-affected tissue analyzed by ELISA. Data are presented as mean ± SD ($n$ = 6). Data are presented as mean ± SD. The significant difference among the groups, $^{*}P < 0.05$, $^{**}P < 0.01$, $^{***}P < 0.001$. Red color intensity indicates upregulation, and blue color intensity indicates the downregulation of gene expression.

## SLIT2 Overexpression Enhances the Infiltration of Macrophages and M1 Macrophage Polarization in Periodontitis

More numbers of macrophages (F4/80 positive cells) were observed in the PAPT section of *Slit2-Tg* mice compared to wild-type mice (**Figure 5A (i)**). Quantitative analysis of infiltrated macrophages from immunohistochemistry images showed 1.3-fold higher numbers of macrophages in PAPT of *Slit2-Tg* mice compared to wild-type mice (**Figure 5A (ii)**). This finding was further verified by the data from flow cytometry analysis (**Figures 5B (i),(ii)**). Flow cytometry analysis revealed 1.4-fold higher numbers of CD11b+F4/80+ cells in the PAPT of *Slit2-Tg* mice compared to wild-type mice (**Figure 5B (ii)**). Prior to the test, cell viability was evaluated and above 95% viability of cells was ensured (data not shown). This finding indicates that the SLIT2 overexpression in periodontitis facilitates the infiltration of macrophages in periodontal tissue.

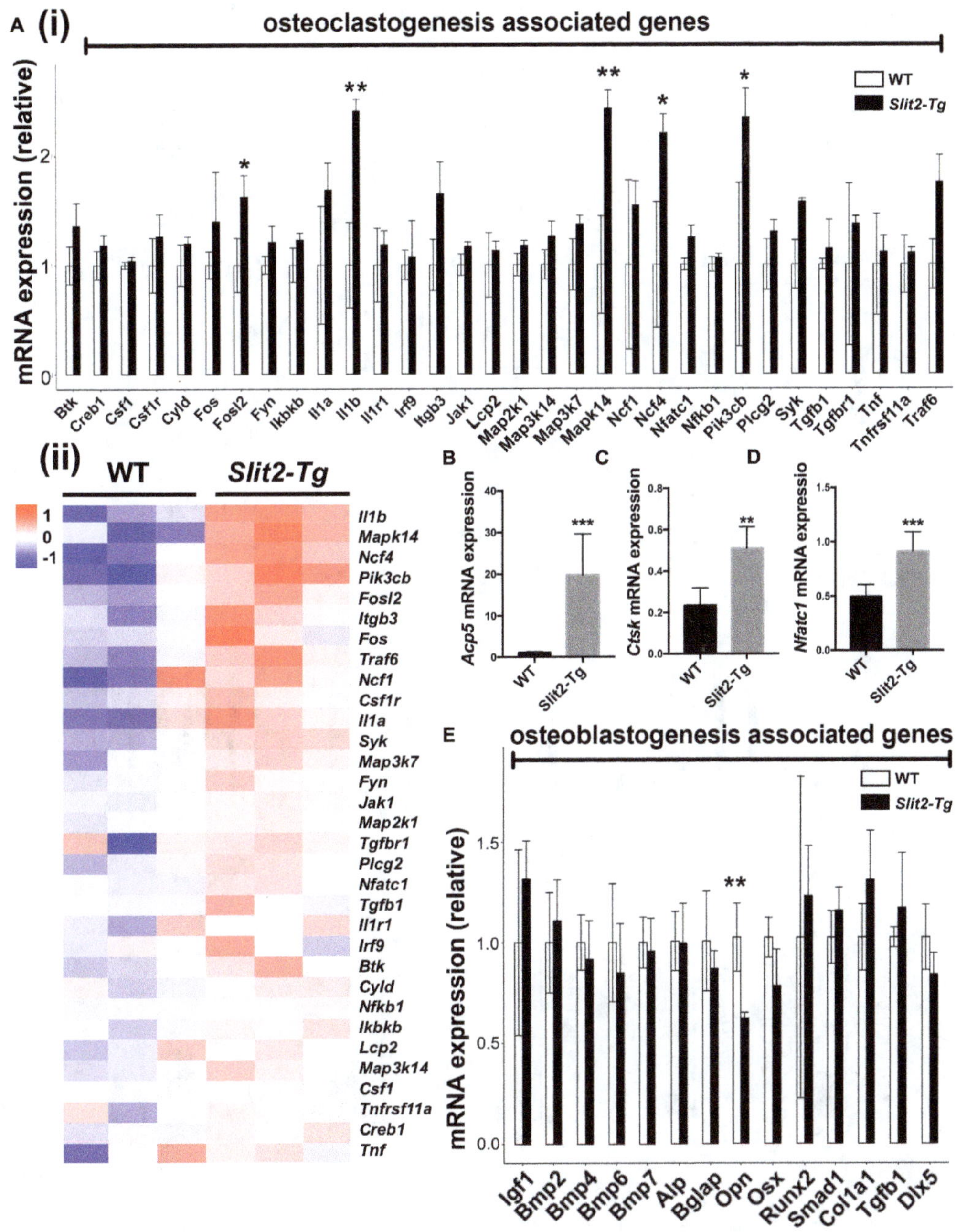


**FIGURE 4 |** SLIT2 overexpression activates osteoclastogenesis-related signaling pathways in periodontitis. **(A (i))** Relative mRNA expression, and **(A (ii))** Heat map showing the differential expression pattern of osteoclastogenesis related genes analyzed by RNA-seq ($n$ = 3). Relative mRNA expression of **(B)** *Acp5*, **(C)** *Ctsk*, and **(D)** *Nfatc1* in periodontal tissue analyzed by RT-qPCR ($n$ = 6). **(E)** Relative mRNA expression of osteoblastogenesis related genes analyzed by RNA sequencing ($n$ = 3). Data are presented as mean ± SD. The significant difference among the groups, $^{*}P < 0.05$, $^{**}P < 0.01$, $^{***}P < 0.001$. WT: wild-type.

Proinflammatory cytokines trigger the M1 macrophage polarization. The relative expression of *Il1β* and *Il8* was upregulated in *Slit2-Tg* PAPT (**Figure 5C**). However, the expression of M2 macrophage polarization related cytokines (such as *Il10* and *Il4*) remained the same in *Slit2-Tg* PAPT and wild-type mice (**Figure 5D**). The protein level of CD16/32, a marker of M1 macrophage polarization, was upregulated (2.8-fold) in PAPT of *Slit2-Tg* mice compared to wild-type mice (**Figure 5E**). Similarly, under inflammatory condition (LPS treatment), cell lysate from *in vitro* cultured macrophages of *Slit2-Tg* mice expressed 4.7-fold higher CD16/32 compared to wild-type mice (**Figure 5F**). Similarly, inflammatory condition upregulated IL-6, IL-1β, and TNF-α expression in *Slit2-Tg* mice macrophages by 3. 6-, 2. 6-, and 1.9-fold, respectively, compared to wild-type mice macrophages (**Figures 5G–I**). This result indicates that SLIT2

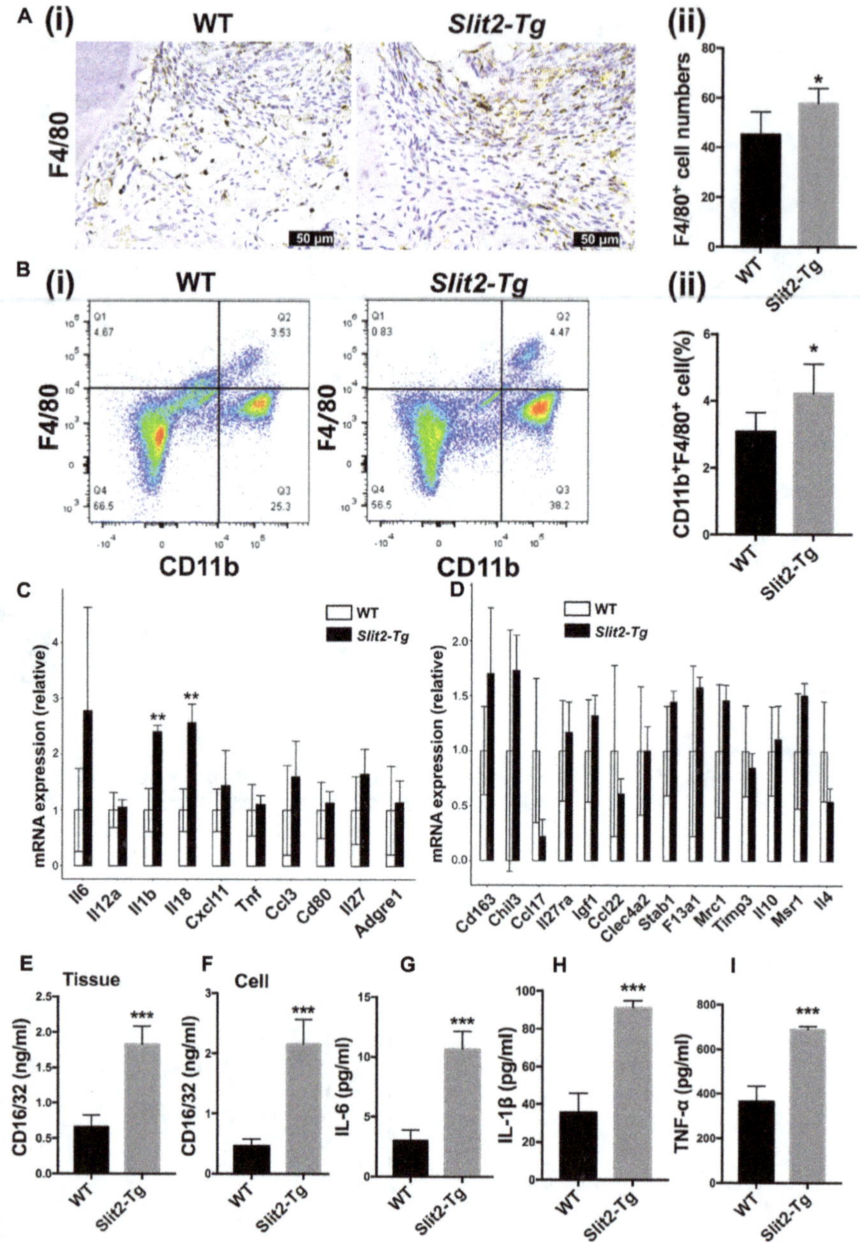

**FIGURE 5 |** SLIT2 overexpression induces M1 macrophage polarization in PAPT. **(A (i))** Representative F4/80 immunohistochemistry images of the PAPT section. **(A (ii))** Quantification of F4/80 expressing cells in a PAPT section from immunohistochemistry images (*n* = 6). **(B (i))** Flow cytometry analysis of F4/80 positive relative frequency of gated populations from PAPT. **(B (ii))** Quantitative analysis of F4/80+ flow cytometry data (*n* = 5). Relative mRNA expression of **(C)** M1, and **(D)** M2 macrophage polarization related genes analyzed by RNA sequencing (*n* = 3). **(E)** Protein level expression of CD16/32 in PAPT (*n* = 6). Protein level expression of, **(F)** CD16/32 in cell lysates of LPS-treated BMMs. Protein expression of **(G)** IL-6, **(H)** IL-1β, and **(I)** TNF-α in conditioned medium of LPS-treated BMMs (*n* = 4). Data are presented as mean ± SD. The significant difference among the groups, $^{*}P < 0.05$, $^{**}P < 0.01$, $^{***}P < 0.001$.

overexpression amplifies macrophage infiltration and M1 macrophage polarization in PAPT.

## SLIT2 Overexpression Upregulates Its Receptor ROBO1

ROBO1, ROBO2, ROBO3, and ROBO4 are 4 receptors of SLIT2 ligand. In RNA-seq heat map, *Robo1* and *Robo2* gene expression were differentially upregulated, and *Robo3* and *Robo4* remained unchanged in *Slit2-Tg* mice PAPT (**Figures 6A–D**). Quantification of RNA-seq data showed 1.5-fold, and RT-qPCR analysis showed a 2.0-fold higher expression of Robo1 in PAPT of *Slit2-Tg* mice compared to wild type mice (**Figure 6A (ii)**). However, the expression of other receptors remained unchanged. This result indicates the possible role of the SLIT2/ROBO1 axis on SLIT2-mediated effects in periodontitis.

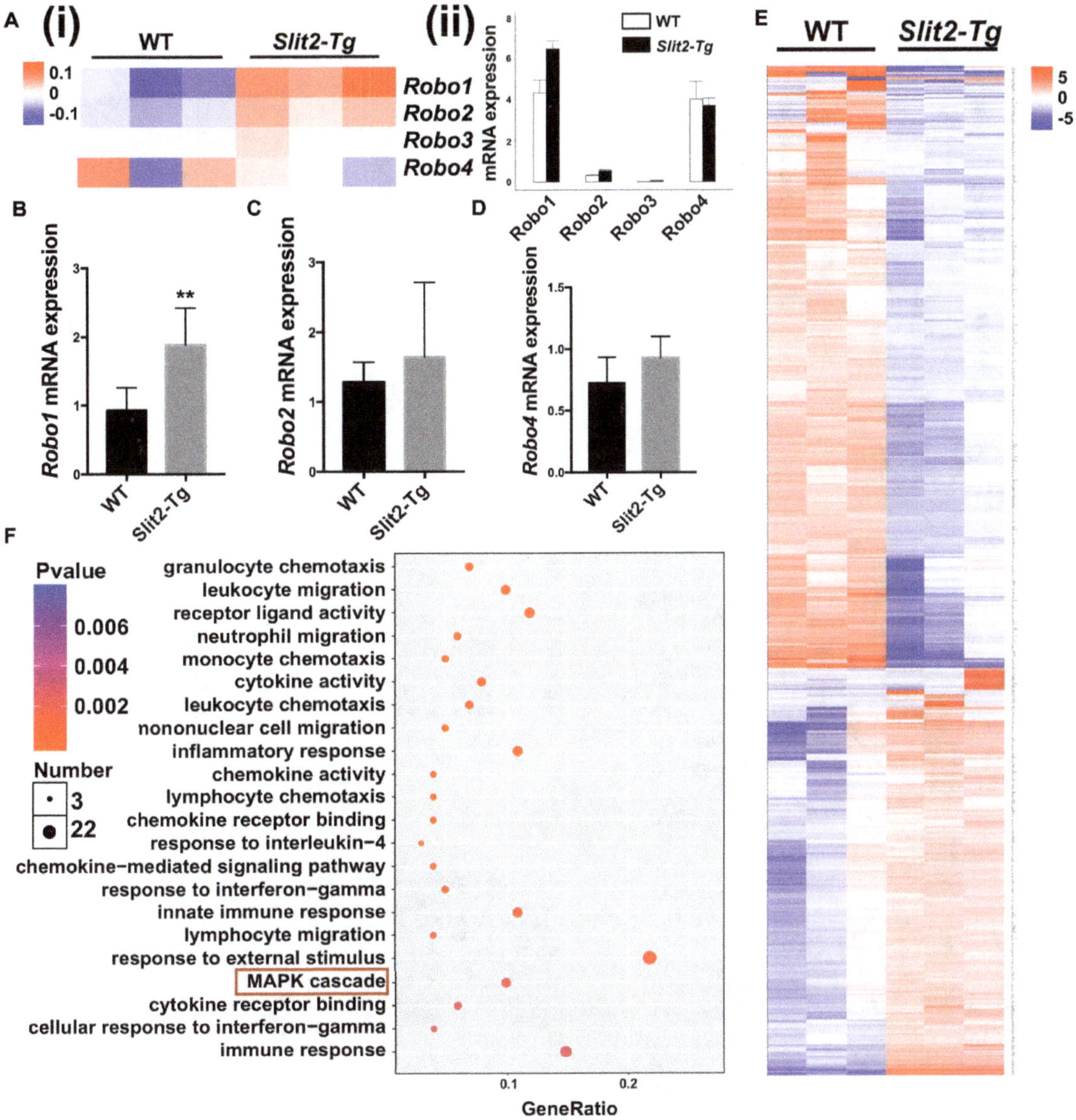


**FIGURE 6 |** SLIT2/ROBO1 signaling possibly regulates the SLIT2-induced inflammation in periodontitis. **(A (i))** Heat map the differential expression of Slit2 receptors *Robo1-4*, and **(A (ii))** Relative mRNA expression of *Robo1*, *Robo2*, *Robo3*, and *Robo4* in PAPT analyzed by RNA sequencing ($n = 3$). Relative mRNA expression of, **(B)** *Robo1*, **(C)** *Robo2*, and **(D)** *Robo4* in PAPT analyzed by RT-qPCR ($n = 6$). **(E)** Heat map of differentially expressed 134 mRNAs in PAPT of *Slit2-Tg* mice to wild-type mice (fdr $< 0.05$,$|FC| > 2$). **(F)** GO pathway enrichment analysis. Data are presented as mean ± SD. The significant difference among the groups, *$P < 0.05$, **$P < 0.01$.

## Activated MAPK Signaling Might Regulates the SLIT2-Mediated Abrogation of Periodontitis

RNA sequencing data detected the expression of total of 53801 genes in mice PAPT (**Supplementary Data S1**). Among those, 134 genes were differentially expressed in *Slit2-Tg* mice. Among 134 genes, 90 were downregulated, and 44 were upregulated (**Figure 6E**). GO pathway enrichment analysis showed the significant changes in expression pattern genes associated with the 22 key signaling pathways related to inflammation, vital cell functions, and others (**Figure 6F**). We further analyzed the expression pattern of various genes associated with the MAPK pathway. RNA-seq data analysis showed a higher expression of *Dusp1, Dusp5, Flna, Hspa1a, Hspa1b, Il1β, MAPK14, Pla2g4b, Pla2g4d*, and *Pla2g4f* in *Slit2-Tg* mice PAPT (**Figure 7A**). Heat map from RNA-seq data of 20 MAPK related genes are shown in **Figure 7B**. Similarly, RT-qPCR result showed 2.1- and 1.6-fold higher expression of *Traf6* and *p38* in PAPT of *Slit2-Tg* mice compared to wild-type mice (**Figures 7B,C**). Western blot analysis showed a 2-fold higher phosphorylation p38 in PAPT of *Slit2-Tg* mice compared to wild-type mice (**Figures 7D (i–iii)**). Our finding indicates the possible role of activated MAPK pathway in SLIT2-mediated effects on periodontitis.

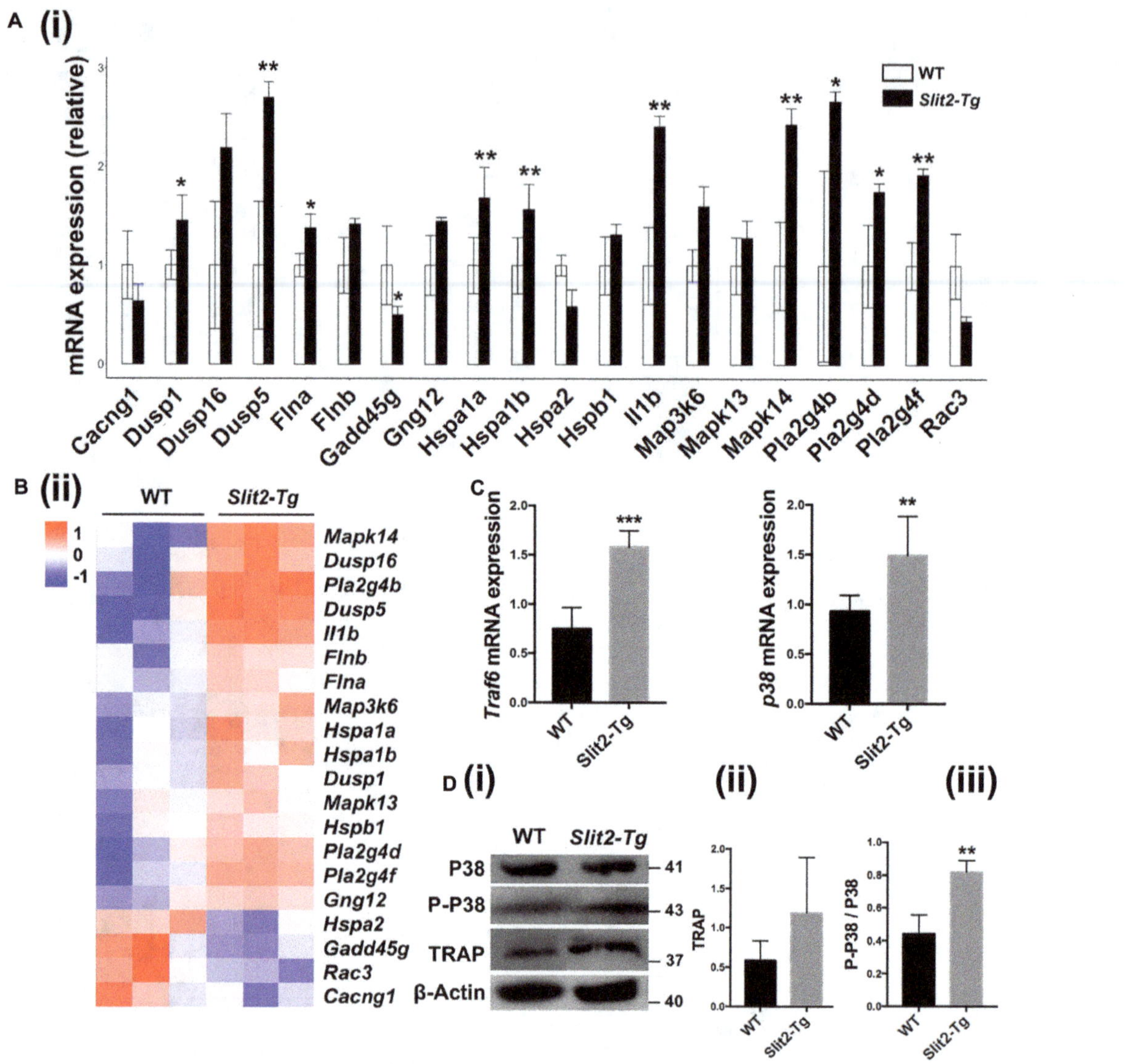


**FIGURE 7 |** SLIT2 overexpression activates MAPK signaling pathway in periodontitis milieu. **(A (i))** Relative mRNA expression ($n = 3$), and **(A (ii))** Heat map of the differential expression pattern of MAPK signaling pathway-related genes in PAPT analyzed by RNA sequencing. Relative mRNA expression of **(B)** *Traf6*, and **(C)** *p38* in PAPT analyzed by RT-qPCR ($n = 6$). **(D (i))** Representative western blot images of MAPK signaling related proteins. **(D (ii), (iii))** Quantitative analysis of TRAP and P-P38 ($n = 4$). Data are presented as mean ± SD. The significant difference among the groups, $^{*}P < 0.05$, $^{**}P < 0.01$, $^{***}P < 0.001$.

## DISCUSSION

Our previous study reported that the higher expression of SLIT2 in cancer tissue of colorectal carcinoma promotes tumor metastasis (Yao et al., 2019). In this study, we found evident upregulation of SLIT2 in periodontitis-affected human gingival tissue, and PAPT of mice, as well as in the serum of periodontitis mice. SLIT2 overexpression did not initiate the periodontitis itself. However, SLIT2 overexpression aggravated the periodontitis and periodontitis-induced alveolar bone loss. SLIT2 intensified the inflammation in PAPT as indicated by higher MVD, and infiltration of leucocytes/macrophages in periodontitis *Slit2*-Tg mice compared to wild-type mice. Expression of proinflammatory markers Cxcr2, IL-18, IL-6, IL-1β, and TNFα were upregulated in PAPT of Slit2-Tg mice. Similarly, PAPT of *Slit2*-Tg mice showed upregulation of osteoclastogenic markers, higher numbers of osteoclasts, and M1 macrophage polarization. SLIT2/ROBO1 axis has been reported to induce proinflammatory properties (Zhao et al., 2014; Yao et al., 2019). ROBO1 receptor was upregulated in PAPT of *Slit2*-Tg mice compared to wild type mice. MAPK signaling is a key regulator of inflammation and osteoclastogenesis (Li et al., 2012; Xu et al., 2020). Expression of MAPK signaling related factors MAPK14 and p-p38 was upregulated in the PAPT of *Slit2*-Tg mice. For the first time, this study reported that the SLIT2 overexpression in periodontal tissue intensifies the periodontitis progression and alveolar bone loss possibly via the activation of MAPK pathway (**Figure 8**).

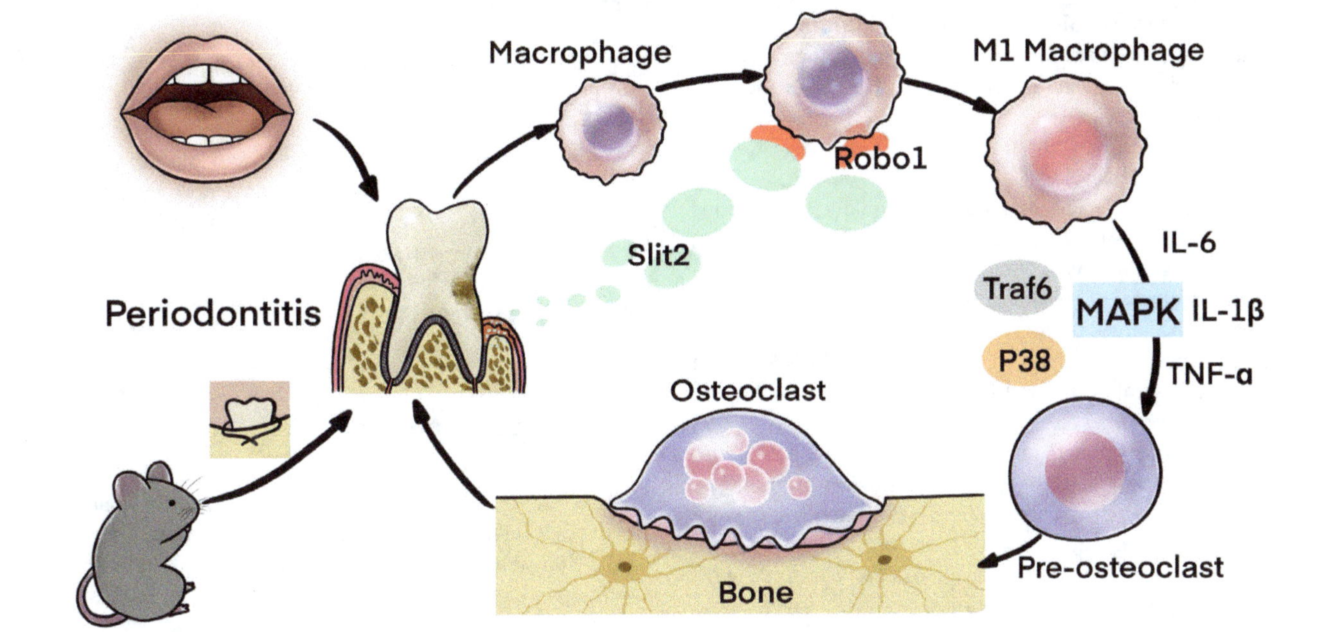


**FIGURE 8 |** Scheme showing the role of SLIT2 overexpression in pathophysiology of periodontitis.

Literature had reported the overexpression of SLIT2 in various cancers, including gastric, colorectal, and osteosarcoma (Shi et al., 2013; Zhao et al., 2018; Yao et al., 2019). However, the expression pattern of SLIT2 in the inflammatory oral disease periodontitis is still unknown. In this study, we unraveled the >4.0-fold upregulation of SLIT2 protein in periodontitis-affected tissue of human and mice compared to healthy tissue. Our recent study showed around 2.0-fold upregulation of SLIT serum levels in colorectal carcinoma patients (Yao et al., 2019). In the present study, serum SLIT2 level in periodontitis mice was upregulated by 5.0-fold compared to healthy mice indicating systemic upregulation. Although periodontitis is an oral inflammatory disease, it has shown various systemic effects (Papapanou, 2015). This result suggests the possible role of overexpressed SLIT2 on the systemic effects of periodontitis. SLIT2 upregulated pathological condition of hepatocellular carcinoma shows a higher expression of ROBO1. Among the 4 ROBO receptors, ROBO1 was robustly upregulated in PAPT (Avci et al., 2008). Moreover, SLIT2/ROBO4 axis has reported to exert anti-inflammatory signaling and SLIT2/ROBO1 has axis been reported to exert proinflammatory signaling (Zhao et al., 2014). In this study, we found that both SLIT2 and ROBO1 were upregulated in periodontitis, suggesting the possible role of SLIT2/ROBO1 axis on escalation of inflammation and disease progression in periodontitis.

SLIT2 promotes angiogenesis (Li et al., 2015), and the migration of specific cancer cells (Zhao et al., 2016; Yao et al., 2019). SLIT2 has been reported to inhibit neutrophil migration, but enhance eosinophil chemotaxis (Tole et al., 2009; Ye et al., 2010). In this study, SLIT2 increased the MVD and leucocyte/macrophage infiltration in PAPT. Pilling et al. (2019) recently reported the SLIT2 isoform-specific neutrophil chemorepellent and chemoattractant functions. The ~140-kDa N-terminal Slit2 fragment (Slit2-N) enhances, and the ~110-kDa N-terminal Slit2 fragment (Slit2-S) inhibits neutrophil migration via binding with same ROBO1 receptor. The neutrophil and macrophage chemoattractant properties of SLIT2 in periodontitis might be the act of Slit2-N fragment. However, further studies illustrating the expression pattern of Slit2-N and Slit2-S and their function on neutrophil/macrophage migration in periodontitis are needed to support this hypothesis.

Disturbed host immune reaction elevates the levels of proinflammatory cytokines such as IL-8, IL-6, IL-1β, and TNF-α in PAPT, creating inflammatory milieu (Pan et al., 2019). These cytokines trigger M1 macrophage polarization, osteoclastogenesis, and immune cell infiltration that escalate inflammation and disease progression in a vicious cycle manner. Overexpression of SLIT2 enhanced the expression of proinflammatory cytokines IL-18, IL-6, IL-1β, and TNF-α. Moreover, PAPT of *Slit2*-Tg mice showed a higher degree of M1 macrophage polarization. Higher numbers of leucocytes and macrophages were infiltrated in PAPT of *Slit2*-Tg mice. Upregulation of osteoclastogenic markers *Acp5*, *Ctsk* and *Nfatc1*, and higher numbers of osteoclasts were observed in PAPT of *Slit2*-Tg mice. We did not witness the direct effect of SLIT2 on osteoblast function during periodontitis. SLIT2 has been reported to inhibit osteoclastogenesis and osteoblast differentiation *in vitro* (Sun et al., 2009; Park et al., 2019). The majority of pathophysiological parameters of the periodontitis were affected by SLIT2 overexpression, indicating the vital role of SLIT2 to on periodontitis progression. Our results suggest that the SLIT2-induced inflammation-mediated osteoclastogenesis might cause alveolar bone loss in periodontitis.

SLIT2 modulates MAPK signaling to regulate the various cell functions (Li et al., 2015; Xu et al., 2018; Zhao et al., 2018). MAPK signaling is a vital regulator of inflammation and pathophysiology of periodontitis (Li et al., 2012; Xu et al., 2020). GO enrichment pathway analysis of top 134 differentially expressed mRNAs in periodontitis-affected tissue of *Slit2*-Tg mice revealed the significant upregulation of MAPK signaling related genes. We further elucidated that the P-p38 was significantly upregulated in PAPT of *Slit2*-Tg mice. Along with MAPK signaling related genes, leucocytes, monocytes, and mononuclear cell chemotaxis/migration-related genes were also significantly upregulated in PAPT of *Slit2*-Tg mice. These findings further support the possible role of MAPK signaling on SLIT2-mediated effects on periodontitis.

In this study, we unraveled the higher expression of the SLIT2 in clinical gingival tissues of periodontitis patients. We further elucidated the higher SLIT2 expression in PAPT and serum of periodontitis mice. This result suggests SLIT2 as a possible diagnostic marker of periodontitis. *Slit2*-Tg periodontitis mice model unveiled the role of SLIT2 on the escalation of disease pathophysiology. This study opens the new research direction in the role of SLIT2 on the pathophysiology of inflammatory diseases. A limitation of this study is that we did not analyze which isotope of SLIT2 regulates the pathophysiology of periodontitis and whether ROBO1 is the key receptor for SLIT2-mediated effect on periodontitis. Another limitation of this study is that we did not meticulously analyze the role of MAPK in SLIT2-mediated escalation of inflammation and osteoclastogenesis. However, our ongoing study on Robo1 knockout periodontitis mice will address these limitations.

## CONCLUSION

SLIT2 was overexpressed during periodontitis. Overexpression of SLIT2 in periodontitis escalated inflammation, lymphocyte/macrophage infiltration, M1 macrophage polarization, osteoclastogenesis, alveolar bone loss, and disease progression. SLIT2 overexpression upregulated Robo1 and MAPK signaling related factors' expression in PAPT during periodontitis. Our results suggest the possible role of SLIT2/ROBO1 signaling of the pathophysiology of periodontitis via activation of MAPK p38 signaling.

## ETHICS STATEMENT

The studies involving human participants were reviewed and approved by The Medical Ethics Committee of the Affiliated Stomatology Hospital of Guangzhou Medical University. The patients/participants provided their written informed consent to participate in this study. The animal study was reviewed and approved by The Experimental Animal Ethics Committee of Guangzhou Medical University. Written informed consent was obtained from the individual(s) for the publication of any potentially identifiable images or data included in this article.

## AUTHOR CONTRIBUTIONS

LG, LJW, LPW, JZ, and JP: study design. JZ, YC, DL, LY, HS, and MZ: experimental conduct. JZ, YC, DL, LY, HS, LHW, LL, SD, YY, and DH: animal work. JZ, JP, YC, DL, LY, and HS: data collection, analysis and interpretation. JZ and JP: manuscript preparation. All authors approved the final version of the manuscript.

## REFERENCES


Abe, T., and Hajishengallis, G. (2013). Optimization of the ligature-induced periodontitis model in mice. *J. Immunol. Methods* 394, 49–54. doi: 10.1016/j.jim.2013.05.002

AlQranei, M. S., and Chellaiah, M. A. (2020). Osteoclastogenesis in periodontal diseases: possible mediators and mechanisms. *J. Oral. Biosci.* doi: 10.1016/j.job.2020.02.002 [Online ahead of print]

Aspriello, S. D., Zizzi, A., Lucarini, G., Rubini, C., Faloia, E., Boscaro, M., et al. (2009). Vascular endothelial growth factor and microvessel density in periodontitis patients with and without diabetes. *J. Periodontol.* 80, 1783–1789. doi: 10.1902/jop.2009.090239

Avci, M. E., Konu, O., and Yagci, T. (2008). Quantification of SLIT-ROBO transcripts in hepatocellular carcinoma reveals two groups of genes with coordinate expression. *BMC Cancer* 8:392. doi: 10.1186/1471-2407-8-392

Chang, J., Lan, T., Li, C., Ji, X., Zheng, L., Gou, H., et al. (2015). Activation of Slit2-Robo1 signaling promotes liver fibrosis. *J. Hepatol.* 63, 1413–1420. doi: 10.1016/j.jhep.2015.07.033

Chaturvedi, S., and Robinson, L. A. (2015). Slit2-Robo signaling in inflammation and kidney injury. *Pediatr. Nephrol.* 30, 561–566. doi: 10.1007/s00467-014-2825-4

Cochran, D. L. (2008). Inflammation and bone loss in periodontal disease. *J. Periodontol.* 79(8 Suppl), 1569–1576. doi: 10.1902/jop.2008.080233

Darveau, R. P. (2010). Periodontitis: a polymicrobial disruption of host homeostasis. *Nat. Rev. Microbiol.* 8, 481–490. doi: 10.1038/nrmicro2337

Fernando, R., Grisolia, A. B. D., Lu, Y., Atkins, S., and Smith, T. J. (2018). Slit2 Modulates the Inflammatory Phenotype of Orbit-Infiltrating Fibrocytes in Graves' Disease. *J. Immunol.* 200, 3942–3949. doi: 10.4049/jimmunol.1800259

Frazee, A. C., Pertea, G., Jaffe, A. E., Langmead, B., Salzberg, S. L., and Leek, J. T. (2015). Ballgown bridges the gap between transcriptome assembly and expression analysis. *Nat. Biotechnol.* 33, 243–246. doi: 10.1038/nbt.3172

Gonzalez, O. A., Novak, M. J., Kirakodu, S., Stromberg, A., Nagarajan, R., Huang, C. B., et al. (2015). Differential gene expression profiles reflecting macrophage polarization in aging and periodontitis gingival tissues. *Immunol. Invest.* 44, 643–664. doi: 10.3109/08820139.2015.1070269

Hajishengallis, G. (2014). Immunomicrobial pathogenesis of periodontitis: keystones, pathobionts, and host response. *Trends Immunol.* 35, 3–11. doi: 10.1016/j.it.2013.09.001

Kassebaum, N. J., Bernabe, E., Dahiya, M., Bhandari, B., Murray, C. J., and Marcenes, W. (2014). Global burden of severe periodontitis in 1990-2010: a systematic review and meta-regression. *J. Dent. Res.* 93, 1045–1053. doi: 10.1177/0022034514552491

Kim, D., Langmead, B., and Salzberg, S. L. (2015). HISAT: a fast spliced aligner with low memory requirements. *Nat. Methods* 12, 357–360. doi: 10.1038/nmeth.3317

Li, C., Yang, G., Lin, L., Xuan, Y., Yan, S., Ji, X., et al. (2019). Slit2 signaling contributes to cholestatic fibrosis in mice by activation of hepatic stellate cells. *Exp. Cell Res.* 385:111626. doi: 10.1016/j.yexcr.2019.111626

Li, Q., Valerio, M. S., and Kirkwood, K. L. (2012). MAPK usage in periodontal disease progression. *J. Signal. Transduct* 2012:308943. doi: 10.1155/2012/308943

Li, S., Huang, L., Sun, Y., Bai, Y., Yang, F., Yu, W., et al. (2015). Slit2 promotes angiogenic activity via the Robo1-VEGFR2-ERK1/2 pathway in both in vivo and in vitro studies. *Invest. Ophthalmol. Vis. Sci.* 56, 5210–5217. doi: 10.1167/iovs-14-16184

Liu, J., Hou, W., Guan, T., Tang, L., Zhu, X., Li, Y., et al. (2018). Slit2/Robo1 signaling is involved in angiogenesis of glomerular endothelial cells exposed to a diabetic-like environment. *Angiogenesis* 21, 237–249. doi: 10.1007/s10456-017-9592-3

Martin, M. (2011). Cutadapt removes adapter sequences from high-throughput sequencing reads. *EMBnet.journal* 17, 10–12.

Mizraji, G., Segev, H., Wilensky, A., and Hovav, A. H. (2013). Isolation, processing and analysis of murine gingival cells. *J. Vis. Exp.* 77:e50388. doi: 10.3791/50388

Pan, W., Wang, Q., and Chen, Q. (2019). The cytokine network involved in the host immune response to periodontitis. *Int. J. Oral Sci.* 11:30. doi: 10.1038/s41368-019-0064-z

Papapanou, P. N. (2015). Systemic effects of periodontitis: lessons learned from research on atherosclerotic vascular disease and adverse pregnancy outcomes. *Int. Dent. J.* 65, 283–291. doi: 10.1111/idj.12185

Park, S. J., Lee, J. Y., Lee, S. H., Koh, J. M., and Kim, B. J. (2019). SLIT2 inhibits osteoclastogenesis and bone resorption by suppression of Cdc42 activity. *Biochem. Biophys. Res. Commun.* 514, 868–874. doi: 10.1016/j.bbrc.2019.05.046

Pertea, M., Pertea, G. M., Antonescu, C. M., Chang, T. C., Mendell, J. T., and Salzberg, S. L. (2015). StringTie enables improved reconstruction of a transcriptome from RNA-seq reads. *Nat. Biotechnol.* 33, 290–295. doi: 10.1038/nbt.3122

Pilling, D., Chinea, L. E., Consalvo, K. M., and Gomer, R. H. (2019). Different isoforms of the neuronal guidance molecule slit2 directly cause chemoattraction or chemorepulsion of human neutrophils. *J. Immunol.* 202, 239–248. doi: 10.4049/jimmunol.1800681

Richards, D. (2014). Review finds that severe periodontitis affects 11% of the world population. *Evid. Based Dent.* 15, 70–71. doi: 10.1038/sj.ebd.6401037

Rodriguez, J. C., Gonzalez, G. A., Fresno, C., Llera, A. S., and Fernandez, E. A. (2016). Improving information retrieval in functional analysis. *Comput. Biol. Med.* 79, 10–20. doi: 10.1016/j.compbiomed.2016.09.017

Schmid, B. C., Rezniczek, G. A., Fabjani, G., Yoneda, T., Leodolter, S., and Zeillinger, R. (2007). The neuronal guidance cue Slit2 induces targeted migration and may play a role in brain metastasis of breast cancer cells. *Breast Cancer Res. Treat.* 106, 333–342. doi: 10.1007/s10549-007-9504-0

Shi, R., Liu, W., Liu, B., Xu, Z., Chen, L., and Zhang, Z. (2013). Slit2 expression and its correlation with subcellular localization of beta-catenin in gastric cancer. *Oncol. Rep.* 30, 1883–1889. doi: 10.3892/or.2013.2662

Spiller, K. L., Wrona, E. A., Romero-Torres, S., Pallotta, I., Graney, P. L., Witherel, C. E., et al. (2016). Differential gene expression in human, murine, and cell line-derived macrophages upon polarization. *Exp. Cell Res.* 347, 1–13. doi: 10.1016/j.yexcr.2015.10.017

Sun, H., Dai, K., Tang, T., and Zhang, X. (2009). Regulation of osteoblast differentiation by slit2 in osteoblastic cells. *Cells Tissues Organs* 190, 69–80. doi: 10.1159/000178020

Tole, S., Mukovozov, I. M., Huang, Y. W., Magalhaes, M. A., Yan, M., Crow, M. R., et al. (2009). The axonal repellent, Slit2, inhibits directional migration of circulating neutrophils. *J. Leukoc. Biol.* 86, 1403–1415. doi: 10.1189/jlb.0609391

Wang, B., Xiao, Y., Ding, B. B., Zhang, N., Yuan, X., Gui, L., et al. (2003). Induction of tumor angiogenesis by Slit-Robo signaling and inhibition of cancer growth by blocking Robo activity. *Cancer Cell* 4, 19–29. doi: 10.1016/s1535-6108(03)00164-8

Wang, L., Guan, N., Jin, Y., Lin, X., and Gao, H. (2015). Subcutaneous vaccination with Porphyromonas gingivalis ameliorates periodontitis by modulating Th17/Treg imbalance in a murine model. *Int. Immunopharmacol.* 25, 65–73. doi: 10.1016/j.intimp.2015.01.007

Wang, L. J., Zhao, Y., Han, B., Ma, Y. G., Zhang, J., Yang, D. M., et al. (2008). Targeting Slit-Roundabout signaling inhibits tumor angiogenesis in chemical-induced squamous cell carcinogenesis. *Cancer Sci.* 99, 510–517. doi: 10.1111/j.1349-7006.2007.00721.x

Wong, K., Park, H. T., Wu, J. Y., and Rao, Y. (2002). Slit proteins: molecular guidance cues for cells ranging from neurons to leukocytes. *Curr. Opin. Genet. Dev.* 12, 583–591. doi: 10.1016/s0959-437x(02)00343-x

Wu, J. Y., Feng, L., Park, H. T., Havlioglu, N., Wen, L., Tang, H., et al. (2001). The neuronal repellent Slit inhibits leukocyte chemotaxis induced by chemotactic factors. *Nature* 410, 948–952. doi: 10.1038/35073616

Xiao, E., Mattos, M., Vieira, G. H. A., Chen, S., Correa, J. D., Wu, Y., et al. (2017). Diabetes Enhances IL-17 expression and alters the oral microbiome to increase its pathogenicity. *Cell Host Microbe* 22:120-128.e4. doi: 10.1016/j.chom.2017.06.014

Xu, R., Qin, N., Xu, X., Sun, X., Chen, X., and Zhao, J. (2018). Inhibitory effect of SLIT2 on granulosa cell proliferation mediated by the CDC42-PAKs-ERK1/2 MAPK pathway in the prehierarchical follicles of the chicken ovary. *Sci. Rep.* 8:9168. doi: 10.1038/s41598-018-27601-z

Xu, W., Chen, X., Wang, Y., Fan, B., Guo, K., Yang, C., et al. (2020). Chitooligosaccharide inhibits RANKL-induced osteoclastogenesis and ligation-induced periodontitis by suppressing MAPK/ c-fos/NFATC1 signaling. *J. Cell. Physiol.* 235, 3022–3032. doi: 10.1002/jcp.29207

Yang, X. M., Han, H. X., Sui, F., Dai, Y. M., Chen, M., and Geng, J. G. (2010). Slit-Robo signaling mediates lymphangiogenesis and promotes tumor lymphatic metastasis. *Biochem. Biophys. Res. Commun.* 396, 571–577. doi: 10.1016/j.bbrc.2010.04.152

Yao, Y., Zhou, Z., Li, L., Li, J., Huang, L., Li, J., et al. (2019). Activation of Slit2/Robo1 Signaling Promotes Tumor Metastasis in Colorectal Carcinoma through Activation of the TGF-beta/Smads Pathway. *Cells* 8:635. doi: 10.3390/cells8060635

Ye, B. Q., Geng, Z. H., Ma, L., and Geng, J. G. (2010). Slit2 regulates attractive eosinophil and repulsive neutrophil chemotaxis through differential srGAP1 expression during lung inflammation. *J. Immunol.* 185, 6294–6305. doi: 10.4049/jimmunol.1001648

Yu, T., Zhao, L., Huang, X., Ma, C., Wang, Y., Zhang, J., et al. (2016). Enhanced Activity of the Macrophage M1/M2 Phenotypes and Phenotypic Switch to M1 in periodontal infection. *J. Periodontol.* 87, 1092–1102. doi: 10.1902/jop.2016.160081

Yuan, W., Zhou, L., Chen, J. H., Wu, J. Y., Rao, Y., and Ornitz, D. M. (1999). The mouse SLIT family: secreted ligands for ROBO expressed in patterns that suggest a role in morphogenesis and axon guidance. *Dev. Biol.* 212, 290–306. doi: 10.1006/dbio.1999.9371

Zhang, Z., Yuan, W., Deng, J., Wang, D., Zhang, T., Peng, L., et al. (2020). Granulocyte colony stimulating factor (G-CSF) regulates neutrophils infiltration and periodontal tissue destruction in an experimental periodontitis. *Mol. Immunol.* 117, 110–121. doi: 10.1016/j.molimm.2019.11.003

Zhao, H., Anand, A. R., and Ganju, R. K. (2014). Slit2-Robo4 pathway modulates lipopolysaccharide-induced endothelial inflammation and its expression is dysregulated during endotoxemia. *J. Immunol.* 192, 385–393. doi: 10.4049/jimmunol.1302021

Zhao, S. J., Shen, Y. F., Li, Q., He, Y. J., Zhang, Y. K., Hu, L. P., et al. (2018). SLIT2/ROBO1 axis contributes to the Warburg effect in osteosarcoma through activation of SRC/ERK/c-MYC/PFKFB2 pathway. *Cell Death Dis.* 9:390. doi: 10.1038/s41419-018-0419-y

Zhao, Y., Su, Y., and Ye, L. (2012). Slit-Robo: a potential way to treat periodontitis. *Med. Hypotheses* 79, 186–188. doi: 10.1016/j.mehy.2012.04.030

Zhao, Y., Zhou, F. L., Li, W. P., Wang, J., and Wang, L. J. (2016). Slit2Robo1 signaling promotes the adhesion, invasion and migration of tongue carcinoma cells via upregulating matrix metalloproteinases 2 and 9, and downregulating Ecadherin. *Mol. Med. Rep.* 14, 1901–1906. doi: 10.3892/mmr.2016.5518

Zhou, L. N., Bi, C. S., Gao, L. N., An, Y., Chen, F., and Chen, F. M. (2019). Macrophage polarization in human gingival tissue in response to periodontal disease. *Oral Dis.* 25, 265–273. doi: 10.1111/odi.12983

Zhou, W. J., Geng, Z. H., Chi, S., Zhang, W., Niu, X. F., Lan, S. J., et al. (2011). Slit-Robo signaling induces malignant transformation through Hakai-mediated E-cadherin degradation during colorectal epithelial cell carcinogenesis. *Cell Res.* 21, 609–626. doi: 10.1038/cr.2011.17

Zhou, X., Yao, Q., Sun, X., Gong, X., Yang, Y., Chen, C., et al. (2017). Slit2 ameliorates renal inflammation and fibrosis after hypoxia-and lipopolysaccharide-induced epithelial cells injury in vitro. *Exp. Cell Res.* 352, 123–129. doi: 10.1016/j.yexcr.2017.02.001

Zhu, L. F., Li, L., Wang, X. Q., Pan, L., Mei, Y. M., Fu, Y. W., et al. (2019). M1 macrophages regulate TLR4/AP1 via paracrine to promote alveolar bone destruction in periodontitis. *Oral Dis.* 25, 1972–1982. doi: 10.1111/odi.13167

10

# Obesity and Bone Health: A Complex Link

*Jing Hou[1], Chen He[1], Wenzhen He[1], Mi Yang[1,2,3], Xianghang Luo[1,2,3] and Changjun Li[1,2,3]**

*[1] Department of Endocrinology, Endocrinology Research Center, The Xiangya Hospital of Central South University, Changsha, China, [2] National Clinical Research Center for Geriatric Disorders (Xiangya Hospital), Changsha, China, [3] Key Laboratory of Organ Injury, Aging and Regenerative Medicine of Hunan Province, Changsha, China*

***Correspondence:***
*Changjun Li*
*lichangjun@csu.edu.cn*

So far, the connections between obesity and skeleton have been extensively explored, but the results are inconsistent. Obesity is thought to affect bone health through a variety of mechanisms, including body weight, fat volume, bone formation/resorption, proinflammatory cytokines together with bone marrow microenvironment. In this review, we will mainly describe the effects of adipokines secreted by white adipose tissue on bone cells, as well as the interaction between brown adipose tissue, bone marrow adipose tissue, and bone metabolism. Meanwhile, this review also reviews the evidence for the effects of adipose tissue and its distribution on bone mass and bone-related diseases, along with the correlation between different populations with obesity and bone health. And we describe changes in bone metabolism in patients with anorexia nervosa or type 2 diabetes. In summary, all of these findings show that the response of skeleton to obesity is complex and depends on diversified factors, such as mechanical loading, obesity type, the location of adipose tissue, gender, age, bone sites, and secreted cytokines, and that these factors may exert a primary function in bone health.

**Keywords: obesity, adipose tissue, bone health, bone remodeling, bone-related diseases**

## INTRODUCTION

Bone is a living tissue with metabolic functions. The size and shape of bones are accurately modeled and reshaped over a lifetime to ensure skeletal structure and integrity (Xie et al., 2014; Li et al., 2017). During bone remodeling, bone can coordinate the activities of osteoblasts, osteocytes, and osteoclasts, thus maintaining the dynamic coupling balance of bone metabolism, in which osteoblasts (bone formation) and osteoclasts (bone resorption) play pivotal roles in bone metabolism. Bone marrow mesenchymal stem cells (BMSCs) have the ability to differentiate into osteoblasts and adipocytes, which is also a dynamic balance (Li et al., 2015; Li C.J. et al., 2018). In addition, bones exhibit the characteristics of endocrine organs, which secrete a variety of hormones to participate in the endocrine cycle throughout the body. For instance, bone can secrete estrogen, androgens, follicle suppressant and other sex hormones to participate in the reproductive process, cellular senescence, and osteoporosis (OP). Moreover, bone marrow fat cells can also secrete a series of adipokine including adiponectin, leptin through autocrine, and paracrine, which play an important regulatory role in local and systemic metabolism of bone marrow. There are however many metabolic osteopathy, including OP, bone tumor, and inflammatory arthritis, where this fine equilibrium is disrupted (Sun et al., 2019).

Overweight and obesity are identified as abnormal or excessive fat accumulation that can lead to impaired health. Body mass index (BMI) is a simple ratio of height to weight that is often used to distinguish between overweight and obesity adults. The WHO defines overweight as having a BMI of 25 to $<30$ kg/m$^2$ and obesity as $\geq 30$ kg/m$^2$. In addition, obesity can be divided into three grades, namely obese class I (30 to $<35$ kg/m$^2$), class II (35 to $<40$ kg/m$^2$), and class III ($\geq 40$ kg/m$^2$) (Barba et al., 2004; Di Angelantonio et al., 2016). However, the diversity of Asian countries is mainly manifested in ethnic and cultural subgroups, degree of urbanization, social and economic conditions, and nutritional transformation. And compared with white people of the same age, sex, and BMI, Asians typically have a higher percentage of body fat. Therefore, the BMI cut-off points for overweight and obesity may be more applicable in Asian countries (Barba et al., 2004). Overweight and obesity are associated with risk and prognosis for certain disease states (Dalamaga and Christodoulatos, 2015).

The prevalence of obesity and obesity-related diseases is on the rise worldwide due to the socioeconomic and demographic transitions. The link between adiposity and bone health has been extensively studied, but the impact of obesity on bones has long been a subject of debate. This review will discuss the correlation between adiposity and bone-related diseases from multiple perspectives.

## EXTRAMEDULLARY ADIPOSE TISSUE AND BONE

Adipose tissue consists mainly of fat cells that have accumulated in large numbers, which are divided into fat lobules by thin layers of loose connective tissue and widely distributed in the subcutaneous and around the internal organs. It is not only involved in body construction and energy storage, but is also a vital endocrine organ. Adipose tissue has an effect on insulin sensitivity, blood pressure level, endothelial function, fibrinolytic activity and inflammatory response, and participates in a variety of important pathophysiological processes.

Adipose tissue exerts a primary function in obesity and related diseases. According to different functions, adipose tissue can be divided into white adipose tissue (WAT), brown adipose tissue (BAT), and beige adipose tissue. WAT is an energy-storing tissue that regulates energy metabolism by secreting cytokines and hormones. Excessive accumulation of WAT in the body can cause obesity and obesity-related diseases. BAT, however, is an energy-consuming organization that is involved in non-shivering heat and diet-induced heat production. Both thermogenic mechanisms are due to the exclusive expression of uncoupled protein-1 (UCPl) in the mitochondria of brown fat cells, resulting in the uncoupling of fatty acids and ATP oxidation, ultimately causing energy dissipation in the form of heat (Del Mar Gonzalez-Barroso et al., 2001; Carobbio et al., 2017; Huang et al., 2020). Thus, BAT can be capable of fighting obesity. Beige fat is more widely distributed than the typical brown fat, which is concentrated in the interscapular storage of rodents and in the supraclavicular and mediastinal areas of humans (Frontini and Cinti, 2010; Wiedmann et al., 2017). Beige fat also possesses an innate ability to metabolize energy as heat release by non-shivering thermogenesis (Zhang et al., 2018).

### Leptin Secreted by White Adipose Tissue and Bone

White adipose tissue has a main endocrine function secreting many adipokines, especially leptin and adiponectin. These latest findings suggest that adipokines are closely related to metabolic diseases such as obesity, insulin resistance and diabetes, and play an important regulatory role in bone disease (Conde et al., 2011). Particularly, leptin and adiponectin have been shown to act directly on certain bone cells, including BMSCs, osteoblasts, and osteoclasts. Consistent evidence suggests that leptin has a direct anabolic effect on osteoblasts. Astudillo et al. (2007) observed that leptin can promote the proliferation of bone marrow stromal cells, differentiation into osteoblasts, and form mineralized nodules, but prevent the differentiation into adipocytes. Thomas (1999) have also shown that leptin leads to dose-dependent increases in mRNA and protein levels of alkaline phosphatase (ALP), osteocalcin (OC), and type I collagen. Gordeladze et al. (2002) found that continuous exposure of leptin to ilium osteoblasts contributed to collagen synthesis, cell differentiation, and *in vitro* mineralization, together with cell survival and transition to preosseous cells.

Additionally, leptin may increase local bone mass and may contribute to the link between bone formation and bone resorption. Holloway et al. (2002) found that after adding human macrophage colony stimulating factor (HM-CSF) and human soluble NF-Kappab ligand receptor activator (sRANKL) to bone culture, leptin can inhibit the formation of human peripheral blood mononuclear cells (PBMCs) and mouse spleen cells to osteoclasts. Leptin increased mRNA and protein expression of osteoprotegerin (OPG, a protein that inhibits osteoclast formation) in PBMC, suggesting that its inhibition may be realized through the RANKL/RANK/OPG pathway (Holloway et al., 2002). Leptin effectively attenuated trabecular bone loss, trabecular structure change and periosteal bone formation. Leptin also significantly reduced RANKL mRNA levels which mainly regulates osteoclast development in cultured human bone marrow stromal cells (Burguera et al., 2001; Reid et al., 2018).

In addition to having a direct anabolic effect on osteoblasts, leptin also indirectly affects bones. Numerous studies have shown that in mice lacking leptin or leptin receptors, spinal trabecular volume increases, vertebral bone mass increases, while femur bone mass decreases and femur bone marrow fat increases sharply (Ducy et al., 2000; Steppan et al., 2000; Hamrick et al., 2004). Remarkably, Steppan et al. (2000) found, compared with the control group, leptin administration significantly increased femur length, systemic bone area, bone mineral density (BMD) and bone mineral content in leptin-deficient mice (ob/ob mice). This conclusion has been confirmed in other studies as well (Hamrick et al., 2005; Bartell et al., 2011; Philbrick et al., 2017). In summary, the role of leptin in skeleton remains a highly controversial area.

## Adiponectin Secreted by White Adipose Tissue and Bone

Adiponectin, the most common adipokine in plasma, has important metabolic and anti-inflammatory effects and is rapidly becoming a valuable marker for treatment in metabolic diseases. The role of adiponectin in certain bone cells including osteoblasts and osteoclasts, has been extensively studied. Human adiponectin promoted bone formation of primary human maxillary BMSCs through the APPL1-P38 MAPK pathway (Pu et al., 2016). Also, adiponectin induced osteogenesis of MSCs through adipoR1-mediated phosphorylation of P38 MAPK. Then, p38 MAPK phosphorylated c-Jun, which enhanced COX-2 (cyclooxygenase-2) expression and ultimately lead to an increase in BMP2 expression (bone morphogenetic protein 2, a strong osteogenic cytokine) (Lee et al., 2009; Huang et al., 2010). Similarly, Luo et al. (2005) demonstrated that adiponectin promoted osteoblastic proliferation, leading to increased alkaline phosphatase (ALP) activity, generation of type I collagen and OC, and increase in mineralized substrates in a dose-dependent and time-dependent manner. The increase of ALP, type I collagen, and OC is a marker of osteoblast differentiation and maturation, while matrix mineralization is a marker of osteoblastic phenotype. This study also provided evidence that adiponectin induced the proliferation and differentiation of human osteoblasts, which was realized through AdipoR/JNK pathway, while the differentiation was realized through AdipoR/P38 pathway (Sowa et al., 2002; Nöth et al., 2003; Luo et al., 2005).

Adiponectin also directly regulates osteoclast function. Adiponectin down-regulated expression of osteoclast regulators such as acid tartrate – resistant phosphatase and cathepsin K. Adiponectin also enhanced osteoclast apoptosis and reduced osteoclast precursor cells survival/proliferation (Tu et al., 2011; Pal China et al., 2018).

Significantly, like leptin, *in vivo* studies showed that the regulation of bone metabolism by adiponectin is also contradictory. Several studies reported that compared with wild-type mice, adiponectin knockout mice showed lower bone mineralization and bone density (Shinoda et al., 2006; Naot et al., 2016). But, others have shown that lack of adiponectin exert a protective effect on skeleton. Pal China et al. (2018) found KO mice prevented trabecular bone loss in mice caused by ovariectomy, and showed better bone quality (Williams et al., 2009). Taken together, the data from *in vitro* and *in vivo* studies fail to provide any definitive conclusions about the relationship between leptin, adiponectin and bone. And, white adipocytes can not only synthesize and secrete hormones including adiponectin and leptin, but also secrete proinflammatory factors such as TNF-α, IL-6, which may negatively regulate bone metabolism, further complicating the relationship between obesity and bone (Fruhbeck et al., 2001).

## Brown Adipose Tissue and Bone

It is well known that BAT not only exists in newborns, but also exists in adults, and gradually decreases with age. In fact, Ponrartana et al. (2012) have observed a significant correlation between BAT volume and cross-sectional bone size, regardless of gender. Moreover, recent findings suggest that BAT activity is positively correlated with skeletal metabolism. In contrast, some previous studies have shown that BAT can secrete fibroblast growth factor 21 (FGF21) and increase plasma FGF21 levels. Wei et al. showed that in animal models, transgenic mice overexpressing FGF21 had a lower bone mass phenotype, while mice given the drug dose of FGF21 also had a lower bone mass, because of reduced bone formation and significantly increased bone absorption (Wei et al., 2012). Also, Fazeli et al. (2015) found that FGF21 was negatively correlated with trabecular microstructural parameters, such as trabecular number (TbN), in patients with anorexia nervosa (AN). Recently, plasma FGF21 level was found to be negatively correlated with bone density in femoral neck and Ward's triangle of hip region (Hao et al., 2018). Taken together, these data reveal that FGF21 is a major negative regulator of bone mass.

Interestingly, as an endocrine organ, bone can also secrete a variety of bioactive substances to control energy metabolism in adipose tissue. OC, a small molecular protein secreted by osteoblasts, is a classic indicator of bone formation. Li Q. et al. (2018) verified the specific role of OC in thermogenesis of brown adipocytes. Their study showed that the OC signaling pathway directly promoted the activation of the Gprc6a Tcf7 Ucp1 promoter through the positive feedback of the interaction between the Wnt3a Tcf7 and the WNT/β-catenin pathway (Li Q. et al., 2018).

In addition, bone regulates browning and energy metabolism via the expression of peroxisome proliferator-activated receptor (PPAR) in mature osteoblasts and osteocytes. Several studies have confirmed that, in bone, PPAR plays a negative regulatory role in bone formation by inhibiting osteoblast generation and promoting osteoclast activity. Specific ablation of PPAR in mature osteoblasts and osteocyte mice (OCY-PPAR-/-) was found to induce high-bone mass and low fat mass phenotypes, as well as increase fat browning and energy comsumption. Moreover, Ocy-PPARγ-/- could partly prevent the dysmetabolism caused by high fat intake (Brun et al., 2017). Interestingly, BMP7 levels were also higher in Ocy-PPARγ-/- mice in conditioned medium and serum. BMP7, derived from osteocytes, is believed to promote browning and reduce steatosis through endocrine mechanisms (Kinoshita et al., 2007; Sugimoto et al., 2007; Tseng et al., 2008; Boon et al., 2013).

Collectively, these results indicate that bone and adipose tissue can interact to regulate bone metabolism and energy metabolism, which provides a new idea for the exploration and development of treatment methods for bone-related diseases.

# BONE MARROW ADIPOCYTES AND BONE

Bone marrow adipose tissue (BMAT), which accounts for about 8% of total fat mass, is an important fat depot in the adult body and exerts a significant function in bone homeostasis and energy metabolism throughout the body (Tencerova et al., 2019). BMAT is thought to be negatively correlated with bone density and bone integrity, so it may be an important regulator of bone turnover

(Fazeli et al., 2013). Studies have shown that BMAT in the lumbar spine is an independent predictive factor of fracture (Wehrli et al., 2000). BMAT is distinct from WAT and BAT. Excessive accumulation of lipids interferes with the normal function of cells and tissues, a condition known as lipotoxicity (Carobbio et al., 2017; Piccolis et al., 2019). Lipotoxicity is caused primarily by bone marrow fat through the secretion of adipokines and free fatty acids (mainly palmitate). In bone marrow, lipotoxicity is mainly manifested by the toxic effect of palmitate on bone cells, especially osteoblasts (Al Saedi et al., 2020). Exposure to adipocyte secretory factors can reduce the ability of BMSC to differentiate into bone cells, but also promote fat formation, a phenomenon that may be explained by a variety of mechanisms, including oxidative stress and proinflammatory mediators (TNF-α and IL-6) and adipokines (Horowitz et al., 2017; Singh et al., 2018). Furthermore, Elbaz et al. (2010) observed that, by co-culturing normal human osteoblasts (NHOst) with pre-differentiation adipocytes in the absence of a fatty acids synthase inhibitor (cerulenin), the differentiation and functional levels of NHOst were significantly reduced due to the lower mineralization and decreased expression of ALP, osterix, OC, and Runx2 (Elbaz et al., 2010). Actually, some evidences, indicates that palmitate has negative effects on osteoblast differentiation, bone nodule formation and mineralization.

Apart from BMSC and osteoblasts, osteoclasts are also affected by bone marrow fat to increase bone resorption and decrease bone mass (Singh et al., 2018). Takeshita et al. (2014) found that, during the differentiation of marrow stromal cells into adipocytes, RANKL expression was induced, along with the down-regulation of osteoprotegerin. The early adipogenic transcription factors C/EBPβ and C/EBPδ could bind to the RANKL promoter and ultimately stimulate RANKL gene transcription (Takeshita et al., 2014; Paccou et al., 2015; Hardouin et al., 2016).

Overall, these findings point to metabolic differences between bone marrow fat and peripheral fat that may be related to the development of therapeutic strategies for metabolic bone disease.

## ANOREXIA NERVOSA, OBESITY, AND BONE

Anorexia nervosa is a major mental disorder that mainly affects women. Patients are unable to maintain normal weight due to extreme self-imposed starvation, which is typical of chronic malnutrition (Kaye et al., 2020). Bone loss is almost the most common feature in many comorbidities associated with this disease.

Interestingly, compared with normal-weight women, anorexic patients showed less subcutaneous adipose tissue (SAT) and visceral adipose tissue (VAT), but more BMAT (Bredella et al., 2009). Previous studies have shown that increased BMAT level has clinical significance and is related to bone density and bone strength. In the above content, we mentioned that bone marrow fat can inhibit bone formation and promote bone resorption. In addition, marrow fat content increased in elderly patients with OP and was inversely correlated with bone density in healthy white women, and also in obese women (Justesen et al., 2001; Shen et al., 2007; Bredella et al., 2011b). Similarly, in ovariectomy animals, loss of bone mass was often accompanied by abnormal accumulation of bone marrow fat (Bredella et al., 2009; Li S. et al., 2018; Beekman et al., 2019). Given the negative correlation between marrow fat and BMD, BMAT may be an important risk factor for low bone density and increased fracture risk in patients with AN. For example, increased BMAT and decreased bone density and bone strength were observed in AN in women and adolescents (Singhal et al., 2018; Fazeli et al., 2019). Moreover, bone marrow fat in L4 vertebral body, femoral metaphyseal and diaphyseal increased markedly in women with AN. Importantly, marrow fat content had a highly significant negative association with BMD in multiple bone sites including the lumbar spine, hip and whole body (Bredella et al., 2009). One reason may be that osteoblasts and fat cells are derived from the mesenchymal stem cells in the bone marrow, the increased adipogenic differentiation may lead to a decreased osteogenic differentiation in BMSCs.

However, studies have shown that in patients recovering from AN, BMAT levels in L4 vertebrae are similar to those in healthy controls (Fazeli et al., 2012). BMAT positively correlated with VAT in overweight/obese women, while no such association was observed in underweight women (Bredella et al., 2011b; Polineni et al., 2020). These data may indicate that BMAT is a dynamic depot, which may play different roles under the condition of insufficient and adequate nutrition. In addition, since hypercortisolemia and hypoestrogenism are both characteristics of AN, these factors may result in marrow adiposity (Putignano et al., 2001). In summary, during chronic starvation, while other fat stores are used as energy sources, this adipose tissue storage is retained, suggesting that it may have significant functions. And, studying this paradox may lead to a better understanding of the function of bone marrow fat.

## TYPE 2 DIABETES, OBESITY AND BONE

Diabetes is a chronic disease characterized by neuropathy, nephropathy and retinopathy, with type 2 diabetes mellitus (T2DM) as the predominant type. The patient presents primarily with insulin resistance, and relative insulin deficiency (Compston, 2018; Su et al., 2019). This has been accompanied by a sharp rise in the incidence of obesity, an important determinant of type 2 diabetes. Abnormal accumulation of fat both inside and outside adipose tissue not only results in structural and functional disorders (insulin resistance) of adipose tissue itself, but also affects muscles, liver, and pancreas (Tsatsoulis et al., 2013; de Araujo et al., 2017). The bone disease of type 2 diabetes remains a mystery because the mechanism by which diabetes affects the bone is multifactorial, including factors such as obesity, hyperinsulinemia and insulin-like growth factors (IGFs). The effect of insulin on bone metabolism is controversial. Studies *in vitro* have reported that insulin signals in osteoblasts can promote bone absorption (Ferron et al., 2010). Consistent with *in vitro* results, Srikanthan et al. also confirmed that insulin resistance, especially hyperinsulinemia, may adversely affect femoral neck strength (Srikanthan et al., 2014). However, other *in vivo* studies show that insulin stimulates osteoblasts to proliferate and increases the histologic markers of bone formation (Shanbhogue et al., 2016). Furthermore, in the early stages of diabetes, obesity and hyperinsulinemia often occur together, and it is challenging to identify the unique contribution of obesity and hyperinsulinemia to bone health.

It is believed that IGFs is associated with the pathogenesis of diabetic complications. In addition, serum IGF-I level was decreased in patients with poor blood glucose control (Thrailkill, 2000; Kanazawa et al., 2012). IGF I is thought to have anabolic effects on bone. Circulating IGF-I activates bone remodeling and plays an anabolic role in bone tissue (Johansson et al., 1992; Zhang et al., 2002). Some clinical studies have suggested that low serum IGF-I level is related to a higher risk of fractures independent of BMD in patients with type 2 diabetes (Ardawi et al., 2013; Miyake et al., 2017). Serum IGF-I level was found to be significantly negatively correlated with the prevalence of vertebral fractures in postmenopausal women with type 2 diabetes (Kanazawa et al., 2011, 2018). Based on the above evidence, the reduced serum IGF-I may be involved in diabetes-induced bone fragility and can be used to assess the risk of fracture in patients with T2DM.

In addition to the factors described above, the effects of hypoglycemic drugs on bone metabolism should also be taken into account. Most studies have shown that sulfonylureas and metformin have protective or neutral effects on fracture risk (Vestergaard et al., 2005; Kahn et al., 2006; Monami et al., 2008; Borges et al., 2011). In contrast, thiazolidinediones activate PPARγ, which in turn stimulate adipogenesis and inhibit osteogenesis (Gimble et al., 1996; Lecka-Czernik, 2017). Studies have reported an increased risk of fracture in patients taking thiazolidinedione (Dormuth et al., 2009; Zhu et al., 2014). Incretin hormones are considered to have the potential to treat type 2 diabetes. For instance, glucagon-like peptide-1 (GLP-1) targets primarily pancreatic β cells, where it stimulates insulin production, which helps control blood glucose levels (Baggio and Drucker, 2007). More recently, there has been growing evidence that incretins may also be beneficial for skeletal strength. GLP-1 plays a key role in bone homeostasis, inhibiting bone resorption and stimulating bone formation in response to nutrient intake (Shanbhogue et al., 2016). Indeed, GLP-1 receptor knockdown in mice can result in dramatic changes in trabecular and cortical microstructures, as well as adverse effects on bone tissue material properties (Mabilleau et al., 2013; Mansur et al., 2015, 2016). Thus, the effect on bone health should be considered when selecting hypoglycemic drugs to avoid inducing or exacerbating fractures and bone diseases in patients.

## OBESITY AND BONE-RELATED DISEASES

### Osteoporosis

Osteoporosis is a skeletal metabolic disorder with multiple causes, characterized by bone loss, microstructure degeneration, increased brittleness, reduced bone strength, and increased risk of fracture. Therefore, OP seriously affects the quality of life and living standards of patients (Khaliq et al., 2016; Pagnotti et al., 2019; Yang et al., 2019).

Bone mineral density is a commonly used indicator in the diagnosis of OP, which is performed by dual energy X-ray bone absorptiometry (DEXA). In addition, BMD can also be used to track changes in OP and evaluate the efficacy of OP drugs.

Numerous studies strongly suggest that, abdominal obesity, hypertension, dyslipidemia and dysglycemia are all considered as components of metabolic syndrome (MS) and are closely related to OP (Muka et al., 2015). Obesity may lead to an increase in bone density because it is associated with higher 17β-estradiol levels and higher mechanical loads, which may protect bones (Nelson and Bulun, 2001). Qiao et al. (2020) observed that adult obese patients had higher BMD in the lumbar spine and femoral neck than those of healthy weight. In general, obesity is negatively correlated with femoral neck OP, suggesting that obesity is a protective factor for OP (Qiao et al., 2020). Kim et al. (2010) found, however, that after adjusting for confounders, bone density was significantly lower in men over 40 and in postmenopausal women with MS. Moreover, the BMD decreased with the increase of MS components. Among MS indicators, waist circumference as a diagnostic criterion for abdominal obesity is the most critical factor leading to this negative correlation. Waist circumference was an important contributor in this association, suggesting that visceral fat may contribute to bone loss. The negative correlation between fat mass and bone density further supports this hypothesis, especially in men (Kim et al., 2010). Furthermore, pro-inflammatory molecules TNF- and IL-6 released from visceral fat play a key role in regulating bone resorption and participating in the pathogenesis of OP (Nanes, 2004; Roy et al., 2016).

Vitamin D is known to play a major role in the development and maintenance of bones and muscles in the body because of its ability to regulate the absorption of calcium and phosphorus. Low levels of vitamin D in the body are considered a potential risk factor for OP and bone fractures. Serum vitamin D deficiency prevents the intestinal tract from absorbing $Ca^{2+}$ from diet, eventually leading to elevated levels of parathyroid hormone (PTH) secretion. Oversecretion of PTH induces osteoclast formation, inhibits osteogenesis, and maintains optimal blood calcium and phosphorus levels required for metabolic processes and neuromuscular function (Roy, 2013). Recent studies have found that the serum 25(OH)D of obese people is lower than that of normal weight people, which is negatively correlated with body weight, BMI, and fat mass (Fassio et al., 2018).

It is worth noting that recently, Li et al. proposed that obesity may lead to low serum 25(OH)D, high serum leptin and high bone density (Snijder et al., 2005; Konradsen et al., 2008; Felson, 2010). In this context, femoral neck and spine BMD were positively correlated with BMI and fat mass index. Recombinant human (Rh) leptin in the treatment of BMSCs significantly facilitated bone formation. In addition, leptin down-regulated CYP24A1 and up-regulated CYP27B1, CYP27A1, and VDR, all of which play key roles in vitamin D metabolism In summary, this study confirmed the relationship between obesity, vitamin D metabolism and osteoblastic development, and the direct effect of leptin on vitamin D metabolism and osteoblastic differentiation of BMSCs may protect bone under the effect of low serum 25(OH)D in obese people (Lim et al., 2019; Li J. et al., 2020).

## Fractures

Osteoporosis, sarcopenia, and obesity are commonly associated with aging. Obviously, fall-related injuries and fractures are the major causes of disability and death among the elderly, seriously affecting their quality of life and survival (Rapp et al., 2010; Sanchez-Riera et al., 2014).

Studies have shown that fat accumulation may contribute to the deterioration of muscle and bone, thereby promoting the development of sarcopenia and OP (Ilich et al., 2014). Additionally, more and more studies have confirmed that sarcopenia is not only closely related to low bone density, but also an important risk factor for fractures (Tarantino et al., 2015).

Obesity was previously deemed to be a protective factor for OP or brittle fractures because patients affected by obesity have more soft tissue to protect bone tissue. That is, the positive impact of mechanical load caused by body weight. But recent research suggests that obesity may increase the risk of certain fractures types (Cao and Picklo, 2015; Scott et al., 2016). Obesity may be a protective factor for hip fracture in adults and significantly reduce the risk of hip fracture (Tang et al., 2013). This view was driven in part by the positive correlation between BMD and BMI. Similar results were seen in obese patients with proximal femoral and vertebral fractures (De Laet et al., 2005).

The association between obesity and fracture in postmenopausal women may be site-dependent. Compared with normal/underweight women, obesity may prevent hip and pelvic fractures, but it increases the risk of proximal humerus fractures. Some non-spinal fractures, such as proximal humerus fractures, upper leg fractures, and ankle fractures, are at higher risk (Compston et al., 2011; Prieto-Alhambra et al., 2012).

In principle, obesity does not completely prevent fractures, and there are some specific site effects on fractures. In fact, obese people are more likely to fall and break bones than people of normal weight. Especially when BMI is over 30, obesity has limited protection against fractures and may even increase the risk of fractures (Kang et al., 2015).

## Osteoarthritis

Osteoarthritis (OA) is the most common degenerative joint disease that affects any joint in the elderly, especially the knee joint. OA is characterized by the progressive deterioration of articular cartilage and structural changes throughout synovial joints, such as synovial membrane, knee meniscus, adipose tissue, periarticular ligaments, and subchondral bone (Brandt, 2006; Loeser et al., 2012; Hunter and Bierma-Zeinstra, 2019). Clinical and animal studies have revealed that age-related OA is related to many factors including age, sex, trauma, and obesity. Among these factors, obesity is one of the most influential and modifiable risk factors (Bijlsma et al., 2011).

Actually, a growing body of evidence suggests a strong link between obesity and inflammation. Adipose tissue has been shown to regulate inflammatory immune responses in cartilage People and animals affected by obesity exhibit higher serum levels of TNF-α, IL-1 and IL-6, all from macrophages in adipose tissue (Park et al., 2005; Ding, 2011). In parallel, the levels of TNF-α, IL-1 and IL-6 in synovial fluid, synovial membrane, subchondral bone and cartilage in patients with OA were increased, confirming their important roles in the pathogenesis of OA TNF-α, IL-6, and IL-1 are the cytokines produced by adipose tissue to directly and negatively regulate cartilage. In addition, TNF-α, IL-1, and IL-6 can promote the formation of other factors, matrix metalloproteinases (MMPs) and prostaglandins, while restrain the synthesis of proteoglycans and type II collagen. Therefore, they play an important role in OA cartilage matrix degradation and bone resorption. Moreover, TNF-α, IL-1, and IL-6 may indirectly cause OA by regulating adiponectin and leptin secreted by fat cells (Koskinen et al., 2011; Wang and He, 2018; Tu et al., 2019).

Reyes et al. (2016) subsequently found that being overweight or obese increased the risk of OA in all three joint areas (knees, hips, and hands), especially the knees. Overweight, class I obesity and class II obesity increased the risk of knee OA by 2-, 3. 1-, and 4.7-fold, respectively (Reyes et al., 2016).

Adipokines represent a new class of compounds that are currently considered to be key molecules involved in the pathogenesis of rheumatic diseases (Felson and Chaisson, 1997; Scotece et al., 2011; Gremese et al., 2014; Feng et al., 2019). Resistin is an adipokines closely related to obesity, local low-level inflammation and MS (Rong et al., 2019). Alissa et al. (2020) recently found that serum resistin levels were higher in patients with primary knee arthritis than in healthy controls. In addition, elevated serum resistin levels were positively correlated with indicators of obesity, markers of inflammation, and WOMAC Index (an indicator of the severity of OA symptoms) (Alissa et al., 2020). Furthermore, Koskinen et al. (2011) believed that the combination of leptin and IL-1 could promote the production of MMP-1, MMP-3, and MMP-13 in human OA cartilage. The effect of leptin on MMP-1, MMP-3, and MMP-13 was mediated by transcription factor NF-κβ, and protein kinase C and MAP kinase pathways. Leptin concentration in synovial fluid was also positively correlated with MMP-1 and MMP-3 levels in patients with OA (Koskinen et al., 2011). The results showed that leptin had catabolic effect on OA joints by increasing the production of MMP in cartilage (Bao et al., 2010).

In addition, adiponectin has been reported to be involved in the pathophysiological process of OA. Kang et al. (2010) reported that the total amount of nitric oxide (NO) and the levels of MMP-1, MMP-3, and MMP-13 were increased in adiponectin stimulated OA chondrocytes compared with unstimulated cells. NO is one of the main mediators of pro-inflammatory cytokines acting on chondrocytes and also regulates different cartilage functions, including chondrocyte phenotypic loss, apoptosis, and extracellular matrix degradation (Otero et al., 2007). In this study, adiponectin increased the expression of MMPs and iNOS in human OA chondrocytes through AMPK and JNK pathways, leading to the degradation of OA cartilage matrix (Kang et al., 2010).

In summary, obesity not only increases the incidence of OA, especially in weight-bearing joints such as knee joints, but also is related to non-weight-bearing joints such as finger joints and wrist OA, suggesting that these metabolic mediators lead to an increase in the incidence of OA in obese patients. This may be because obesity increases the mechanical load of articular cartilage, leading to its degradation, and fatty tissue secretes metabolic factors (such as IL-1, TNF-A, adiponectin, and leptin), leading to an increased prevalence of OA in obese people (Oliveria et al., 1999; Grotle et al., 2008; Kalichman and Kobyliansky, 2009).

### Rheumatoid Arthritis

Rheumatoid arthritis (RA), the most common form of inflammatory arthritis, is a chronic systemic autoimmune disease characterized by aggressive symmetrical inflammation of multiple joints (Kobayashi et al., 2010; Miossec, 2013; Minamino et al., 2020). Epidemiological studies have shown that about 90% of RA patients develop bone erosion within 2 years of onset, resulting in joint deformity or even disability. Therefore, RA has brought a heavy burden and great pain to affected families, patients and even the whole society (Nam et al., 2017).

Overweight/obesity is associated with higher rates of chronic autoimmune diseases and inflammatory diseases, including type 2 diabetes and RA (Zhang et al., 2014). There is evidence that an increase in BMI is associated with an increased risk of RA (Feng et al., 2019). As mentioned above, adipokines such as adiponectin and visfatin have also been reported to play a key role in the pathophysiology of autoimmune diseases (Coelho et al., 2013). It has now been well established that patients with RA show higher plasma adiponectin, leptin, and visfatin levels compared with healthy controls (Otero et al., 2006). Visfatin is a proinflammatory mediator that induces the production of TNF-α, IL-1, IL-6, IL-8, and MMPs, which are typical manifestations of RA joint inflammation (Brentano et al., 2007). Similarly, adiponectin stimulated fibroblast-like synoviocytes (FLS) in patients with RA to produce IL-6, IL-8, and PGE2 (Choi et al., 2009; Lee and Bae, 2018). In addition, adiponectin increased the production of VEGF and MMPs in RA FLS, which may induce inflammation and joint destruction (Lee et al., 2014; Choi et al., 2020; **Figure 1**).

Previous studies have shown that the frequency of circulating T follicular helper cells (Tfh) is significantly increased in RA patients, which is positively correlated with disease activity and anti-CCP autoantibody levels (Liu et al., 2012, 2015). RA FLSs stimulated by AD (adiponectin) promoted the production of Tfh cells. In addition, intra-articular injection of AD aggravated synovitis and increased the frequency of Tfh cells in CIA mice treated with AD (Nurieva et al., 2008; Liu et al., 2020).

Obesity is not only prevalent in RA patients, but also associated with disease activity. Obesity reduces the chance of RA remission and negatively affects disease activity and outcomes reported by patients during treatment (Liu et al., 2017). Lee and Bae (2018) observed that the levels of circulating adiponectin and visfatin in RA patients were significantly higher than those in the control group. The levels of visfatin in 28 joints were positively correlated with disease activity score and CRP level (Lee and Bae, 2018).

## OBESITY TYPE AND BONE

On the one hand, obesity is divided into peripheral obesity and abdominal obesity according to the distribution of fat in the body. Abdominal fat is made up of abdominal wall fat (SAT) and abdominal fat (VAT), also known as central obesity, visceral obesity. Previous studies have shown that adipokins are associated with bone metabolism, and that central obesity can lead to osteopenia or OP because bone density decreases with an increase in waist-to-hip ratio, an index of central obesity (Mitsuyo et al., 2007). In one study, whole body bone mineral content was positively correlated with HOMA-IR and negatively correlated with the percentage of trunk fat, which is a good representative of visceral fat, suggesting that abdominal obesity may have an adverse effect on systemic bone parameters (Krishnan et al., 2018).

Local fat is increasingly recognized as a determinant of bone density, and this association may be mediated by adipocytokines (Vicente et al., 2009). Russell et al. (2010) proposed that VAT was a negative predictor of spine BMD, apparent BMD, systemic BMD and bone mineral content for obese adolescent girls aged 12–18 years (Katzmarzyk et al., 2012). Importantly, VAT/SAT, adipokines, cytokines, E-selectin, and adiponectin were negative predictors of bone density, while leptin was positive. Consequently, VAT is an independent negative determining factor of bone density in obesity (Jurimae et al., 2008; Agbaht et al., 2009; Russell et al., 2010; Bredella et al., 2011a).

On the other hand, according to the different obesity phenotypes, it can be divided into normal metabolic healthy BMI, metabolic healthy obesity and metabolic abnormal obesity (Karelis et al., 2004; Dobson et al., 2016). Marques Loureiro et al. (2019) observed significantly increased deficiencies of calcium, phosphorus, vitamin D, and PTH in the metabolically unhealthy obese (MUHO) group compared to the metabolically healthy obese (MHO) group. In summary, the MUHO phenotype presents a higher risk of bone metabolism-related changes, which may contribute to the development of metabolic bone disease (Marques Loureiro et al., 2019; **Figure 2**).

## DIFFERENT POPULATIONS WITH OBESITY AND BONE

### Children and Adolescents

While childhood obesity has always been a major health problem, its prevalence has been on the rise. In addition, childhood obesity may be associated with multiple complications, such as hyperinsulinemia, hypertension, MS, and non-alcoholic fatty liver disease (NAFLD; Oh et al., 2016). Childhood obesity may affect the growth patterns of children and adolescents, according to several studies Children influenced by obesity may develop accelerated skeletal maturity and advanced bone age beyond their actual age (Johnson et al., 2012; Marcovecchio and Chiarelli, 2013). A study of 232 children (aged 6–15 years) found that the prevalence of advanced bone age increased significantly with increased body weight, height, BMI, and waist circumference percentiles (Oh et al., 2020).

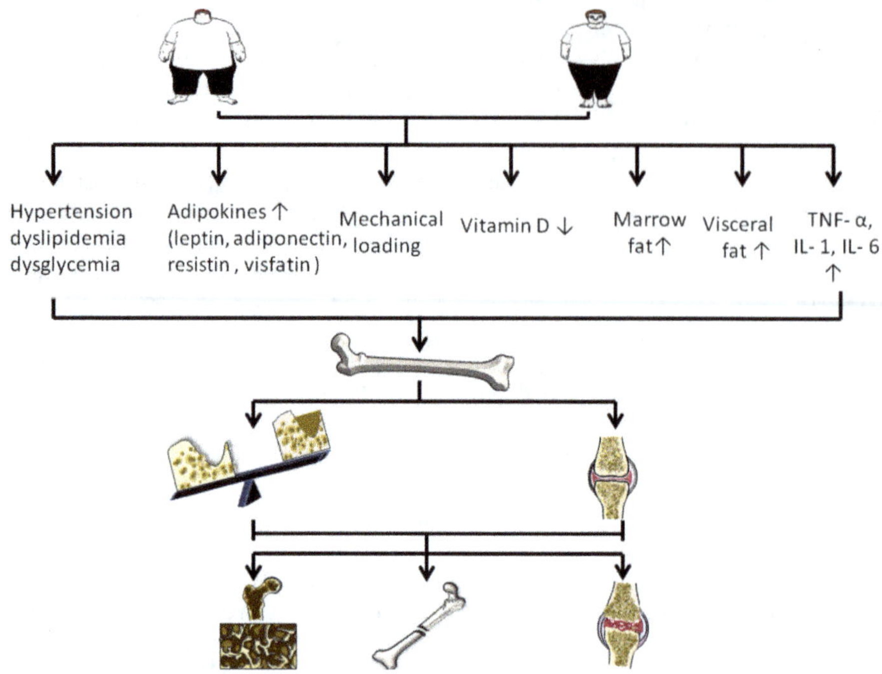


**FIGURE 1 |** Changes of various factors caused by obesity on the regulation of bone disease. Obesity can increase mechanical load, visceral fat and bone marrow fat. In addition, obesity is associated with increased adipokines, increased TNF – or, IL-1, IL- 6, decreased vitamin D, and accompanied by hypertension, dyslipidemia, and dysglycemia. They regulate bone disease by affecting bone formation, bone resorption, and cartilage.

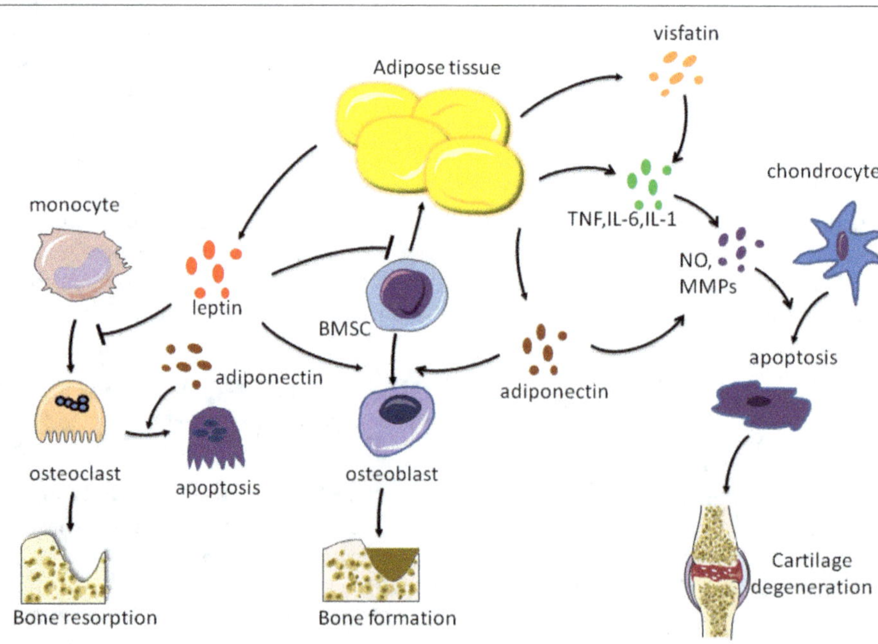


**FIGURE 2 |** Effects of factors secreted by adipose tissue on bone metabolism. Adipose tissue can secrete leptin, adiponectin, visfatin, TNF-*a*, IL-6, and IL-1 These factors act on chondrocytes, osteoblasts, osteoclasts, respectively, to regulate bone formation and resorption, as well as cartilage degradation.

Instead, a study of young people with an average age of 10–17 confirmed that obese children and adolescents had higher bone mass and density than their normal-weight peers (Chaplais et al., 2018).

Notably, Zhao et al. (2020) recently found that obesity had no benefit for BMD in Chinese children aged 0-5 years. t BMD was positively correlated with age, height/length, and inversely with BMI. The BMD gradually increased in the range within 21.2kg, but began to gain slowly and even decreased when the body weight exceeded 21.2kg (Zhao et al., 2020).

As noted above, although there have been several studies on the effects of fat mass on skeletal health in normal weight and obese adolescents, the results remain controversial.

### Postmenopausal Women

Osteoporosis is considered a major public health problem for postmenopausal women. Low estrogen levels lead to rapid bone loss in women five to seven years after menopause (Kanis et al., 2008). Actually, some evidences, indicated that age and BMI were important factors influencing BMD. The BMD of obese postmenopausal women was higher than that of normal size women, and the reduction of BMD of obese women can be delayed by weight bearing (Méndez et al., 2013).

At the same time, Cherif et al. also observed that the left femur, right femur, total hip joint, and overall bone density were higher in obese women (Cherif et al., 2018).

In addition, adipokines secreted by fat are considered as potential pathophysiological factors of OP. Several studies have shown that leptin has significant effects on bone growth and bone metabolism through central and peripheral pathways, and may be involved in the occurrence of various bone diseases (Chen and Yang, 2015). Studies have shown a positive correlation between leptin levels and BMI. And higher BMI is associated with higher bone density. However, obesity had no effect on adiponectin and resistin secretion in postmenopausal women with OP, so leptin was the only one of the adipokines studied to be considered as a protective factor for bone tissue in postmenopausal women (Pasco et al., 2001; Glogowska-Szelag et al., 2019).

Thus, the above results indicate that, adiposity may be beneficial to bone density in postmenopausal women. The protective effect of high body weight and BMI may be due to hormonal influences in the body. Postmenopausal women affected by obesity have more adipose tissue and more estrogen conversion, resulting in higher estrogen levels in their bodies.

### Elderly Patients With Obesity

Obesity, sarcopenia, and OP are common chronic diseases in the elderly. Sarcopenia is a newly discovered age-related disease related to lipid metabolism and insulin resistance. The main diagnostic criteria for sarcopenia are reduced skeletal muscle mass, muscle strength, and function. Older people continue to lose muscle mass as they age, while body fat, especially visceral fat, tends to rise, known as "sarcopenic obesity" (SO; Stenholm et al., 2008; Arango-Lopera et al., 2013). A recent study found that women with SO were more easy to show elevated blood glucose, while men with SO were more likely to present with OP and dyslipidemia (Du et al., 2019). On the other hand, muscles secrete a set of cytokines called myokines, thereby regulating bone metabolism. Myostatin, as a key myokine, has been reported for its effect on bone. Myostatin can inhibit osteogenic differentiation of BMSCs, as well as osteoblast differentiation and mineralization (Hamrick et al., 2007; Chen et al., 2017). Likewise, myostatin may inhibit osteogenesis by activating the RANKL signaling pathway, thus showing an adverse impact on bone mass (Saad, 2020). In addition, myostatin itself is an important autocrine/paracrine factor that inhibits skeletal muscle growth (Rodriguez et al., 2014; Cui et al., 2020). Thus, inhibition or blocking of the myostatin signaling pathway may provide potential therapeutic targets for a number of diseases, particularly in sarcopenia and OP.

Several studies have reported the links between BMD and body fat and lean mass. When body weight was stratified into lean body mass and fat mass, the increase in BMD was more pronounced for lean body mass, whereas fat mass was only beneficial for men and premenopausal women. Santos et al. also observed a more direct relationship between lean body mass and bone density (total bone density, femur, and spine), while sarcopenia was associated with OP. Obesity was more likely to be a protective factor for OP in old subjects aged 80 and over (Santos et al., 2018). At the same time, Barrera et al. demonstrated the beneficial effects of high BMI on femoral neck bone density in older adults. Men and women with a BMI of more than 30 kg/m$^2$ had about a 33% risk of bone mass loss compared to those with a normal BMI (Barrera et al., 2004). In particular, obese people were reported to have higher bone density, but they also showed damaged bone microstructures and different fall patterns (Compston, 2013; Ilich et al., 2016).

## HIGH-FAT DIET INDUCED OBESITY AND BONE

Conclusions about the relationship between obesity and bone in humans rely on statistical correlations or models, rather than controlled trials. Therefore, the establishment of obesity mouse model is helpful to study the effect of high-fat diet (HFD)-induced obesity on bone metabolism. Studies have shown that obese animals burn the same amount of energy, no matter how much fat is in their diet (Brown et al., 2003; Tortoriello et al., 2004; Relling et al., 2006). The mice provided a model for studying the relationship between body size, obesity and skeletal characteristics. High fat intake in rodents leads to obesity, and several studies have shown a strong link between bone size, strength and body size. However, mice are not always reliable indicators of human pathophysiology. Human can enjoy more colorful life style, more abundant food and more complicated living environment. Moreover, patients with obesity often have multiple complications, not just weight gain. These factors make the relationship between obesity and bone more complex in humans than in mice.

### Cancellous Bone

The effects of a high-fat diet on cancellous bone in rodents have been shown to be harmful. Previous studies have reported that after 4, 8, and 12 weeks of HFD treatment, the trabecular density of 6-week-old male C57BL/6J mice decreased with the increase of adipocytes and trabecular degeneration. In addition, in obese mice, serum leptin levels were associated with bone trabeculae, but not cortical bone density, while adiponectin and total cholesterol levels were not associated with bone mass (Fujita et al., 2012). Scheller et al. (2016) also noted that bone trabecular volume fraction, bone mineral content, and quantity decreased after 12, 16, or 20 weeks of high-fat feeding compared with normal rat chow (ND) controls, and only partial recovery after weight loss.

In addition, Inzana et al. (2013) found that femoral cancellous metaphyseal bones were more susceptible to adverse effects of high-fat diet before bone maturation, and had poor recovery ability after dietary correction (low-fat diet, LFD).

A recent study conducted by Tian et al. showed that the bone mass of femoral trabecular bone in C57BL/6J mice increased significantly after 8 weeks of HFD, but decreased significantly at 16 and 24 weeks (Tian et al., 2017). In other words, after short-term feeding, HFD may show a positive effect on bone mass, however, after long-term feeding, bone mass was significantly decreased in HFD mice.

## Cortical Bone

However, the effects of diet induced obesity on cortical bone in rodents are less clear, with positive, negative, and neutral results reported. The femoral cortical thickness and cross-sectional area of 4-week old male mice were increased after feeding HFD-DAG (Diacylglycerol). HFD-DAG had obvious promoting effect on bone and bone metabolism (Choi et al., 2015). In addition, Silva et al. recently suggested that a high-fat diet had beneficial effects on most femoral size and skeletal mechanical properties, as well as radius size and stiffness (Silva et al., 2019). However, Ionova-Martin et al. found that femur strength, hardness, and toughness were significantly lower in both young and adult mice fed HFD than in the control group (Ionova-Martin et al., 2011).

In contrast, Cao et al. concluded that feeding mice HFD for 14 weeks reduced proximal tibial cancellous bone mass in young mice, but had no effect on cortical bone mass (Cao et al., 2009). Halade et al. (2011) also revealed that mice fed corn oil (CO) for 6 months showed a 66% reduction in distal femoral trabecular volume fraction, with no significant effect on cortical bone. To sum up, in the above studies, the effect of HFD on cortical bone was not as significant as that on cancellous bone.

It is generally believed that age-related OP has three main processes. The first and most important process is reduction of trabecular bone, the second is continuous bone resorption on the cortical surface, and the third is cortical bone loss (Chen et al., 2009). Similarly, the above studies indicate that the most significant change in obesity-related bone loss is the reduction of femoral trabecular bone Combined, these results suggest that HFD could regulate the changes of trabecular and cortical bone in different ways. This may be due to the fact that cancellous bone generally responds more strongly to diet or drug therapy, physiological conditions, or aging than cortical bone, because cancellous bone is more active in remodeling because of its larger surface to volume ratio than cortical bone (Morgan et al., 2008). On the other hand, bearing capacity and mechanical stress are important factors in determining cortical bone mass, while trabecular bone density is affected by sex maturation related hormones (Mora et al., 1994).

## Bone Formation/Resorption

In addition to affecting bone structure, HFD can also have significant effects on cell function. Bone mass reflects the balance between bone formation and bone resorption and is involved in the coordination and regulation of the number and activity of osteoblasts and osteoclasts at the cellular level. The RANKL/RANK/OPG signaling pathway plays a major role in this regulation. A previous study showed that the expression of RANKL, the ratio of RANKL to OPG, and the level of serum TRAP in osteoblasts from HFD mice were increased, suggesting that HFD can promote osteoclast activity and bone resorption (Cao et al., 2009). Notably, Halade et al. reported that in mice fed HFD, the accumulation of bone marrow adipocytes resulted in significantly higher levels of pro-inflammatory factors, leading to increased bone resorption. In addition, increased expression of osteoclast-specific cathepsin K and RANKL and decreased osteoblast-specific RUNX2/Cbfa1 in CO-feeding mice also supported bone resorption (Halade et al., 2011).

Furthermore, Shu et al. (2015) revealed that the lower trabecular volume, but increased osteoclast numbers could be found in the femoral metaphyseal sections of HFD-fed mice after 3, 6, and 12 weeks. The elevated osteoclast precursor frequency, increased osteoclast formation, and bone resorption activity, along with increased osteoclastogenic regulators such as RANKL, TNF, and PPARγ were seen in bone marrow cells from HFD-fed mice. But, osteoblast function was also increased after 12 weeks of HFD (Shu et al., 2015). A possible explanation is that mechanical load of body weight stimulates bone formation, reduces apoptosis, and enhances proliferation and differentiation of osteoblasts and osteocytes. Therefore, it was not surprising that bone formation rates and osteoblast numbers increased in this study, since HFD mice were significantly heavier than the control group (Bonewald and Johnson, 2008). In conclusion, it is reasonable to believe that the bone loss caused by HFD is mainly related to the promotion of osteoclast differentiation and activity by changing the bone marrow microenvironment.

Based on these findings, the effect of HFD is bipolar and may be the result of a combination of body weight, fat mass, bone formation/absorption, pro-inflammatory mediators and bone marrow microenvironment. Obesity initially has a beneficial effect on bones, possibly due to anabolic effects that increase mechanical load. However, due to the development of metabolic complications including systemic inflammation, the second stage is followed by a reduction in bone formation (Lecka-Czernik et al., 2015). As mentioned above, these results may support the idea that as obesity rises, the benefits for bone health are diminishing.

# CONCLUSION

In conclusion, obesity or overweight is strictly related to bone metabolism, although the correlation has not yet been fully unified. Adipose tissue interacts with bone by secreting various cytokines, so as to regulate bone health. Meanwhile BMAT also exerts a crucial impact on bone density and bone microstructure.

In addition, human obesity is a complex problem that involves not only excessive fat intake but also other nutrient consumption imbalances such as vitamin D, calcium and phosphorus, which are known to affect bone metabolism, further making it difficult to determine the impact of obesity on human bone health. Moreover, while BMI is closely related to the gold standard of body fat, it does not distinguish between lean and fat mass, nor does it provide an indication of the distribution of body fat. The loss of muscle mass in the elderly means that BMI is also less accurate at predicting body fat in this group. Therefore, determining whether obesity causes changes in bone mass based on BMI is less accurate. Central obesity measures, including waist circumference, waist-to-height ratio and waist-to-hip ratio, are better predictors of visceral obesity, bone-related disease and mortality than BMI. Simply put, all of these findings indicate that skeletal response to obesity has either a positive or negative effect on bone, suggesting that the influence of obesity on bone metabolism is intricate and depend on diverse factors, such as mechanical load by the weight, obesity type, the location of adipose tissue, gender, age, and bone sites, along with secreted cytokines, these factors may play a major function for bone health. The effects of obesity on bone metabolism and bone microstructure involve these multiple factors, which may exert different regulatory mechanisms and ultimately affect the skeletal health. The investigation of the relationship between obesity and bone is conducive to finding new targets for the treatment of bone-related diseases, including OP, fractures, RA, and OA.

## AUTHOR CONTRIBUTIONS

JH wrote the manuscript. CH, WH, and MY revised the manuscript. CL and XL were responsible for the guidance and supervision. All authors contributed to the article and approved the submitted version.

## REFERENCES


Agbaht, K., Gurlek, A., Karakaya, J., and Bayraktar, M. (2009). Circulating adiponectin represents a biomarker of the association between adiposity and bone mineral density. *Endocrine* 35, 371–379. doi: 10.1007/s12020-009-9158-2

Al Saedi, A., Goodman, A. C., Myers, D. E., Hayes, A., and Duque, G. (2020). Rapamycin affects palmitate-induced lipotoxicity in osteoblasts by modulating apoptosis and autophagy. *J. Gerontol. A Biol. Sci. Med. Sci.* 75, 58–63. doi: 10.1093/gerona/glz149

Alissa, E. M., Alzughaibi, L. S., and Marzouki, Z. M. (2020). Relationship between serum resistin, body fat and inflammatory markers in females with clinical knee osteoarthritis. *Knee* 27, 45–50. doi: 10.1016/j.knee.2019.12.009

Arango-Lopera, V. E., Arroyo, P., Gutierrez-Robledo, L. M., Perez-Zepeda, M. U., and Cesari, M. (2013). Mortality as an adverse outcome of sarcopenia. *J. Nutr. Health Aging* 17, 259–262. doi: 10.1007/s12603-012-0434-0

Ardawi, M. S., Akhbar, D. H., Alshaikh, A., Ahmed, M. M., Qari, M. H., Rouzi, A. A., et al. (2013). Increased serum sclerostin and decreased serum IGF-1 are associated with vertebral fractures among postmenopausal women with type-2 diabetes. *Bone* 56, 355–362. doi: 10.1016/j.bone.2013.06.029

Astudillo, P., Ríos, S., Pastenes, L., Pino, A. M., and Rodríguez, J. P. (2007). Increased adipogenesis of osteoporotic human-mesenchymal stem cells (MSCs) characterizes by impaired leptin action . *J. Cell. Biochem.* 103, 1054–1065. doi: 10.1002/jcb.21516

Baggio, L. L., and Drucker, D. J. (2007). Biology of incretins: GLP-1 and GIP. *Gastroenterology* 132, 2131–2157. doi: 10.1053/j.gastro.2007.03.054

Bao, J. P., Chen, W. P., Feng, J., Hu, P. F., Shi, Z. L., and Wu, L. D. (2010). Leptin plays a catabolic role on articular cartilage. *Mol. Biol. Rep.* 37, 3265–3272. doi: 10.1007/s11033-009-9911-x

Barba, C., Cavalli-Sforza, T., Cutter, J., Darnton-Hill, I., Deurenberg, P., Deurenberg-Yap, M., et al. (2004). Appropriate body-mass index for Asian populations and its implications for policy and intervention strategies. *Lancet* 363, 157–163. doi: 10.1016/s0140-6736(03)15268-3

Barrera, G., Bunout, D., Gattas, V., de la Maza, M. P., Leiva, L., and Hirsch, S. (2004). A high body mass index protects against femoral neck osteoporosis in healthy elderly subjects. *Nutrition* 20, 769–771. doi: 10.1016/j.nut.2004.05.014

Bartell, S. M., Rayalam, S., Ambati, S., Gaddam, D. R., Hartzell, D. L., Hamrick, M., et al. (2011). Central (ICV) leptin injection increases bone formation, bone mineral density, muscle mass, serum IGF-1, and the expression of osteogenic genes in leptin-deficient ob/ob mice. *J. Bone Miner. Res.* 26, 1710–1720. doi: 10.1002/jbmr.406

Beekman, K. M., Zwaagstra, M., Veldhuis-Vlug, A. G., van Essen, H. W., den Heijer, M., Maas, M., et al. (2019). Ovariectomy increases RANKL protein expression in bone marrow adipocytes of C3H/HeJ mice. *Am. J. Physiol. Endocrinol. Metab.* 317, E1050–E1054.

Bijlsma, J. W. J., Berenbaum, F., and Lafeber, F. P. J. G. (2011). Osteoarthritis: an update with relevance for clinical practice. *Lancet* 377, 2115–2126. doi: 10.1016/s0140-6736(11)60243-2

Bonewald, L. F., and Johnson, M. L. (2008). Osteocytes, mechanosensing and Wnt signaling. *Bone* 42, 606–615. doi: 10.1016/j.bone.2007.12.224

Boon, M. R., van den Berg, S. A., Wang, Y., van den Bossche, J., Karkampouna, S., Bauwens, M., et al. (2013). BMP7 activates brown adipose tissue and reduces diet-induced obesity only at subthermoneutrality. *PLoS One* 8:e74083. doi: 10.1371/journal.pone.0074083

Borges, J. L., Bilezikian, J. P., Jones-Leone, A. R., Acusta, A. P., Ambery, P. D., Nino, A. J., et al. (2011). A randomized, parallel group, double-blind, multicentre study comparing the efficacy and safety of Avandamet (rosiglitazone/metformin) and metformin on long-term glycaemic control and bone mineral density after 80 weeks of treatment in drug-naive type 2 diabetes mellitus patients. *Diabetes Obes. Metab.* 13, 1036–1046. doi: 10.1111/j.1463-1326.2011.01461.x

Brandt, K. D. (2006). Yet more evidence that osteoarthritis is not a cartilage disease. *Ann. Rheum. Dis.* 65, 1261–1264. doi: 10.1136/ard.2006.058347

Bredella, M. A., Fazeli, P. K., Miller, K. K., Misra, M., Torriani, M., Thomas, B. J., et al. (2009). Increased bone marrow fat in anorexia nervosa. *J. Clin. Endocrinol. Metab.* 94, 2129–2136. doi: 10.1210/jc.2008-2532

Bredella, M. A., Torriani, M., Ghomi, R. H., Thomas, B. J., Brick, D. J., Gerweck, A. V., et al. (2011a). Determinants of bone mineral density in obese premenopausal women. *Bone* 48, 748–754. doi: 10.1016/j.bone.2010.12.011

Bredella, M. A., Torriani, M., Ghomi, R. H., Thomas, B. J., Brick, D. J., Gerweck, A. V., et al. (2011b). Vertebral bone marrow fat is positively associated with visceral fat and inversely associated with IGF-1 in obese women. *Obesity (Silver Spring)* 19, 49–53. doi: 10.1038/oby.2010.106

Brentano, F., Schorr, O., Ospelt, C., Stanczyk, J., Gay, R. E., Gay, S., et al. (2007). Pre-B cell colony-enhancing factor/visfatin, a new marker of inflammation in rheumatoid arthritis with proinflammatory and matrix-degrading activities. *Arthritis Rheum.* 56, 2829–2839. doi: 10.1002/art.22833

Brown, J. L., Spicer, M. T., and Spicer, L. J. (2003). Effect of high-fat diet on body composition and hormone responses to glucose tolerance tests. *Endocrine* 19, 327–332. doi: 10.1385/endo:19:3:327

Brun, J., Berthou, F., Trajkovski, M., Maechler, P., Foti, M., and Bonnet, N. (2017). Bone regulates browning and energy metabolism through mature osteoblast/osteocyte PPARgamma expression. *Diabetes* 66, 2541–2554. doi: 10.2337/db17-0116

Burguera, B., Hofbauer, L. C., Thomas, T., Gori, F., Evans, G. L., Khosla, S., et al. (2001). Leptin reduces ovariectomy-induced bone loss in rats. *Endocrinology* 142, 3546–3553. doi: 10.1210/endo.142.8.8346

Cao, J. J., and Picklo, M. J. Sr. (2015). Involuntary wheel running improves but does not fully reverse the deterioration of bone structure of obese rats despite decreasing adiposity. *Calcif. Tissue Int.* 97, 145–155. doi: 10.1007/s00223-015-9992-6

Cao, J. J., Gregoire, B. R., and Gao, H. (2009). High-fat diet decreases cancellous bone mass but has no effect on cortical bone mass in the tibia in mice. *Bone* 44, 1097–1104. doi: 10.1016/j.bone.2009.02.017

Carobbio, S., Pellegrinelli, V., and Vidal-Puig, A. (2017). Adipose tissue function and expandability as determinants of lipotoxicity and the metabolic syndrome. *Adv. Exp. Med. Biol.* 960, 161–196. doi: 10.1007/978-3-319-48382-5_7

Chaplais, E., Naughton, G., Greene, D., Dutheil, F., Pereira, B., Thivel, D., et al. (2018). Effects of interventions with a physical activity component on bone health in obese children and adolescents: a systematic review and meta-analysis. *J. Bone Miner. Metab.* 36, 12–30. doi: 10.1007/s00774-017-0858-z

Chen, H., Zhou, X., Emura, S., and Shoumura, S. (2009). Site-specific bone loss in senescence-accelerated mouse (SAMP6): a murine model for senile osteoporosis. *Exp. Gerontol.* 44, 792–798. doi: 10.1016/j.exger.2009.09.009

Chen, X. X., and Yang, T. (2015). Roles of leptin in bone metabolism and bone diseases. *J. Bone Miner. Metab.* 33, 474–485. doi: 10.1007/s00774-014-0569-7

Chen, Y. S., Guo, Q., Guo, L. J., Liu, T., Wu, X. P., Lin, Z. Y., et al. (2017). GDF8 inhibits bone formation and promotes bone resorption in mice. *Clin. Exp. Pharmacol. Physiol.* 44, 500–508. doi: 10.1111/1440-1681.12728

Cherif, R., Mahjoub, F., Sahli, H., Cheour, E., Vico, L., Sakly, M., et al. (2018). Positive Association of Obesity and insulin resistance with bone mineral density in Tunisian postmenopausal women. *J. Clin. Densitom.* 21, 163–171. doi: 10.1016/j.jocd.2017.05.015

Choi, H. M., Doss, H. M., and Kim, K. S. (2020). Multifaceted physiological roles of adiponectin in inflammation and diseases. *Int. J. Mol. Sci.* 21:1219. doi: 10.3390/ijms21041219

Choi, H. M., Lee, Y. A., Lee, S. H., Hong, S. J., Hahm, D. H., Choi, S. Y., et al. (2009). Adiponectin may contribute to synovitis and joint destruction in rheumatoid arthritis by stimulating vascular endothelial growth factor, matrix metalloproteinase-1, and matrix metalloproteinase-13 expression in fibroblast-like synoviocytes more than proinflammatory mediators. *Arthritis Res. Ther.* 11:R161.

Choi, H. S., Park, S. J., Lee, Z. H., and Lim, S. K. (2015). The effects of a high fat diet containing diacylglycerol on bone in C57BL/6J mice. *Yonsei Med. J.* 56, 951–960. doi: 10.3349/ymj.2015.56.4.951

Coelho, M., Oliveira, T., and Fernandes, R. (2013). Biochemistry of adipose tissue: an endocrine organ. *Arch. Med. Sci.* 9, 191–200. doi: 10.5114/aoms.2013.33181

Compston, J. (2013). Obesity and fractures. *Joint Bone Spine* 80, 8–10. doi: 10.1016/j.jbspin.2012.07.016

Compston, J. (2018). Type 2 diabetes mellitus and bone. *J. Intern. Med.* 283, 140–153.

Compston, J. E., Watts, N. B., Chapurlat, R., Cooper, C., Boonen, S., Greenspan, S., et al. (2011). Obesity is not protective against fracture in postmenopausal women: GLOW. *Am. J. Med.* 124, 1043–1050. doi: 10.1016/j.amjmed.2011.06.013

Conde, J., Scotece, M., Gomez, R., Lopez, V., Gomez-Reino, J. J., and Gualillo, O. (2011). Adipokines and osteoarthritis: novel molecules involved in the pathogenesis and progression of disease. *Arthritis* 2011:203901.

Cui, Y., Yi, Q., Sun, W., Huang, D., Zhang, H., Duan, L., et al. (2020). Molecular basis and therapeutic potential of myostatin on bone formation and metabolism in orthopedic disease. *Biofactors* 71, 4361–4371.

Dalamaga, M., and Christodoulatos, G. S. (2015). Adiponectin as a biomarker linking obesity and adiposopathy to hematologic malignancies. *Horm. Mol. Biol. Clin. Investig.* 23, 5–20.

de Araujo, I. M., Salmon, C. E., Nahas, A. K., Nogueira-Barbosa, M. H., Elias, J. Jr., and de Paula, F. J. (2017). Marrow adipose tissue spectrum in obesity and type 2 diabetes mellitus. *Eur. J. Endocrinol.* 176, 21–30. doi: 10.1530/eje-16-0448

De Laet, C., Kanis, J. A., Oden, A., Johanson, H., Johnell, O., Delmas, P., et al. (2005). Body mass index as a predictor of fracture risk: a meta-analysis. *Osteoporos. Int.* 16, 1330–1338.

Del Mar Gonzalez-Barroso, M., Ricquier, D., and Cassard-Doulcier, A. M. (2001). The human uncoupling protein−1 gene (UCP1): present status and perspectives in obesity research. *Obes. Rev.* 1, 61–72. doi: 10.1046/j.1467-789x.2000.00009.x

Di Angelantonio, E., Bhupathiraju, S. N., Wormser, D., Gao, P., Kaptoge, S., de Gonzalez, A. B., et al. (2016). Body-mass index and all-cause mortality: individual-participant-data meta-analysis of 239 prospective studies in four continents. *Lancet* 388, 776–786.

Ding, C. (2011). Metabolic triggered inflammation in osteoarthritis. *Osteoarthritis Cartilage* 41, 90–91. doi: 10.1016/j.semarthrit.2011.06.009

Dobson, R., Burgess, M. I., Sprung, V. S., Irwin, A., Hamer, M., Jones, J., et al. (2016). Metabolically healthy and unhealthy obesity: differential effects on myocardial function according to metabolic syndrome, rather than obesity. *Int. J. Obes. (Lond.)* 40, 153–161. doi: 10.1038/ijo.2015.151

Dormuth, C. R., Carney, G., Carleton, B., Bassett, K., and Wright, J. M. (2009). Thiazolidinediones and fractures in men and women. *Arch. Intern. Med.* 169, 1395–1402. doi: 10.1001/archinternmed.2009.214

Du, Y., Wang, X., Xie, H., Zheng, S., Wu, X., Zhu, X., et al. (2019). Sex differences in the prevalence and adverse outcomes of sarcopenia and sarcopenic obesity in community dwelling elderly in East China using the AWGS criteria. *BMC Endocr. Disord.* 19:109. doi: 10.1186/s12902-019-0432-x

Ducy, P., Amling, M., Takeda, S., Priemel, M., Schilling, A. F., Beil, F. T., et al. (2000). Leptin inhibits bone formation through a hypothalamic relay: a central control of bone mass. *Cell* 100, 197–207. doi: 10.1016/s0092-8674(00)81558-5

Elbaz, A., Wu, X., Rivas, D., Gimble, J. M., and Duque, G. (2010). Inhibition of fatty acid biosynthesis prevents adipocyte lipotoxicity on human osteoblasts in vitro. *J. Cell. Mol. Med.* 14, 982–991. doi: 10.1111/j.1582-4934.2009.00751.x

Fassio, A., Idolazzi, L., Rossini, M., Gatti, D., Adami, G., Giollo, A., et al. (2018). The obesity paradox and osteoporosis. *Eat. Weight Disord.* 23, 293–302.

Fazeli, P. K., Bredella, M. A., Freedman, L., Thomas, B. J., Breggia, A., Meenaghan, E., et al. (2012). Marrow fat and preadipocyte factor-1 levels decrease with recovery in women with anorexia nervosa. *J. Bone Miner. Res.* 27, 1864–1871. doi: 10.1002/jbmr.1640

Fazeli, P. K., Faje, A. T., Bredella, M. A., Polineni, S., Russell, S., Resulaj, M., et al. (2019). Changes in marrow adipose tissue with short-term changes in weight in premenopausal women with anorexia nervosa. *Eur. J. Endocrinol.* 180, 189–199. doi: 10.1530/eje-18-0824

Fazeli, P. K., Faje, A. T., Cross, E. J., Lee, H., Rosen, C. J., Bouxsein, M. L., et al. (2015). Serum FGF-21 levels are associated with worsened radial trabecular bone microarchitecture and decreased radial bone strength in women with anorexia nervosa. *Bone* 77, 6–11. doi: 10.1016/j.bone.2015.04.001

Fazeli, P. K., Horowitz, M. C., MacDougald, O. A., Scheller, E. L., Rodeheffer, M. S., Rosen, C. J., et al. (2013). Marrow fat and bone–new perspectives. *J. Clin. Endocrinol. Metab.* 98, 935–945.

Felson, D. T., and Chaisson, C. E. (1997). Understanding the relationship between body weight and osteoarthritis. *Baillieres Clin. Rheumatol.* 11, 671–681. doi: 10.1016/s0950-3579(97)80003-9

Felson, T. (2010). Effect of weight and body mass index on bone mineral density in men and women: the Framingham study. *J. Bone Miner. Res.* 8, 567–573. doi: 10.1002/jbmr.5650080507

Feng, X., Xu, X., Shi, Y., Liu, X., Liu, H., Hou, H., et al. (2019). Body mass index and the risk of rheumatoid arthritis: an updated dose-response meta-analysis. *Biomed. Res. Int.* 2019:3579081.

Ferron, M., Wei, J., Yoshizawa, T., Fattore, A. Del, DePinho, R. A., Teti, A., et al. (2010). Insulin signaling in osteoblasts integrates bone remodeling and energy metabolism. *Cell* 142, 296–308. doi: 10.1016/j.cell.2010.06.003

Frontini, A., and Cinti, S. (2010). Distribution and development of brown adipocytes in the murine and human adipose organ. *Cell Metab.* 11, 253–256. doi: 10.1016/j.cmet.2010.03.004

Fruhbeck, G., Gomez-Ambrosi, J., Muruzabal, F. J., and Burrell, M. A. (2001). The adipocyte: a model for integration of endocrine and metabolic signaling in energy metabolism regulation. *Am. J. Physiol. Endocrinol. Metab.* 280, E827–E847.

Fujita, Y., Watanabe, K., and Maki, K. (2012). Serum leptin levels negatively correlate with trabecular bone mineral density in high-fat diet-induced obesity mice. *J. Musculoskelet. Neuronal Interact.* 12, 84–94.

Gimble, J. M., Robinson, C. E., Wu, X., Kelly, K. A., Rodriguez, B. R., Kliewer, S. A., et al. (1996). Peroxisome proliferator-activated receptor-gamma activation by thiazolidinediones induces adipogenesis in bone marrow stromal cells. *Mol. Pharmacol.* 50, 1087–1094.

Glogowska-Szelag, J., Kos-Kudla, B., Marek, B., Nowak, M., and Sieminska, L. (2019). Assessment of selected adipocytokines in obese women with postmenopausal osteoporosis. *Endokrynol. Pol.* 70, 478–483. doi: 10.5603/ep.a2019.0043

Gordeladze, J. O., Drevon, C. A., Syversen, U., and Reseland, J. E. (2002). Leptin stimulates human osteoblastic cell proliferation, de novo collagen synthesis, and mineralization: impact on differentiation markers, apoptosis, and osteoclastic signaling. *J. Cell. Biochem.* 85, 825–836. doi: 10.1002/jcb.10156

Gremese, E., Tolusso, B., Gigante, M. R., and Ferraccioli, G. (2014). Obesity as a risk and severity factor in rheumatic diseases (autoimmune chronic inflammatory diseases). *Front. Immunol.* 5:576. doi: 10.3389/fimmu.2014.00576

Grotle, M., Hagen, K. B., Natvig, B., Dahl, F. A., and Kvien, T. K. (2008). Obesity and osteoarthritis in knee, hip and/or hand: an epidemiological study in the general population with 10 years follow-up. *BMC Musculoskelet. Disord.* 9:132. doi: 10.1186/1471-2474-9-132

Halade, G. V., Jamali, A. El, Williams, P. J., Fajardo, R. J., and Fernandes, G. (2011). Obesity-mediated inflammatory microenvironment stimulates osteoclastogenesis and bone loss in mice. *Exp. Gerontol.* 46, 43–52. doi: 10.1016/j.exger.2010.09.014

Hamrick, M. W., Della-Fera, M. A., Choi, Y. H., Pennington, C., Hartzell, D., and Baile, C. A. (2005). Leptin treatment induces loss of bone marrow adipocytes and increases bone formation in leptin-deficient ob/ob mice. *J. Bone Miner. Res.* 20, 994–1001. doi: 10.1359/jbmr.050103

Hamrick, M. W., Pennington, C., Newton, D., Xie, D., and Isales, C. (2004). Leptin deficiency produces contrasting phenotypes in bones of the limb and spine. *Bone* 34, 376–383. doi: 10.1016/j.bone.2003.11.020

Hamrick, M. W., Shi, X., Zhang, W., Pennington, C., Thakore, H., Haque, M., et al. (2007). Loss of myostatin (GDF8) function increases osteogenic differentiation of bone marrow-derived mesenchymal stem cells but the osteogenic effect is ablated with unloading. *Bone* 40, 1544–1553. doi: 10.1016/j.bone.2007.02.012

Hao, R. H., Gao, J. L., Li, M., Huang, W., Zhu, D. L., Thynn, H. N., et al. (2018). Association between fibroblast growth factor 21 and bone mineral density in adults. *Endocrine* 59, 296–303. doi: 10.1007/s12020-017-1507-y

Hardouin, P., Rharass, T., and Lucas, S. (2016). Bone marrow adipose tissue: to be or not to be a typical adipose tissue? *Front. Endocrinol. (Lausanne)* 7:85. doi: 10.3389/fendo.2016.00085

Holloway, W. R., Collier, F. M., Aitken, C. J., Myers, D. E., Hodge, J. M., Malakellis, M., et al. (2002). Leptin inhibits osteoclast generation. *J. Bone Miner. Res.* 17, 200–209. doi: 10.1359/jbmr.2002.17.2.200

Horowitz, M. C., Berry, R., Holtrup, B., Sebo, Z., Nelson, T., Fretz, J. A., et al. (2017). Bone marrow adipocytes. *Adipocyte* 6, 193–204.

Huang, C. Y., Lee, C. Y., Chen, M. Y., Tsai, H. C., Hsu, H. C., and Tang, C. H. (2010). Adiponectin increases BMP-2 expression in osteoblasts via AdipoR receptor signaling pathway. *J. Cell. Physiol.* 224, 475–483. doi: 10.1002/jcp.22145

Huang, Y., Xiao, Y., Liu, Y., Guo, M., Guo, Q., Zhou, F., et al. (2020). MicroRNA-188 regulates aging-associated metabolic phenotype. *Aging Cell* 19:e13077.

Hunter, D. J., and Bierma-Zeinstra, S. (2019). Osteoarthritis. *Lancet* 393, 1745–1759.

Ilich, J. Z., Kelly, O. J., and Inglis, J. E. (2016). Osteosarcopenic obesity syndrome: what is it and how can it be identified and diagnosed? *Curr. Gerontol. Geriatr. Res.* 2016:7325973.

Ilich, J. Z., Kelly, O. J., Inglis, J. E., Panton, L. B., Duque, G., and Ormsbee, M. J. (2014). Interrelationship among muscle, fat, and bone: connecting the dots on cellular, hormonal, and whole body levels. *Ageing Res. Rev.* 15, 51–60. doi: 10.1016/j.arr.2014.02.007

Inzana, J. A., Kung, M., Shu, L., Hamada, D., Xing, L. P., Zuscik, M. J., et al. (2013). Immature mice are more susceptible to the detrimental effects of high fat diet on cancellous bone in the distal femur. *Bone* 57, 174–183. doi: 10.1016/j.bone.2013.08.003

Ionova-Martin, S. S., Wade, J. M., Tang, S., Shahnazari, M., Ager, J. W. III, Lane, N. E., et al. (2011). Changes in cortical bone response to high-fat diet from adolescence to adulthood in mice. *Osteoporos. Int.* 22, 2283–2293. doi: 10.1007/s00198-010-1432-x

Johansson, A. G., Lindh, E., and Ljunghall, S. (1992). Insulin-like growth factor I stimulates bone turnover in osteoporosis. *Lancet* 339:1619. doi: 10.1016/0140-6736(92)91889-g

Johnson, W., Stovitz, S. D., Choh, A. C., Czerwinski, S. A., Towne, B., and Demerath, E. W. (2012). Patterns of linear growth and skeletal maturation from birth to 18 years of age in overweight young adults. *Int. J. Obes. (Lond.)* 36, 535–541.

Jurimae, J., Jurimae, T., Leppik, A., and Kums, T. (2008). The influence of ghrelin, adiponectin, and leptin on bone mineral density in healthy postmenopausal women. *J. Bone Miner. Metab.* 26, 618–623. doi: 10.1007/s00774-008-0861-5

Justesen, J., Stenderup, K., Ebbesen, E. N., Mosekilde, L., Steiniche, T., and Kassem, M. (2001). Adipocyte tissue volume in bone marrow is increased with aging and in patients with osteoporosis. *Biogerontology* 2, 165–171.

Kahn, S. E., Haffner, S. M., Heise, M. A., Herman, W. H., Holman, R. R., Jones, N. P., et al. (2006). Glycemic durability of rosiglitazone, metformin, or glyburide monotherapy. *N. Engl. J. Med.* 355, 2427–2443. doi: 10.1056/nejmoa066224

Kalichman, L., and Kobyliansky, E. (2009). Hand osteoarthritis in Chuvashian population: prevalence and determinants. *Rheumatol. Int.* 30, 85–92. doi: 10.1007/s00296-009-0920-9

Kanazawa, I., Notsu, M., Miyake, H., Tanaka, K., and Sugimoto, T. (2018). Assessment using serum insulin-like growth factor-I and bone mineral density is useful for detecting prevalent vertebral fractures in patients with type 2 diabetes mellitus. *Osteoporos. Int.* 29, 2527–2535. doi: 10.1007/s00198-018-4638-y

Kanazawa, I., Yamaguchi, T., and Sugimoto, T. (2011). Serum insulin-like growth factor-I is a marker for assessing the severity of vertebral fractures in postmenopausal women with type 2 diabetes mellitus. *Osteoporos. Int.* 22, 1191–1198. doi: 10.1007/s00198-010-1310-6

Kanazawa, I., Yamaguchi, T., and Sugimoto, T. (2012). Effects of intensive glycemic control on serum levels of insulin-like growth factor-I and dehydroepiandrosterone sulfate in type 2 diabetes mellitus. *J. Endocrinol. Invest.* 35, 469–472.

Kang, D. H., Guo, L. F., Guo, T., Wang, Y., Liu, T., Feng, X. Y., et al. (2015). Association of body composition with bone mineral density in northern Chinese men by different criteria for obesity. *J. Endocrinol. Invest.* 38, 323–331. doi: 10.1007/s40618-014-0167-5

Kang, E. H., Lee, Y. J., Kim, T. K., Chang, C. B., Chung, J. H., Shin, K., et al. (2010). Adiponectin is a potential catabolic mediator in osteoarthritis cartilage. *Arthritis Res. Ther.* 12:R231.

Kanis, J. A., Burlet, N., Cooper, C., Delmas, P. D., Reginster, J. Y., Borgstrom, F., et al. (2008). European guidance for the diagnosis and management of osteoporosis in postmenopausal women. *Osteoporos. Int.* 19, 399–428. doi: 10.1007/s00198-008-0560-z

Karelis, A. D., Brochu, M., and Rabasa-Lhoret, R. (2004). Can we identify metabolically healthy but obese individuals (MHO)? *Diabetes Metab.* 30, 569–572. doi: 10.1016/s1262-3636(07)70156-8

Katzmarzyk, P. T., Barreira, T. V., Harrington, D. M., Staiano, A. E., Heymsfield, S. B., and Gimble, J. M. (2012). Relationship between abdominal fat and bone mineral density in white and African American adults. *Bone* 50, 576–579. doi: 10.1016/j.bone.2011.04.012

Kaye, W. H., Wierenga, C. E., Bischoff-Grethe, A., Berner, L. A., Ely, A. V., Bailer, U. F., et al. (2020). Neural insensitivity to the effects of hunger in women remitted from anorexia nervosa. *Am. J. Psychiatry.* 177, 601–610. doi: 10.1176/appi.ajp.2019.19030261

Khaliq, A., Sayed, S. A., and Mahmood, A. (2016). Evaluating the risk of osteoporosis through bone mass density. *J. Ayub Med. Coll. Abbottabad* 28, 730–733.

Kim, H. Y., Choe, J. W., Kim, H. K., Bae, S. J., Kim, B. J., Lee, S. H., et al. (2010). Negative association between metabolic syndrome and bone mineral density in Koreans, especially in men. *Calcif. Tissue Int.* 86, 350–358. doi: 10.1007/s00223-010-9347-2

Kinoshita, K., Iimuro, Y., Otogawa, K., Saika, S., Inagaki, Y., Nakajima, Y., et al. (2007). Adenovirus-mediated expression of BMP-7 suppresses the development of liver fibrosis in rats. *Gut* 56, 706–714. doi: 10.1136/gut.2006.092460

Kobayashi, H., Giles, J. T., Polak, J. F., Blumenthal, R. S., Leffell, M. S., Szklo, M., et al. (2010). Increased prevalence of carotid artery atherosclerosis in rheumatoid arthritis is artery-specific. *J. Rheumatol.* 37, 730–739. doi: 10.3899/jrheum.090670

Konradsen, S., Ag, H., Lindberg, F., Hexeberg, S., and Jorde, R. (2008). Serum 1,25-dihydroxy vitamin D is inversely associated with body mass index. *Eur. J. Nutr.* 47, 87–91. doi: 10.1007/s00394-008-0700-4

Koskinen, A., Vuolteenaho, K., Nieminen, R., Moilanen, T., and Moilanen, E. (2011). Leptin enhances MMP-1, MMP-3 and MMP-13 production in human osteoarthritic cartilage and correlates with MMP-1 and MMP-3 in synovial fluid from OA patients. *Clin. Exp. Rheumatol.* 29, 57–64.

Krishnan, S., Anderson, M. P., Fields, D. A., and Misra, M. (2018). Abdominal obesity adversely affects bone mass in children. *World J. Clin. Pediatr.* 7, 43–48. doi: 10.5409/wjcp.v7.i1.43

Lecka-Czernik, B. (2017). Diabetes, bone and glucose-lowering agents: basic biology. *Diabetologia* 60, 1163–1169. doi: 10.1007/s00125-017-4269-4

Lecka-Czernik, B., Stechschulte, L. A., Czernik, P. J., and Dowling, A. R. (2015). High bone mass in adult mice with diet-induced obesity results from a combination of initial increase in bone mass followed by attenuation in bone formation; implications for high bone mass and decreased bone quality in obesity. *Mol. Cell. Endocrinol.* 410, 35–41. doi: 10.1016/j.mce.2015.01.001

Lee, H. W., Sang, Y. K., Kim, A. Y., Lee, E. J., Choi, J. Y., and Kim, J. B. (2009). Adiponectin stimulates osteoblast differentiation through induction of COX2 in mesenchymal progenitor cells. *Stem Cells* 27, 2254–2262. doi: 10.1002/stem.144

Lee, Y. A., Ji, H. I., Lee, S. H., Hong, S. J., Yang, H. I., Yoo, M. Chul, et al. (2014). The role of adiponectin in the production of IL-6, IL-8, VEGF and MMPs in human endothelial cells and osteoblasts: implications for arthritic joints. *Exp. Mol. Med.* 46:e72. doi: 10.1038/emm.2013.141

Lee, Y. H., and Bae, S.-C. (2018). Circulating adiponectin and visfatin levels in rheumatoid arthritis and their correlation with disease activity: a meta-analysis. *Int. J. Rheum. Dis.* 21, 664–672. doi: 10.1111/1756-185x.13038

Li, C. J., Chai, Y., Wang, L., Gao, B., Chen, H., Gao, P., et al. (2017). Programmed cell senescence in skeleton during late puberty. *Nat. Commun.* 8:1312.

Li, C. J., Cheng, P., Liang, M. K., Chen, Y. S., Lu, Q., Wang, J. Y., et al. (2015). MicroRNA-188 regulates age-related switch between osteoblast and adipocyte differentiation. *Sci. Found. China* 125, 22–22.

Li, C. J., Xiao, Y., Yang, M., Su, T., Sun, X., Guo, Q., et al. (2018). Long noncoding RNA Bmncr regulates mesenchymal stem cell fate during skeletal aging. *J. Clin. Invest.* 128, 5251–5266. doi: 10.1172/jci99044

Li, J., Gao, Y., Yu, T., Lange, J. K., LeBoff, M. S., Gorska, A., et al. (2020). Obesity and leptin influence vitamin D metabolism and action in human marrow stromal cells. *J. Steroid. Biochem. Mol. Biol.* 198:105564. doi: 10.1016/j.jsbmb.2019.105564

Li, Q., Hua, Y., Yang, Y., He, X., Zhu, W., Wang, J., et al. (2018). T cell factor 7 (TCF7)/TCF1 feedback controls osteocalcin signaling in brown adipocytes independent of the wnt/beta-catenin pathway. *Mol. Cell. Biol.* 38:e00562-17.

Li, S., Jiang, H., Wang, B., Gu, M., Zhang, N., Liang, W., et al. (2018). Effect of leptin on marrow adiposity in ovariectomized rabbits assessed by proton magnetic resonance spectroscopy. *J. Comput. Assist. Tomogr.* 42, 588–593. doi: 10.1097/rct.0000000000000725

Lim, H. S., Byun, D. W., Suh, K. I., Park, H. K., Kim, H. J., Kim, T. H., et al. (2019). Is there a difference in serum vitamin D levels and bone mineral density according to body mass index in young adult women? *J. Bone Metab.* 26, 145–150. doi: 10.11005/jbm.2019.26.3.145

Liu, R., Li, X., Zhang, Z., Zhou, M., Sun, Y., Su, D., et al. (2015). Allogeneic mesenchymal stem cells inhibited T follicular helper cell generation in rheumatoid arthritis. *Sci. Rep.* 5:12777.

Liu, R., Wu, Q., Su, D., Che, N., Chen, H., Geng, L., et al. (2012). A regulatory effect of IL-21 on T follicular helper-like cell and B cell in rheumatoid arthritis. *Arthritis Res. Ther.* 14:R255.

Liu, R., Zhao, P., Zhang, Q., Che, N., Xu, L., Qian, J., et al. (2020). Adiponectin promotes fibroblast-like synoviocytes producing IL-6 to enhance T follicular helper cells response in rheumatoid arthritis. *Clin. Exp. Rheumatol.* 38, 11–18.

Liu, Y., Hazlewood, G. S., Kaplan, G. G., Eksteen, B., and Barnabe, C. (2017). Impact of obesity on remission and disease activity in rheumatoid arthritis: a systematic review and meta-analysis. *Arthritis Care Res. (Hoboken)* 69, 157–165. doi: 10.1002/acr.22932

Loeser, R. F., Goldring, S. R., Scanzello, C. R., and Goldring, M. B. (2012). Osteoarthritis: a disease of the joint as an organ. *Arthritis Rheum.* 64, 1697–1707. doi: 10.1002/art.34453

Luo, X. H., Guo, L. J., Yuan, L. Q., Xie, H., and Liao, E. Y. (2005). Adiponectin stimulates human osteoblasts proliferation and differentiation via the MAPK signaling pathway. *Chin. J. Osteoporos.* 309, 99–109. doi: 10.1016/j.yexcr.2005.05.021

Mabilleau, G., Mieczkowska, A., Irwin, N., Flatt, P. R., and Chappard, D. (2013). Optimal bone mechanical and material properties require a functional glucagon-like peptide-1 receptor. *J. Endocrinol.* 219, 59–68. doi: 10.1530/joe-13-0146

Mansur, S. A., Mieczkowska, A., Bouvard, B., Flatt, P. R., Chappard, D., Irwin, N., et al. (2015). Stable incretin mimetics counter rapid deterioration of bone quality in type 1 diabetes mellitus. *J. Cell. Physiol.* 230, 3009–3018. doi: 10.1002/jcp.25033

Mansur, S. A., Mieczkowska, A., Flatt, P. R., Bouvard, B., Chappard, D., Irwin, N., et al. (2016). A new stable GIP-oxyntomodulin hybrid peptide improved bone strength both at the organ and tissue levels in genetically-inherited type 2 diabetes mellitus. *Bone* 87, 102–113. doi: 10.1016/j.bone.2016.04.001

Marcovecchio, M. L., and Chiarelli, F. (2013). Obesity and growth during childhood and puberty. *World Rev. Nutr. Diet.* 106, 135–141. doi: 10.1159/000342545

Marques Loureiro, L., Lessa, S., Mendes, R., Pereira, S., Saboya, C. J., and Ramalho, A. (2019). Does the metabolically healthy obese phenotype protect adults with class III obesity from biochemical alterations related to bone metabolism? *Nutrients* 11:2125. doi: 10.3390/nu11092125

Méndez, J. P., Rojano-Mejía, D., Pedraza, J., Coral-Vázquez, R. M., Soriano, R., García-García, E., et al. (2013). Bone mineral density in postmenopausal Mexican-Mestizo women with normal body mass index, overweight, or obesity. *Menopause* 20, 568–572.

Minamino, H., Katsushima, M., Yoshida, T., Hashimoto, M., Fujita, Y., Shirakashi, M., et al. (2020). Increased circulating adiponectin is an independent disease activity marker in patients with rheumatoid arthritis: a cross-sectional study using the KURAMA database. *PLoS One* 15:e0229998. doi: 10.1371/journal.pone.0229998

Miossec, P. (2013). Rheumatoid arthritis: still a chronic disease. *Lancet* 381, 884–886. doi: 10.1016/s0140-6736(12)62192-8

Mitsuyo, K., Soko, S., and Solomon, D. H. (2007). Bone mineral density in adults with the metabolic syndrome: analysis in a population-based U.S. sample. *J. Clin. Endocrinol. Metab.* 92, 4161–4164. doi: 10.1210/jc.2007-0757

Miyake, H., Kanazawa, I., and Sugimoto, T. (2017). Decreased serum insulin-like growth factor-i is a risk factor for non-vertebral fractures in diabetic postmenopausal women. *Intern. Med.* 56, 269–273. doi: 10.2169/internalmedicine.56.7416

Monami, M., Cresci, B., Colombini, A., Pala, L., Balzi, D., Gori, F., et al. (2008). Bone fractures and hypoglycemic treatment in type 2 diabetic patients: a case-control study. *Diabetes Care* 31, 199–203. doi: 10.2337/dc07-1736

Mora, S., Goodman, W. G., Loro, M. L., Roe, T. F., Sayre, J., and Gilsanz, V. (1994). Age-related changes in cortical and cancellous vertebral bone density in girls: assessment with quantitative CT. *AJR Am. J. Roentgenol.* 162, 405–409. doi: 10.2214/ajr.162.2.8310936

Morgan, E. F., Barnes, G. L., and Einhorn, T. A. (2008). "Chapter 1-the bone organ system : form and function," in *Osteoporosis*, eds R. Marcus, D. Feldman, and J. Kelsey (Boston, MA: Elsevier Academic Press).

Muka, T., Trajanoska, K., Jong, K. D., Ling, O., Uitterlinden, A. G., Hofman, A., et al. (2015). The association between metabolic syndrome, bone mineral density, hip bone geometry and fracture risk: the Rotterdam study. *PLoS One* 10:e0129116. doi: 10.1371/journal.pone.0129116

Nam, J. L., Takase-Minegishi, K., Ramiro, S., Chatzidionysiou, K., Smolen, J. S., van der Heijde, D., et al. (2017). Efficacy of biological disease-modifying antirheumatic drugs: a systematic literature review informing the 2016 update of the EULAR recommendations for the management of rheumatoid arthritis. *Ann. Rheum. Dis.* 76, 1113–1136. doi: 10.1136/annrheumdis-2016-210713

Nanes, M. S. (2004). Tumor necrosis factor-alpha: molecular and cellular mechanisms in skeletal pathology. *Gene* 321, 1–15. doi: 10.1016/s0378-1119(03)00841-2

Naot, D., Watson, M., Callon, K. E., Tuari, D., Musson, D. S., Choi, A. J., et al. (2016). Reduced bone density and cortical bone indices in female adiponectin-knockout mice. *Endocrinology* 157, 3550–3561. doi: 10.1210/en.2016-1059

Nelson, L. R., and Bulun, S. E. (2001). Estrogen production and action. *J. Am. Acad. Dermatol.* 45(Suppl. 3), S116–S124.

Nöth, U., Tuli, R., Seghatoleslami, R., Howard, M., Shah, A., Hall, D. J., et al. (2003). Activation of p38 and Smads mediates BMP-2 effects on human trabecular bone-derived osteoblasts. *Exp. Cell Res.* 291, 201–211. doi: 10.1016/s0014-4827(03)00386-0

Nurieva, R. I., Chung, Y., Hwang, D., Yang, X. O., Kang, H. S., Ma, L., et al. (2008). Generation of T follicular helper cells is mediated by interleukin-21 but independent of T helper 1, 2, or 17 cell lineages. *Immunity* 29, 138–149. doi: 10.1016/j.immuni.2008.05.009

Oh, M. S., Kim, S., Jang, J. H., Park, J. Y., Kang, H. S., Lee, M. S., et al. (2016). Associations among the degree of nonalcoholic fatty liver disease, metabolic syndrome, degree of obesity in children, and parental obesity. *Pediatr. Gastroenterol. Hepatol. Nutr.* 19, 199–206. doi: 10.5223/pghn.2016.19.3.199

Oh, M. S., Kim, S., Lee, J., Lee, M. S., Kim, Y. J., and Kang, K. S. (2020). Factors associated with advanced bone age in overweight and obese children. *Pediatr. Gastroenterol. Hepatol. Nutr.* 23, 89–97. doi: 10.5223/pghn.2020.23.1.89

Oliveria, S. A., Felson, D. T., Cirillo, P. A., Reed, J. I., and Walker, A. M. (1999). Body weight, body mass index, and incident symptomatic osteoarthritis of the hand, hip, and knee. *Epidemiology* 10, 161–166. doi: 10.1097/00001648-199903000-00013

Otero, M., Lago, R., Gomez, R., Lago, F., Dieguez, C., Gomez-Reino, J. J., et al. (2006). Changes in plasma levels of fat-derived hormones adiponectin, leptin, resistin and visfatin in patients with rheumatoid arthritis. *Ann. Rheum. Dis.* 65, 1198–1201. doi: 10.1136/ard.2005.046540

Otero, M., Lago, R., Gomez, R., Lago, F., Gomez-Reino, J. J., and Gualillo, O. (2007). Phosphatidylinositol 3-kinase, MEK-1 and p38 mediate leptin/interferon-gamma synergistic NOS type II induction in chondrocytes. *Life Sci.* 81, 1452–1460. doi: 10.1016/j.lfs.2007.09.007

Paccou, J., Hardouin, P., Cotten, A., Penel, G., and Cortet, B. (2015). The role of bone marrow fat in skeletal health: usefulness and perspectives for clinicians. *J. Clin. Endocrinol. Metab.* 100, 3613–3621. doi: 10.1210/jc.2015-2338

Pagnotti, G. M., Styner, M., Uzer, G., Patel, V. S., Wright, L. E., Ness, K. K., et al. (2019). Combating osteoporosis and obesity with exercise: leveraging cell mechanosensitivity. *Nat. Rev. Endocrinol.* 15, 339–355. doi: 10.1038/s41574-019-0170-1

Pal China, S., Sanyal, S., and Chattopadhyay, N. (2018). Adiponectin signaling and its role in bone metabolism. *Cytokine* 112, 116–131. doi: 10.1016/j.cyto.2018.06.012

Park, H. S., Park, J. Y., and Yu, R. (2005). Relationship of obesity and visceral adiposity with serum concentrations of CRP, TNF-alpha and IL-6. *Diabetes Res. Clin. Pract.* 69, 29–35. doi: 10.1016/j.diabres.2004.11.007

Pasco, J. A., Henry, M. J., Kotowicz, M. A., Collier, G. R., Ball, M. J., Ugoni, A. M., et al. (2001). Serum leptin levels are associated with bone mass in nonobese women. *J. Clin. Endocrinol. Metab.* 86, 1884–1887. doi: 10.1210/jc.86.5.1884

Philbrick, K. A., Wong, C. P., Branscum, A. J., Turner, R. T., and Iwaniec, U. T. (2017). Leptin stimulates bone formation in ob/ob mice at doses having minimal impact on energy metabolism. *J. Endocrinol.* 232, 461–474. doi: 10.1530/joe-16-0484

Piccolis, M., Bond, L. M., Kampmann, M., Pulimeno, P., Chitraju, C., Jayson, C. B. K., et al. (2019). Probing the global cellular responses to lipotoxicity caused by saturated fatty acids. *Mol. Cell* 74, 32–44.e8.

Polineni, S., Resulaj, M., Faje, A. T., Meenaghan, E., Bredella, M. A., Bouxsein, M., et al. (2020). Red and white blood cell counts are associated with bone marrow adipose tissue, bone mineral density, and bone microarchitecture in premenopausal women. *J. Bone Miner. Res.* 35, 1031–1039. doi: 10.1002/jbmr.3986

Ponrartana, S., Aggabao, P. C., Hu, H. H., Aldrovandi, G. M., Wren, T. A., and Gilsanz, V. (2012). Brown adipose tissue and its relationship to bone structure in pediatric patients. *J. Clin. Endocrinol. Metab.* 97, 2693–2698. doi: 10.1210/jc.2012-1589

Prieto-Alhambra, D., Premaor, M. O., Avilés, F. Fina, Hermosilla, E., Martinez-Laguna, D., Carbonell-Abella, C., et al. (2012). The association between fracture and obesity is site-dependent: a population-based study in postmenopausal women. *J. Bone Min. Res.* 27, 294–300. doi: 10.1002/jbmr.1466

Pu, Y., Wu, H., Lu, S., Hu, H., Li, D., Wu, Y., et al. (2016). Adiponectin promotes human jaw bone marrow stem cell osteogenesis. *J. Dent. Res.* 95, 769–775. doi: 10.1177/0022034516636853

Putignano, P., Dubini, A., Toja, P., Invitti, C., Bonfanti, S., Redaelli, G., et al. (2001). Salivary cortisol measurement in normal-weight, obese and anorexic women: comparison with plasma cortisol. *Eur. J. Endocrinol.* 145, 165–171. doi: 10.1530/eje.0.1450165

Qiao, D., Li, Y., Liu, X., Zhang, X., Qian, X., Zhang, H., et al. (2020). Association of obesity with bone mineral density and osteoporosis in adults: a systematic review and meta-analysis. *Public Health* 180, 22–28. doi: 10.1016/j.puhe.2019.11.001

Rapp, K., Cameron, I. D., Kurrle, S., Klenk, J., Kleiner, A., Heinrich, S., et al. (2010). Excess mortality after pelvic fractures in institutionalized older people. *Osteoporos. Int.* 21, 1835–1839. doi: 10.1007/s00198-009-1154-0

Reid, I. R., Baldock, P. A., and Cornish, J. (2018). Effects of Leptin on the skeleton. *Endocr. Rev.* 39, 938–959. doi: 10.1210/er.2017-00226

Relling, D. P., Esberg, L. B., Fang, C. X., Johnson, W. T., Murphy, E. J., Carlson, E. C., et al. (2006). High-fat diet-induced juvenile obesity leads to cardiomyocyte dysfunction and upregulation of Foxo3a transcription factor independent of lipotoxicity and apoptosis. *J. Hypertens.* 24, 549–561. doi: 10.1097/01.hjh.0000203846.34314.94

Reyes, C., Leyland, K. M., Peat, G., Cooper, C., Arden, N. K., and Prieto-Alhambra, D. (2016). Association between overweight and obesity and risk of clinically diagnosed knee, hip, and hand osteoarthritis: a population-based Cohort study. *Arthritis Rheumatol.* 68, 1869–1875. doi: 10.1002/art.39707

Rodriguez, J., Vernus, B., Chelh, I., Cassar-Malek, I., Gabillard, J. C., Hadj Sassi, A., et al. (2014). Myostatin and the skeletal muscle atrophy and hypertrophy signaling pathways. *Cell. Mol. Life Sci.* 71, 4361–4371. doi: 10.1007/s00018-014-1689-x

Rong, B., Feng, R., Liu, C., Wu, Q., and Sun, C. (2019). Reduced delivery of epididymal adipocyte-derived exosomal resistin is essential for melatonin ameliorating hepatic steatosis in mice. *J. Pineal Res.* 66:e12561. doi: 10.1111/jpi.12561

Roy, B. (2013). Biomolecular basis of the role of diabetes mellitus in osteoporosis and bone fractures. *World J. Diabetes* 4, 101–113. doi: 10.4239/wjd.v4.i4.101

Roy, B., Curtis, M. E., Fears, L. S., Nahashon, S. N., and Fentress, H. M. (2016). Molecular mechanisms of obesity-induced osteoporosis and muscle atrophy. *Front. Physiol.* 7:439. doi: 10.3389/fphys.2016.00439

Russell, M., Mendes, N., Miller, K. K., Rosen, C. J., Lee, H., Klibanski, A., et al. (2010). Visceral fat is a negative predictor of bone density measures in obese adolescent girls. *J. Clin. Endocrinol. Metab.* 95, 1247–1255. doi: 10.1210/jc.2009-1475

Saad, F. A. (2020). Novel insights into the complex architecture of osteoporosis molecular genetics. *Ann. N. Y. Acad. Sci.* 1462, 37–52. doi: 10.1111/nyas.14231

Sanchez-Riera, L., Carnahan, E., Vos, T., Veerman, L., Norman, R., Lim, S. S., et al. (2014). The global burden attributable to low bone mineral density. *Ann. Rheum. Dis.* 73, 1635–1645.

Santos, V. R. D., Christofaro, D. G. D., Gomes, I. C., Junior, I. F. F., and Gobbo, L. A. (2018). Relationship between obesity, sarcopenia, sarcopenic obesity, and bone mineral density in elderly subjects aged 80 years and over. *Rev. Bras. Ortop.* 53, 300–305. doi: 10.1016/j.rboe.2017.09.002

Scheller, E. L., Khoury, B., Moller, K. L., Wee, N. K. Y., Khandaker, S., Kozloff, K. M., et al. (2016). Changes in skeletal integrity and marrow adiposity during high-fat diet and after weight loss. *Front. Endocrinol.* 7:102. doi: 10.3389/fendo.2016.00102

Scotece, M., Conde, J., Gomez, R., Lopez, V., Lago, F., Gomez-Reino, J. J., et al. (2011). Beyond fat mass: exploring the role of adipokines in rheumatic diseases. *ScientificWorldJournal* 11, 1932–1947. doi: 10.1100/2011/290142

Scott, D., Chandrasekara, S. D., Laslett, L. L., Cicuttini, F., Ebeling, P. R., and Jones, G. (2016). Associations of sarcopenic obesity and dynapenic obesity with bone mineral density and incident fractures over 5-10 years in community-dwelling older adults. *Calcif. Tissue Int.* 99, 30–42. doi: 10.1007/s00223-016-0123-9

Shanbhogue, V. V., Mitchell, D. M., Rosen, C. J., and Bouxsein, M. L. (2016). Type 2 diabetes and the skeleton: new insights into sweet bones. *Lancet Diabetes Endocrinol.* 4, 159–173. doi: 10.1016/s2213-8587(15)00283-1

Shen, W., Chen, J., Punyanitya, M., Shapses, S., Heshka, S., and Heymsfield, S. B. (2007). MRI-measured bone marrow adipose tissue is inversely related to DXA-measured bone mineral in Caucasian women. *Osteoporos. Int.* 18, 641–647. doi: 10.1007/s00198-006-0285-9

Shinoda, Y., Yamaguchi, M., Ogata, N., Akune, T., Kubota, N., Yamauchi, T., et al. (2006). Regulation of bone formation by adiponectin through autocrine/paracrine and endocrine pathways. *J. Cell. Biochem.* 99, 196–208. doi: 10.1002/jcb.20890

Shu, L., Beier, E., Sheu, T., Zhang, H., Zuscik, M. J., Puzas, E. J., et al. (2015). High-fat diet causes bone loss in young mice by promoting osteoclastogenesis through alteration of the bone marrow environment. *Calcif. Tissue Int.* 96, 313–323. doi: 10.1007/s00223-015-9954-z

Silva, M. J., Eekhoff, J. D., Patel, T., Kenney-Hunt, J. P., Brodt, M. D., Steger-May, K., et al. (2019). Effects of high-fat diet and body mass on bone morphology and mechanical properties in 1100 advanced intercross mice. *J. Bone Miner. Res.* 34, 711–725. doi: 10.1002/jbmr.3648

Singh, L., Tyagi, S., Myers, D., and Duque, G. (2018). Good, bad, or ugly: the biological roles of bone marrow fat. *Curr. Osteoporos. Rep.* 16, 130–137. doi: 10.1007/s11914-018-0427-y

Singhal, V., Tulsiani, S., Campoverde, K. J., Mitchell, D. M., Slattery, M., Schorr, M., et al. (2018). Impaired bone strength estimates at the distal tibia and its determinants in adolescents with anorexia nervosa. *Bone* 106, 61–68. doi: 10.1016/j.bone.2017.07.009

Snijder, M. B., Dam, R. M. V., Visser, M., Deeg, D. J. H., and Lips, P. (2005). Adiposity in relation to vitamin D status and parathyroid hormone levels: a population-based study in older men and women. *J. Clin. Endocrinol. Metab.* 90, 4119–4123. doi: 10.1210/jc.2005-0216

Sowa, H., Kaji, H., Yamaguchi, T., Sugimoto, T., and Chihara, K. (2002). Smad3 promotes alkaline phosphatase activity and mineralization of osteoblastic MC3T3-E1 cells. *J. Bone Miner. Res.* 17, 1190–1199. doi: 10.1359/jbmr.2002.17.7.1190

Srikanthan, P., Crandall, C. J., Miller-Martinez, D., Seeman, T. E., Greendale, G. A., Binkley, N., et al. (2014). Insulin resistance and bone strength: findings from the study of midlife in the United States. *J. Bone Miner. Res.* 29, 796–803. doi: 10.1002/jbmr.2083

Stenholm, S., Harris, T. B., Rantanen, T., Visser, M., Kritchevsky, S. B., and Ferrucci, L. (2008). Sarcopenic obesity: definition, cause and consequences. *Curr. Opin. Clin. Nutr. Metab. Care* 11, 693–700. doi: 10.1097/mco.0b013e328312c37d

Steppan, C. M., Crawford, D. T., Chidsey-Frink, K. L., Ke, H. Z., and Swick, A. G. (2000). Leptin is a potent stimulator of bone growth in ob/ob mice. *Regul. Pept.* 92, 73–78. doi: 10.1016/s0167-0115(00)00152-x

Su, T., Xiao, Y., Xiao, Y., Guo, Q., Li, C., Huang, Y., et al. (2019). Bone marrow mesenchymal stem cells-derived exosomal mir-29b-3p regulates aging-associated insulin resistance. *ACS Nano* 13, 2450–2462.

Sugimoto, H., Yang, C., Lebleu, V. S., Soubasakos, M. A., and Kalluri, R. (2007). BMP-7 functions as a novel hormone to facilitate liver regeneration. *FASEB J.* 21, 256–264. doi: 10.1096/fj.06-6837com

Sun, X., Guo, Q., Wei, W., Robertson, S., Yuan, Y., and Luo, X. (2019). Current progress on microRNA-based gene delivery in the treatment of osteoporosis and osteoporotic fracture. *Int. J. Endocrinol.* 2019:6782653.

Takeshita, S., Fumoto, T., Naoe, Y., and Ikeda, K. (2014). Age-related marrow adipogenesis is linked to increased expression of RANKL. *J. Biol. Chem.* 289, 16699–16710. doi: 10.1074/jbc.m114.547919

Tang, X., Liu, G., Kang, J., Hou, Y., Jiang, F., Yuan, W., et al. (2013). Obesity and risk of hip fracture in adults: a meta-analysis of prospective cohort studies. *PLoS One* 8:e55077. doi: 10.1371/journal.pone.0055077

Tarantino, U., Piccirilli, E., Fantini, M., Baldi, J., Gasbarra, E., and Bei, R. (2015). Sarcopenia and fragility fractures: molecular and clinical evidence of the bone-muscle interaction. *J. Bone Joint Surg. Am.* 97, 429–437. doi: 10.2106/jbjs.n.00648

Tencerova, M., Okla, M., and Kassem, M. (2019). Insulin signaling in bone marrow adipocytes. *Curr. Osteoporos. Rep.* 17, 446–454. doi: 10.1007/s11914-019-00552-8

Thomas, T. (1999). Leptin acts on human marrow stromal cells to enhance differentiation to osteoblasts and to inhibit differentiation to adipocytes. *Endocrinology* 140, 1630–1638. doi: 10.1210/endo.140.4.6637

Thrailkill, K. M. (2000). Insulin-like growth factor-I in diabetes mellitus: its physiology, metabolic effects, and potential clinical utility. *Diabetes Technol. Ther.* 2, 69–80. doi: 10.1089/152091599316775

Tian, L., Wang, C., Xie, Y., Wan, S., Zhang, K., and Yu, X. (2017). High fructose and high fat exert different effects on changes in trabecular bone micro-structure. *J. Nutr. Health Aging* 22, 361–370. doi: 10.1007/s12603-017-0933-0

Tortoriello, D. V., McMinn, J., and Chua, S. C. (2004). Dietary-induced obesity and hypothalamic infertility in female DBA/2J mice. *Endocrinology* 145, 1238–1247. doi: 10.1210/en.2003-1406

Tsatsoulis, A., Mantzaris, M. D., Bellou, S., and Andrikoula, M. (2013). Insulin resistance: an adaptive mechanism becomes maladaptive in the current environment - an evolutionary perspective. *Metabolism* 62, 622–633. doi: 10.1016/j.metabol.2012.11.004

Tseng, Y. H., Kokkotou, E., Schulz, T. J., Huang, T. L., Winnay, J. N., Taniguchi, C. M., et al. (2008). New role of bone morphogenetic protein 7 in brown adipogenesis and energy expenditure. *Nature* 454, 1000–1004. doi: 10.1038/nature07221

Tu, M., Yang, M., Yu, N., Zhen, G., Wan, M., Liu, W., et al. (2019). Inhibition of cyclooxygenase-2 activity in subchondral bone modifies a subtype of osteoarthritis. *Bone Res.* 7:29.

Tu, Q., Zhang, J., Dong, L. Q., Saunders, E., Luo, E., Tang, J., et al. (2011). Adiponectin inhibits osteoclastogenesis and bone resorption via APPL1-mediated suppression of Akt1. *J. Biol. Chem.* 286, 12542–12553. doi: 10.1074/jbc.m110.152405

Vestergaard, P., Rejnmark, L., and Mosekilde, L. (2005). Relative fracture risk in patients with diabetes mellitus, and the impact of insulin and oral antidiabetic medication on relative fracture risk. *Diabetologia* 48, 1292–1299. doi: 10.1007/s00125-005-1786-3

Vicente, G., James, C., Mo, A. O., Lee, D. C., Dorey, F. J., and Mittelman, S. D. (2009). Reciprocal relations of subcutaneous and visceral fat to bone structure and strength. *J. Clin. Endocrinol. Metab.* 94, 3387–3393. doi: 10.1210/jc.2008-2422

Wang, T., and He, C. (2018). Pro-inflammatory cytokines: the link between obesity and osteoarthritis. *Cytokine Growth Factor Rev.* 44, 38–50. doi: 10.1016/j.cytogfr.2018.10.002

Wehrli, F. W., Hopkins, J. A., Hwang, S. N., Song, H. K., and Haddad, J. G. (2000). Cross-sectional study of osteopenia with quantitative MR imaging and bone densitometry. *Radiology* 217, 527–538. doi: 10.1148/radiology.217.2.r00nv20527

Wei, W., Dutchak, P. A., Wang, X., Ding, X., Wang, X., Bookout, A. L., et al. (2012). Fibroblast growth factor 21 promotes bone loss by potentiating the effects of peroxisome proliferator-activated receptor gamma. *Proc. Natl. Acad. Sci. U.S.A.* 109, 3143–3148. doi: 10.1073/pnas.1200797109

Wiedmann, N. M., Stefanidis, A., and Oldfield, B. J. (2017). Characterization of the central neural projections to brown, white, and beige adipose tissue. *FASEB J.* 31, 4879–4890. doi: 10.1096/fj.201700433r

Williams, G. A., Wang, Y., Callon, K. E., Watson, M., Lin, J. M., Lam, J. B., et al. (2009). In vitro and in vivo effects of adiponectin on bone. *Endocrinology* 150, 3603–3610.

Xie, H., Cui, Z., Wang, L., Xia, Z., Hu, Y., Xian, L., et al. (2014). PDGF-BB secreted by preosteoclasts induces CD31hiEmcnhi vessel subtype in coupling osteogenesis. *Nat. Med.* 20, 1270–1278. doi: 10.1038/nm.3668

Yang, M., Guo, Q., Peng, H., Xiao, Y. Z., Xiao, Y., Huang, Y., et al. (2019). Kruppel-like factor 3 inhibition by mutated lncRNA Reg1cp results in human high bone mass syndrome. *J. Exp. Med.* 216, 1944–1964. doi: 10.1084/jem.20181554

Zhang, F., Hao, G., Shao, M., Nham, K., An, Y., Wang, Q., et al. (2018). An adipose tissue atlas: an image-guided identification of human-like bat and beige depots in rodents. *Cell Metab.* 27, 252–262.e3.

Zhang, M., Xuan, S., Bouxsein, M. L., von Stechow, D., Akeno, N., Faugere, M. C., et al. (2002). Osteoblast-specific knockout of the insulin-like growth factor (IGF) receptor gene reveals an essential role of IGF signaling in bone matrix mineralization. *J. Biol. Chem.* 277, 44005–44012. doi: 10.1074/jbc.m208265200

Zhang, Y., Liu, J., Yao, J., Ji, G., Qian, L., Wang, J., et al. (2014). Obesity: pathophysiology and intervention. *Nutrients* 6, 5153–5183.

Zhao, Y., Qin, R., Ma, X., Qin, Z., Yang, Z., Hong, H., et al. (2020). Adiposity is not beneficial to bone mineral density in 0-5 year old Chinese children: the Jiangsu bone health study. *Obes. Res. Clin. Pract.* 14, 39–46. doi: 10.1016/j.orcp.2019.10.011

Zhu, Z. N., Jiang, Y. F., and Ding, T. (2014). Risk of fracture with thiazolidinediones: an updated meta-analysis of randomized clinical trials. *Bone* 68, 115–123. doi: 10.1016/j.bone.2014.08.010

11

# Conditional Knockout of PKC-δ in Osteoclasts Favors Bone Mass Accrual in Males Due to Decreased Osteoclast Function

*Shangfu Li[1,2,3*†], Tianwei He[1,2,3†], Depeng Wu[1,2,3†], Liangming Zhang[1,2,3], Ruiqiang Chen[1,2,3], Bin Liu[1,2,3], Jinbo Yuan[4], Jennifer Tickner[4], An Qin[5], Jiake Xu[4] and Limin Rong[1,2,3*]*

*[1] Department of Spine Surgery, The Third Affiliated Hospital of Sun Yat-sen University, Guangzhou, China, [2] Guangdong Provincial Center for Quality Control of Minimally Invasive Spine Surgery, Guangzhou, China, [3] Guangdong Provincial Center for Engineering and Technology Research of Minimally Invasive Spine Surgery, Guangzhou, China, [4] School of Biomedical Sciences, The University of Western Australia, Perth, WA, Australia, [5] Shanghai Key Laboratory of Orthopedic Implants, Department of Orthopedic Surgery, Shanghai Ninth People's Hospital, Shanghai Jiao Tong University School of Medicine, Shanghai, China*

***Correspondence:**
*Limin Rong*
*ronglm@mail.sysu.edu.cn*
*Shangfu Li*
*lishangfu@mail.sysu.edu.cn*

*†These authors have contributed equally to this work*

Protein kinase C delta (PKC-δ) functions as an important regulator in bone metabolism. However, the precise involvement of PKC-δ in the regulation of osteoclasts remains elusive. We generated an osteoclast specific PKC-δ knockout mouse strain to investigate the function of PKC-δ in osteoclast biology. Bone phenotype was investigated using microcomputed tomography. Osteoclast and osteoblast parameters were assessed using bone histomorphometry, and analysis of osteoclast formation and function with osteoclastogensis and hydroxyapatite resorption assays. The molecular mechanisms by which PKC-δ regulated osteoclast function were dissected by Western Blotting, TUNEL assay, transfection and transcriptome sequencing. We found that ablation of PKC-δ in osteoclasts resulted in an increase in trabecular and cortical bone volume in male mice, however, the bone mass phenotype was not observed in female mice. This was accompanied by decreased osteoclast number and surface, and Cathepsin-K protein levels *in vivo*, as well as decreased osteoclast formation and resorption *in vitro* in a male-specific manner. PKC-δ regulated androgen receptor transcription by binding to its promoter, moreover, PKC-δ conditional knockout did not increase osteoclast apoptosis but increased MAPK signaling and enhanced androgen receptor transcription and expression, finally leding to significant alterations in gene expression and signaling changes related to extracellular matrix proteins specifically in male mice. In conclusion, PKC-δ plays an important role in osteoclast formation and function in a male-specific manner. Our work reveals a previously unknown target for treatment of gender-related bone diseases.

**Keywords: protein kinase C delta, osteoclast, sex difference, androgen receptor, apoptosis, transcriptome sequencing**

## INTRODUCTION

Protein kinase C delta is a member of the highly homologous serine and threonine PKC family, it was the first novel PKC isoform to be identified by screening of mammalian cDNA libraries (Ono et al., 1988). PKC-δ is expressed ubiquitously among cells and tissues, and it is activated in a diacylglycerol and phosphatidylserine dependent but $Ca^{2+}$ independent manner (Steinberg, 2008).

Various lines of evidence have shown that PKC-δ, activated in distinct ways, plays a critical role in regulating multiple cellular functions including growth, differentiation, apoptosis, and survival (Roffey et al., 2009).

Bone is maintained by a coupled process called bone remodeling which is characterized by the coordinated activity of bone-forming OBs and bone-resorbing OCs (Iaquinta et al., 2019), and involves a complex series of sequential steps that are highly regulated (Zaidi, 2007). In recent years, extended studies have been carried out to investigate the interrelationship between PKC-δ and skeletal diseases. It is reported that parathyroid hormone activates PKC-δ and regulates osteoblastic differentiation via a PLC-independent pathway (Yang et al., 2006). By using PKC-δ null mice, Cremasco et al. (2012) reported that PKC-δ deficiency perturbs bone homeostasis by selective uncoupling of CTSK secretion and ruffled border formation in OCs via PKC-δ-myristoylated alanine-rich C-kinase substrate (the actin bundling protein) pathway. In addition, further study revealed that global loss of PKC-δ protects against LPS-induced osteolysis owing to an intrinsic defect in osteoclastic bone resorption (Khor et al., 2013). However, the precise involvement of PKC-δ in the regulation of OC biology and bone homeostasis remains elusive.

Here, we generated a mouse strain in which PKC-δ is completely inactivated only in resorbing OCs by breeding mice carrying CTSK promoter-regulated Cre-recombinase with mice possessing loxP recombination sites flanking exon 7 of the PKC-δ gene. Our study aimed to comprehensively characterize the bone phenotype of mice with selective ablation of PKC-δ in OCs; we aimed to dissect the molecular mechanisms by which PKC-δ regulates OC differentiation and function. This study will potentially identify novel molecular targets for OC-associated bone diseases.

## MATERIALS AND METHODS

### Animal Procedures and Animal Care

All transgenic mice were generated on a C57BL/6J and C57BL/6N genetic background. Mice were group-housed under standard conditions: 12-h light/dark cycle, standard diet containing 1% calcium and 0.76% phosphate, and water *ad libitum* in standard cages. All mice were produced and maintained at the National Resource Center for Mutant Mice Model Animal Research Center of Nanjing University in China according to institutional guidelines. Seven mice per group for both sexes were used for the analysis of bone phenotype using Micro-CT and subsequent histology.

### Generation of Osteoclast-Specific PKC-δ Conditional Knockout Mice

LoxP mice were obtained from RIKEN BioResource Research Center (Stock Number: RBRC06462, Strain Name: C57BL/6-Prkcd<tm1shb>, 3-1-1 Koyadai, Tsukuba, Ibaraki, Japan). CTSK-Cre mice were kindly provided by Professor Jiake Xu from School of Biomedical Sciences, The University of Western Australia. Mice with an OC-cKO of the PKC-δ (PKC-δ cKO) were generated by crossing mice heterozygous for a floxed exon 7 PKC-δ allele (PKC-δ $(ex7)^{flox/wt}$) with CTSK-Cre mice heterozygously carrying a cyclization recombinase of which the expression is controlled by the CTSK promoter (CTSK-$Cre^{+}$PKC-$\delta^{flox/wt}$). Offspring were genotyped and the presence of the CTSK-Cre transgene was determined on genomic DNA (gDNA) via PCR with primer sequences presented in **Supplementary Table S1**. In all the experiments described below, we analyzed CTSK-$Cre^{+}$PKC-$\delta^{flox/flox}$ mice that lack PKC-δ in OCs, and CTSK-$Cre^{-}$PKC-$\delta^{flox/flox}$ littermates as controls.

### Micro-CT Scanning

Micro structure of bone in mice was measured by high-resolution Micro-CT using a Scanco μCT100 scanner (Brüttisellen, Zurich, Switzerland). Micro-CT analysis was performed on fixed right tibia isolated from euthanized mice scanned with a fixed isotropic voxel size of 10 μm, 100 slices, 70 kV at 200 μA and 300 ms integration time. Standard parameters were then evaluated in the trabecular region of the proximal tibia, commencing at a distance of 0.5 mm from the growth plate and extending a further 1.5 mm distally. Measured parameters included BV/TV (%), trabecular number (Tb.N, $mm^{-1}$), trabecular thickness (Tb.Th, mm) and trabecular separation (Tb.Sp, mm). Cortical bone was analyzed starting at a distance of 2.75 mm from the growth plate and extending 0.5 mm distally to determine total cortical area (Tt.Ar, $mm^2$), cortical bone area (Ct.Ar, $mm^2$), cortical area fraction (Ct.Ar/Tt.Ar, %) and cortical thickness (Ct.Th, μm).

### Bone Histomorphometry and Immunohistochemistry

Left tibia were fixed overnight in 10% buffered formalin, decalcified with 14% EDTA for 7 days, embedded in paraffin and sectioned (3 μm) for staining. Trabecular bone and *in vivo* OB parameters were analyzed using hematoxylin and eosin (HE) stained sections, while *in vivo* OC parameters were determined from TRAP stained sections as previously described (Yao et al., 2014). Histomorphometric analysis was performed by quantifying parameters including osteoclast surface per bone surface (Oc.S/BS), number of osteoclasts per bone perimeter (N.Oc/B.Pm), osteoblast surface per bone surface (Ob.S/BS)

**Abbreviations:** Acta2, actin alpha 2; AR, androgen receptor; α-MEM, alpha modified Minimal Essential Medium; Bgn, biglycan; BMM, bone marrow macrophage; BV/TV, bone volume/total volume; cKO, conditional knockout; Col1a1, collagen type I alpha 1 chain; Col1a2, collagen type I alpha 2 chain; Col5a2, collagen type V alpha 2 chain; Col6a3, collagen type VI alpha 3 chain; Ct.Ar, cortical bone area; Ct.Ar/Tt.Ar, cortical area fraction; CTSK, cathepsin K; Ct.Th, cortical thickness; DMEM, Dulbecco's modified Eagle's medium; DEG, differentially expressed gene; ECM, extracellular matrix; ER, estrogen receptor; ERK, extracellular signal-regulated kinase; Fn1, fibronectin 1; GAPDH, glyceraldehyde-3-phosphate dehydrogenase; GO, Gene Ontology; IHC, Immunohistochemistry; JNK, c-Jun amino-terminal kinase; LNCaP, lymph node carcinoma of the prostate; MAPK, mitogen-activated protein kinase; MAR, mineral apposition rate; M-CSF, macrophage colony stimulating factor; Micro-CT, microcomputed tomography; Mmp12, matrix metallopeptidase 12; N.Ob/B.Pm, number of osteoblast per bone perimeter; N.Oc/B.Pm, number of osteoclasts per bone perimeter; OB, osteoblast; Ob.S/BS, osteoblast surface per bone surface; OC, osteoclast; Oc.S/BS, osteoclast surface per bone surface; PKC-δ, protein kinase C delta; RANKL, receptor activator of NF-κB ligand; Serpine 1, serpin family E member 1; Serpinh 1, serpin family H member 1; Sparc, secreted protein acidic and cysteine rich; Tb.N, trabecular number; Tb.Sp, trabecular separation; Tb.Th, trabecular thickness; Thbs1, thrombospondin 1; Tnc, tenascin C; TRAP, tartrate-resistant acid phosphatase; Tt.Ar, total cortical area.

and number of osteoblast per bone perimeter (N.Ob/B.Pm) using an Olympus microscope and the BIOQUANT OSTEO software (BIOQUANT OSTEO 2013 Ver.13.20.6, Nashville, United States). We counted the numbers of positively stained cells in five sequential sections per mouse in each group. Safranin O Fast Green Staining, Massons trichrome staining and Von Kossa staining (in un-decalcified sections) were used to assess chondrocytes, organic and inorganic matrix components in the tibia, respectively. Cartilage thickness was measured in the middle of tibia as previously described (Tong et al., 2019) by using ImageJ software (NIH, Bethesda, MD, United States).

For the un-decalcified bone samples, femoral were dissected, fixed in 70% ethanol, dehydrated and embedded in methyl methacrylate, sagittal sections at 5 μm thickness were undergone von Kossa staining. Trabecular bone volume fraction was analyzed using ImageJ software. For dynamic histomorphometry and bone fluorescent-labeling studies, mice were injected intraperitoneally with calcein (Sigma, 20 mg/kg body weight) and alizarin red complexon (Sigma, 50 mg/kg body weight) at 9 and 2 days, respectively, before sacrifice. The MAR (μm/day) was measured in unstained sections under a fluorescence microscope (Olympus BX-63, Japan) and used to calculate the bone formation rate relative to the bone surface (BFR/BS, $\mu m^3/\mu m^2$/year) in the trabecular bone.

For CTSK IHC staining, antigen retrieval was carried out by incubating specimens with bone tissue specific antigen-retrieval solutions (SBT100013, Showbio, Shanghai, China) for 60 min at 37°C. Non-specific binding was blocked with goat serum before incubation with primary antibody against mouse CTSK (ab19027, Abcam, Cambridge, United Kingdom) at 4°C overnight. For detection, sections were treated with HRP-conjugated secondary antibody (GK500505A, Dako, Carpinteria, CA, United States) for 30 min at 37°C, followed by DAB substrate (ZLI-9017, ZSGB-Bio, Beijing, China) for 30 s, counter-stained with Maye's hematoxylin, dehydrated, and mounted. Semi-quantitative evaluation was performed as previously described (Da et al., 2009) in five random trabecular regions of each section. Two experienced pathologists scored each section which was blinded to them and the final scores were evaluated by consensus.

## Macrophage Isolation From Mouse Bone Marrow, Culture, Osteoclast Differentiation, and TRAP Staining

Bone marrow macrophage from tibia and femur of WT and cKO mice were prepared as previously described (He et al., 2019). BMMs were then seeded on to 96-well plate ($6 \times 10^3$ cells/well) and cultured in α-MEM supplemented with 30 ng/mL M-CSF (416-ML, R&D system, Minneapolis, MN, United States), and 100 ng/mL RANKL (462-TEC, R&D system). The media was replaced every 2 days and after 7 days of culture the cells were fixed and stained with Acid Phosphatase Staining kit (387A, Sigma-Aldrich, St. Louis, MO, United States) according to the protocol of the manufacturer. TRAP positive multinucleated cells with more than three nuclei were counted as OCs.

## Western Blotting Assay

For short time course signaling pathways, BMMs at $3 \times 10^5$ cells/well were seeded into 6-well plates and incubated in complete medium with 30 ng/ml MCSF and 100 ng/ml RANKL for 4 days to allow PKC-δ deletion in OCs. In the next day, cells were starved for 4 h and then 100 ng/ml RANKL were added. Cells were harvested at the time points of 0, 5, 10, 20, 30 and 60 min. For long time periods, BMMs were stimulated with RANKL and MCSF for 0, 1, 3, 5, 7 days. Cells were lysed in RIPA buffer at indicated times for 30 min on ice for protein extraction. An equal amount of proteins (30 μg/lane) were resolved by SDS-polyacrylamide gel electrophoresis and then transferred to a polyvinylidene difluoride membrane (Millipore). The membrane was probed with the indicated primary antibody (in details in **Supplementary Table S2**), detected using horseradish peroxidase-conjugated secondary antibodies and visualized with ECL reagents (Amersham). α-tubulin was detected on the same membrane and used as a loading control.

## Real-Time RT-PCR Assay

Total RNA from BMMs was extracted with RNAiso Plus (D9108A, Takara, Japan) and reverse transcription was carried out using 1 μg of total RNA with the PrimeScript RT reagent Kit and gDNA Eraser (DRR047A, Takara) in a volume of 20 μl. One microliter of cDNA was amplified with the specific primers (Invitrogen, sequences in **Supplementary Table S1**) and were quantified on a Light Cycler 480II (Roche) using SYBR green dye (DRR820A, Takara), normalizing with GAPDH. The Ct value of the reference gene GAPDH was subtracted from the Ct value of the target genes (ΔCt), and the average ΔCt value of the triplicates was taken. Relative expression levels of each gene were obtained by using the $2^{-\Delta\Delta Ct}$ method. All the experiments were repeated three times.

## TUNEL Assay

Apoptosis in OCs was identified by using the *In Situ* Cell Death Detection Kit, Fluorescein (11684795910, Roche Diagnostics GmbH, Germany) according to the manufacturer's instructions. Briefly, after 5 and 7 days of RANKL induction in 35 mm and high glass bottom μ-Dish (81158, Ibidi, Germany), samples were fixed in 4% paraformaldehyde for 1 h at 20°C and permeabilized with 0.1% Triton X-100 solution for 2 min on ice. Then the TUNEL reaction mixtures were added to the samples and incubated for 60 min at 37°C in the dark. Finally the samples were visualized under confocal microscope by using an excitation wavelength of 488 nm and detection in the range of 515–565 nm (green). The actin was detected by phalloidin staining (red).

## Hydroxyapatite Resorption Assay

BMMs ($6 \times 10^3$ cells/well) were directly seeded into a 96 well Corning Osteo Assay Surface plate (3989, Corning Life Sciences, Tewksbury, MA, United States) to begin the differentiation process. Plates were incubated with a differentiation medium (30 ng/ml M-CSF combined 100 ng/ml RANKL), which was changed every 2 days. After 5 and 7 days, the plates were stripped with 1.2% sodium hypochlorite solution for 5 min to remove cells and air-dried prior to imaging. Overlapping images of the entire well were taken at 20× magnification and these were then used to produce a composite image using Image Composite Editor (ICE 2.0, Microsoft, United States). The total resorption area was measured in the composite image using Image-Pro Plus (version 6.0, Media Cybernetics Company, Rockville, MD, United States).

## Transfection, Transcriptional and Luciferase Assay

Prostate adenocarcinoma cell line (LNCaP, CRL1740) and 293T cell line (CRL3216) were purchased from ATCC. LNCaP cells were maintained in phenol red-free RPMI 1640 supplemented with 10% FBS. 293-T cells were maintained in DMEM supplemented with 10% FBS. Plasmids were obtained from Genomeditech Co., Ltd (Shanghai, China). Cells were transfected with AR firefly luciferase reporter (pGMAR-Lu) plasmid and control renilla luciferase reporter (pGMR-TK) plasmid using Lipofectamine$^{TM}$ 2000 Transfection Reagent (#11668019, Life Technologies) according to the manufacturer's instruction. Cells were transferred to a 96-well plate 24 h after transfection and were further transfected with PKC-δ plasmid for another 48 h. Finally, luciferase activity was assessed using the Dural-Luciferase® Reporter Assay System (#E1910, Promega, United States) according to the manufacturer's instructions.

## Transcriptome Sequencing and Bioinformatics Analysis

Total RNA was extracted using RNeasy Mini kit (QIAGEN, Germany) following the manufacturer's instructions. The quality and integrity of RNA was assessed using the RNA Nano 6000 Assay Kit of the Bioanalyzer 2100 system (Agilent Technologies, CA, United States). A total amount of 3 μg RNA per sample was used for mRNA-Seq library construction using NEBNext Ultra$^{TM}$ RNA Library Prep Kit for Illumina (NEB, United States) according to manufacturer's recommendations. Heatmap was generated by pheatmap package in R. DEGs analysis was performed using the edgeR R package (3.18.1). The *p*-value was adjusted using the Benjamini and Hochberg method, corrected *p*-value of 0.05 and absolute fold change of 2 was set as the threshold for significantly differential expression. GO enrichment analysis of DEGs was implemented by the clusterProfiler R package, in which gene length bias were corrected, GO terms with corrected *p*-value less than 0.05 were considered significantly enriched by DEGs. KEGG database[1] was used for KEGG pathway enrichment analysis of DEGs, and clusterProfiler R package was used to test the statistical enrichment of DEGs in KEGG pathways. The RNA-seq data were analyzed by wcgene biotech (shanghai, china).

## Statistical Analysis

All data was pooled from at least three independent experiments. Descriptive statistics included means and standard deviations for continuous variables and percentages for categorical ones. Normality of distribution was assessed by Kolmogorov–Smirnov test. Differences were examined by two tailed Student's *t*-test for comparing two groups and by one- or two-way analysis of variance (ANOVA) test for comparing multiple groups. When significant differences were indicated by ANOVA, Turkey's *post hoc* test was used to compare the differences between groups. All data analysis was performed with SPSS 20.0 Package (SPSS software 20.0; SPSS, Chicago, IL, United States). All statistical tests were two-sided and values of *p* smaller than 0.05 were considered significant.

# RESULTS

## Mice With PKC-δ cKO in Osteoclasts Exhibit Increased Bone Mass With Changes in Micro-Structure in a Sex Dependent Manner

Firstly, we confirmed the CTSK-driven PKC-δ deletion in OCs in mice. To analyze a direct effect of PKC-δ deficiency on OCs and bone homeostasis, we used the conditional PKC-δ allele in which exons 7 are flanked by loxP sites. Cre-mediated deletion of exons 7 results in a frame shift and a PKC-δ null allele (**Supplementary Figure S1A**). For specific deletion in OCs, we crossed the conditional PKC-δ allele to CTSK-Cre mice, efficiency of Cre-mediated deletion of PKC-δ exons 7 and consequent loss of PKC-δ expression in OCs was confirmed by gDNA PCR for the deleted and floxed alleles (**Supplementary Figure S1B**), together with the significant decrease of PKC-δ mRNA expression (**Supplementary Figure S1C**, BMMs stimulated with RANKL for 5 days) and protein expression (**Supplementary Figure S1D**, co-culture with RANKL for 7 days).

To determine the biological consequences of PKC-δ cKO in OCs in skeletal development, we analyzed the bone phenotype of PKC-δ cKO mice *in vivo*. Interestingly, 3-month-old male cKO mice were smaller than WT littermates, in addition, their body weight was lighter (30.5.4 ± 2.2 g vs. 26.8 ± 2.4 g) and statistical difference was found ($p < 0.05$). In contrast, there were no significant changes in female mice regarding their size and body weight (23.5 ± 2.1 g vs. 23.1 ± 2.5 g) (**Figure 1A**). We further examined the bone micro-structure using Micro-CT and found that male PKC-δ cKO mice exhibited increased trabecular and cortical bone compared to their WT littermates (**Figures 1B,C**). In the trabecular bone, with statistically significant changes ($p < 0.05$), the percentage of trabecular bone volume versus total volume was about 45% increased in male cKO mice compared to WT (BV/TV, 9.48% vs. 13.87%, **Figure 1Bii**). Moreover, there were trend of increase in trabecular number (Tb.N, 4.12/mm vs. 4.41/mm, **Figure 1Biii**) and thickness (Tb.Th, 0.047 mm vs. 0.054 mm, **Figure 1Biv**) and approximately 10% reduction in trabecular separation (Tb.Sp, 0.25 mm vs. 0.22 mm, **Figure 1Bv**). However, there were no significant changes in trabecular bone in female cKO mice when compared with the WT controls (**Figure 1B**). In the cortical bone, statistical differences of increased changes were found in male mice regarding cortical area fraction (Ct.Ar/Tt.Ar, 88.7% vs. 90.0%, **Figure 1Civ**) and cortical thickness (Ct.Th, 0.156 mm vs. 0.174 mm, **Figure 1Cv**).

[1]http://www.genome.jp/kegg/

While trend of increase were found in total cortical area (Tt.Ar, 0.95 $mm^2$ vs. 1.02 $mm^2$, **Figure 1Cii**) and cortical bone area (Ct.Ar, 0.85 $mm^2$ vs. 0.89 $mm^2$, **Figure 1Ciii**). As expected, the cortical changes were mild and negligible in cortical bone in female mice (**Figure 1C**). Taken together, these results revealed an increase in trabecular and cortical bone volume due to ablation of PKC-δ specifically in OCs in a sex dependent maner in male mice.

## Increased Bone Fraction and Decreased Osteoclast in Trabecular Bone of PKC-δ Conditional Knockout Mice

Based on the moderate osteopetrotic phenotype observed by Micro-CT, we further explored the specific *in vivo* cellular changes at the trabecular bone surface of PKC-δ cKO mice. Because bone remodeling is highly coordinated by OC bone resorption and OB bone formation, we determined the effects of PKC-δ deletion in OCs on bone structure, OB and OC parameters. To this end, HE, TRAP and CTSK stained histological sections of tibias from 12 weeks old PKC-δ cKO and WT mice were used for histomorphometric analysis (**Figure 2**). HE staining displayed increased trabecular bone in PKC-δ cKO male mice (**Figure 2A**, indicated by yellow arrow), further confirming the Micro-CT findings (**Figure 1B**). Analysis of TRAP staining revealed a reduction in OC number and surface after PKC-δ ablation specifically in OCs (**Figures 2Bi,ii**). No significant differences were observed in OB surface and number of OBs in PKC-δ cKO mice when compared to WT littermates (**Figures 2Biii,iv**). We further verified our finding by CTSK (a specific protein expressed in mature OCs) IHC staining. As expected, semi-quantitative analysis showed decreased CTSK protein levels after inactivation of PKC-δ in OCs (**Figure 2Bv**).

It was reported that non-cannonical Wnt signaling through G protein-linked PKC-δ activation promoted bone formation (Tu et al., 2007). In addition, studies have shown that PKC-δ is an important regulator of osteochondral plasticity at the interface between articular cartilage and the osteochondral junction using PKC-δ null mice (Yang et al., 2015). To exclude the influence of osteoblast formation and cartilage changes on the bone phenotype after PKC-δ cKO in OCs, we performed bone formation and bone component analysis in the proximal tibia of 12-week-old WT and PKC-δ cKO mice. Representative images of fluorescence double labeling (**Supplementary Figures S2Ai–iv**) and histomorphometric analysis of the MAR (**Supplementary Figure S2Av**) and the bone formation rate with a bone surface referent (BFR/BS, **Supplementary Figure S2Avi**) indicated that PKC-δ cKO did not affect bone formation either in male or female mice. Bone is a dynamic organ composed of organic and inorganic elements, we used von Kossa staining (for inorganic components) and Masson's trichrome staining (for organic components) to investigate the effect of ablation of PKC-δ specifically in OCs on bone composition. Representative images showed increased inorganic contents in trabecular bone in male mice but not in female mice (**Supplementary Figure S2Bi**, indicate by yellow arrows) and semi-quantitative analysis revealed increased trabecular bone volume fraction (**Supplementary Figure S2Bii**). No changes to organic components were observed in either male or female mice (**Supplementary Figure S2C**). We examined cartilage using Safranin O Fast Green Staining (**Supplementary Figure S2Di**) and no significant differences of cartilage thickness (**Supplementary Figure S2Dii**, 126 ± 23 μm vs. 134 ± 18 μm for female and 141 ± 27 μm vs. 145 ± 22 μm for male) were found in both sexes.

Collectively, these data supported the notion that PKC-δ cKO mice exhibited moderate osteopetrosis predominately owing to changes in OC parameters.

## Decreased Osteoclastogenesis and Bone Resorption in Bone Marrow Monocytes From Male PKC-δ cKO Mice

In addition to the decreased OCs observed in PKC-δ cKO male mice *in vivo*, we further investigated the effects of PKC-δ ablation selectively in OCs on osteoclastogenesis and bone resorption *in vitro*. As shown in **Figures 3A–C**, BMMs from male PKC-δ cKO produced significantly less OCs than WT littermates after stimulating with RANKL for 5 days (**Figures 3A,C**) and 7 days (**Figures 3B,C**), whereas there were no differences in OC number between female mice and WT controls (**Figures 3A–C**). Interestingly, as indicated by yellow arrows (**Figure 3A**), we found that male PKC-δ cKO OCs displayed morphology changes (be much more easily to lysis which likes a morphology change of apoptosis). Consistent with OC formation, by using Hydroxyapatite resorption assay, we demonstrated that bone resorption area was also significantly reduced in BMMs of male PKC-δ cKO after incubating with RANKL for both 5 days (**Figures 3D,F**) and 7 days (**Figures 3E,F**).

## Enhanced Androgen Receptor Transcription and Expression and Increased MAPK Signaling During Osteoclastogenesis in Male PKC-δ cKO Mice

Osteoclast apoptosis is associated with cell morphology changes. As we observed obvious morphology changes in OCs during osteoclastogenesis in male PKC-δ cKO mice, we tested whether selective deletion of PKC-δ in OCs affected OC apoptosis. Interestingly, using TUNEL assay, we did not observe significant fluorescence intensity changes during osteoclastogenesis after stimulating with RANKL for 5 days (**Figures 4A,B**) and 7 days (**Figures 4C,D**) in either male or female PKC-δ cKO mice. To confirm this finding we further detected protein expression changes characteristic of apoptosis. As shown in **Figure 5A**, cleaved Caspase-3, Caspase-3, cleaved PARP and PARP protein expression levels in PKC-δ cKO mice were similar to that of WT controls during osteoclastogenesis (**Figure 5B**), further confirming that ablation of PKC-δ selectively in OC does not promote OC apoptosis.

Because AR is abundantly expressed in male OC and can potently suppress osteoclastogenesis and bone resorption (Huber et al., 2001; Kawano et al., 2003), to further explore the molecular basis for gender dependent changes during OC differentiation and function, we theorized that PKC-δ regulated

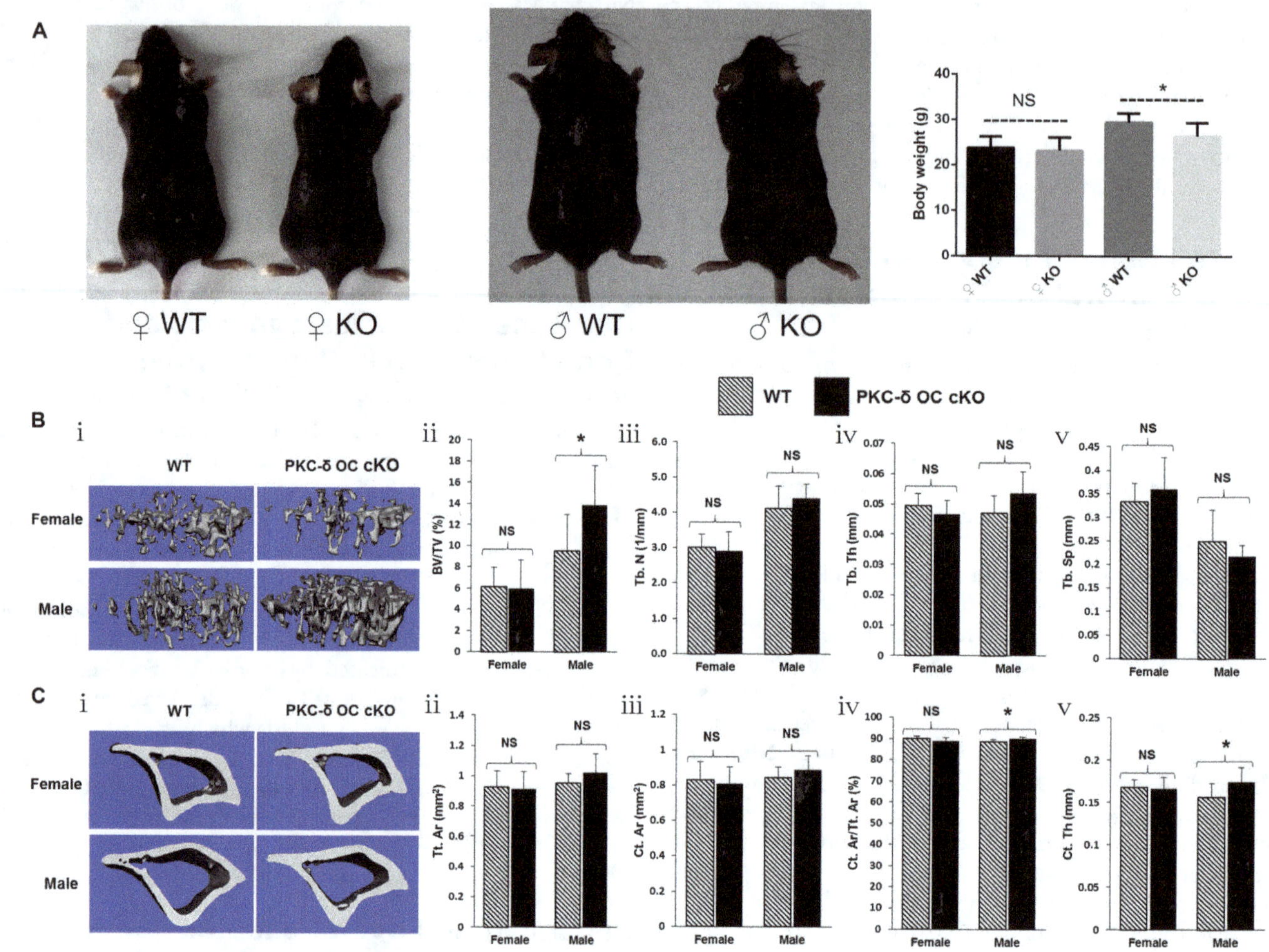

**FIGURE 1 |** Conditional knockout of PKC-δ in osteoclast resulted in bone mass accrual in 12-week old male mice. **(A)** Representative images and body weight of the pups at 12 weeks of age (WT wild type, KO knockout). **(B,C)** Representative 3D reconstructions of trabecular **(Bi)** and cortical **(Ci)** bone and bone parameters assessed by Micro-CT in proximal tibia in age- and sex-matched WT and PKC-δ conditional knockout mice, respectively ($n = 7$ per group). Trabecular bone parameters **(Bii–v)** are shown as trabecular bone volume fraction (BV/TV, %; **Bii**), trabecular number (Tb.N, 1/mm; **Biii**), trabecular thickness (Tb.Th, mm; **Biv**) and trabecular separation (Tb.Sp, mm; **Bv**). Micro-CT analysis of cortical bone parameters **(Cii–v)** are shown as total cortical area (Tt.Ar, $mm^2$; **Cii**), cortical bone area (Ct.Ar, $mm^2$; **Ciii**), cortical area fraction (Ct.Ar/Tt.Ar, %; **Civ**) and cortical thickness (Ct.Th, μm; **Cv**). Data are presented as mean/fold change ± SD. NS, non-significant, $^*p < 0.05$ compared with WT control group by two-way ANOVA with Tukey's *post hoc* test.

AR transcription and expression by binding to its promoter. Therefore, we firstly examined the effect of PKC-δ on AR transcriptional activity by transfection and luciferase assay. LNCaP and 293T cells were transfected with AR reporter plasmids. As expected, luciferase activity was dramatically increased after co-transfection with PKC-δ plasmid in both cell lines (**Figure 5C**), indicating that PKC-δ regulated AR transcription by binding to its promoter. Based on this finding, we further investigated the AR RNA and protein expression changes during osteoclastogenesis in PKC-δ cKO mice (**Figures 5D–F**). Interestingly, RT-PCR semi-quantification analysis revealed that selective ablation of PKC-δ in OC could greatly enhance AR transcription during osteoclastogenesis both in 3 days and 5 days after RANKL induction only in male mice (**Figure 5D**). Furthermore, optical density analysis shown that AR protein expression was also significantly elevated at all the time-points (1/3/5/7 days) following RANKL stimulation in male mice but not in female mice (**Figures 5E,F**).

Since members of the MAPK signaling (including ERK, JNK and P38) and NF-κB signaling pathways play a crucial role in OC survival, differentiation and function (Abu-Amer, 2013; Lee et al., 2018). We further investigated these signaling at 0, 5, 10, 20, 30, 60 min after RANKL stimulation in PKC-δ cKO and wild type mice. As shown in **Figure 6**, in female mice, although significant changes were found in some time points of p-P38 (0 and 5 min), p-ERK (60 min), and p-JNK (0, 5, 30, and 60 min), the trend of changes was not consistent. Moreover, no significant differences of IκB-α expression were found in cKO mice (**Figures 6A,B**). By contrast, the phosphorylation of P38 and ERK was remarkably enhanced at all the time points while the phosphorylation of JNK was significantly increased at 0, 5, 10, 20, and 60 min after RANKL treatment in male mice of PKC-δ cKO. However, the

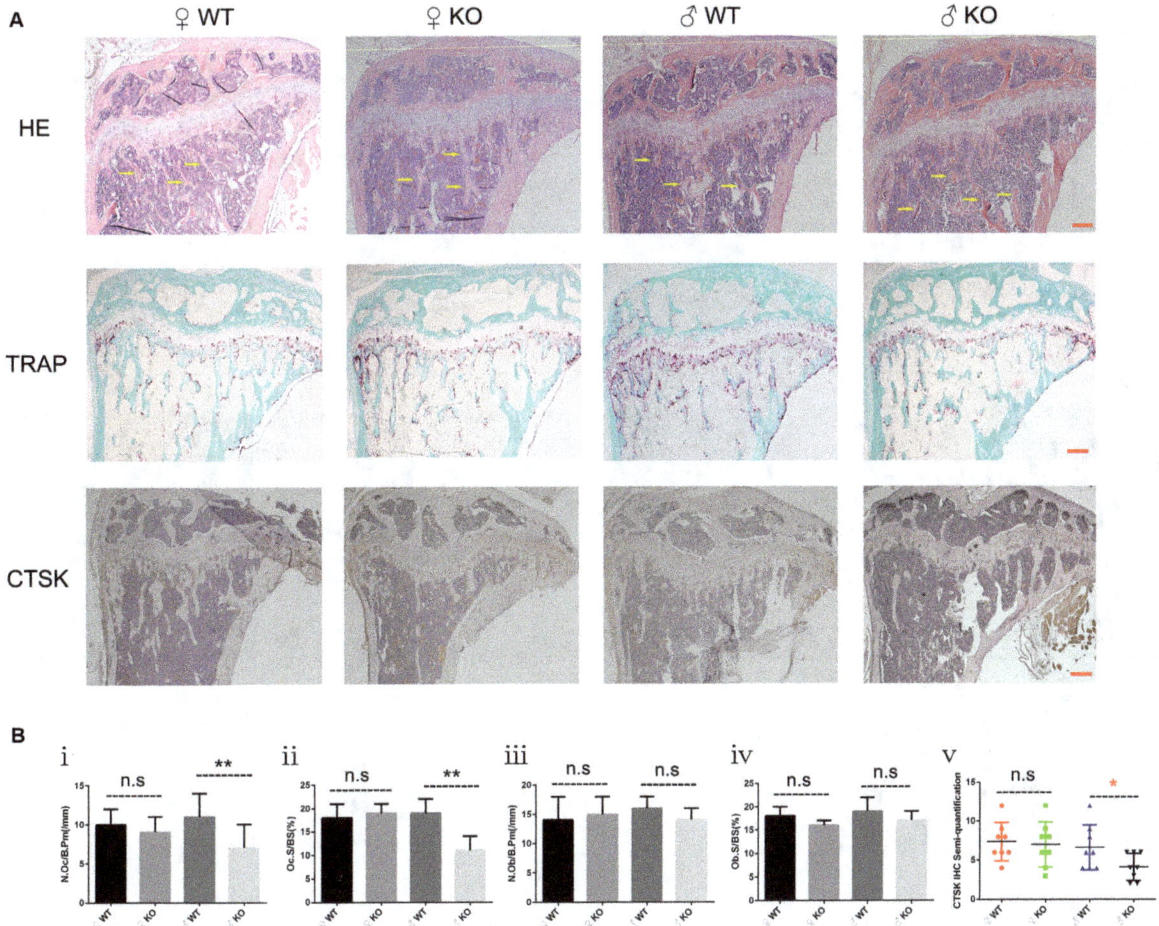

**FIGURE 2 |** Increased bone fraction and decreased osteoclast number in the trabecular bone of male PKC-δ cKO mice. Analysis of proximal tibia sections of 3-month-old PKC-δ cKO and age-sex matched wild type mice using histology ($n = 7$ per group). **(A)** Representative images of HE/TRAP/CTSK stained tibia sections. Arrows indicate trabecular bone within the tibia. Magnification = 40×, bar represents 200 μm. **(B)** Quantitative histomorphometric analysis of bone parameters: **(Bi)** Number of osteoclasts relative to bone surface (N.Oc/B.Pm, $mm^{-1}$); **(Bii)** Osteoclast surface relative to bone surface (Oc.S/BS, %); **(Biii)** Number of osteoblasts (N.Ob/B.Pm, $mm^{-1}$); **(Biv)** Osteoblast surface (Ob.S/BS, %); **(Bv)** Semi-quantification of CTSK IHC staining. Bar charts represent mean ± SD. n.s. no statistical significance, $^*p < 0.05$, $^{**}p < 0.01$ compared with WT control group by two-way ANOVA with Tukey's *post hoc* test.

expression levels of IκB-α were not changed (**Figures 6C,D**). These findings suggested that PKC-δ cKO enhanced the RANKL-induced MAKP signaling pathway only in male mice, especially the expression of p-P38 and p-ERK.

Taken together, our data clearly demonstrated that inactivation of PKC-δ specifically in OCs had no effect on OC apoptosis but enhanced AR transcription and expression and increased MAPK signaling during osteoclastogenesis in a sex dependent manner in male mice.

## Conditional Inactivation of PKC-δ in Osteoclasts Led to Significant Gene Expression and Signaling Changes Related to Extracellular Matrix Proteins Only in Male Mice

To further address the issue of gender differences after PKC-δ cKO, we investigated the gene expression differences in BMMs after stimulating with RANKL by transcriptomics sequencing and bioinformatics analysis. RNA-seq-based expression heat map of PKC-δ cKO mice BMM-derived OCs showed that the lack of PKC-δ altered the expression of many genes much more dramatically in male mice (**Figure 7A**). We further identified the DEGs responsible for the gender differences by using Volcano plot (**Figure 7B**): There were 14 up-regulated DEGs and 2 down-regulated DEGs in male mice when compared with WT controls (**Figure 7C** and **Table 1**). In contrast, there is only one DEG in female mice (**Figure 7C**). To reveal the most likely pathways and genes responsible for the sex differences, we performed the GO enrichment analysis (**Figure 7D**). It is noticeable that most of the DEGs are located in the cellular components of extracellular region and the molecular functions are mainly collagen binding and peptidase regulator activity. We further explored the underlying molecular mechanisms for the gender differences of PKC-δ cKO on OC differentiation and function by KEGG pathway enrichment analysis (**Figures 7E,F**).

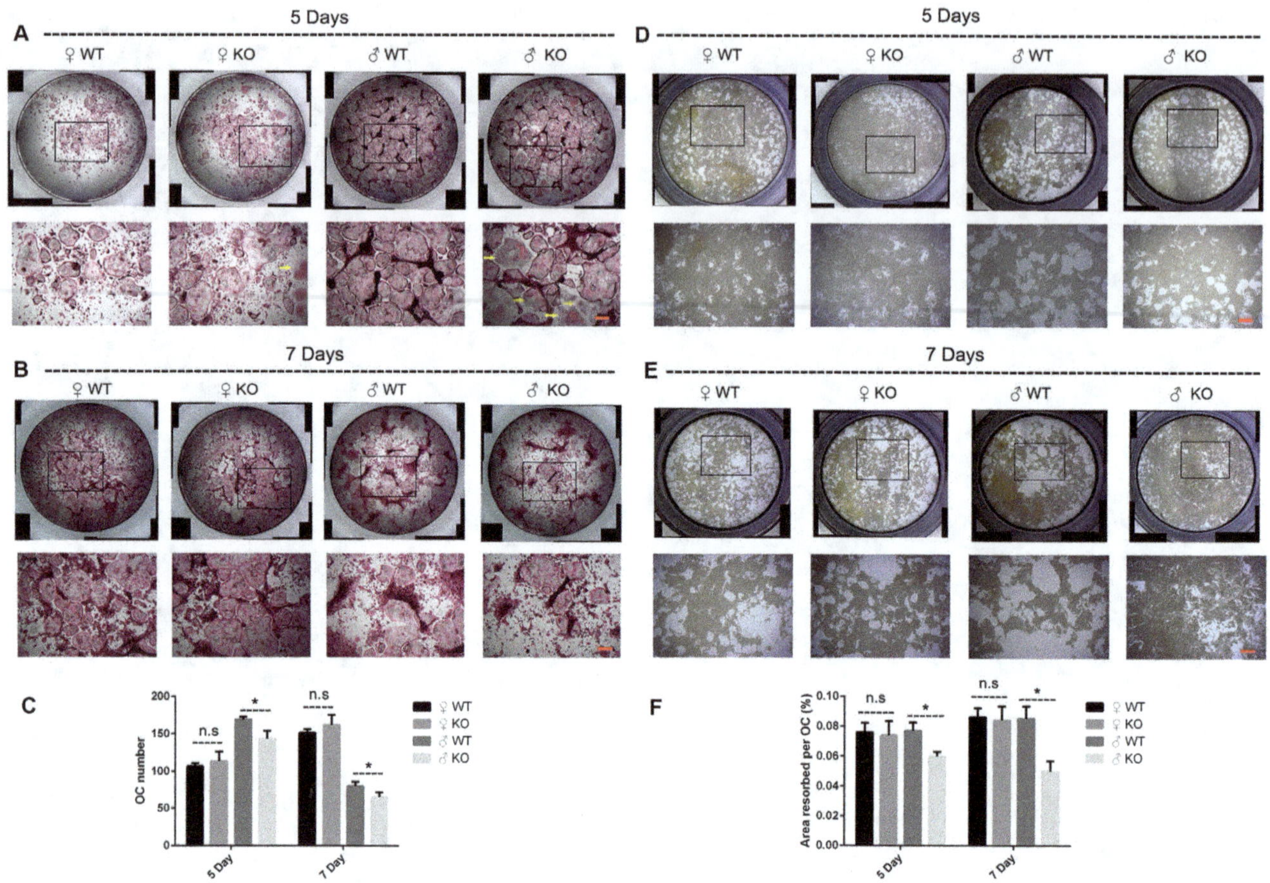


**FIGURE 3 |** Ablation of PKC-δ specifically in osteoclasts decreased osteoclastogenesis and bone resorption in male mice. **(A,B)** Representative images of osteoclasts with TRAP staining after RANKL (100 ng/ml) induction for 5 days **(A)** and 7 days **(B)**, the square in the upper images of each well indicated where the lower images were captured, the yellow arrow shows unusual morphology of OC in male PKC-δ cKO mice. Magnification = 50×, bar represents 200 μm. **(C)** The number of TRAP positive multinucleated cells (>3 nuclei) per well was quantified. **(D,E)** Representative images of eroded areas after RANKL (100 ng/ml) stimulation for 5 days **(D)** and 7 days **(E)**, the square in the upper images of each well indicated where the lower images were captured. Magnification = 50×, bar represents 200 μm. **(F)** Quantitative analysis of the resorbed proportion per osteoclast by measuring the area of the mineral coating removal. WT wild type, KO knockout. Experiments were carried out in triplicate and results are presented as mean ± SD. Bar represents 200 μm, n.s. no statistical significance, $^*p < 0.05$ vs. WT control group by two-way ANOVA with Tukey's *post hoc* test.

The enriched KEGG pathway scatterplot showed that most of the up-regulated DEGs were related to focal adhesion and ECM–receptor interaction (**Figure 7E**), while the down-regulated DEGs are mainly responsible for OC differentiation and lysosomes (**Figure 7F**).

Collectively, all these results indicated that deletion of PKC-δ specifically in OCs led to alteration of many DEGs and significant signaling changes only in male mice.

## DISCUSSION

In this study, we found that PKC-δ deficiency in OCs favors bone mass accrual in a sex-dependent manner in male mice. Histological analysis revealed increased bone fraction and decreased OCs in the trabecular bone of male mice after cKO. Furthermore, our work suggests that PKC-δ cKO decreased osteoclastogenesis and OC function only in male mice. Finally, deletion of PKC-δ selectively in OCs did not increase OC apoptosis but enhanced AR transcription and expression and increased MAPK signaling in addition to alteration of expression of many genes and signaling changes related to ECM biology during osteoclastogenesis in male mice. Hence, these data clearly showed that ablation of PKC-δ specifically in OCs contibuted to an osteopetrotic phenotype in a sex-dependent fasion in male mice. More importantly, this work revealed the gender differences at both cellular and molecular levels. Our work displayed PKC-δ as an important regulator in OC biology and revealed a previously unknown target for treatment of sex-related bone disease.

The observed effect of loss of PKC-δ resulting in increased trabecular bone is consistent with the previous studies displayed by Cremasco et al. (2012) and Khor et al. (2013). However, there is a discrepancy that the sex differences demonstrated in

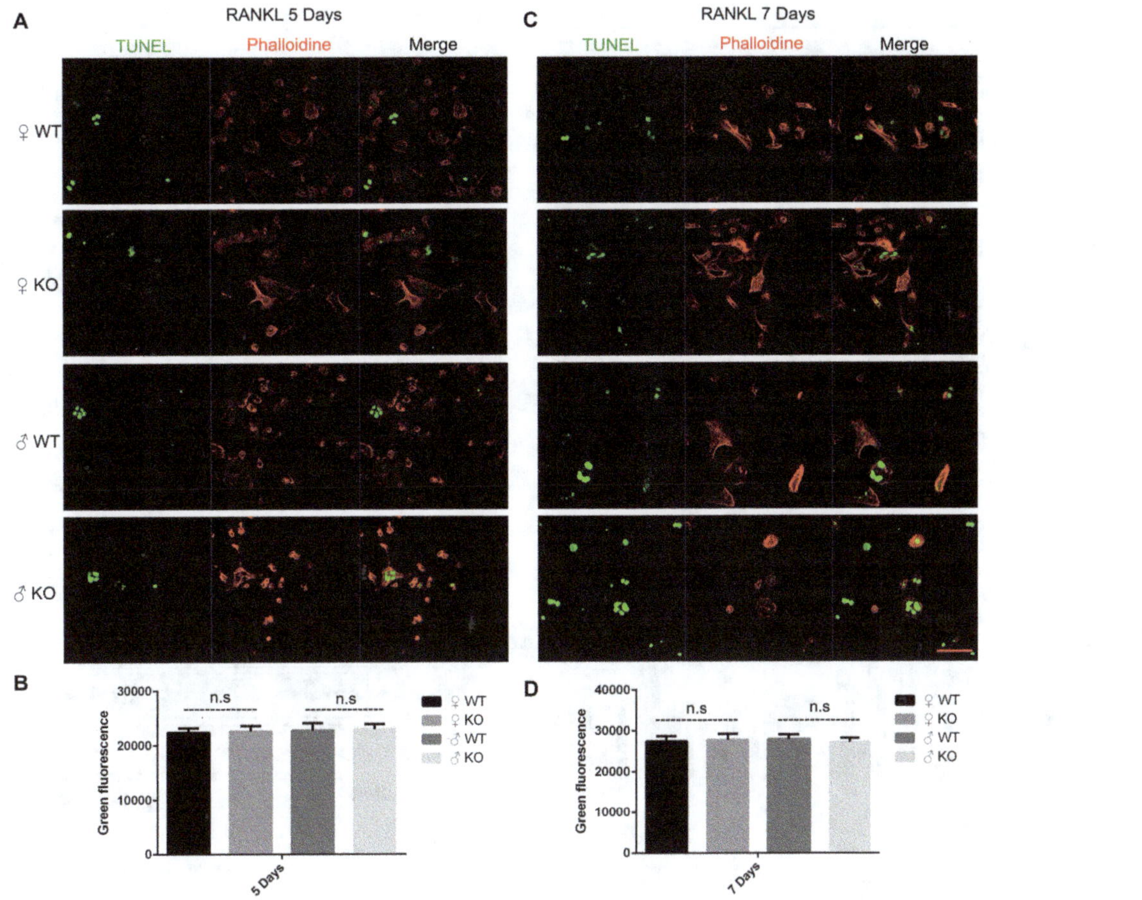


**FIGURE 4 |** Deletion of PKC-δ selectively in osteoclasts did not increase osteoclast apoptosis during osteoclastogenesis. **(A,C)** Osteoclasts on μ-Dish were immunofluorescently stained with TUNEL and phalloidin to visualize apoptosis and actin by confocal microscopy after RANKL induction for 5 days **(A)** and 7 days **(C)**. Magnification = 400×, bar represents 50 μm. **(B,D)** Semi-quantification of osteoclasts apoptosis was measured in a fluorescence microplate reader after stimulating with RANKL for 5 days **(B)** and 7 days **(D)**. Bar charts represent mean ± SD. Data are representative of three experiments. n.s. no statistical significance compared with WT control group by one-way ANOVA with Tukey's *post hoc* test.

our study was not observed in their papers on the global KO mice. In addition, the exact role of PKC-δ in OC formation and bone resorption is debatable. It is controversial that both PKC activators (Wang et al., 2003) and inhibitors (Yao et al., 2015) are able to inhibit osteoclastogenesis and bone resorption. PKC-δ was identified as the predominant isoform expressed in OCs among all PKC family (Khor et al., 2013), Khor et al. (2013) found enhanced osteoclastogenesis in PKC-δ null mice, and surmised that this is an attempt to compensate for an intrinsic bone resorption defect in these mice. In contrast, Cremasco et al. (2012) showed that PKC-δ deficiency did not impair OC differentiation in PKC-δ null mice. With respect to the role of PKC-δ on OC function, Cremasco et al. (2012) found that PKC-δ was required for CTSK exocytosis and genetic disruption of PKC-δ profoundly impaired OC bone resorption in bone slices and significantly decreased collagen type I fragment concentration in the culture medium. However, PKC-δ ablation did not impair ruffled border formation or trafficking of lysosomes containing v-ATPase (acidification), leading to no resorption changes in osteologic hydroxyapatite-coated slices in PKC-δ null mice. In contrast, others showed that rottlerin, a PKC-δ specific inhibitor, potently inhibited lysosomal acidification in human OCs (Sorensen et al., 2010). To investigate the exact role of PKC-δ in OC formation and function, we inactivated PKC-δ specifically in OCs by using the Cre-loxp system and found decreased osteoclastogenesis and bone resorption in PKC-δ cKO BMMs in a sex dependent manner in male mice. Consistent with our work, Khor et al. (2013) also showed that inhibition of PKC-δ and knock out of PKC-δ resulted in impaired osteoclastic bone resorption *in vitro*. These conflicting results are indicative that PKC-δ has dual roles in bone remodeling, where it may modulate both bone formation and resorption ultimately influencing the bone turnover process. Because bone is a dynamic organ with complex micro-enviroment, understanding the exact role of PKC-δ in OC biology is critical to dissecting its role in other bone cells, such as osteoblasts, osteocytes, chondrocytes and endothelial cells.

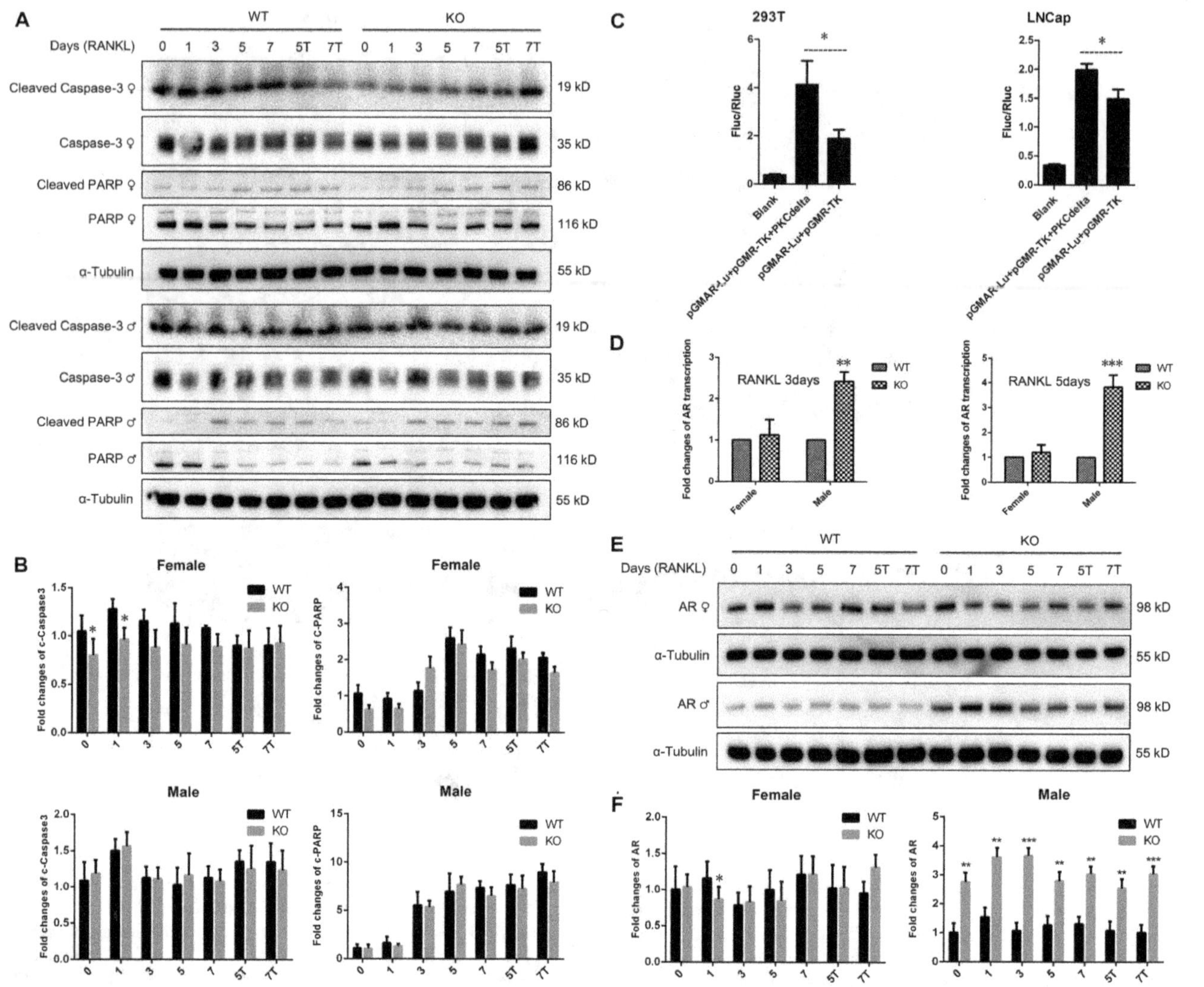

**FIGURE 5 |** No changes of apoptosis protein expression and significant up-regulation of androgen receptor transcription and expression in male PKC-δ deficient osteoclasts. **(A,B)** Western Blot analysis of characteristic apoptosis proteins (cleaved Caspase-3, Caspase-3, cleaved PARP and PARP) by detecting total protein from WT and PKC-δ cKO BMMs stimulated with RANKL on the indicated days **(A)**; Quantitative analysis of protein expression relative to WT littermate, as measured by densitometry of Western Blot images **(B)**. T $10^{-8}$ M testosterone, α-Tubulin was probed as a loading control. Statistical analysis was performed by comparing to WT in each time point for male and female, respectively. **(C)** AR transcriptional activity was significantly enhanced by PKC-δ in 293-T and LNCaP cells by transfection and luciferase assay. pGMAR-Lu AR firefly luciferase reporter, pGMR-TK control renilla luciferase reporter. **(D)** RT-PCR shown that AR transcriptional activity was significantly increased in PKC-δ cKO male mice after stimulating with 100 ng/ml RANKL for 3 days and 5 days, respectively. **(E,F)** Western Blot analysis of AR protein expression by detecting total protein from PKC-δ cKO and WT BMMs stimulated with RANKL on the indicated days **(E)**; Quantitative analysis of AR expression in cKO mice relative to WT littermate by measuring densitometry of Western Blot images **(F)**. T $10^{-8}$ M testosterone, α-Tubulin was probed as a loading control. Experiments were repeated three times. $^{*}p < 0.05$, $^{**}p < 0.01$, $^{***}p < 0.001$ vs. control group by two tailed Student's *t*-test **(C)** and by two-way ANOVA with Tukey's *post hoc* test **(B,D,F)**.

Another contradictory result was that the MAPK signaling was enhanced after PKC-δ ablation selectively in OCs. There may be two reasons for decreased OC differentiation and function accompanied paradoxically with increased MAPK signaling. Firstly, because ERK is responsible for OC survival (Miyazaki et al., 2000) while JNK signaling mediates an anti-apoptotic effect of RANKL in OCs (Ikeda et al., 2008). We assumed that the enhanced survival and anti-apoptotic signaling in OCs may be due to an attempt to compensate for the decreased OC function. Secondly, the MAPK signaling may be not the main signaling after PKC-δ deletion specifically in OCs.

An interesting outcome of our studies is the clear sex differences in bone phenotype and OC differentiation and function after deletion of PKC-δ selectively in OCs. It is an unknown phenomenon and not well described in the hormone-related-gene deficient mice. One example of differences between male and female mice has been found in aromatase-deficient mice, where the female aromatase-ablation mice had an increase in bone turnover resembling early postmenopausal

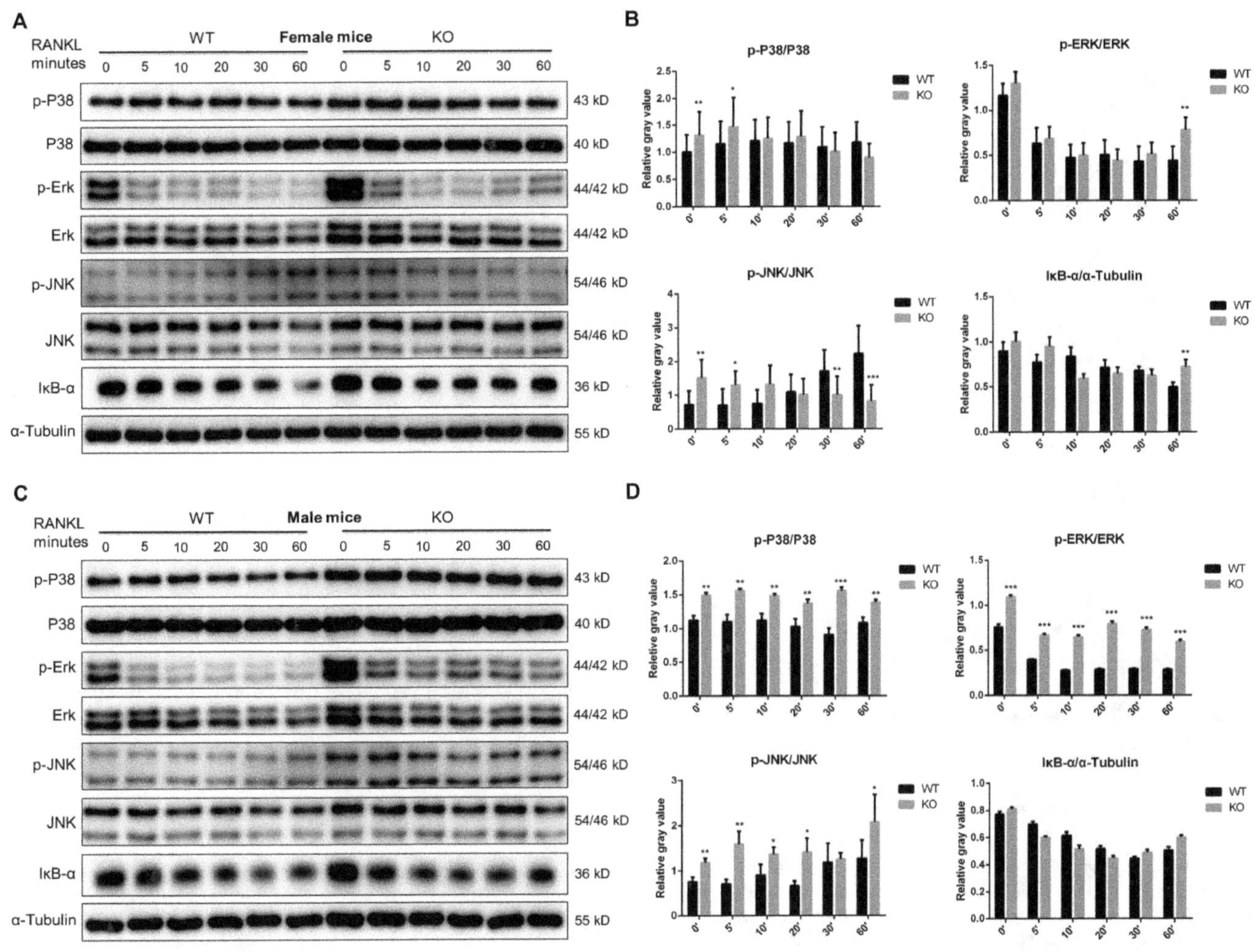


**FIGURE 6 |** PKC-δ conditional knockout in osteoclasts enhanced RANKL-induced MAPK signaling pathway during osteoclastogenesis in male mice. **(A,C)** Representative Western Blot images of p-JNK, JNK, p-ERK, ERK, p-P38, P-38, IκB-α and α-tubulin at 0, 5, 10, 20, 30, 60 min stimulated by 100 ng/ml RANKL in pre-osteoclasts from PKC-δ cKO and wild type female **(A)** and male **(C)** mice. **(B,D)** The relative ratios of phosphorylated proteins to unphosphorylated proteins or IκB-α to internal control were quantitatively determined in female **(B)** and male **(D)** mice, respectively. The data in the Figures represent the means ± SD. α-Tubulin was used as internal control. Experiments were carried out in triplicate. Significant differences between the cKO and wild type groups are indicated as $^{*}p < 0.05$, $^{**}p < 0.01$, $^{***}p < 0.001$ by two-way ANOVA with Tukey's *post hoc* test **(B,D)**.

osteoporosis, whereas the male aromatase-deficient mice showed decreases in both osteoblastic and osteoclastic surfaces similar to age-related osteopenia compared with WT littermates (Oz et al., 2000). Another example of a sex difference has been found in the ER knockout mice. where the female mice have decreased bone resorption and increased trabecular bone volume, whereas the bones of the male mice were unaffected by the ablation of the ER gene (Sims et al., 2002). However, we have identified two potential explanations that may account for the observed sex differences in PKC-δ cKO mice. Firstly, the presence of functional ARs in OCs (Almeida et al., 2017) indicates that OCs are able to respond directly to androgen through the AR (Pederson et al., 1999), resulting in a suppressive effect on bone resorption (Kawano et al., 2003). The sex-specific effects of androgen on gene expression in human monocyte-derived OCs indicate that AR function is indispensable for male bone formation and remodeling (Wang and Stern, 2011). Moreover, androgens regulated PKC-δ transcription and modulated its apoptotic function in prostate cancer cells (Gavrielides et al., 2006), and prenatal testosterone exposure induces hypertension in adult females via an AR-dependent PKC-δ-mediated mechanism (Blesson et al., 2015). These studies and our results suggest that PKC-δ has a direct interaction with the AR promoter. The studies above lead us to speculate that deletion of PKC-δ in OCs may suppress OC function through increasing AR expression. By using qPCR-based array, Wang and Stern (2011) showed that although OCs from both male and female mice responded to 17β-estradiol and testosterone, the effects of both estrogen and androgen differ in the two sexes, highlighting the importance

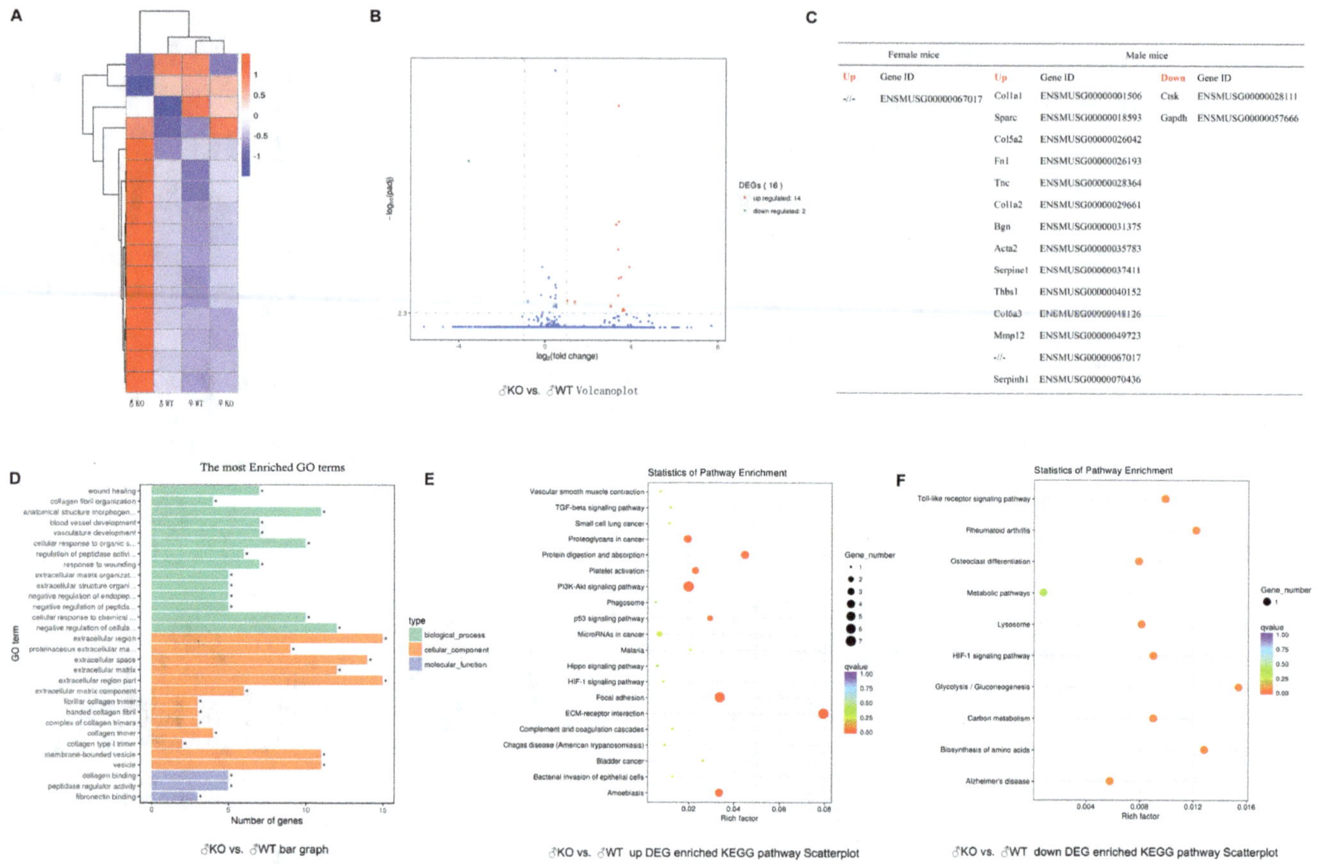


**FIGURE 7 |** Inactivation of PKC-δ specifically in osteoclasts led to significant alteration of differentially expressed genes (DEGs) and signaling changes only in male mice. **(A)** Heat map of DEGs up and down in 12-week-old PKC-δ cKO mice BMMs derived osteoclasts. **(B)** Volcano plot of data set showing the DEGs in the BMMs stimulating with RANKL for 3 days. Dots with red and green color represented the up-regulated and down-regulated DEGs, respectively, between PKC-δ cKO and WT male mice. **(C)** List of up-regulated and down-regulated DEGs extracted from **(A,B)** with Gene ID and presented in details in **Table 1**. **(D)** Bar graph of GO enrichment analysis of DEGs showing the most enriched GO terms compared between PKC-δ cKO and WT male mice by two tailed Student's *t*-test. **(E)** Gene set enrichment analysis of BMMs from KEGG database revealed the most likely up-regulated pathways responsible for the gender differences. **(F)** Scatterplot of KEGG pathway enrichment analysis of DEGs showed the down-regulated pathways comparing PKC-δ cKO and WT male mice. RNA-seq data from three biological replicates per group were used.

of considering gender in the design of therapeutics. This study further supports our findings of sex specific effects of PKC-δ. Secondly, transcriptome sequencing and bioinformatics analysis showed that inactivation of PKC-δ specifically in OCs led to up-regulation of only one pseudogene without function in female mice. In contrast, many genes were altered (Colla1, Colla2, Col5a2, Col6a3, Thbs1, Bgn, Tnc, Sparc, Fn1, Acta2, Serpine1, Mmp12, Serpinh1 were up-regulated while Ctsk and Gapdh were down-regulated) during osteoclastogenesis after PKC-δ ablation in male mice. It should be noted that these DEGs are mainly responsible for ECM and collagen synthesis, degradation and signaling [for example Thbs1 (Amend et al., 2015), Bgn (Shirakura et al., 2017), Sparc (Rosset and Bradshaw, 2016), Fn1 (Magnan et al., 2018), and Serpinh1 (Mimura et al., 2016)]. Interestingly, most of these DEGs play important roles in OC biology (especially Col6a3 (Mullin et al., 2018), Bgn (Bi et al., 2006; Kram et al., 2017), Thbs1 (Kukreja et al., 2009; Amend et al., 2015; Koduru et al., 2018), Tnc (Baniwal et al., 2012), Sparc (Ma et al., 2017), and Acta2 (Mullin et al., 2014)] and also displayed sexual dimorphism in regulating many cellular processes. With respect to collagen related genes, postnatal changes and sexual dimorphism were found in collagen expression in mouse skin. Colla1 and Colla2 mRNAs increased noticeably at day 30 and remained at high levels until day 120 in male mice, Col3a1mRNA also showed significantly high levels at day 120 in male mice as compared to female. Moreover, testosterone and its effect on collagen expression are responsible for the skin sexual dimorphism (Arai et al., 2017). Intriguingly, the Col5a1 gene is associated with increased risk of anterior cruciate ligament ruptures only in female participants (Posthumus et al., 2009). Bgn-deficient mice are resistant to OVX-induced trabecular bone loss and there is a gender difference in response to Bgn deficiency (Nielsen et al., 2003). For Fn1 and Tnc, tendon of the female mice had approximately twofold elevations in ECM proteins such as Fn1 and Tnc compared with male

**TABLE 1** | Genes differentially expressed during osteoclastogenesis in male PKC-δ conditional knockout mice ($n = 3$).

| Gene symbol | Gene name | Fold changes (cKO vs. WT, $log_2$) | *p*-value |
|---|---|---|---|
| Col1a1 | Collagen type I alpha 1 chain | 3.427 | 1.04E-21 |
| Col1a2 | Collagen type I alpha 2 chain | 3.389 | 5.27E-17 |
| Col5a2 | Collagen type V alpha 2 chain | 3.640 | 1.70E-06 |
| Col6a3 | Collagen type VI alpha 3 chain | 3.687 | 2.73E-06 |
| Sparc | Secreted protein acidic and cysteine rich | 3.915 | 5.38E-14 |
| Fn1 | Fibronectin 1 | 3.404 | 4.37E-41 |
| Tnc | Tenascin C | 3.396 | 6.15E-09 |
| Bgn | Biglycan | 3.045 | 5.38E-07 |
| Acta2 | Actin alpha 2 | 3.423 | 6.69E-12 |
| Serpine 1 | Serpin family E member 1 | 3.539 | 3.45E-12 |
| Thbs1 | Thrombospondin 1 | 3.293 | 3.59E-21 |
| Mmp12 | Matrix metallopeptidase 12 | 1.042 | 4.71E-08 |
| Serpinh 1 | Serpin family H member 1 | 3.612 | 3.40E-06 |
| Ctsk | Cathepsin K | −1.099 | 0 |
| Gapdh | Glyceraldehyde-3-phosphate dehydrogenase | −3.541 | 8.60E-32 |

mice (Sarver et al., 2017). For Acta2, male MDR2 knockout mice tended to have a more pronounced reversal of liver fibrosis than females treated with corticosterone (Petrescu et al., 2017). For Mmp9, less elastin in the aneurysm wall in women than that in men, and the simultaneous higher level of Mmp-9, suggesting differences in the elastolytic process in abdominal aortic aneurysms between the sexes (Villard et al., 2014); in addition, male mucopolysaccharidosis type I mice have an increased incidence of aortic insufficiency associated with an increase in MMP-12 aortic arch content (Tolar et al., 2009). For CTSK, sexual dimorphism existed in MAPK-Activated protein kinase-2 regulation of RANKL-induced osteoclastogenesis in OC progenitor subpopulations (Herbert et al., 2015). Collectively, all these DEGs are closely related to the ECM and the majority display sexual dimorphism. It is reasonable to assume that the gender difference found in the studies above also could be found in other deficient mice; herein it is important to examine the phenotype of both sexes. Although the precise role of PKC-δ in ECM-related gene signaling is complex and remains to be elucidated, it is possible that PKC-δ may regulate AR activity through the DEGs above. However, the underlying molecular mechanisms of the differential expression and the role of these genes in sex related differences in OC functions need to be further investigated.

Limitations of our study should be acknowledged. First, it is reported that CTSK-Cre caused unexpected germline deletion of genes in mice which was found to be due to the expression of CTSK in both testis and ovary (Winkeler et al., 2012). This illustrates that we need to be alert to potential germline recombination which may confound our results regarding the changes of size and androgen signaling. It is reported that lack of PKC-δ (PKC-δ null mice) disrupts fertilization and embryonic development in both males and females (Ma et al., 2015). Testis and ovary dysfunction and hypogonadism are always accompanied with osteopenia (Watts et al., 2012; Karakas and Surampudi, 2018). However, in our study, we found that PKC-δ deficiency in OCs favored bone mass accrual and enhanced AR transcription and expression during osteoclastogenesis only in male mice, furthermore, the reproduction function was not affected after PKC-δ cKO in OCs (unpublished data), suggesting that the proposed effects resulting from germline deletion of PKC-δ are contradictory to our results. In addition, CTSK is mainly expressed in OCs, the expression levels of CTSK in other tissues are much lower than that in bone (Soderstrom et al., 1999). Taken together, we speculate that the CTSK expression in gonads may not confound our results. Although many of the OC-targeted Cre-deleter strains, including CTSK, TRAP and *LysM*, are imperfect and each model has its own limitations (Dallas et al., 2018), the CTSK-Cre mouse is the most widely used Cre transgenic mouse line for the *in vivo* study of OCs, their careful use will continue to provide key advances in our understanding of OC function in bone health and disease. Second, it is difficult to transfect pre-OC of the RAW264.7 cell line and BMMs with plasmids, hence the lack of evidence showing direct interaction between PKC-δ and AR in OC. However, many lines of evidence from other cell lines, such as mesenteric artery smooth muscle cells (Blesson et al., 2015), 293-T and LNCaP cells, support our findings. Clinical and genetic studies of PKC-δ gene mutations in humans are important to confirm these pre-clinical studies in mice, blood and bone samples from patients with PKC-δ deficiency will provide further information to address this issue (Belot et al., 2013; Kuehn et al., 2013; Salzer et al., 2013; Kiykim et al., 2015).

In summary, our data clearly demonstrate sex differences in the function of PKC-δ in mice. More importantly, we provide compelling evidence demonstrating that the sex differences are closely related to AR, MAPK, and ECM related signaling, unveiling an important role for PKC-δ in the pathogenesis of osteoporosis in animal models, cell culture, and molecular interactions. This work contributes to our understanding of the role of PKC-δ in OC bone resorption and might aid in the discovery of novel therapeutic targets for treatment of gender-related bone disorders.

## ETHICS STATEMENT

All the experiments were approved by the Institutional Animal Care and Use Committee of the Third Affiliated Hospital of Sun Yat-sen University (Approval No: IACUC-F3-18-1202) and were performed according to EU Directive 2010/63/EU.

## AUTHOR CONTRIBUTIONS

SL and LR conceived the ideas. SL, JX, and AQ planned experiments. SL, TH, DW, and JY performed experiments and analyzed the data. JX and AQ contributed reagents. SL wrote the manuscript. JT and JX revised manuscript content. All authors reviewed the manuscript.

## REFERENCES


Abu-Amer, Y. (2013). NF-kappaB signaling and bone resorption. *Osteoporos. Int.* 24, 2377–2386. doi: 10.1007/s00198-013-2313-x

Almeida, M., Laurent, M. R., Dubois, V., Claessens, F., O'Brien, C. A., Bouillon, R., et al. (2017). Estrogens and androgens in skeletal physiology and pathophysiology. *Physiol. Rev.* 97, 135–187. doi: 10.1152/physrev.00033.2015

Amend, S. R., Uluckan, O., Hurchla, M., Leib, D., Novack, D. V., Silva, M., et al. (2015). Thrombospondin-1 regulates bone homeostasis through effects on bone matrix integrity and nitric oxide signaling in osteoclasts. *J. Bone Miner. Res.* 30, 106–115. doi: 10.1002/jbmr.2308

Arai, K. Y., Hara, T., Nagatsuka, T., Kudo, C., Tsuchiya, S., Nomura, Y., et al. (2017). Postnatal changes and sexual dimorphism in collagen expression in mouse skin. *PLoS One* 12:e0177534. doi: 10.1371/journal.pone.0177534

Baniwal, S. K., Shah, P. K., Shi, Y., Haduong, J. H., Declerck, Y. A., Gabet, Y., et al. (2012). Runx2 promotes both osteoblastogenesis and novel osteoclastogenic signals in ST2 mesenchymal progenitor cells. *Osteoporos. Int.* 23, 1399–1413. doi: 10.1007/s00198-011-1728-5

Belot, A., Kasher, P. R., Trotter, E. W., Foray, A. P., Debaud, A. L., Rice, G. I., et al. (2013). Protein kinase cdelta deficiency causes mendelian systemic lupus erythematosus with B cell-defective apoptosis and hyperproliferation. *Arthritis Rheum.* 65, 2161–2171. doi: 10.1002/art.38008

Bi, Y., Nielsen, K. L., Kilts, T. M., Yoon, A., Karsdal, M. A., Wimer, H. F., et al. (2006). Biglycan deficiency increases osteoclast differentiation and activity due to defective osteoblasts. *Bone* 38, 778–786. doi: 10.1016/j.bone.2005.11.005

Blesson, C. S., Chinnathambi, V., Hankins, G. D., Yallampalli, C., and Sathishkumar, K. (2015). Prenatal testosterone exposure induces hypertension in adult females via androgen receptor-dependent protein kinase Cdelta-mediated mechanism. *Hypertension* 65, 683–690. doi: 10.1161/HYPERTENSIONAHA.114.04521

Cremasco, V., Decker, C. E., Stumpo, D., Blackshear, P. J., Nakayama, K. I., Nakayama, K., et al. (2012). Protein kinase C-delta deficiency perturbs bone homeostasis by selective uncoupling of cathepsin K secretion and ruffled border formation in osteoclasts. *J. Bone Miner. Res.* 27, 2452–2463. doi: 10.1002/jbmr.1701

Da, C. L., Xin, Y., Zhao, J., and Luo, X. D. (2009). Significance and relationship between Yes-associated protein and survivin expression in gastric carcinoma and precancerous lesions. *World J. Gastroenterol.* 15, 4055–4061. doi: 10.3748/wjg.15.4055

Dallas, S. L., Xie, Y., Shiflett, L. A., and Ueki, Y. (2018). Mouse cre models for the study of bone diseases. *Curr. Osteoporos. Rep.* 16, 466–477. doi: 10.1007/s11914-018-0455-7

Gavrielides, M. V., Gonzalez-Guerrico, A. M., Riobo, N. A., and Kazanietz, M. G. (2006). Androgens regulate protein kinase Cdelta transcription and modulate its apoptotic function in prostate cancer cells. *Cancer Res.* 66, 11792–11801. doi: 10.1158/0008-5472.can-06-1139

He, L., Hong, G., Zhou, L., Zhang, J., Fang, J., He, W., et al. (2019). Asiaticoside, a component of *Centella asiatica* attenuates RANKL-induced osteoclastogenesis via NFATc1 and NF-kappaB signaling pathways. *J. Cell. Physiol.* 234, 4267–4276. doi: 10.1002/jcp.27195

Herbert, B. A., Valerio, M. S., Gaestel, M., and Kirkwood, K. L. (2015). Sexual dimorphism in MAPK-activated protein kinase-2 (MK2) regulation of RANKL-induced osteoclastogenesis in osteoclast progenitor subpopulations. *PLoS One* 10:e0125387. doi: 10.1371/journal.pone.0125387

Huber, D. M., Bendixen, A. C., Pathrose, P., Srivastava, S., Dienger, K. M., Shevde, N. K., et al. (2001). Androgens suppress osteoclast formation induced by RANKL and macrophage-colony stimulating factor. *Endocrinology* 142, 3800–3808. doi: 10.1210/endo.142.9.8402

Iaquinta, M. R., Mazzoni, E., Bononi, I., Rotondo, J. C., Mazziotta, C., Montesi, M., et al. (2019). Adult stem cells for bone regeneration and repair. *Front. Cell. Dev. Biol.* 7:268. doi: 10.3389/fcell.2019.00268

Ikeda, F., Matsubara, T., Tsurukai, T., Hata, K., Nishimura, R., and Yoneda, T. (2008). JNK/c-Jun signaling mediates an anti-apoptotic effect of RANKL in osteoclasts. *J. Bone Miner. Res.* 23, 907–914. doi: 10.1359/jbmr.080211

Karakas, S. E., and Surampudi, P. (2018). New biomarkers to evaluate hyperandrogenemic women and hypogonadal men. *Adv. Clin. Chem.* 86, 71–125. doi: 10.1016/bs.acc.2018.06.001

Kawano, H., Sato, T., Yamada, T., Matsumoto, T., Sekine, K., Watanabe, T., et al. (2003). Suppressive function of androgen receptor in bone resorption. *Proc. Natl. Acad. Sci. U.S.A.* 100, 9416–9421. doi: 10.1073/pnas.1533500100

Khor, E. C., Abel, T., Tickner, J., Chim, S. M., Wang, C., Cheng, T., et al. (2013). Loss of protein kinase C-delta protects against LPS-induced osteolysis owing to an intrinsic defect in osteoclastic bone resorption. *PLoS One* 8:e70815. doi: 10.1371/journal.pone.0070815

Kiykim, A., Ogulur, I., Baris, S., Salzer, E., Karakoc-Aydiner, E., Ozen, A. O., et al. (2015). Potentially beneficial effect of hydroxychloroquine in a patient with a novel mutation in protein kinase cdelta deficiency. *J. Clin. Immunol.* 35, 523–526. doi: 10.1007/s10875-015-0178-9

Koduru, S. V., Sun, B. H., Walker, J. M., Zhu, M., Simpson, C., Dhodapkar, M., et al. (2018). The contribution of cross-talk between the cell-surface proteins CD36 and CD47-TSP-1 in osteoclast formation and function. *J. Biol. Chem.* 293, 15055–15069. doi: 10.1074/jbc.RA117.000633

Kram, V., Kilts, T. M., Bhattacharyya, N., Li, L., and Young, M. F. (2017). Small leucine rich proteoglycans, a novel link to osteoclastogenesis. *Sci. Rep.* 7:12627. doi: 10.1038/s41598-017-12651-6

Kuehn, H. S., Niemela, J. E., Rangel-Santos, A., Zhang, M., Pittaluga, S., Stoddard, J. L., et al. (2013). Loss-of-function of the protein kinase C delta (PKCdelta) causes a B-cell lymphoproliferative syndrome in humans. *Blood* 121, 3117–3125. doi: 10.1182/blood-2012-12-469544

Kukreja, A., Radfar, S., Sun, B. H., Insogna, K., and Dhodapkar, M. V. (2009). Dominant role of CD47-thrombospondin-1 interactions in myeloma-induced fusion of human dendritic cells: implications for bone disease. *Blood* 114, 3413–3421. doi: 10.1182/blood-2009-03-211920

Lee, K., Seo, I., Choi, M. H., and Jeong, D. (2018). Roles of mitogen-activated protein kinases in osteoclast biology. *Int. J. Mol. Sci.* 19:3004. doi: 10.3390/ijms19103004

Ma, J., Gao, S., Xie, X., Sun, E., Zhang, M., Zhou, Q., et al. (2017). SPARC inhibits breast cancer bone metastasis and may be a clinical therapeutic target. *Oncol. Lett.* 14, 5876–5882. doi: 10.3892/ol.2017.6925

Ma, W., Baumann, C., and Viveiros, M. M. (2015). Lack of protein kinase C-delta (PKCdelta) disrupts fertilization and embryonic development. *Mol. Reprod. Dev.* 82, 797–808. doi: 10.1002/mrd.22528

Magnan, L., Labrunie, G., Marais, S., Rey, S., Dusserre, N., Bonneu, M., et al. (2018). Characterization of a cell-assembled extracellular matrix and the effect of the devitalization process. *Acta Biomater.* 82, 56–67. doi: 10.1016/j.actbio.2018.10.006

Mimura, H., Takaya, T., Matsuda, S., Nakano, K., Muraoka, R., Tomida, M., et al. (2016). Functional role of HSP47 in the periodontal ligament subjected to occlusal overload in mice. *Int. J. Med. Sci.* 13, 248–254. doi: 10.7150/ijms.14129

Miyazaki, T., Katagiri, H., Kanegae, Y., Takayanagi, H., Sawada, Y., Yamamoto, A., et al. (2000). Reciprocal role of ERK and NF-kappaB pathways in survival and activation of osteoclasts. *J. Cell Biol.* 148, 333–342. doi: 10.1083/jcb.148.2.333

Mullin, B. H., Mamotte, C., Prince, R. L., and Wilson, S. G. (2014). Influence of ARHGEF3 and RHOA knockdown on ACTA2 and other genes in osteoblasts and osteoclasts. *PLoS One* 9:e98116. doi: 10.1371/journal.pone.0098116

Mullin, B. H., Zhu, K., Xu, J., Brown, S. J., Mullin, S., Tickner, J., et al. (2018). Expression quantitative trait locus study of bone mineral density GWAS variants in human osteoclasts. *J. Bone Miner. Res.* 33, 1044–1051. doi: 10.1002/jbmr.3412

Nielsen, K. L., Allen, M. R., Bloomfield, S. A., Andersen, T. L., Chen, X. D., Poulsen, H. S., et al. (2003). Biglycan deficiency interferes with ovariectomy-induced bone loss. *J. Bone Miner. Res.* 18, 2152–2158. doi: 10.1359/jbmr.2003.18.12.2152

Ono, Y., Fujii, T., Ogita, K., Kikkawa, U., Igarashi, K., and Nishizuka, Y. (1988). The structure, expression, and properties of additional members of the protein kinase C family. *J. Biol. Chem.* 263, 6927–6932.

Oz, O. K., Zerwekh, J. E., Fisher, C., Graves, K., Nanu, L., Millsaps, R., et al. (2000). Bone has a sexually dimorphic response to aromatase deficiency. *J. Bone Miner. Res.* 15, 507–514. doi: 10.1359/jbmr.2000.15.3.507

Pederson, L., Kremer, M., Judd, J., Pascoe, D., Spelsberg, T. C., Riggs, B. L., et al. (1999). Androgens regulate bone resorption activity of isolated osteoclasts in vitro. *Proc. Natl. Acad. Sci. U.S.A.* 96, 505–510. doi: 10.1073/pnas.96.2.505

Petrescu, A. D., Grant, S., Frampton, G., Kain, J., Hadidi, K., Williams, E., et al. (2017). Glucocorticoids cause gender-dependent reversal of hepatic fibrosis in the MDR2-knockout mouse model. *Int. J. Mol. Sci.* 18:E2389. doi: 10.3390/ijms18112389

Posthumus, M., September, A. V., O'Cuinneagain, D., van der Merwe, W., Schwellnus, M. P., and Collins, M. (2009). The COL5A1 gene is associated with increased risk of anterior cruciate ligament ruptures in female participants. *Am. J. Sports Med.* 37, 2234–2240. doi: 10.1177/0363546509338266

Roffey, J., Rosse, C., Linch, M., Hibbert, A., McDonald, N. Q., and Parker, P. J. (2009). Protein kinase C intervention: the state of play. *Curr. Opin. Cell Biol.* 21, 268–279. doi: 10.1016/j.ceb.2009.01.019

Rosset, E. M., and Bradshaw, A. D. (2016). SPARC/osteonectin in mineralized tissue. *Matrix Biol.* 52–54, 78–87. doi: 10.1016/j.matbio.2016.02.001

Salzer, E., Santos-Valente, E., Klaver, S., Ban, S. A., Emminger, W., Prengemann, N. K., et al. (2013). B-cell deficiency and severe autoimmunity caused by deficiency of protein kinase C delta. *Blood* 121, 3112–3116. doi: 10.1182/blood-2012-10-460741

Sarver, D. C., Kharaz, Y. A., Sugg, K. B., Gumucio, J. P., Comerford, E., and Mendias, C. L. (2017). Sex differences in tendon structure and function. *J. Orthop. Res.* 35, 2117–2126. doi: 10.1002/jor.23516

Shirakura, M., Kram, V., Robinson, J., Sikka, S., Kilts, T. M., Wadhwa, S., et al. (2017). Extracellular matrix mediates BMP-2 in a model of temporomandibular joint osteoarthritis. *Cells Tissues Organs* 204, 84–92. doi: 10.1159/000464102

Sims, N. A., Dupont, S., Krust, A., Clement-Lacroix, P., Minet, D., Resche-Rigon, M., et al. (2002). Deletion of estrogen receptors reveals a regulatory role for estrogen receptors-beta in bone remodeling in females but not in males. *Bone* 30, 18–25. doi: 10.1016/s8756-3282(01)00643-3

Soderstrom, M., Salminen, H., Glumoff, V., Kirschke, H., Aro, H., and Vuorio, E. (1999). Cathepsin expression during skeletal development. *Biochim. Biophys. Acta* 1446, 35–46. doi: 10.1016/s0167-4781(99)00068-8

Sorensen, M. G., Karsdal, M. A., Dziegiel, M. H., Boutin, J. A., Nosjean, O., and Henriksen, K. (2010). Screening of protein kinase inhibitors identifies PKC inhibitors as inhibitors of osteoclastic acid secretion and bone resorption. *BMC Musculoskelet. Disord.* 11:250. doi: 10.1186/1471-2474-11-250

Steinberg, S. F. (2008). Structural basis of protein kinase C isoform function. *Physiol. Rev.* 88, 1341–1378. doi: 10.1152/physrev.00034.2007

Tolar, J., Braunlin, E., Riddle, M., Peacock, B., McElmurry, R. T., Orchard, P. J., et al. (2009). Gender-related dimorphism in aortic insufficiency in murine mucopolysaccharidosis type I. *J. Heart Valve Dis.* 18, 524–529.

Tong, W., Zeng, Y., Chow, D. H. K., Yeung, W., Xu, J., Deng, Y., et al. (2019). Wnt16 attenuates osteoarthritis progression through a PCP/JNK-mTORC1-PTHrP cascade. *Ann. Rheum. Dis.* 78, 551–561. doi: 10.1136/annrheumdis-2018-214200

Tu, X., Joeng, K. S., Nakayama, K. I., Nakayama, K., Rajagopal, J., Carroll, T. J., et al. (2007). Noncanonical Wnt signaling through G protein-linked PKCdelta activation promotes bone formation. *Dev. Cell* 12, 113–127. doi: 10.1016/j.devcel.2006.11.003

Villard, C., Eriksson, P., Swedenborg, J., and Hultgren, R. (2014). Differences in elastin and elastolytic enzymes between men and women with abdominal aortic aneurysm. *Aorta* 2, 179–185. doi: 10.12945/j.aorta.2014.14-017

Wang, C., Steer, J. H., Joyce, D. A., Yip, K. H., Zheng, M. H., and Xu, J. (2003). 12-O-tetradecanoylphorbol-13-acetate (TPA) inhibits osteoclastogenesis by suppressing RANKL-induced NF-kappaB activation. *J. Bone Miner. Res.* 18, 2159–2168. doi: 10.1359/jbmr.2003.18.12.2159

Wang, J., and Stern, P. H. (2011). Sex-specific effects of estrogen and androgen on gene expression in human monocyte-derived osteoclasts. *J. Cell. Biochem.* 112, 3714–3721. doi: 10.1002/jcb.23297

Watts, N. B., Adler, R. A., Bilezikian, J. P., Drake, M. T., Eastell, R., Orwoll, E. S., et al. (2012). Osteoporosis in men: an endocrine society clinical practice guideline. *J. Clin. Endocrinol. Metab.* 97, 1802–1822. doi: 10.1210/jc.2011-3045

Winkeler, C. L., Kladney, R. D., Maggi, L. B. Jr., and Weber, J. D. (2012). Cathepsin K-Cre causes unexpected germline deletion of genes in mice. *PLoS One* 7:e42005. doi: 10.1371/journal.pone.0042005

Yang, D., Guo, J., Divieti, P., and Bringhurst, F. R. (2006). Parathyroid hormone activates PKC-delta and regulates osteoblastic differentiation via a PLC-independent pathway. *Bone* 38, 485–496. doi: 10.1016/j.bone.2005.10.009

Yang, X., Teguh, D., Wu, J. P., He, B., Kirk, T. B., Qin, S., et al. (2015). Protein kinase C delta null mice exhibit structural alterations in articular surface, intra-articular and subchondral compartments. *Arthritis Res. Ther.* 17:210. doi: 10.1186/s13075-015-0720-4

Yao, J., Li, J., Zhou, L., Cheng, J., Chim, S. M., Zhang, G., et al. (2015). Protein kinase C inhibitor, GF109203X attenuates osteoclastogenesis, bone resorption and RANKL-induced NF-kappaB and NFAT activity. *J. Cell. Physiol.* 230, 1235–1242. doi: 10.1002/jcp.24858

Yao, Z., Li, Y., Yin, X., Dong, Y., Xing, L., and Boyce, B. F. (2014). NF-kappaB RelB negatively regulates osteoblast differentiation and bone formation. *J. Bone Miner. Res.* 29, 866–877. doi: 10.1002/jbmr.2108

Zaidi, M. (2007). Skeletal remodeling in health and disease. *Nat. Med.* 13, 791–801. doi: 10.1038/nm1593

# 12

# The Role of Bone-Derived Exosomes in Regulating Skeletal Metabolism and Extraosseous Diseases

*Huili Lyu, Ye Xiao, Qi Guo, Yan Huang and Xianghang Luo**

*Endocrinology Research Center, Department of Endocrinology, Xiangya Hospital of Central South University, Changsha, China*

***Correspondence:***
*Xianghang Luo*
*xianghangluo@sina.com;*
*xianghangluo@hotmail.com*

Bone-derived exosomes are naturally existing nano-sized extracellular vesicles secreted by various cells, such as bone marrow stromal cells, osteoclasts, osteoblasts, and osteocytes, containing multifarious proteins, lipids, and nucleic acids. Accumulating evidence indicates that bone-derived exosomes are involved in the regulation of skeletal metabolism and extraosseous diseases through modulating intercellular communication and the transfer of materials. Following the development of research, we found that exosomes can be considered as a potential candidate as a drug delivery carrier thanks to its ability to transport molecules into targeted cells with high stability, safety, and efficiency. This review aims to discuss the emerging role of bone-derived exosomes in skeletal metabolism and extraosseous diseases as well as their potential role as candidate biomarkers or for developing new therapeutic strategies.

**Keywords: exosome, skeletal metabolism, extraosseous diseases, bone tissue engineering, biomarker**

## THE INTRODUCTION OF EXOSOMES

Exosomes, first discovered in the 1980s, refer to extracellular vesicles with a diameter of 30–100 nm, and they were thought to be involved in the selective release of the transferrin receptor during maturation of sheep reticulocytes (Pan and Johnstone, 1983; Johnstone et al., 1987). Despite existing in reticulocytes, exosomes were found to be released by a variety of other cells, including lymphocytes (Guay et al., 2019), dendritic cells, platelets, mast cells (Cheung et al., 2016), neurons, macrophages (Bourdonnay et al., 2015), mesenchymal stem cells (MSCs), intestinal epithelial cells (IECs), and so on (van Niel et al., 2001; Clayton et al., 2005; Taylor and Gerçel-Taylor, 2005; Raposo and Stoorvogel, 2013). Exosomes initiate formation when the inner membrane of the endosomes bud inwardly to form luminal vesicles, which then transform into multivesicular bodies (MVBs). These MVBs can either be fused with lysosomes to degrade themselves, or they can release vesicles, named exosomes, after fusion with the plasma membranes (**Figure 1**) (Simons and Raposo, 2009). It was indicated that lipids are enriched on the surfaces of exosomes, including cholesterol, sphingomyelin, and ceramides. Furthermore, exosomes contain numerous biological molecules, such as proteins, enzymes, and microRNAs (miRNAs) (Valadi et al., 2007), which mediate intercellular communication and play an important role in the physiological and pathological processes (Kowal et al., 2014; Janas et al., 2015). Exosomes secrete complex

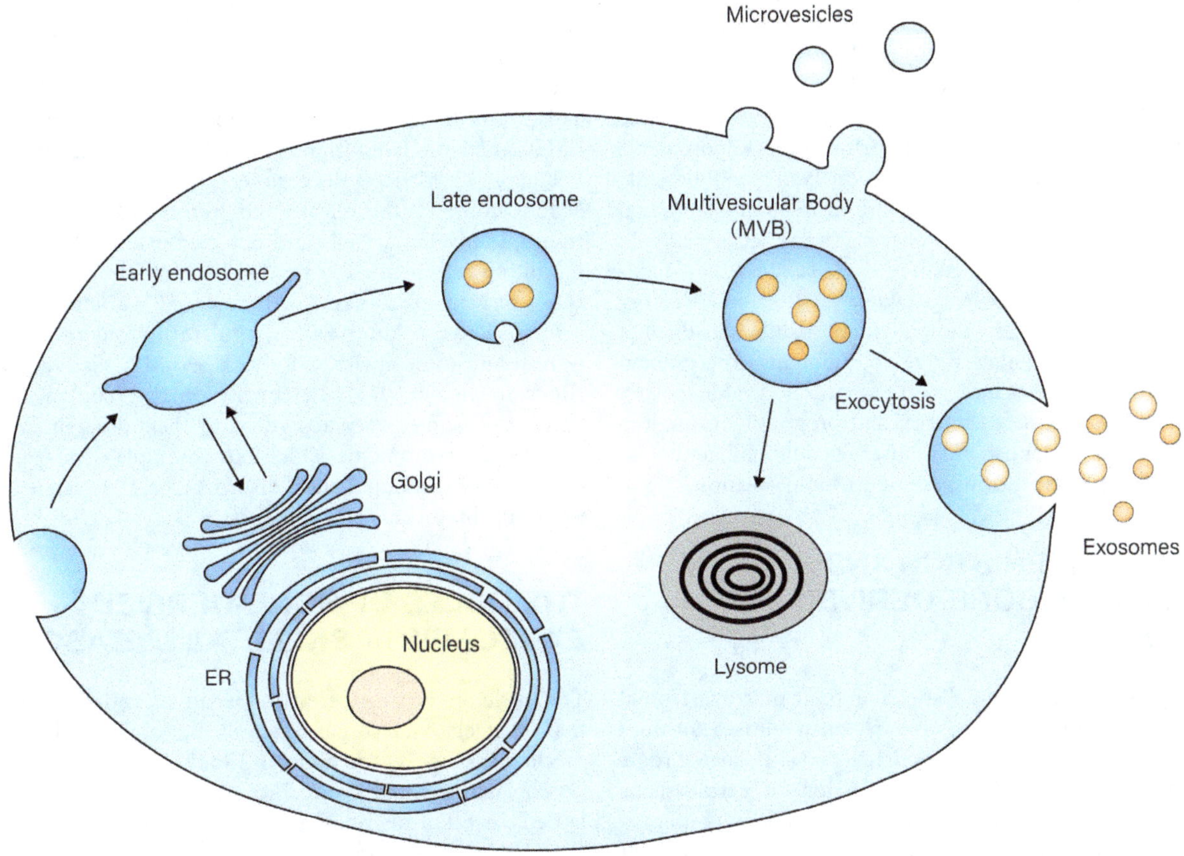


**FIGURE 1 |** Exosome biogenesis and secretion The membrane of the late endosome buds inwardly to form luminal vesicles, which then transform into multi-vesicle bodies (MVBs). MVBs then fuse with the plasma membrane and release vesicles named exosomes into the extracellular space. MVBs can also be fused with lysosomes, and they degrade vesicles inside.

content that depends not only on the cell type but also the microenvironment, such as mechanical properties, cellular PH, biochemical stimuli, and hypoxia (Choudhry and Harris, 2018). While previous research has shown that exosomes originating from different cells contain a specific subset of endosome-related proteins, they are involved in MVE biogenesis (e.g., Alix and Tsg101), membrane transport, and fusion (e.g., Rab GTPases, Annexins, and flotillin) (Colombo et al., 2014); among these actions, ubiquitous proteins like tetraspanins (CD9 and CD81), heat shock proteins (HSP70 and HSP90), and tumor-susceptibility gene 101 (Tsg101) are frequently used as markers of exosomes (Bjørge et al., 2017).

Exosomes have been widely investigated because of their multiple functions in diverse physiological process and diseases. As one of the most important factors in the paracrine regulation mechanism, exosomes can directly participate in signaling communication between cells. Dai et al. (2019) elucidated that prostate cancer (PCa)-derived exosomes could promote tumor growth and premetastatic niche formation in bone through transforming PKM2 into BMSCs. Alveolar macrophages (AMs) were found to secret exosomes containing the SOCS1 protein, which could be taken up by alveolar epithelial cells (AECs) and can inhibit STAT1 activation, leading to downregulation of inflammatory signaling both *in vitro* and *in vivo* (Bourdonnay et al., 2015). In addition, the microvesicles—released from primary lung epithelial cells induced by hyperoxia—containing hnRNPA2B1-associated miRNAs could be delivered into a macrophage and stimulate inflammation (Lee et al., 2019). Taken together, these experiments illustrated the essential role of exosomes in bilateral actions between AMs and AECs. Besides, the FasL-positive microvesicles released by melanoma cells were proven to induce the apoptosis of Jurkat and lymphoid cells, through which a tumor may escape from the effect of the immune system (Andreola et al., 2002). It can be seen that the exosomes derived from multiple cells are able to transfer different molecules, proteins, RNAs, and therefore have a significant effect on recipient cells.

## TECHNIQUES FOR ISOLATING EXOSOMES

To optimally understand and exploit the biological action and clinical application of exosomes, it is essential to isolate them from cell culture supernatants or primary body fluids. The exosomes originate from a wealth of sources, such as whole blood

(Wu et al., 2017), menstrual blood (Dalirfardouei et al., 2018), urine (Street et al., 2017), cerebrospinal fluid (CSF) (Manek et al., 2018), milk (Leiferman et al., 2019), and so on. So far, a series of methods have been developed to isolate exosomes on the basis of size difference, molecular weight, density, certain surface markers, including differential ultracentrifugation (Raposo et al., 1996), density gradient ultracentrifugation (van der Pol et al., 2012), size based filtration, size-exclusion chromatography (Rood et al., 2010), immunoaffinity isolation (Kang et al., 2017), precipitation (Coumans et al., 2017; Li P. et al., 2017), field-flow fractionation (Zhang and Lyden, 2019), and so on. Generally speaking, every isolation technique exhibits its distinct advantages and disadvantages due to different experimental principles. Since exosomes have great potential and value in early clinical diagnosis, disease treatment, and prognosis evaluation, it is imperative to establish more user-friendly, efficient, and reliable technologies for the purpose of exosome isolation.

## THE CHARACTERISTICS AND CONTENTS OF BONE-DERIVED EXOSOMES

In recent years it has been established that bone marrow stromal cells, osteoclasts, osteoblasts, and osteocytes can release exosomes that can not only regulate bone remodeling and skeletal disorders but can also participate in the progression of extraosseous diseases (Liu et al., 2017). Bone-derived exosomes contain a multitude of molecules, such as proteins and nucleic acids, that vary dynamically according to cell types as well as pathological and physiological conditions. In a recent study, researchers detected a total of 1,536 proteins contained in osteoblast-derived exosomes; they found that several valuable proteins involved in membrane trafficking and signaling pathways might be implicated in human bone diseases, including transforming growth factor beta receptor 3 (TGFBR3), lipoprotein receptor-related protein (LRP)6, bone morphogenetic protein receptor type-1 (BMPR1), and smad ubiquitylation regulatory factor-1 (SMURF1) (Ge et al., 2017). In addition, one proteomics profiling of exosomes from primary mouse osteoblasts revealed the difference in content between osteosomes under various differentiation statuses. To be more specific, 10 of the commonly expressed proteins were found to be increased more than five-fold in mineralizing (D24 osteosomes) primary mouse calvarial osteoblasts compared with proliferating osteoblasts (D0 osteosomes) (Bilen et al., 2017). Xu et al. (2014) tried to figure out the physiological role of exosomal miRNAs in osteoblast differentiation; they detected 79 miRNAs ($\sim$8.84%) in exosomes isolated from BMSC culture supernatants and verified the presence of miRNA in exosomes during BMSCs osteogenic differentiation for the first time. Moreover, this study revealed differential expression of 14 exosomal miRNAs during osteogenic differentiation of human BMSCs; nine miRNAs (let-7a, miR-199b, miR-218, miR-148a, miR-135b, miR-203, miR-219, miR-299-5p, and miR-302b) were upregulated, and four miRNAs (miR-221, miR-155, miR-885-5p, miR-181a, and miR-320c) were downregulated (Xu et al., 2014). Another research study demonstrated that BMSC-derived exosomes could significantly reverse either S100- or LPS/ATP-induced injury in mice and hepatocytes. However, these protective effects were partly abolished with the involvement of the miR-223 inhibitor. This study firstly revealed the role of miRNA transferred by BMSCs-exo on liver injury caused by autoimmune hepatitis (Chen et al., 2018). Roccaro et al. (2013) found that BM-MSCs promoted the release and transfer of exosomes to MM (multiple myeloma) cells and detected a lower level of tumor-inhibiting factor miR-15a in MM BM-MSC versus normal BM-MSC-derived exosomes. Furthermore, a variety of oncogenic proteins and cytokines, which regulate adhesion and migration, were found to be enriched in MM BM-MSC-derived exosomes (Roccaro et al., 2013). In conclusion, the contents of bone-derived exosomes vary according to their different originators and microenvironments, which exert multiple effects on a serious of diseases, including skeletal disorders, prostate cancer, multiple myeloma, breast cancer, and so on.

## THE ROLES OF BONE-DERIVED EXOSOMES IN SKELETAL METABOLISM

The skeleton is considered to be an essential support organ that protects vital organs, stores minerals, and provides a mechanical bracket for body and movement (Han et al., 2018). Osteoblast-mediated bone formation and osteoclast-mediated bone resorption maintain a dynamic balance through signaling proteins, such as asephrin-Eph, which bone remodeling process occurs throughout the lifespan to ensure the integrity of the skeleton and its multiple functions (Zhao et al., 2006; Suchacki et al., 2017). It has also been proposed that osteocytes play essential roles in bone remodeling by affecting the activities of osteoblasts and osteoclasts (Tatsumi et al., 2007).

The molecular regulation mechanism of bone remolding is affected by many factors, such as age (Ambrogini et al., 2010), genes, proteins (Ishijima et al., 2001), hormone levels (Hayashi et al., 2019), enzymes (Jin et al., 2014), amino acids (Yu et al., 2019), and cytokines (Wang et al., 2015). For example, the bone-resorbing activity of osteoclasts was negatively regulated by a signal transducer and activator of transcription 5 (Stat5), which performs its functions through suppressing MAPK activity via regulation of Dusp1 and Dusp2 (Hirose et al., 2014). Researchers found that sphingosine-1-phosphate (S1P) is able to mediate the location of osteoclast (OC) precursors (OPs) between bone and blood through its receptors, and thereby influence the osteoclastogenesis and bone remolding (Ishii et al., 2010). Glucocorticoids are shown to induce bone loss through inhibiting osteoblast function and differentiation by targeting glucocorticoid receptors and suppressing AP-1-dependent cytokines (Rauch et al., 2010). Greenblatt et al. (2015) also found a key regulator of bone turnover—charged multivesicular body protein 5 (CHMP5); it can suppress the RANK-induced NF-κB signaling in osteoclasts and thereby dampen osteoclast differentiation.

An imbalance in bone metabolism regulation can lead to many diseases, including osteoporosis, which is characterized by age-related bone loss and increased fat formation (Moerman et al., 2004), high bone mass (HBM) resulting from abnormally increased bone formation (Yang et al., 2019), osteoarthritis, which is marked by progressive degeneration of articular cartilage (Rahmati et al., 2017), and so on. For example, the follicle-stimulating hormone (FSH) could promote activation of osteoclasts and enhance bone resorption through several signaling pathways, such as NF-kB, thus leading to a high risk of osteoporosis associated with menopause (Sponton and Kajimura, 2017). In recent years, scholars have made remarkable progress in the study of bone remodeling and related diseases as well as the role exosomes play in bone remolding, and this is attracting more and more attention.

## BMSC-Derived Exosomes

There is a class of stromal stem cells with the capacity for autologous renewal in bone marrow named BMSCs. They can differentiate into osteoblasts, chondrocytes, and adipocytes (Fan et al., 2017; Li et al., 2018), and they can thereby influence bone formation, maintenance, and reconstruction (Nakajima et al., 2018). Emerging evidence suggests that BMSCs have the ability to repair bone tissue damage and promote bone regeneration, but the specific mechanism involved in this has not been clarified. It has been reported that transplanted MSCs are not able to exist *in vivo* permanently, but the therapy effect still persists even after MSCs elimination. Recently, scientists have found that this bone-protective effect may be related to paracrine vesicles, much like exosomes secreted by BMSC (Ng et al., 2015).

One study revealed that exosomes isolated from bone-marrow-derived MSCs could rescue the retardation of fracture healing in $CD9^{-/-}$ mice. The mechanism in this process is more than the recruitment of stem cells or progenitor cells by cytokines, but it also involves the induction of osteogenesis and angiogenesis partly regulated by exosomal miRNAs (Furuta et al., 2016). Fang et al. (2019) demonstrated that BMSC Exos significantly reverse the decreased osteogenic differentiation of BMSCs in steroid-induced femoral head necrosis (SFHN), and they then detected a total of 84 genes and 20 differentially expressed genes (DEGs), which consist of 11 upregulated and nine downregulated genes. Among these, DEGs, Bmps, Mmp9, and Sox9, which are related to regulating the immune system processes and the BMP/TGF-β pathway, may play important roles in the pathogenetic process of SFHN (Fang et al., 2019).

The exosomes' potential osteogenic capacity in bone regeneration was declared by Narayanan et al. (2016). They performed a series of studies to investigate how osteogenic exosomes derived from HMSCs could be endocytosed by primary HMSCs and could upregulate the expression of BMP9 and TGF-β1, which are both potent molecules in osteogenic differentiation (Luther et al., 2011; Kuroda et al., 2012). In addition, the *in vivo* experiments also indicated that both the regular exosomes and osteogenic exosomes can promote the osteogenic differentiation of HMSCs and matrix mineralization, while the osteogenic exosomes have a higher potential to induce better vascularization and calcium phosphate nucleation (Narayanan et al., 2016). Qin et al. (2016) found that exosomes isolated from BMSCs could be internalized into osteoblasts and enhance the expression of osteogenic genes. To investigate the mechanism by which exosomes promote osteogenic differentiation, they detected the miRNA in exosomes by miRNA sequencing and found highly expressed miR-27a, miR-206a, and miR-196a, among which miR-196a has the greatest potential in functional testing (Qin et al., 2016). Liu et al. (2015) indicated that transplantation of BMMSCs could rescue osteopenia in Fas-deficient-MRL/lpr mice through secreting exosomes, which were found to transfer Fas to recipient MRL/lpr BMMSCs, reduce their miR29b levels, enhance osteogenic differentiation *in vitro*, and promote bone formation *in vivo*.

Despite the critical effect in bone remolding, several studies have confirmed that BMSC-derived exosomes have the ability to reduce cartilage destruction and promote cartilage repair (Pourakbari et al., 2019). Osteoarthritis (OA) is a kind of rheumatic disease characterized by degeneration of articular cartilage and osteophyte formation (Findlay and Kuliwaba, 2016), and previous research has suggested that bone marrow-derived MSCs could be applied to treating OA and cartilage lesions in animals and humans (Nejadnik et al., 2010; Xie et al., 2012). Recently, accumulating evidence has implied that exosomes isolated from BMSCs function as vital media to elicit protective responses in cartilage. Cosenza et al. (2017) identified that BM-MSCs-derived exosomes could protect cartilage and bone from degradation through reducing apoptosis of chondrocytes, inhibiting macrophage activation, and promoting polarization of the M2 macrophage. Toh et al. (2017) proposed that the mechanism through which MSC exosomes modulate cartilage repair might rely on their ability to restore homeostasis in bioenergetics, cell number, and immunoregulation. Researchers addressed how MSCs are able to secrete miRNA-enriched exosomes to facilitate intercellular communication (Chen et al., 2010), and it is thus reasonable to conclude that exosomal miRNAs may be essential in cartilage differentiation. For instance, exosomal miRNA-23b could induce chondrogenic differentiation of hMSCs via inhibiting the expression of target PKA (Ham et al., 2012). Besides, Ning et al. (2013) found that miR-92a deficiency could cause a reduced number of chondrogenic progenitors, impaired chondrogenic differentiation, and pharyngeal cartilage defects in zebrafish. The mechanisms involved in the effect of miR-92a on chondrogenic differentiation rely on its regulation of Bmp signaling through targeting nog3 mRNA (Ning et al., 2013).

## Osteoclast-Derived Exosomes

Osteoclasts are giant multinucleated cells originating from mononuclear macrophage precursor cells, and they are mainly responsible for bone resorption *in vivo* (Nevius et al., 2015). Osteoclasts participate in the occurrence and development of many bone diseases, such as osteoporosis (Novack, 2007; Hsu et al., 2011), rheumatoid arthritis, and so on. Sun et al. (2016) showed that osteoclasts could secrete miR-214-containing exosomes, which are transferred into osteoblasts via ephrinA2/EphA2 recognition to inhibit osteoblast function (**Figure 2**). Besides, the level of miR-214 is measured to be higher in the serum exosomes of osteoporotic patients and mice compared with healthy ones, which might be a potential

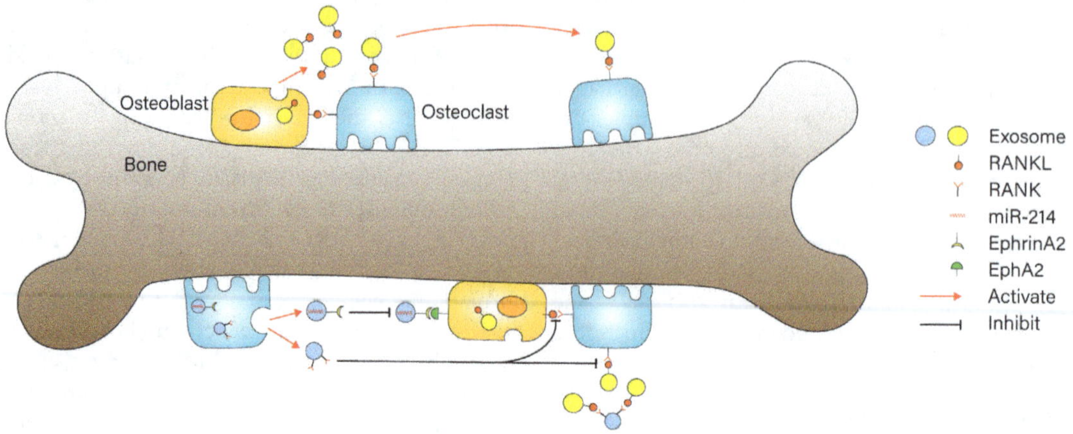


**FIGURE 2** | Exosome-mediated communication between osteoblasts and osteoclasts Osteoblast-derived exosomes containing RANKL could stimulate osteoclast differentiation through binding to RANK on the surface of osteoclasts. RNAK-enriched exosomes from osteoclasts competitively bind to RANKL and prevent activation of the RANK signaling pathway in osteoclasts. miR-214-containing exosomes from osteoclasts could be transferred into osteoblasts via ephrinA2/EphA2 recognition to inhibit osteoblast function.

biomarker for osteoporosis (Sun et al., 2016). Moreover, the work of Zhao et al. (2015) demonstrated that miR-214 plays a catalytic role during RANKL-induced osteoclast differentiation through the PI3K/Akt signaling pathway by targeting phosphatase and tensin homolog (Pten). They also established Acp5-miR-214 transgenic (OC-TG214) mice to explore the effect of miR214 *in vivo*, and the results indicated that the upregulation of miR-214 in osteoclasts induced lower levels of Pten protein, higher activity of osteoclast bone resorbing, and poorer bone mineral density (BMD) (Zhao et al., 2015). Researchers tested the regulation of osteoclast formation in 1,25$(OH)_2D_3$-stimulated mouse marrow; they firstly found that osteoclast precursor-derived exosomes significantly stimulated formation of osteoclasts, while exosomes from mature osteoclasts suppressed osteoclastogenesis. Next, the presence of enriched RANK was found in exosomes from osteoclasts. The RANK depletion of osteoclast-derived exosomes reduced their effect of inhibiting osteoclastogenesis. These results revealed that RNAK contained in exosomes might be the active agent that competitively binds to RANKL and prevents stimulation of the RANK signaling pathway in osteoclasts, and it thus plays a greater inhibitory role in osteoclastogenesis (**Figure 2**) (Huynh et al., 2016). Li et al. (2016) delineated the role of exosomal miR-214-3p in the intercellular communication between osteoclasts and osteoblasts, which could be transferred from osteoclasts to osteoblasts to inhibit osteoblastic bone formation. More importantly, osteoclast-targeted inhibition miR-214-3p effectively reversed the suppression of osteoblast activity and facilitated bone formation, and this is suggestive of which might be a potential therapeutic method for bone loss (Li et al., 2016).

## Osteoblast-Derived Exosomes

Osteoblasts are derived from bone marrow MSCs with multidirectional differentiation potential, and they play a critical role in the synthesis, secretion, and mineralization of the bone matrix through its capacity to secrete glycoprotein and collagen. BMSCs first differentiate into osteoprogenitor cells, then turn into osteoblast precursors, and finally transform into osteoblasts (Garg et al., 2017), and this process is regulated by miRNAs (Li et al., 2009), proteins (Zou et al., 2013), signaling pathways, and so on. One *in vitro* research conducted by Cui et al. (2016) demonstrated the intercellular positive feedback mechanism between mineralizing osteoblasts (MOBs) and bone marrow stromal cells (ST2 cells). Their experiment results indicated that MOB-derived exosomes could be incorporated into ST2 cells and significantly promote their osteogenic differentiation; during this process, 91 miRNAs were detected as being overexpressed and 182 miRNAs were downregulated. Additionally, the analysis of the targeting genes and pathway networks of these miRNAs revealed that the pro-osteogenic function of MOBs-derived exosomes may partially depend on activation of the Wnt signaling pathway through downregulating Axin1 expression and upregulating β-catenin expression (Cui et al., 2016). Ge et al. (2017) identified 1,536 proteins in osteoblast-derived exosomes and sorted out several pivotal proteins that are closely related to bone diseases through network and pathway analyses. Deng et al. (2015) indicated that osteoblast-derived microvesicles can transfer RANKL proteins into osteoclast precursors and promote their differentiation into osteoclasts through activating RANKL–RANK signaling, which revealed a new mechanism involved in communication between osteoblasts and osteoclasts (**Figure 2**). Then, they conducted a series of experiments to further explore the role of microvesicles in bone metabolism by using imipramine, which was found to block microvesicles generation (Bianco et al., 2009). The *in vitro* results showed that inhibition of microvesicles generation from osteoblasts leads to significant suppression of osteoclast differentiation. Besides, the *in vivo* experiments revealed that OVX mice treated with imipramine exhibit superior properties in bone mineral density, bone volume, trabecular number, and thickness, suggesting that imipramine could prevent progression of bone loss caused by estrogen deficiency due to its function of blocking microvesicles generation (Deng et al., 2017). Through literature review and analysis, Xie et al. (2017) summarized the role of a number of mineralizing MC3T3 cell-derived exosomes in bone remolding. To be specific, miR-30d-5p, miR-133b-3p, and miR-140-3p were found to inhibit osteoblast differentiation, while let-7, miR-335-3p, miR-378b can promote osteoblast differentiation (Xie et al., 2017).

### Osteocyte-Derived Exosomes

Bone tissue is formed by the bone matrix and osteocytes originating from osteoblasts, which are widely distributed in the bone matrix and are tightly connected through the bone lacuna–tubule network system (Bonewald, 2007). Sato et al. firstly indicated the relationship between osteocyte exosomes and circulating exosomes in the serum. It was hinted that 12 miRNAs levels were significantly decreased in the circulating exosomes of OL (osteocyte less) mice plasma in contrast with control mice plasma. Therefore, it could be concluded that osteocytes release exosomes containing specific miRNAs that are transferred into circulating (Sato et al., 2017). The osteocyte-derived exosomes have been proven to mediate muscle–bone communication, and Qin et al. (2017) established that osteocyte-derived exosomes, which express the downregulation of miR-218 after myostatin treatment, can be incorporated into ostoblastic cells and suppress osteoblastic differentiation through downregulation of Wnt signaling; this can be reversed by expression of exogenous miR-218, suggesting the therapeutic potential of miR-218 in osteocytes for the treatment of bone disorders. In addition, the work of Zhang et al. (2014) confirmed the relationship between miR-218 and Wnt/β-catenin signaling in the osteogenic differentiation of human adipose tissue-derived stem cells (hASCs). Their *in vitro* experiments elucidated that overexpression of miR-218 activates the Wnt signaling pathway via directly downregulating SFRP2/DKK2 levels and then promotes hASCs osteogenic differentiation, whereas upregulation of Wnt/β-catenin signal can enhance the expression of miR-218 (Zhang et al., 2014). It has been proven that Wnt signaling acts as a positive regulator in osteoblast differentiation and regulation of bone mass (Esen et al., 2013). Taken together, miR-218 functions as a signal amplifier in the complex feed-forward regulatory circuit to activate hASCs osteogenic differentiation (Zhang et al., 2014), which further demonstrated the potential application prospect of exosomal miR-218 in bone regeneration.

## THE EFFECT OF BONE-DERIVED EXOSOMES IN EXTRAOSSEOUS DISEASES

Recent studies have shown that bone-derived exosomes not only participate in regulating bone remodeling in the bone microenvironment but also act as vital communication media in multiple biological processes, including antigen presentation, apoptosis, inflammation, cancer progression, and so on (Gurunathan et al., 2019). As a result, the multiple roles of bone-derived exosomes in distant tissues and extraosseous systems attracted much attention.

### Role of Bone-Derived Exosomes in Cancer

So far, people have tried many ways to explore the mechanism of cancer and conquer oncotherapy. There is no denying that we have a deeper understanding of cancer in multiple areas, such as immune responses (Fritz and Lenardo, 2019), inflammation (Ritter and Greten, 2019), lipid metabolism (Snaebjornsson et al., 2020), and so on, but there is still no proper method that could cure cancer without side effects. It is therefore interesting that bone-derived exosomes were found to participate in the progression of cancer in terms of regulating gene expression, angiogenesis, migration, and proliferation. The work of Naseri et al. (2018) indicated that BMSCs-derived exosomes (MSCs-Exo), which are loaded with LNA-anti-miR-142-3p, can deliver their cargos into 4T1 and TUBO breast cancer cells—leading to downregulation of miR-142-3p and overexpression of tumor suppressor genes—and thereby exert an efficient anti-tumor function. Additionally, their *in vivo* experiments revealed that the mice treated with LNA-miR-142-3p inhibitor-loaded MSCs-Exos showed reduced tumor volume and growth rate. These results confirmed the efficiency of transferring anti-miR molecules like LNA-anti-miR-142-3p into target tissues via MSCs-Exos and also provided new outlooks in terms of oncotherapy (Naseri et al., 2018). In another study, researchers explored how exosomes isolated from human bone marrow mesenchymal stem cells (hBMSCs) can promote migration and proliferation of osteosarcoma and gastric cancer cells through activating the Hedgehog signaling pathway (Qi et al., 2017). Additionally, it is reported that the Hedgehog signaling pathway, an essential regulator in maintaining tissue polarity and cell differentiation, plays a significant role in multiple cancers, including most basal cell carcinomas (BCCs) and extracutaneous tumors (Yang et al., 2010). Bliss et al. (2016) tried to investigate the mechanisms by which MSCs communicate with BCCs (breast cancer cells) and promote dormancy of human breast cancer cells in bone marrow. They demonstrated that MSCs primed by cancer cells can release exosomes containing miR-222/223, which in turn favor their survival and enhance drug resistance. Moreover, the treatment of MSCs transfected with anti-miR222/223 facilitated chemosensitivity of dormant BCCs in mice (Bliss et al., 2016).

Zhu et al. (2012) figured out another mechanism by which BMSCs-derived exosomes promote tumor growth *in vivo*. They detected higher expression of VEGF and CXCR4 in tumor cells treated with BMSC-exosomes, suggesting that BMSC-exosomes could enhance angiogenesis and provide tumors with a richer blood supply and therefore promote their proliferation and growth. However, the results of another experiment are different from these. Bruno et al. (2013) found that human hepatocellular carcinoma cells (HepG2), human ovarian cancer cells (Skov-3), and Kaposi's sarcoma cells incubated with BMSC-derived microvesicles exhibited lower proliferation ability, higher expression of negative regulators of the cell cycle, and an increased number of cells staying in the G0/G1 phase. They also observed the effect of microvesicles on growth of implanted tumors in mice, and the data indicated that BMSC-derived microvesicles could inhibit tumor growth and increase necrosis areas in tumors (Bruno et al., 2013). These opposing conclusions could be derived due to the occasion of MSCs or microvesicles treatment (Klopp et al., 2011). The injection of BMSC-derived extracellular vesicles (EVs) into established tumors could inhibit tumor growth, while the growth of tumors in the early stages treated with EVs could be facilitated.

## Role of Bone-Derived Exosomes in Neurologic Diseases

Researchers demonstrated that exosomes isolated from MSCs can mediate the transfer of miR-133b into astrocytes and neurons, inducing increased axonal plasticity and neurite remodeling in the ischemic boundary zone (IBZ), and thereby lead to functional recovery in rats subjected to middle cerebral artery occlusion (MCAo) (Xin et al., 2012, 2013). Besides, miR-133b + MSC treatment dramatically downregulated the expression of the connective tissue growth factor (CTGF) and the Ras homolog gene family member A (RhoA) (Xin et al., 2013), which are relevant to central nervous system (CNS) repair, post-injury restructuring (Hertel et al., 2000) and regulation of axonogenesis (Hall and Lalli, 2010). In another study, Nakano et al. (2016) found that rat BM-MSC-derived exosomes can ameliorate learning and memory impairment in STZ-diabetic mice through suppressing oxidative stress and recovering decreased synapse numbers, and this process might rely on the internalization of exosomes into astrocytes and neurons, causing recovery of damaged astrocytes and neurons. To further investigate the specific miRNAs or proteins that participated in improving diabetes-induced cognitive impairment, they conducted a series of experiments. The results proposed that the oversecretion of exosomal miR-146a due to endogenous bone marrow-derived MSCs within the condition of an enriched environment (EE) plays a key role in restraining astrocytic inflammation and preventing cognitive impairment in diabetic rats (Kubota et al., 2018). Mead and Tomarev (2017) demonstrated that BMSC-derived exosomes can be efficiently integrated into target retinal ganglion cells (RGC), thus promoting the recovery of the RGC function followed by optic nerve crush (ONC) through enhanced regeneration of RGC axons and inhibiting RGC loss in an miRNA-dependent manner. It is worth mentioning that the neuroprotective effect of BMSC-derived exosomes on RGC after ONC is significantly more potent than simple BMSC treatment (Mead et al., 2013; Mesentier-Louro et al., 2014), and this is probably due to their capacity to integrate into the retina and retain high doses. In conclusion, BMSC-derived exosomes exert a significant effect on promoting nerve repair and functional recovery, indicating their potential in the field of regeneration and remodeling of nervous system (Qing et al., 2018).

## Role of Bone-Derived Exosomes in Nephropathy

It has been reported in previous researches that BM-MSCs play a key role in protecting kidney from injury (Morigi and De Coppi, 2014), although the mechanisms are not entirely elucidated. Recently, several reports have demonstrated the critical roles of BM-MSC-derived exosomes in renal injury. Wang et al. (2019b) elucidated that BMSC exosomes protect renal tubular epithelial cells (NRK-52E) against apoptosis caused by ischemia reperfusion at the early reperfusion stage through transfer of exosomal miR-199a-5p from BMSCs into NRK-52E, leading to the suppression of endoplasmic reticulum (ER) stress in target cells by targeting the binding immunoglobulin protein (BIP) (Wang et al., 2019b). In another experiment, exosomes derived from MSC-CM were found to play a significant role in preventing diabetic nephropathy by inhibiting apoptosis of tubular epithelial cells (TECs) and reversing decreased tight junction protein ZO-1, thereby enhancing the barrier function of renal tubules (Nagaishi et al., 2016). In the model of kidney injury induced by ischemia reperfusion, BMSC-derived exosomes could inhibit the apoptosis of tubular cells and enhance their proliferation, thus protecting the kidney against AKI and CKD (Gatti et al., 2011).

Bruno et al. (2009) reported that the incorporation of exosomes isolated from bone marrow MSCs into tubular epithelial cells (TECs) can exert proliferative and antiapoptotic effects *in vitro* and significantly alleviate lesions of glycerol-induced AKI in SCID mice. Moreover, they provided evidence that the effects mentioned above were completely abolished by RNase treatment, indicating that the horizontal transfer of mRNAs contained in exosomes appears to be a requirement of their protective functions (Bruno et al., 2009). Similarly, one study revealed that BM-MSC-derived exosomes have a positive effect on renal PTECs (proximal tubular epithelial cells) after ATP depletion injury, which could inhibit PTECs apoptosis and enhance transespithelial resistance (TER), at least partly, via miRNAs transfer or through transcription modulation stimulated by exosomes. The GO analysis of modulated miRNAs confirmed that several upregulated genes in the condition of ATP depletion injury were suppressed after exosome treatment, including SHC1 (Src homology 2 domain containing transforming protein 1), caspase-3, caspase-7, and SMAD4 (SMAD family member 4) genes (Lindoso et al., 2014).

## Role of Bone-Derived Exosomes in Cardiac Diseases

Previous studies have proposed that BMSCs can protect cardiomyocytes from apoptosis and prevent LV (left ventricular) remodeling after MI through paracrine signaling (Uemura et al., 2006), suggesting the potential role of BMSCs in cardiac diseases. Researchers have carried out numerous experiments to investigate the underlying mechanism involved in their cardioprotective effects. Recent studies turned to focus on exosomes which are known as key transporters of paracrine factors (Gartz and Strande, 2018) and revealed the emerging role of exosomes as candidate for treatment of cardiac diseases. One research completed by Ma et al. (2018) confirmed that BMSC-derived exosomes loaded with miR-132 could be taken up by HUVECs (Human umbilical venous endothelial cells), causing overexpression of miR-132 in HUVECs, and they could thereby enhance angiogenesis *in vitro* and promote recovery of cardiac function in an AMI (acute myocardial infarction) model. To clarify the mechanism by which miR-132 exosomes modulate angiogenesis, they further measured miR-132 target gene RASA1 (Lei et al., 2015). Their data indicated that downregulated RASA1, in response to increased miR-132, can stimulate neovascularization and maintain the cardiac function *in vivo* (Ma et al., 2018). Feng et al. (2014) demonstrated that BMSC-derived exosomes could mediate the transfer of highly expressed miR-22 in the condition of ischemic preconditioning (IPC) from BMSCs into cardiomyocytes, leading to reduced apoptosis and cardiac fibrosis after myocardial infarction by downregulating the expression level of target Mecp2. Shao et al. (2017) compared the efficiency of bone marrow-derived MSCs and MSC-Exo in myocardial infarction recovery for the first time. The results displayed that MSC-Exo gained an advantage over MSCs in preserving myocardial function after infarction through inhibiting inflammation, suppressing fibrosis, promoting proliferation, and reducing apoptosis. Moreover, the sequencing analysis of miRNA indicated that MSC-Exo and MSCs possessed a similar miRNA profile, including downregulated miR-130, miR-378, and miR-34 as well as upregulated miR-29 and miR-24, suggesting that MSC-Exo could be considered as the replacement for MSCs to develop innovative therapies for myocardial infarction.

### Role of Bone-Derived Exosomes in Cutaneous Repair

During the cutaneous repair process, a variety of cells, growth factors, and the extracellular matrix cooperate to replace dead cells and reconstruct damaged tissues, in which the proliferation of fibroblasts, angiogenesis, skin cell proliferation, and re-epithelization are extremely critical (Wu et al., 2018). In a study conducted by McBride et al. (2017), Wnt3a was detected as being tethered with human BM-MSC exosomes exteriorly. Their *in vitro* results further implied that BM-MSC exosomes significantly promoted dermal fibroblast proliferation, migration, and angiogenesis, which simulative function depends heavily on CD63+ exosomes and Wnt co-receptor lipoprotein-related proteins (LRP6) (McBride et al., 2017). Shabbir et al. (2015) found that BM-MSC exosomes can be incorporated into fibroblasts and stimulate their growth and migration in a normal and diabetic chronic wound; they could also be uptaken by HUVEC cells and enhanced endothelial angiogenesis *in vitro*. Furthermore, BM-MSC exosomes can activate several pathways that play important roles in skin wound healing, such as AKT, ERK 1/2, and STAT3, and enhance the expression of various growth factors (Shabbir et al., 2015). Considering the important role of STAT3 signaling in wound healing (Dauer et al., 2005), they further investigated the content of exosomes and finally found STAT3 DNA binding activity in BMSC-derived exosomes.

### Role of Bone-Derived Exosomes in Metabolic Diseases

Nowadays, patients suffering from metabolic diseases are increasingly widespread through the world, including diabetes, obesity, hyperlipidemia, and so on (Ling and Rönn, 2019; Warshauer et al., 2020). Dysfunction of metabolism is found to greatly promote the occurrence and progression of these diseases (Newgard, 2017). For example, it is already known that the function of the pancreatic islet α cell is extremely important to glucostasis, and researchers have demonstrated that the a kind of pancreatic lncRNA called Paupar could activate Pax6 α-cell target genes and help to maintain glucose homeostasis; the deletion of Paupar in mice resulted in damaged α-cell function (Singer et al., 2019). Recently, researchers have demonstrated that exosomes isolated from BM-MSCs in aged mice could be incorporated into adipocytes, myocytes, and hepatocytes and reduce their insulin sensitivity through targeting SIRT1 (sirtuin 1). They also conducted miRNA microarray analysis and detected extremely high expression of miR-29b- 3p in exosomes from BM-MSCs of old mice. The injection of nanocomplexes mediating BM-MSCs-specific inhibition of miR-29b-3p could alleviate the aging-associated insulin resistance in mice, suggesting the potential therapeutic role of exosomal miR-29b-3p in aging-associated insulin resistance (Su et al., 2019).

## BONE-DERIVED EXOSOMES AS A SOURCE OF BIOMARKERS FOR DISEASE DIAGNOSIS

The content in exosomes are alterative according to the physiological and pathological state of cells; exosomes can thus reflect the physiological condition and disease development to some extent. For example, researchers analyzed human plasma EV proteomes in rest and exercise, and they found 322 differently expressed proteins, suggesting transient release of EVs into circulation in the condition of exercise (Whitham et al., 2018). Besides, exosomes can be easily collected because of their existence in blood, urine, milk, and so on (Mori et al., 2019). In previous studies, researchers have discovered the clinical value of miRNAs as potential biomarkers in some diseases. For example, the contents of two miRNAs that are elevated during osteoclastogenesis, miR16 and miR378, are found to be correspondingly higher in mice with a heavy bone metastatic tumor burden or in breast cancer patients, suggesting their potential as indicators for bone metastasis progression (Eii et al., 2013). At present, the proteins and nucleic acids contained in exosomes have been widely researched for their potential as biomarkers in clinical disease diagnosis (Wang et al., 2018).

Sato et al. (2017) firstly revealed the positive correlation between osteocytes and 12 miRNAs contained in circulating plasma exosomes, suggesting that osteocytes released exosomes that then transferred into blood. Muntión et al. (2016) isolated BM-MSC-derived exosomes from MDS patients and healthy donors (HD) and then performed microRNA expression arrays. The results demonstrated that 21 microRNAs in exosomes from MDS patients were overexpressed compared with HDs, among which the microR-10a and miR-15a were extremely high (Muntión et al., 2016). In MM patients, BMSCs release exosomes and deliver them into MM cells to regulate tumor progression. Compared with normal humans, exosomes isolated from patients' BMSCs contain lower levels of tumor suppressor gene miR-15a and higher levels of oncogenic proteins, cytokines, and adhesion molecules (Roccaro et al., 2013). It has also been reported that elevated serum exosomal miR-214-3p is closely associated with reduced bone formation in elderly women with fractures and OVX mice, suggesting that there is great potential for the use of exosomal miR-214-3p in the diagnosis of osteoporosis (Li et al., 2016). Barrera-Ramirez et al. (2017) compared miRNA profiling of hMSC-derived exosomes from patients with acute myeloid leukemia (AML) patients and healthy people. They identified five differentially expressed miRNAs, including upregulated miR-26a-5p and miR-101-3p as well as downregulated miR-23b-5p, miR-339-3p, and miR-425-5p in AML-derived samples (Barrera-Ramirez et al., 2017); these candidate miRNAs might serve as biomarkers of AML and provide new insight into the pathogenesis and treatment of AML.

In addition, exosomes can be used as markers of diseases progression. Researchers reported exosome profiling in human ES (exudative seroma) for the first time, which was obtained from the lymphatic drainage implanted after lymphadenectomy in melanoma patients. They found that ES-derived exosomes have richer proteins compared with serum derived exosomes, including HSP90B, Annexin A1, and S100 A4, which are related to antigen presentation, the ER–phagosome pathway, and G2/M transition. In comparison with N1a patients, the number of ES-derived exosomes as well as the proteins associated with melanoma tumor cells significantly increased. Finally, they detected BRAFV600E mutation in ES-derived exosomal nucleic acids, which could serve as a factor to evaluate the risk of relapse in patients (García-Silva et al., 2019). In addition, Broggi et al. (2019) also analyzed the lymphatic exudate of metastatic melanoma patients undergoing lymphadenectomy (LAN) and demonstrated that exosomes carrying melanoma-related miRNAs or proteins could be applied as indicators of nodal metastatic spread.

## APPLICATION OF MSC-DERIVED EXOSOMES IN BONE TISSUE ENGINEERING

Many clinical diseases can lead to bone defects and reduced bone formation, including fractures (Matsumoto et al., 2010), bone tumors (Waning et al., 2019), osteoporosis (Cao et al., 2012), and so on. The commonly used treatments, such as bone transplantation, are still very limited. How to promote bone formation and repair bone defects has therefore always been a challenge faced by clinicians. Based on the cytobiology and materialogy, bone tissue engineering—now a significant research problem—is focused on promoting bone tissue regeneration by using seed cells, biological scaffolds, and bioactive factors (Bose et al., 2012). Previous studies have reported the important role MSCs play in repairing damaged organs and tissues through multiple mechanisms (Caplan and Dennis, 2006; Cao et al., 2012). BMSCs are most commonly used cells in stem cell researches due to their abundant sources and convenient separation methods (Morikawa et al., 2009). Recently scientists found that MSC-derived exosomes—the microvesicles mediating intercellular communication—have great potential in bone tissue engineering.

Zhang et al. demonstrated that MSC-Exosome/β-TCP complex scaffolds have a better repair effect on rat skull defects in comparison with pure β-TCP scaffolds. They found that the MSC-Exosomes could be internalized into HMBSs and promote their proliferation, migration, and differentiation *in vitro*. They then examined the gene expression in hBMSCs induced by exosomes, and the results suggested that the underlying mechanism by which exosomes stimulate osteogenic differentiation partly rely on the activation of the PI3K/Akt pathway (Zhang et al., 2016). Qi et al. (2016) indicated that hiPSC-MSC-Exos could upregulate the expression of RUNX2, COL1, and ALP and activate the differentiation of osteoblasts *in vitro*. They also conducted an *in vivo* experiment in mice with calvarial defects, and the results showed that hiPSC-MSC-Exos could stimulate bone formation in osteoporotic conditions. Moreover, the three-dimensional micro-CT images showed higher neovascularization in β-TCP + Exos group compared with β-TCP group. Taken together, these works suggested the potential application of MSC-Exos + β-TCP scaffolds in bone defects due to their effect of facilitating angiogenesis and osteogenesis (Qi et al., 2016). In another study, researchers produced two same-sized calvarial bone defects in SD rats and treated them with hydrogel and hydrogel + exosomes; the results showed that exosomes from BMSCs could significantly enhance the bone formation in rats in the aspects of micro-CT, histological examinations, HE, and Masson staining (Qin et al., 2016).

In addition to bone remodeling, angiogenesis is also extremely important for the maintenance of bone homeostasis and bone regeneration (Saran et al., 2014; Xie et al., 2014). Angiogenesis refers to the formation of blood vessels from microvascular endothelial cells through budding, bridging, and microvascular fusion, all of which aid the transportation of necessary oxygen, nutrients, and inorganic salts to bone via extensive networks (Adams and Alitalo, 2007). Previous studies have reported that MSCs-derived exosomes play a role in promoting angiogenesis in heart (Bian et al., 2014), renal injury, cutaneous repair (Zhang et al., 2015), skeletal muscle regeneration (Nakamura et al., 2015), limb ischemia repair, and so on. Likewise, in the process of fracture healing, new blood vessels can provide nutritional support, accelerate local metabolic rate, as well as improve the efficiency of bone reconstruction and the speed of fracture healing (Deschaseaux et al., 2009; Seebach et al., 2012). For example, MSC-derived exosomes could rescue delayed fracture healing in $CD9^{-/-}$ mice and facilitate fracture healing in wild type mice; the mechanism is partly depended on the effect of MCP-1, -3, SDF-1, angiogenic factors and miRNAs (Furuta et al., 2016). In ischemic femoral head necrosis, it is also significant to promote angiogenesis and restrain ischemic necrosis areas (Glueck et al., 2007). Li H. et al. (2017) indicated that BMSC-ExosMU (exosomes secreted from HIF-1α-overexpressing BMSCs) could promote osteogenic differentiation of BMSCs through enhancing the expression of OCN and ALP *in vitro*. The MTT assay and cell-scratched wound evaluation also found that BMSC-ExosMU could promote proliferation, migration, and tube formation of HUVECs. Next, they conducted an *in vivo* experiment, and the results revealed that the SANFH (steroid-induced avascular necrosis of femoral head) model treated with BMSC-ExosMU was detected higher vessel density and denser trabecular tissue generation compared with the control group, suggesting the significant role of BMSC-ExosMU in promoting osteogenesis and angiogenesis (Li H. et al., 2017).

## EXOSOMES AS TARGETED DELIVERY VEHICLES FOR THERAPY IN SKELETAL AND EXTRAOSSEOUS DISORDERS

In recent years, the application of pharmaceutical carriers in clinical diseases has received extensive attention, and this has particularly applied to nanoscale pharmaceutical carriers, such as liposomes, microparticles, nanoparticles, etc. They have several characteristics that contribute to their high delivery efficiency, including the capacity to encapsulate hydrophobic drugs, improve drug bioavailability, transport molecules with high specificity, and so on (Tan et al., 2010). Despite the advantages mentioned above, the artificial nano drug-loading systems still face many problems. For example, the carrier molecules are easily removed by antibodies as well as complement and coagulation factors. Besides, a toxic reaction cannot be avoided due to their synthetic lipid membranes. As natural endogenous nano-microvesicles, exosomes play important roles in intercellular signal transmission and material exchange. In contrast, exosomes can overcome multiple limitations of artificial nano delivery systems and are more suitable candidates for delivery vehicles. Firstly, the exosomes have higher security because they can evade the immune detection system; in this case the immune rejection is eliminated. They also have better tolerance, which helps to protect cargo from destruction, thus leading to a longer circulating half-life. Secondly, exosomes have a natural targeting capacity depending on their cell sources. Thirdly, the membrane of exosomes can be artificially modified to enhance their functions. Finally, exosomes can penetrate cytomembranes and biological barriers easily due to their nanometer size and specific surface molecules (Ei Andaloussi et al., 2013; Jiang and Gao, 2017).

### Exosome as Compounds Delivery System

At present, some chemotherapeutic drugs, such as doxorubicin and paclitaxel, can be effectively loaded into exosomes. Tian et al. (2014) indicated that exosome-encapsulated Dox (doxorubicin) can be integrated into breast cancer cells with high efficiency and significantly enhanced the therapeutic effect of Dox. They also evaluated the cardiac toxicity in tumor-bearing mice, a dose-dependent side effect of Dox (Minotti et al., 2004), and found that intravenously injected iExos-Dox has weaker cardiotoxicity compared with free Dox, suggesting that exsomes are ideal drug delivery vehicles with high safety and efficiency for targeted tumor therapy. Another study revealed that the PTX (Paclitaxel) incorporated into exosomes by mild sonication can maintain stability at various conditions for over a month and has significantly enhanced drug cytotoxicity compared with PTX alone (Kim et al., 2016). In addition to transporting chemotherapeutic drugs to target cells with high efficiency, exosomes can also greatly increase the effects of other drugs, such as anti-inflammatory agents. For example, Sun et al. (2010) found that the binding of curcumin to naturally existing nanoparticle exosomes can significantly enhance the curcumin's anti-inflammatory activity through increasing its delivery into targeted macrophages, which leads to an improved anti-shock function in mice treated with LPS.

### Exosome as siRNA Delivery System

Currently, siRNA technology has been widely used in gene function research, clinical therapy, and other fields for the reason that it can induce targeted mRNA degradation and lead to post-transcriptional gene silencing (Burnett and Rossi, 2012; Crooke et al., 2018). However, siRNA-based gene treatment still faces many challenges, such as the poor cellular uptake and low stability in the circulating system. There is much evidence to suggest that the nanocarrier exosomes facilitate siRNA uptake into the targeted cells and improve its pharmacokinetics (Ozcan et al., 2015; Wang et al., 2017). It was reported that the exosome/TRPP2 siRNA complex can efficiently deliver TRPP2 (transient receptor potential polycystic 2) siRNA into FaDu cells and suppress its expression, resulting in the inhibition of the EMT (epithelial-mesenchymal transition) process and reduced invasion of FaDu cells (Wang et al., 2019a). Shokrollahi et al. (2019) treated human neuroblastoma cells (SH-SY5Y) with exosomes transfected by Hsp27 siRNA and evaluated the maturation of the human neuroblastoma cells. The data showed that the uptake of exosomes carrying siRNA HSP-27 by SH-SY5Y cells significantly inhibited their survival, clonogenic activity, and differentiation toward neuronal lineage (Shokrollahi et al., 2019). Shtam et al. (2013) used siRNA-loading exosomes to deliver RAD51-siRNA into HeLa cells and induce gene silencing, thereby inhibiting cell survival and proliferation. Exosomes can also be engineered into more suitable nanocarriers for carrying siRNA through modification. To enhance the targeting ability, Alvarez-Erviti et al. (2011) remolded the exosomes through attaching a neuron-specific RVG peptide to Lamp2b expressed on the exosomal membrane. The result revealed that the RVG exosomes were able to transport GAPDH siRNA into targeted neurons, microglia, and oligodendrocytes, and this resulted in downregulation of BACE1 gene expression, which plays a key role in Alzheimer's disease (Alvarez-Erviti et al., 2011).

### Exosome as miRNA Delivery System

miRNAs are a group of non-coding single-stranded RNAs of approximately 22 nucleotides that exist in plant and animal cells (Bartel, 2004). A series of studies have shown that miRNAs can participate in cellular gene network regulation by silencing target mRNA, and they therefore play important roles in cell proliferation, differentiation, and apoptosis (Beavers et al., 2015). It has also been summarized that miRNAs play key roles in bone formation and may serve as the new breakthrough in the treatment of skeletal diseases (Hu et al., 2010). As previously mentioned, an exosome can transfer its cargo, such as miRNAs, into targeted cells and regulate their growth and differentiation (Thomou et al., 2017). For instance, brown fat-derived exosomes carrying specific miRNA could regulate liver through targeting Fgf21 (Chen and Pfeifer, 2017). It has been proposed that the exosome can be used as a vehicle for transporting functional miRNAs and exerting therapeutic action. The miRNAs have been proven to be involved in the pathogenesis of several neurodegenerative diseases, such as Alzheimer's disease, Parkinson's disease, etc. The delivery of miRNAs packed by exosomes to central nervous system is therefore widely used for the improvement of neurological functions (Ridolfi and Abdel-Haq, 2017). Katakowski et al. (2013) obtained exosomes carrying miR-146b through plasmid transfection, and they found that miR-146b can be delivered into tumor cells via exosomes, suppressing expression of EGFR and NF-jB proteins and leading to inhibition of glioma growth *in vitro*. They also demonstrated that M146-exo can significantly reduce tumor growth in the rat brain (Katakowski et al., 2013). Chen et al. (2018) demonstrated that the miR-223 transferred by BMSCs-exo can greatly protect hepatocytes from injury in autoimmune hepatitis. One study conducted by Yu et al. (2015) revealed that anti-apoptotic miRNAs like miR-19a can be delivered into cardiomyocytes via $MSC^{GATA-4}$ (MSC overexpressing GATA-4)-derived exosomes and promote cardiac protection, which effect is connected with the inhibition of miR-19a target PTEN as well as activation of the Akt and ERK signaling pathway.

## CONCLUSION AND PERSPECTIVE

Since the first discovery of exosomes released by mature erythrocytes in 1983, this topic has attracted much attention from researchers because of their inherent properties. Exosomes are a class of extracellular vesicles sized 30–100 nm that contain cholesterol, sphingomyelin, ceramide, and other lipids on the surface that can be secreted by a variety of cells, including BMSCs, osteoclasts, osteoblasts, osteocytes, dendritic cells, epithelial cells, tumor cells, etc. In the recent years, researchers have developed various techniques to isolate exosomes based on their physical, chemical, and biological properties, and different methods have their unique advantages and disadvantages which may influence the product quality and following analysis.

With the development of molecular biotechnology, many researchers have tended to investigate the bone metabolism and skeletal disorders from a paracrine perspective, among which the exosome-mediated intercellular communication is rapidly gaining increasing attention. Bone-derived exosomes can regulate cell apoptosis, proliferation, and differentiation through multiple pathways, thus exerting important effects during physiological and pathological processes, such as bone remodeling, bone loss, fracture healing, and so on. This review has summarized the role of exosomes derived from BMSCs, osteoclasts, osteoblasts, and osteocytes in skeletal metabolism. The multiple effects of bone-derived exosomal miRNAs in bone remodeling have also been listed in **Table 1**. Besides, the bone-derived exosomes are found to participate in development of extraosseous diseases. For example, bone-derived exosomes could promote or suppress tumor growth through regulating genes expression, signaling pathways, angiogenesis, and so on. There are also numerous experiments illustrating that bone-derived exosomes are able to protect functional cells from apoptosis, thereby facilitating nerve repair, preventing nephropathy, preserving myocardial functions, and so on. It is reasonable to believe that bone-derived exosomes are highly relevant to the exploration of mechanisms of extraosseous diseases based on their ability to reach distant tissues and extraosseous systems.

In recent years, scientists have discovered the important role of exosomes in transmitting information between cells.

**TABLE 1** | The role of bone-derived exosomal miRNAs in bone remolding.

| Exosomal miRNA | Cells | miRNA expression | miRNA function |
|---|---|---|---|
| miR-27a<br>miR-206a<br>miR-196a | BMSCs | High | Promote osteogenic differentiation of osteoblasts (Qin et al., 2016) |
| miR-214 | Osteoclasts | High | Inhibit osteoblasts function Promote RANKL induced osteoclasts differentiation (Zhao et al., 2015; Sun et al., 2016) |
| miR-30d-5p<br>miR-133b-3p<br>miR-140-3p | Mineralizing MC3T3 cells | High | Inhibit osteoblasts differentiation (Xie et al., 2017) |
| let-7<br>miR-335-3p<br>miR-378b | Mineralizing MC3T3 cells | High | Promote osteoblasts differentiation (Xie et al., 2017) |
| miR-218 | Osteocytes | Low | Inhibit osteoblastic differentiation (Zhang et al., 2014; Qin et al., 2017) |
| miR-1192<br>miR-680<br>miR-302a | Mineralizing osteoblasts (MOBs) | High | Promote bone marrow stromal cell (ST2) differentiation to osteoblasts (Cui et al., 2016) |

The contents of the exosomes can reflect the physiological and pathological processes in cells, which can be released into various body fluids and microenvironments, thereby transmitting carried signals to distant tissues and cells (Yoshida et al., 2019). Exosomes can therefore be used for diseases diagnosis. In addition, the microvesicular structure of the exosomes can protect their contents from degradation, which demonstrates their stability in body fluids and enormous potential in the diagnosis and surveillance of diseases (Kourembanas, 2015). Bone-derived exosomes have become a research hotspot in the context of their use as biomarkers for clinical diseases, such as osteoporosis, MDS, AML, and so on; this provides a great opportunity for the development of a novel and sensitive diagnosis method.

BMSCs are one of the most commonly used seed cells in tissue engineering. A series of studies have shown that BMSCs have the ability to repair bone defects (Rackwitz et al., 2012), but there still exist some problems in terms of the immune response, ethics, and so on. Recently, it has been reported that BMSCs release exosomes containing signaling molecules through paracrine mechanisms to promote tissue repair (Liang et al., 2014). Therefore, scientists have started to focus on the application of BMSC-derived exosomes in bone tissue engineering. It has been found that BMSC-derived exosomes have the function of regulating osteoblasts and osteoclasts as well as promoting bone formation and neovascularization, and exosomes thus have great application prospects and research value in the field of bone tissue engineering. In addition, the potential use of exosomes as drug delivery systems for disease treatment has gained significant interest from the scientific community since they are of a nano-size and have strong penetrability and hypotoxicity as well as low immunogenicity and cell targeting properties. However, the clinical application of bone-derived exosomes still faces several challenges. The exosome extraction method currently used is not efficient enough to be applied in clinic; it is therefore imperative to design a strategy to increase the yield and purity of exosomes. Besides, the content and function of exosomes from different sources differ greatly, and the genetic information contained in exosomes is thus still not fully elucidated. There is consequently still a long way to go before exosomes can be widely used in clinic.

In summary, this article has provided an overview of the effect and mechanism of bone-derived exosomes in skeletal metabolism and extraosseous diseases, and it has opened up new perspectives for exosomes serving as biomarkers and drug delivery carriers. We have reason to believe that, with the further development of biotechnology and in-depth exploration of exosomes, the role of bone-derived exosomes in clinical diagnosis, monitoring, and treatment will be fully utilized.

## AUTHOR CONTRIBUTIONS

HL wrote the manuscript and designed the figures. YX, QG, and YH revised the manuscript. XL provided critical feedback and helped to shape the manuscript. All authors listed have made a substantial contribution to the work.

## REFERENCES


Adams, R. H., and Alitalo, K. (2007). Molecular regulation of angiogenesis and lymphangiogenesis. *Nat Rev. Mol. Cell Biol.* 8, 464–478. doi: 10.1038/nrm2183

Alvarez-Erviti, L., Seow, Y., Yin, H., Betts, C., Lakhal, S., and Wood, M. J. (2011). Delivery of siRNA to the mouse brain by systemic injection of targeted exosomes. *Nat. Biotechnol.* 29, 341–345. doi: 10.1038/nbt.1807

Ambrogini, E., Almeida, M., Martin-Millan, M., Paik, J. H., Depinho, R. A., Han, L., et al. (2010). FoxO-mediated defense against oxidative stress in osteoblasts is indispensable for skeletal homeostasis in mice. *Cell Metab.* 11, 136–146. doi: 10.1016/j.cmet.2009.12.009

Andreola, G., Rivoltini, L., Castelli, C., Huber, V., Perego, P., Deho, P., et al. (2002). Induction of lymphocyte apoptosis by tumor cell secretion of FasL-bearing microvesicles. *J. Exp. Med.* 195, 1303–1316. doi: 10.1084/jem.20011624

Barrera-Ramirez, J., Lavoie, J. R., Maganti, H. B., Stanford, W. L., Ito, C., Sabloff, M., et al. (2017). Micro-RNA profiling of exosomes from marrow-derived mesenchymal stromal cells in patients with acute myeloid leukemia: implications in leukemogenesis. *Stem Cell Rev.* 13, 817–825. doi: 10.1007/s12015-017-9762-0

Bartel, D. P. (2004). MicroRNAs: genomics, biogenesis, mechanism, and function. *Cell* 116, 281–297.

Beavers, K. R., Nelson, C. E., and Duvall, C. L. (2015). MiRNA inhibition in tissue engineering and regenerative medicine. *Adv. Drug Deliver. Rev.* 88, 123–137. doi: 10.1016/j.addr.2014.12.006

Bian, S., Zhang, L., Duan, L., Wang, X., Min, Y., and Yu, H. (2014). Extracellular vesicles derived from human bone marrow mesenchymal stem cells promote angiogenesis in a rat myocardial infarction model. *J. Mol. Med.* 92, 387–397. doi: 10.1007/s00109-013-1110-5

Bianco, F., Perrotta, C., Novellino, L., Francolini, M., Riganti, L., Menna, E., et al. (2009). Acid sphingomyelinase activity triggers microparticle release from glial cells. *EMBO J.* 28, 1043–1054. doi: 10.1038/emboj.2009.45

Bilen, M. A., Pan, T., Lee, Y. C., Lin, S. C., Yu, G., Pan, J., et al. (2017). Proteomics profiling of exosomes from primary mouse osteoblasts under proliferation versus mineralization conditions and characterization of their uptake into prostate cancer cells. *J. Proteome Res.* 16, 2709–2728. doi: 10.1021/acs.jproteome.6b00981

Bjørge, I. M., Kim, S. Y., Mano, J. F., Kalionis, B., and Chrzanowski, W. (2017). Extracellular vesicles, exosomes and shedding vesicles in regenerative medicine - a new paradigm for tissue repair. *Biomater. Sci. UK* 6, 60–78. doi: 10.1039/c7bm00479f

Bliss, S. A., Sinha, G., Sandiford, O. A., Williams, L. M., Engelberth, D. J., Guiro, K., et al. (2016). Mesenchymal stem cell-derived exosomes stimulate cycling quiescence and early breast cancer dormancy in bone marrow. *Cancer Res.* 76, 5832–5844. doi: 10.1158/0008-5472.can-16-1092

Bonewald, L. F. (2007). Osteocyte messages from a bony tomb. *Cell Metab.* 5, 410–411. doi: 10.1016/j.cmet.2007.05.008

Bose, S., Roy, M., and Bandyopadhyay, A. (2012). Recent advances in bone tissue engineering scaffolds. *Trends Biotechnol.* 30, 546–554. doi: 10.1016/j.tibtech.2012.07.005

Bourdonnay, E., Zasłona, Z., Penke, L. R., Speth, J. M., Schneider, D. J., Przybranowski, S., et al. (2015). Transcellular delivery of vesicular SOCS proteins from macrophages to epithelial cells blunts inflammatory signaling. *J. Exp. Med.* 212, 729–742. doi: 10.1084/jem.20141675

Broggi, M. A. S., Maillat, L., Clement, C. C., Bordry, N., Corthésy, P., Auger, A., et al. (2019). Tumor-associated factors are enriched in lymphatic exudate compared to plasma in metastatic melanoma patients. *J. Exp. Med.* 216, 1091–1107. doi: 10.1084/jem.20181618

Bruno, S., Collino, F., Deregibus, M. C., Grange, C., Tetta, C., and Camussi, G. (2013). Microvesicles derived from human bone marrow mesenchymal stem cells inhibit tumor growth. *Stem Cells Dev.* 22, 758–771. doi: 10.1089/scd.2012.0304

Bruno, S., Grange, C., Deregibus, M. C., Calogero, R. A., Saviozzi, S., Collino, F., et al. (2009). Mesenchymal stem cell-derived microvesicles protect against acute tubular injury. *J Am. Soc. Nephrol.* 20, 1053–1067. doi: 10.1681/asn.2008070798

Burnett, J. C., and Rossi, J. J. (2012). RNA-based therapeutics: current progress and future prospects. *Chem. Biol.* 19, 60–71. doi: 10.1016/j.chembiol.2011.12.008

Cao, L., Liu, G., Gan, Y., Fan, Q., Yang, F., Zhang, X., et al. (2012). The use of autologous enriched bone marrow MSCs to enhance osteoporotic bone defect repair in long-term estrogen deficient goats. *Biomaterials* 33, 5076–5084. doi: 10.1016/j.biomaterials.2012.03.069

Caplan, A. I., and Dennis, J. E. (2006). Mesenchymal stem cells as trophic mediators. *J. Cell. Biochem.* 98, 1076–1084. doi: 10.1002/jcb.20886

Chen, L., Lu, F. B., Chen, D. Z., Wu, J. L., Hu, E. D., Xu, L. M., et al. (2018). BMSCs-derived miR-223-containing exosomes contribute to liver protection in experimental autoimmune hepatitis. *Mol. Immunol.* 93, 38–46. doi: 10.1016/j.molimm.2017.11.008

Chen, T. S., Lai, R. C., Lee, M. M., Choo, A. B., Lee, C. N., and Lim, S. K. (2010). Mesenchymal stem cell secretes microparticles enriched in pre-microRNAs. *Nucleic Acids Res.* 38, 215–224. doi: 10.1093/nar/gkp857

Chen, Y., and Pfeifer, A. (2017). brown fat-derived exosomes: small vesicles with big impact. *Cell Metab.* 25, 759–760. doi: 10.1016/j.cmet.2017.03.012

Cheung, K. L., Jarrett, R., Subramaniam, S., Salimi, M., Gutowska-Owsiak, D., Chen, Y. L., et al. (2016). Psoriatic T cells recognize neolipid antigens generated by mast cell phospholipase delivered by exosomes and presented by CD1a. *J. Exp. Med.* 213, 2399–2412. doi: 10.1084/jem.20160258

Choudhry, H., and Harris, A. L. (2018). Advances in hypoxia-inducible factor biology. *Cell Metab.* 27, 281–298. doi: 10.1016/j.cmet.2017.10.005

Clayton, A., Turkes, A., Navabi, H., Mason, M. D., and Tabi, Z. (2005). Induction of heat shock proteins in B-cell exosomes. *J. Cell Sci.* 118, 3631–3638. doi: 10.1242/jcs.02494

Colombo, M., Raposo, G., and Théry, C. (2014). Biogenesis, secretion, and intercellular interactions of exosomes and other extracellular vesicles. *Annu. Rev. Cell Dev. Bi.* 30, 255–289. doi: 10.1146/annurev-cellbio-101512-122326

Cosenza, S., Ruiz, M., Toupet, K., Jorgensen, C., and Noël, D. (2017). Mesenchymal stem cells derived exosomes and microparticles protect cartilage and bone from degradation in osteoarthritis. *Sci. Rep. UK* 7:16214. doi: 10.1038/s41598-017-15376-8

Coumans, F. A. W., Brisson, A. R., Buzas, E. I., Dignat-George, F., Drees, E. E. E., Ei-Andaloussi, S., et al. (2017). Methodological guidelines to study extracellular vesicles. *Circ. Res.* 120, 1632–1648. doi: 10.1161/CIRCRESAHA.117.309417

Crooke, S. T., Witztum, J. L., Bennett, C. F., and Baker, B. F. (2018). RNA-targeted therapeutics. *Cell Metab.* 27, 714–739. doi: 10.1016/j.cmet.2018.03.004

Cui, Y., Luan, J., Li, H., Zhou, X., and Han, J. (2016). Exosomes derived from mineralizing osteoblasts promote ST2 cell osteogenic differentiation by alteration of microRNA expression. *FEBS Lett.* 590, 185–192. doi: 10.1002/1873-3468.12024

Dai, J., Escara-Wilke, J., Keller, J. M., Jung, Y., Taichman, R. S., Pienta, K. J., et al. (2019). Primary prostate cancer educates bone stroma through exosomal pyruvate kinase M2 to promote bone metastasis. *J. Exp. Med.* 216, 2883–2899. doi: 10.1084/jem.20190158

Dalirfardouei, R., Jamialahmadi, K., and Mahdipour, E. (2018). A feasible method for the isolation of mesenchymal stem cells from menstrual blood and their exosomes. *Tissue Cell* 55, 53–62. doi: 10.1016/j.tice.2018.09.010

Dauer, D. J., Ferraro, B., Song, L., Yu, B., Mora, L., Buettner, R., et al. (2005). Stat3 regulates genes common to both wound healing and cancer. *Oncogene* 24, 3397–3408. doi: 10.1038/sj.onc.1208469

Deng, L., Peng, Y., Jiang, Y., Wu, Y., Ding, Y., Wang, Y., et al. (2017). Imipramine Protects against Bone Loss by Inhibition of Osteoblast-Derived Microvesicles. *Int. J. Mol. Sci.* 18:E1013. doi: 10.3390/ijms18051013

Deng, L., Wang, Y., Peng, Y., Wu, Y., Ding, Y., Jiang, Y., et al. (2015). Osteoblast-derived microvesicles: a novel mechanism for communication between osteoblasts and osteoclasts. *Bone* 79, 37–42. doi: 10.1016/j.bone.2015.05.022

Deschaseaux, F., Sensébé, L., and Heymann, D. (2009). Mechanisms of bone repair and regeneration. *Trends Mol. Med.* 15, 417–429. doi: 10.1016/j.molmed.2009.07.002

Ei Andaloussi, S., Lakhal, S., Mäger, I., and Wood, M. J. (2013). Exosomes for targeted siRNA delivery across biological barriers. *Adv. Drug Deliver. Rev.* 65, 391–397. doi: 10.1016/j.addr.2012.08.008

Eii, B., Mercatali, L., Ibrahim, T., Campbell, N., Schwarzenbach, H., Pantel, K., et al. (2013). Tumor-induced osteoclast miRNA changes as regulators and biomarkers of osteolytic bone metastasis. *Cancer Cell* 24, 542–556. doi: 10.1016/j.ccr.2013.09.008

Esen, E., Chen, J., Karner, C. M., Okunade, A. L., Patterson, B. W., and Long, F. (2013). WNT-LRP5 signaling induces Warburg effect through mTORC2 activation during osteoblast differentiation. *Cell Metab.* 17, 745–755. doi: 10.1016/j.cmet.2013.03.017

Fan, Y., Hanai, J. I., Le, P. T., Bi, R., Maridas, D., DeMambro, V., et al. (2017). Parathyroid hormone directs bone marrow mesenchymal cell fate. *Cell Metab.* 25, 661–672. doi: 10.1016/j.cmet.2017.01.001

Fang, S., Li, Y., and Chen, P. (2019). Osteogenic effect of bone marrow mesenchymal stem cell-derived exosomes on steroid-induced osteonecrosis of the femoral head. *Drug Design Dev. Ther.* 13, 45–55. doi: 10.2147/DDDT.S178698

Feng, Y., Huang, W., Wani, M., Yu, X., and Ashraf, M. (2014). Ischemic preconditioning potentiates the protective effect of stem cells through secretion of exosomes by targeting Mecp2 via miR-22. *PLoS One* 9:e88685. doi: 10.1371/journal.pone.0088685

Findlay, D. M., and Kuliwaba, J. S. (2016). Bone-cartilage crosstalk: a conversation for understanding osteoarthritis. *Bone Res.* 4:16028. doi: 10.1038/boneres.2016.28

Fritz, J. M., and Lenardo, M. J. (2019). Development of immune checkpoint therapy for cancer. *J. Exp. Med.* 216, 1244–1254. doi: 10.1084/jem.20182395

Furuta, T., Miyaki, S., Ishitobi, H., Ogura, T., Kato, Y., Kamei, N., et al. (2016). Mesenchymal stem cell-derived exosomes promote fracture healing in a mouse model. *Stem Cells Transl Med.* 5, 1620–1630. doi: 10.5966/sctm.2015-0285

García-Silva, S., Benito-Martín, A., Sánchez-Redondo, S., Hernández-Barranco, A., Ximénez-Embún, P., Nogués, L., et al. (2019). Use of extracellular vesicles from lymphatic drainage as surrogate markers of melanoma progression and mutation. *J. Exp. Med.* 216, 1061–1070. doi: 10.1084/jem.20181522

Garg, P., Mazur, M. M., Buck, A. C., Wandtke, M. E., Liu, J., and Ebraheim, N. A. (2017). Prospective review of mesenchymal stem cells differentiation into osteoblasts. *Orthopaedic Surg.* 9, 13–19. doi: 10.1111/os.12304

Gartz, M., and Strande, J. L. (2018). Examining the Paracrine Effects of Exosomes in Cardiovascular Disease and Repair. *J. Am. Heart Assoc.* 7:e007954. doi: 10.1161/JAHA.117.007954

Gatti, S., Bruno, S., Deregibus, M. C., Sordi, A., Cantaluppi, V., Tetta, C., et al. (2011). Microvesicles derived from human adult mesenchymal stem cells protect against ischaemia-reperfusion-induced acute and chronic kidney injury. *Nephrol. Dial. Transplant.* 26, 1474–1483. doi: 10.1093/ndt/gfr015

Ge, M., Wu, Y., Ke, R., Cai, T., Yang, J., and Mu, X. (2017). Value of Osteoblast-Derived Exosomes in Bone Diseases. *J. Craniofac. Surg.* 28, 866–870. doi: 10.1097/SCS.0000000000003463

Glueck, C. J., Freiberg, R. A., Oghene, J., Fontaine, R. N., and Wang, P. (2007). Association between the T-786C eNOS polymorphism and idiopathic osteonecrosis of the head of the femur. *J. Bone Joint surg. Am. Vol.* 89, 2460–2468. doi: 10.2106/jbjs.f.01421

Greenblatt, M. B., Park, K. H., Oh, H., Kim, J. M., Shin, D. Y., Lee, J. M., et al. (2015). CHMP5 controls bone turnover rates by dampening NF-κB activity in osteoclasts. *J. Exp. Med.* 212, 1283–1301. doi: 10.1084/jem.20150407

Guay, C., Kruit, J. K., Rome, S., Menoud, V., Mulder, N. L., Jurdzinski, A., et al. (2019). Lymphocyte-derived exosomal micrornas promote pancreatic β cell death and may contribute to type 1 diabetes development. *Cell Metab.* 29, .348.e6–361.e6. doi: 10.1016/j.cmet.2018.09.011

Gurunathan, S., Kang, M. H., Jeyaraj, M., Qasim, M., and Kim, J. H. (2019). Review of the isolation, characterization, biological function, and multifarious therapeutic approaches of exosomes. *Cells* 8:307. doi: 10.3390/cells8040307

Hall, A., and Lalli, G. (2010). Rho and Ras GTPases in axon growth, guidance, and branching. *Csh. Perspect. Biol.* 2:a001818. doi: 10.1101/cshperspect.a001818

Ham, O., Song, B. W., Lee, S. Y., Choi, E., Cha, M. J., Lee, C. Y., et al. (2012). The role of microRNA-23b in the differentiation of MSC into chondrocyte by targeting protein kinase A signaling. *Biomaterials* 33, 4500–4507. doi: 10.1016/j.biomaterials.2012.03.025

Han, Y., You, X., Xing, W., Zhang, Z., and Zou, W. (2018). Paracrine and endocrine actions of bone-the functions of secretory proteins from osteoblasts, osteocytes, and osteoclasts. *Bone Res.* 6, 16. doi: 10.1038/s41413-018-0019-6

Hayashi, M., Nakashima, T., Yoshimura, N., Okamoto, K., Tanaka, S., and Takayanagi, H. (2019). Autoregulation of Osteocyte Sema3A Orchestrates Estrogen Action and Counteracts Bone Aging. *Cell Metab.* 29, 627.e5–637.e5. doi: 10.1016/j.cmet.2018.12.021

Hertel, M., Tretter, Y., Alzheimer, C., and Werner, S. (2000). Connective tissue growth factor: a novel player in tissue reorganization after brain injury? *Eur. J. Neurosci.* 12, 376–380. doi: 10.1046/j.1460-9568.2000.00930.x

Hirose, J., Masuda, H., Tokuyama, N., Omata, Y., Matsumoto, T., Yasui, T., et al. (2014). Bone resorption is regulated by cell-autonomous negative feedback loop of Stat5-Dusp axis in the osteoclast. *J. Exp. Med.* 211, 153–163. doi: 10.1084/jem.20130538

Hsu, Y. H., Chen, W. Y., Chan, C. H., Wu, C. H., Sun, Z. J., and Chang, M. S. (2011). Anti-IL-20 monoclonal antibody inhibits the differentiation of osteoclasts and protects against osteoporotic bone loss. *J. Exp. Med.* 208, 1849–1861. doi: 10.1084/jem.20102234

Hu, R., Li, H., Liu, W., Yang, L., Tan, Y. F., and Luo, X. H. (2010). Targeting miRNAs in osteoblast differentiation and bone formation. *Expert Opin. Ther. Tar.* 14, 1109–1120. doi: 10.1517/14728222.2010.512916

Huynh, N., VonMoss, L., Smith, D., Rahman, I., Felemban, M. F., Zuo, J., et al. (2016). Characterization of regulatory extracellular vesicles from osteoclasts. *J. Dent. Res.* 95, 673–679. doi: 10.1177/0022034516633189

Ishii, M., Kikuta, J., Shimazu, Y., Meier-Schellersheim, M., and Germain, R. N. (2010). Chemorepulsion by blood S1P regulates osteoclast precursor mobilization and bone remodeling in vivo. *J. Exp. Med.* 207, 2793–2798. doi: 10.1084/jem.20101474

Ishijima, M., Rittling, S. R., Yamashita, T., Tsuji, K., Kurosawa, H., Nifuji, A., et al. (2001). Enhancement of osteoclastic bone resorption and suppression of osteoblastic bone formation in response to reduced mechanical stress do not occur in the absence of osteopontin. *J. Exp. Med.* 193, 399–404. doi: 10.1084/jem.193.3.399

Janas, T., Janas, M. M., Sapoń, K., and Janas, T. (2015). Mechanisms of RNA loading into exosomes. *FEBS Lett.* 589, 1391–1398. doi: 10.1016/j.febslet.2015.04.036

Jiang, X. C., and Gao, J. Q. (2017). Exosomes as novel bio-carriers for gene and drug delivery. *Int. J. Pharmaceut.* 521, 167–175. doi: 10.1016/j.ijpharm.2017.02.038

Jin, Z., Wei, W., Yang, M., Du, Y., and Wan, Y. (2014). Mitochondrial complex I activity suppresses inflammation and enhances bone resorption by shifting macrophage-osteoclast polarization. *Cell Metab.* 20, 483–498. doi: 10.1016/j.cmet.2014.07.011

Johnstone, R. M., Adam, M., Hammond, J. R., Orr, L., and Turbide, C. (1987). Vesicle formation during reticulocyte maturation. Association of plasma membrane activities with released vesicles (exosomes). *J Biol. Chem.* 262, 9412–9420.

Kang, Y. T., Kim, Y. J., Bu, J., Cho, Y. H., Han, S. W., and Moon, B. I. (2017). High-purity capture and release of circulating exosomes using an exosome-specific dual-patterned immunofiltration (ExoDIF) device. *Nanoscale* 9, 13495–13505. doi: 10.1039/c7nr04557c

Katakowski, M., Buller, B., Zheng, X., Lu, Y., Rogers, T., Osobamiro, O., et al. (2013). Exosomes from marrow stromal cells expressing miR-146b inhibit glioma growth. *Cancer Lett.* 335, 201–204. doi: 10.1016/j.canlet.2013.02.019

Kim, M. S., Haney, M. J., Zhao, Y., Mahajan, V., Deygen, I., Klyachko, N. L., et al. (2016). Development of exosome-encapsulated paclitaxel to overcome MDR in cancer cells. *Nanomedicine* 12, 655–664. doi: 10.1016/j.nano.2015.10.012

Klopp, A. H., Gupta, A., Spaeth, E., Andreeff, M., and Marini, F. (2011). Concise review: dissecting a discrepancy in the literature: do mesenchymal stem cells support or suppress tumor growth? *Stem Cells* 29, 11–19. doi: 10.1002/stem.559

Kourembanas, S. (2015). Exosomes: vehicles of intercellular signaling, biomarkers, and vectors of cell therapy. *Annu. Rev. Physiol.* 77, 13–27. doi: 10.1146/annurev-physiol-021014-071641

Kowal, J., Tkach, M., and Théry, C. (2014). Biogenesis and secretion of exosomes. *Curr. Opin. Cell Biol.* 29, 116–125. doi: 10.1016/j.ceb.2014.05.004

Kubota, K., Nakano, M., Kobayashi, E., Mizue, Y., Chikenji, T., Otani, M., et al. (2018). An enriched environment prevents diabetes-induced cognitive impairment in rats by enhancing exosomal miR-146a secretion from endogenous bone marrow-derived mesenchymal stem cells. *PLoS One* 13:e0204252. doi: 10.1371/journal.pone.0204252

Kuroda, S., Sumner, D. R., and Virdi, A. S. (2012). Effects of TGF-β1 and VEGF-A transgenes on the osteogenic potential of bone marrow stromal cells in vitro and in vivo. *J. Tissue Eng.* 3, 2041731412459745. doi: 10.1177/2041731412459745

Lee, H., Li, C., Zhang, Y., Zhang, D., Otterbein, L. E., and Jin, Y. (2019). Caveolin-1 selectively regulates microRNA sorting into microvesicles after noxious stimuli. *J. Exp. Med.* 216, 2202–2220. doi: 10.1084/jem.20182313

Lei, Z., van Mil, A., Brandt, M. M., Grundmann, S., Hoefer, I., Smits, M., et al. (2015). MicroRNA-132/212 family enhances arteriogenesis after hindlimb ischaemia through modulation of the Ras-MAPK pathway. *J. Cell. Mol. Med.* 19, 1994–2005. doi: 10.1111/jcmm.12586

Leiferman, A., Shu, J., Upadhyaya, B., Cui, J., and Zempleni, J. (2019). Storage of extracellular vesicles in human milk, and MicroRNA profiles in human milk exosomes and infant formulas. *J. Pediatr. Gastr. Nutr.* 69, 235–238. doi: 10.1097/MPG.0000000000002363

Li, C. J., Xiao, Y., Yang, M., Su, T., Sun, X., Guo, Q., et al. (2018). Long noncoding RNA Bmncr regulates mesenchymal stem cell fate during skeletal aging. *J. Clin. Invest.* 128, 5251–5266. doi: 10.1172/JCI99044

Li, D., Liu, J., Guo, B., Liang, C., Dang, L., Lu, C., et al. (2016). Osteoclast-derived exosomal miR-214-3p inhibits osteoblastic bone formation. *Nat. Commun.* 7:10872. doi: 10.1038/ncomms10872

Li, H., Liu, D., Li, C., Zhou, S., Tian, D., Xiao, D., et al. (2017). Exosomes secreted from mutant-HIF-1α-modified bone-marrow-derived mesenchymal stem cells attenuate early steroid-induced avascular necrosis of femoral head in rabbit. *Cell Biol. Int.* 41, 1379–1390. doi: 10.1002/cbin.10869

Li, H., Xie, H., Liu, W., Hu, R., Huang, B., Tan, Y. F., et al. (2009). A novel microRNA targeting HDAC5 regulates osteoblast differentiation in mice and contributes to primary osteoporosis in humans. *J. Clin. Invest.* 119, 3666–3677. doi: 10.1172/JCI39832

Li, P., Kaslan, M., Lee, S. H., Yao, J., and Gao, Z. (2017). Progress in exosome isolation techniques. *Theranostics* 7, 789–804. doi: 10.7150/thno.18133

Liang, X., Ding, Y., Zhang, Y., Tse, H. F., and Lian, Q. (2014). Paracrine mechanisms of mesenchymal stem cell-based therapy: current status and perspectives. *Cell Transplant.* 23, 1045–1059. doi: 10.3727/096368913X667709

Lindoso, R. S., Collino, F., Bruno, S., Araujo, D. S., Sant'Anna, J. F., Tetta, C., et al. (2014). Extracellular vesicles released from mesenchymal stromal cells modulate miRNA in renal tubular cells and inhibit ATP depletion injury. *Stem Cells Dev.* 23, 1809–1819. doi: 10.1089/scd.2013.0618

Ling, C., and Rönn, T. (2019). Epigenetics in human obesity and type 2 diabetes. *Cell Metab.* 29, 1028–1044. doi: 10.1016/j.cmet.2019.03.009

Liu, J., Li, D., Wu, X., Dang, L., Lu, A., and Zhang, G. (2017). Bone-derived exosomes. *Curr. Opin. Pharmacol.* 34, 64–69. doi: 10.1016/j.coph.2017.08.008

Liu, S., Liu, D., Chen, C., Hamamura, K., Moshaverinia, A., Yang, R., et al. (2015). MSC transplantation improves osteopenia via epigenetic regulation of notch signaling in lupus. *Cell Metab.* 22, 606–618. doi: 10.1016/j.cmet.2015.08.018

Luther, G., Wagner, E. R., Zhu, G., Kang, Q., Luo, Q., Lamplot, J., et al. (2011). BMP-9 induced osteogenic differentiation of mesenchymal stem cells: molecular mechanism and therapeutic potential. *Curr. Gene Ther.* 11, 229–240.

Ma, T., Chen, Y., Chen, Y., Meng, Q., Sun, J., Shao, L., et al. (2018). MicroRNA-132, delivered by mesenchymal stem cell-derived exosomes, promote angiogenesis in myocardial infarction. *Stem Cells Int.* 2018:3290372. doi: 10.1155/2018/3290372

Manek, R., Moghieb, A., Yang, Z., Kumar, D., Kobessiy, F., Sarkis, G. A., et al. (2018). Protein Biomarkers and Neuroproteomics Characterization of Microvesicles/Exosomes from Human Cerebrospinal Fluid Following Traumatic Brain Injury. *Mol. Neurobiol.* 55, 6112–6128. doi: 10.1007/s12035-017-0821-y

Matsumoto, T., Ii, M., Nishimura, H., Shoji, T., Mifune, Y., Kawamoto, A., et al. (2010). Lnk-dependent axis of SCF-cKit signal for osteogenesis in bone fracture healing. *J. Exp. Med.* 207, 2207–2223. doi: 10.1084/jem.20100321

McBride, J. D., Rodriguez-Menocal, L., Guzman, W., Candanedo, A., Garcia-Contreras, M., and Badiavas, E. V. (2017). Bone marrow mesenchymal stem cell-derived CD63 exosomes transport wnt3a exteriorly and enhance dermal fibroblast proliferation, migration, and angiogenesis in vitro. *Stem Cells Dev.* 26, 1384–1398. doi: 10.1089/scd.2017.0087

Mead, B., Logan, A., Berry, M., Leadbeater, W., and Scheven, B. A. (2013). Intravitreally transplanted dental pulp stem cells promote neuroprotection and axon regeneration of retinal ganglion cells after optic nerve injury. *Invest. Ophth. Vis. Sci.* 54, 7544–7556. doi: 10.1167/iovs.13-13045

Mead, B., and Tomarev, S. (2017). Bone marrow-derived mesenchymal stem cells-derived exosomes promote survival of retinal ganglion cells through miRNA-dependent mechanisms. *Stem Cell. Transl. Med.* 6, 1273–1285. doi: 10.1002/sctm.16-0428

Mesentier-Louro, L. A., Zaverucha-do-Valle, C., Da Silva-Junior, A. J., Nascimento-Dos-Santos, G., Gubert, F., de Figueirêdo, A. B., et al. (2014). Distribution of mesenchymal stem cells and effects on neuronal survival and axon regeneration after optic nerve crush and cell therapy. *PLoS One* 9:e110722. doi: 10.1371/journal.pone.0110722

Minotti, G., Menna, P., Salvatorelli, E., Cairo, G., and Gianni, L. (2004). Anthracyclines: molecular advances and pharmacologic developments in antitumor activity and cardiotoxicity. *Pharmacol. Rev.* 56, 185–229. doi: 10.1124/pr.56.2.6

Moerman, E. J., Teng, K., Lipschitz, D. A., and Lecka-Czernik, B. (2004). Aging activates adipogenic and suppresses osteogenic programs in mesenchymal marrow stroma/stem cells: the role of PPAR-gamma2 transcription factor and TGF-beta/BMP signaling pathways. *Aging Cell* 3, 379–389. doi: 10.1111/j.1474-9728.2004.00127.x

Mori, M. A., Ludwig, R. G., Garcia-Martin, R., Brandão, B. B., and Kahn, C. R. (2019). Extracellular miRNAs: from biomarkers to mediators of physiology and disease. *Cell Metab.* 30, 656–673. doi: 10.1016/j.cmet.2019.07.011

Morigi, M., and De Coppi, P. (2014). Cell therapy for kidney injury: different options and mechanisms–mesenchymal and amniotic fluid stem cells. *Nephron. Exp. Nephrol.* 126:59. doi: 10.1159/000360667

Morikawa, S., Mabuchi, Y., Kubota, Y., Nagai, Y., Niibe, K., Hiratsu, E., et al. (2009). Prospective identification, isolation, and systemic transplantation of multipotent mesenchymal stem cells in murine bone marrow. *J. Exp. Med.* 206, 2483–2496. doi: 10.1084/jem.20091046

Muntión, S., Ramos, T. L., Diez-Campelo, M., Rosón, B., Sánchez-Abarca, L. I., Misiewicz-Krzeminska, I., et al. (2016). Microvesicles from mesenchymal stromal cells are involved in hpc-microenvironment crosstalk in myelodysplastic patients. *PLoS One* 11:e0146722. doi: 10.1371/journal.pone.0146722

Nagaishi, K., Mizue, Y., Chikenji, T., Otani, M., Nakano, M., Konari, N., et al. (2016). Mesenchymal stem cell therapy ameliorates diabetic nephropathy via the paracrine effect of renal trophic factors including exosomes. *Sci. Rep. UK* 6:34842. doi: 10.1038/srep34842

Nakajima, K., Kunimatsu, R., Ando, K., Ando, T., Hayashi, Y., Kihara, T., et al. (2018). Comparison of the bone regeneration ability between stem cells from human exfoliated deciduous teeth, human dental pulp stem cells and human bone marrow mesenchymal stem cells. *Biochem. Bioph. Res. Co.* 497, 876–882. doi: 10.1016/j.bbrc.2018.02.156

Nakamura, Y., Miyaki, S., Ishitobi, H., Matsuyama, S., Nakasa, T., Kamei, N., et al. (2015). Mesenchymal-stem-cell-derived exosomes accelerate skeletal muscle regeneration. *FEBS Lett.* 589, 1257–1265. doi: 10.1016/j.febslet.2015.03.031

Nakano, M., Nagaishi, K., Konari, N., Saito, Y., Chikenji, T., Mizue, Y., et al. (2016). Bone marrow-derived mesenchymal stem cells improve diabetes-induced cognitive impairment by exosome transfer into damaged neurons and astrocytes. *Sci. Rep. UK* 6:24805. doi: 10.1038/srep24805

Narayanan, R., Huang, C. C., and Ravindran, S. (2016). Hijacking the cellular mail: exosome mediated differentiation of mesenchymal stem cells. *Stem Cells Int.* 2016:3808674. doi: 10.1155/2016/3808674

Naseri, Z., Oskuee, R. K., Jaafari, M. R., and Forouzandeh Moghadam, M. (2018). Exosome-mediated delivery of functionally active miRNA-142-3p inhibitor reduces tumorigenicity of breast cancer in vitro and in vivo. *Int. J. Nanomed.* 13, 7727–7747. doi: 10.2147/IJN.S182384

Nejadnik, H., Hui, J. H., Feng Choong, E. P., Tai, B. C., and Lee, E. H. (2010). Autologous bone marrow-derived mesenchymal stem cells versus autologous chondrocyte implantation: an observational cohort study. *Am. J. Sports Med.* 38, 1110–1116. doi: 10.1177/0363546509359067

Nevius, E., Pinho, F., Dhodapkar, M., Jin, H., Nadrah, K., Horowitz, M. C., et al. (2015). Oxysterols and EBI2 promote osteoclast precursor migration to bone surfaces and regulate bone mass homeostasis. *J. Exp. Med.* 212, 1931–1946. doi: 10.1084/jem.20150088

Newgard, C. B. (2017). Metabolomics and metabolic diseases: where do we stand? *Cell Metab.* 25, 43–56. doi: 10.1016/j.cmet.2016.09.018

Ng, K. S., Kuncewicz, T. M., and Karp, J. M. (2015). beyond hit-and-run: stem cells leave a lasting memory. *Cell Metab.* 22, 541–543. doi: 10.1016/j.cmet.2015.09.019

Ning, G., Liu, X., Dai, M., Meng, A., and Wang, Q. (2013). MicroRNA-92a upholds Bmp signaling by targeting noggin3 during pharyngeal cartilage formation. *Dev. Cell* 24, 283–295. doi: 10.1016/j.devcel.2012.12.016

Novack, D. V. (2007). Estrogen and bone: osteoclasts take center stage. *Cell Metab.* 6, 254–256. doi: 10.1016/j.cmet.2007.09.007

Ozcan, G., Ozpolat, B., Coleman, R. L., Sood, A. K., and Lopez-Berestein, G. (2015). Preclinical and clinical development of siRNA-based therapeutics. *Adv. Drug Deliver. Rev.* 87, 108–119. doi: 10.1016/j.addr.2015.01.007

Pan, B. T., and Johnstone, R. M. (1983). Fate of the transferrin receptor during maturation of sheep reticulocytes in vitro: selective externalization of the receptor. *Cell* 33, 967–978. doi: 10.1016/0092-8674(83)90040-5

Pourakbari, R., Khodadadi, M., Aghebati-Maleki, A., Aghebati-Maleki, L., and Yousefi, M. (2019). The potential of exosomes in the therapy of the cartilage and bone complications; emphasis on osteoarthritis. *Life Sci.* 236:116861. doi: 10.1016/j.lfs.2019.116861

Qi, J., Zhou, Y., Jiao, Z., Wang, X., Zhao, Y., Li, Y., et al. (2017). Exosomes Derived from Human Bone Marrow Mesenchymal Stem Cells Promote Tumor Growth Through Hedgehog Signaling Pathway. *Cell. Physiol. Biochem.* 42, 2242–2254. doi: 10.1159/000479998

Qi, X., Zhang, J., Yuan, H., Xu, Z., Li, Q., Niu, X., et al. (2016). Exosomes secreted by human-induced pluripotent stem cell-derived mesenchymal stem cells repair critical-sized bone defects through enhanced angiogenesis and osteogenesis in osteoporotic rats. *Int. J. Biol. Sci.* 12, 836–849. doi: 10.7150/ijbs.14809

Qin, Y., Peng, Y., Zhao, W., Pan, J., Ksiezak-Reding, H., Cardozo, C., et al. (2017). Myostatin inhibits osteoblastic differentiation by suppressing osteocyte-derived exosomal microRNA-218: a novel mechanism in muscle-bone communication. *J. Biol. Chem.* 292, 11021–11033. doi: 10.1074/jbc.M116.770941

Qin, Y., Wang, L., Gao, Z., Chen, G., and Zhang, C. (2016). Bone marrow stromal/stem cell-derived extracellular vesicles regulate osteoblast activity and differentiation in vitro and promote bone regeneration in vivo. *Sci. Rep. UK* 6:21961. doi: 10.1038/srep21961

Qing, L., Chen, H., Tang, J., and Jia, X. (2018). Exosomes and their MicroRNA cargo: new players in peripheral nerve regeneration. *Neurorehab. Neural Re.* 32, 765–776. doi: 10.1177/1545968318798955

Rackwitz, L., Eden, L., Reppenhagen, S., Reichert, J. C., Jakob, F., Walles, H., et al. (2012). Stem cell- and growth factor-based regenerative therapies for avascular necrosis of the femoral head. *Stem Cell Res. Ther.* 3:7. doi: 10.1186/scrt98

Rahmati, M., Nalesso, G., Mobasheri, A., and Mozafari, M. (2017). Aging and osteoarthritis: central role of the extracellular matrix. *Ageing Res. Rev.* 40, 20–30. doi: 10.1016/j.arr.2017.07.004

Raposo, G., Nijman, H. W., Stoorvogel, W., Liejendekker, R., Harding, C. V., Melief, C. J., et al. (1996). B lymphocytes secrete antigen-presenting vesicles. *J. Exp. Med.* 183, 1161–1172. doi: 10.1084/jem.183.3.1161

Raposo, G., and Stoorvogel, W. (2013). Extracellular vesicles: exosomes, microvesicles, and friends. *J Cell Biol.* 200, 373–383. doi: 10.1083/jcb.201211138

Rauch, A., Seitz, S., Baschant, U., Schilling, A. F., Illing, A., Stride, B., et al. (2010). Glucocorticoids suppress bone formation by attenuating osteoblast differentiation via the monomeric glucocorticoid receptor. *Cell Metab.* 11, 517–531. doi: 10.1016/j.cmet.2010.05.005

Ridolfi, B., and Abdel-Haq, H. (2017). Neurodegenerative disorders treatment: the MicroRNA role. *Curr. Gene Ther.* 17, 327–363. doi: 10.2174/1566523218666180119120726

Ritter, B., and Greten, F. R. (2019). Modulating inflammation for cancer therapy. *J. Exp. Med.* 216, 1234–1243. doi: 10.1084/jem.20181739

Roccaro, A. M., Sacco, A., Maiso, P., Azab, A. K., Tai, Y. T., Reagan, M., et al. (2013). BM mesenchymal stromal cell-derived exosomes facilitate multiple myeloma progression. *J. Clin. Invest.* 123, 1542–1555. doi: 10.1172/jci66517

Rood, I. M., Deegens, J. K., Merchant, M. L., Tamboer, W. P., Wilkey, D. W., Wetzels, J. F., et al. (2010). Comparison of three methods for isolation of urinary microvesicles to identify biomarkers of nephrotic syndrome. *Kidney Int.* 78, 810–816. doi: 10.1038/ki.2010.262

Saran, U., Gemini Piperni, S., and Chatterjee, S. (2014). Role of angiogenesis in bone repair. *Arch. Biochem. Biophys.* 561, 109–117. doi: 10.1016/j.abb.2014.07.006

Sato, M., Suzuki, T., Kawano, M., and Tamura, M. (2017). Circulating osteocyte-derived exosomes contain miRNAs which are enriched in exosomes from MLO-Y4 cells. *Biomed. Rep.* 6, 223–231. doi: 10.3892/br.2016.824

Seebach, C., Henrich, D., Wilhelm, K., Barker, J. H., and Marzi, I. (2012). Endothelial progenitor cells improve directly and indirectly early vascularization of mesenchymal stem cell-driven bone regeneration in a critical bone defect in rats. *Cell Transplant.* 21, 1667–1677. doi: 10.3727/096368912X638937

Shabbir, A., Cox, A., Rodriguez-Menocal, L., Salgado, M., and Van Badiavas, E. (2015). Mesenchymal stem cell exosomes induce proliferation and migration of normal and chronic wound fibroblasts, and enhance angiogenesis in vitro. *Stem Cells Dev.* 24, 1635–1647. doi: 10.1089/scd.2014.0316

Shao, L., Zhang, Y., Lan, B., Wang, J., Zhang, Z., Zhang, L., et al. (2017). MiRNA-sequence indicates that mesenchymal stem cells and exosomes have similar mechanism to enhance cardiac repair. *Biomed Res. Int.* 2017:4150705. doi: 10.1155/2017/4150705

Shokrollahi, E., Nourazarian, A., Rahbarghazi, R., Salimi, L., Karbasforush, S., Khaksar, M., et al. (2019). Treatment of human neuroblastoma cell line SH-SY5Y with HSP27 siRNA tagged-exosomes decreased differentiation rate into mature neurons. *J. Cell. Physiol.* 234, 21005–21013. doi: 10.1002/jcp.28704

Shtam, T. A., Kovalev, R. A., Varfolomeeva, E. Y., Makarov, E. M., Kil, Y. V., and Filatov, M. V. (2013). Exosomes are natural carriers of exogenous siRNA to human cells in vitro. *Cell Commun. Signal.* 11:88. doi: 10.1186/1478-811X-11-88

Simons, M., and Raposo, G. (2009). Exosomes–vesicular carriers for intercellular communication. *Curr. Opin. Cell Biol.* 21, 575–581. doi: 10.1016/j.ceb.2009.03.007

Singer, R. A., Arnes, L., Cui, Y., Wang, J., Gao, Y., Guney, M. A., et al. (2019). The long noncoding RNA paupar modulates PAX6 regulatory activities to promote alpha cell development and function. *Cell Metab.* 30, 1091.e8–1106.e8. doi: 10.1016/j.cmet.2019.09.013

Snaebjornsson, M. T., Janaki-Raman, S., and Schulze, A. (2020). Greasing the wheels of the cancer machine: the role of lipid metabolism in cancer. *Cell Metab.* 31, 62–76. doi: 10.1016/j.cmet.2019.11.010

Sponton, C. H., and Kajimura, S. (2017). Burning fat and building bone by FSH blockade. *Cell Metab.* 26, 285–287. doi: 10.1016/j.cmet.2017.07.018

Street, J. M., Koritzinsky, E. H., Glispie, D. M., and Yuen, P. S. T. (2017). Urine exosome isolation and characterization. *Methods Mol. Biol.* 1641, 413–423. doi: 10.1007/978-1-4939-7172-5_23

Su, T., Xiao, Y. Z., Xiao, Y., Guo, Q., Li, C., Huang, Y., et al. (2019). Bone marrow mesenchymal stem cells-derived exosomal MiR-29b-3p regulates aging-associated insulin resistance. *ACS Nano* 13, 2450–2462. doi: 10.1021/acsnano.8b09375

Suchacki, K. J., Roberts, F., Lovdel, A., Farquharson, C., Morton, N. M., MacRae, V. E., et al. (2017). Skeletal energy homeostasis: a paradigm of endocrine discovery. *J. Endocrinol.* 234, R67–R79. doi: 10.1530/JOE-17-0147

Sun, D., Zhuang, X., Xiang, X., Liu, Y., Zhang, S., Liu, C., et al. (2010). A novel nanoparticle drug delivery system: the anti-inflammatory activity of curcumin is enhanced when encapsulated in exosomes. *Mol. Ther.* 18, 1606–1614. doi: 10.1038/mt.2010.105

Sun, W., Zhao, C., Li, Y., Wang, L., Nie, G., Peng, J., et al. (2016). Osteoclast-derived microRNA-containing exosomes selectively inhibit osteoblast activity. *Cell Discov.* 2:16015. doi: 10.1038/celldisc.2016.15

Tan, M. L., Choong, P. F., and Dass, C. R. (2010). Recent developments in liposomes, microparticles and nanoparticles for protein and peptide drug delivery. *Peptides* 31, 184–193. doi: 10.1016/j.peptides.2009.10.002

Tatsumi, S., Ishii, K., Amizuka, N., Li, M., Kobayashi, T., Kohno, K., et al. (2007). Targeted ablation of osteocytes induces osteoporosis with defective mechanotransduction. *Cell Metab.* 5, 464–475. doi: 10.1016/j.cmet.2007.05.001

Taylor, D. D., and Gerçel-Taylor, C. (2005). Tumour-derived exosomes and their role in cancer-associated T-cell signalling defects. *Brit. J. Cancer* 92, 305–311. doi: 10.1038/sj.bjc.6602316

Thomou, T., Mori, M. A., Dreyfuss, J. M., Konishi, M., Sakaguchi, M., Wolfrum, C., et al. (2017). Adipose-derived circulating miRNAs regulate gene expression in other tissues. *Nature* 542, 450–455. doi: 10.1038/nature21365

Tian, Y., Li, S., Song, J., Ji, T., Zhu, M., Anderson, G. J., et al. (2014). A doxorubicin delivery platform using engineered natural membrane vesicle exosomes for targeted tumor therapy. *Biomaterials* 35, 2383–2390. doi: 10.1016/j.biomaterials.2013.11.083

Toh, W. S., Lai, R. C., Hui, J. H. P., and Lim, S. K. (2017). MSC exosome as a cell-free MSC therapy for cartilage regeneration: implications for osteoarthritis treatment. *Semin. Cell Dev. Biol.* 67, 56–64. doi: 10.1016/j.semcdb.2016.11.008

Uemura, R., Xu, M., Ahmad, N., and Ashraf, M. (2006). Bone marrow stem cells prevent left ventricular remodeling of ischemic heart through paracrine signaling. *Circ. Res.* 98, 1414–1421. doi: 10.1161/01.res.0000225952.61196.39

Valadi, H., Ekström, K., Bossios, A., Sjöstrand, M., Lee, J. J., and Lötvall, J. O. (2007). Exosome-mediated transfer of mRNAs and microRNAs is a novel mechanism of genetic exchange between cells. *Nat. Cell Biol.* 9, 654–659. doi: 10.1038/ncb1596

van der Pol, E., Böing, A. N., Harrison, P., Sturk, A., and Nieuwland, R. (2012). Classification, functions, and clinical relevance of extracellular vesicles. *Pharmacol. Rev.* 64, 676–705. doi: 10.1124/pr.112.005983

van Niel, G., Raposo, G., Candalh, C., Boussac, M., Hershberg, R., Cerf-Bensussan, N., et al. (2001). Intestinal epithelial cells secrete exosome-like vesicles. *Gastroenterology* 121, 337–349. doi: 10.1053/gast.2001.26263

Wang, C., Chen, L., Huang, Y., Li, K., Jinye, A., Fan, T., et al. (2019a). Exosome-delivered TRPP2 siRNA inhibits the epithelial-mesenchymal transition of FaDu cells. *Oncol. Lett.* 17, 1953–1961. doi: 10.3892/ol.2018.9752

Wang, C., Zhu, G., He, W., Yin, H., Lin, F., Gou, X., et al. (2019b). BMSCs protect against renal ischemia-reperfusion injury by secreting exosomes loaded with miR-199a-5p that target BIP to inhibit endoplasmic reticulum stress at the very early reperfusion stages. *FASEB J.* 33, 5440–5456. doi: 10.1096/fj.201801821R

Wang, J., Liu, Y., Sun, W., Zhang, Q., Gu, T., and Li, G. (2018). Plasma exosomes as novel biomarker for the early diagnosis of gastric cancer. *Cancer Biomark. Sec. A of Dis. Mark.* 21, 805–812. doi: 10.3233/CBM-170738

Wang, T., Shigdar, S., Shamaileh, H. A., Gantier, M. P., Yin, W., Xiang, D., et al. (2017). Challenges and opportunities for siRNA-based cancer treatment. *Cancer Lett.* 387, 77–83. doi: 10.1016/j.canlet.2016.03.045

Wang, X., Wei, W., Krzeszinski, J. Y., Wang, Y., and Wan, Y. (2015). A liver-bone endocrine relay by igfbp1 promotes osteoclastogenesis and mediates fgf21-induced bone resorption. *Cell Metab.* 22, 811–824. doi: 10.1016/j.cmet.2015.09.010

Waning, D. L., Guise, T. A., and Mohammad, K. S. (2019). A "Connexin" responsible for the fatal attraction of cancer to bone. *Cell Metab.* 29, 6–8. doi: 10.1016/j.cmet.2018.12.014

Warshauer, J. T., Bluestone, J. A., and Anderson, M. S. (2020). New frontiers in the treatment of type 1 diabetes. *Cell Metab.* 31, 46–61. doi: 10.1016/j.cmet.2019.11.017

Whitham, M., Parker, B. L., Friedrichsen, M., Hingst, J. R., Hjorth, M., Hughes, W. E., et al. (2018). Extracellular vesicles provide a means for tissue crosstalk during exercise. *Cell Metab* 27, 237–251. doi: 10.1016/j.cmet.2017.12.001

Wu, M., Ouyang, Y., Wang, Z., Zhang, R., Huang, P. H., Chen, C., et al. (2017). Isolation of exosomes from whole blood by integrating acoustics and microfluidics. *Proc. Natl. Acad. Sci. U.S.A.* 114, 10584–10589. doi: 10.1073/pnas.1709210114

Wu, P., Zhang, B., Shi, H., Qian, H., and Xu, W. (2018). MSC-exosome: a novel cell-free therapy for cutaneous regeneration. *Cytotherapy* 20, 291–301. doi: 10.1016/j.jcyt.2017.11.002

Xie, H., Cui, Z., Wang, L., Xia, Z., Hu, Y., Xian, L., et al. (2014). PDGF-BB secreted by preosteoclasts induces angiogenesis during coupling with osteogenesis. *Nat. Med.* 20, 1270–1278. doi: 10.1038/nm.3668

Xie, X., Wang, Y., Zhao, C., Guo, S., Liu, S., Jia, W., et al. (2012). Comparative evaluation of MSCs from bone marrow and adipose tissue seeded in PRP-derived scaffold for cartilage regeneration. *Biomaterials* 33, 7008–7018. doi: 10.1016/j.biomaterials.2012.06.058

Xie, Y., Chen, Y., Zhang, L., Ge, W., and Tang, P. (2017). The roles of bone-derived exosomes and exosomal microRNAs in regulating bone remodelling. *J. Cell. Mol. Med.* 21, 1033–1041. doi: 10.1111/jcmm.13039

Xin, H., Li, Y., Buller, B., Katakowski, M., Zhang, Y., Wang, X., et al. (2012). Exosome-mediated transfer of miR-133b from multipotent mesenchymal stromal cells to neural cells contributes to neurite outgrowth. *Stem Cells* 30, 1556–1564. doi: 10.1002/stem.1129

Xin, H., Li, Y., Liu, Z., Wang, X., Shang, X., Cui, Y., et al. (2013). MiR-133b promotes neural plasticity and functional recovery after treatment of stroke with multipotent mesenchymal stromal cells in rats via transfer of exosome-enriched extracellular particles. *Stem Cells* 31, 2737–2746. doi: 10.1002/stem.1409

Xu, J. F., Yang, G. H., Pan, X. H., Zhang, S. J., Zhao, C., Qiu, B. S., et al. (2014). Altered microRNA expression profile in exosomes during osteogenic differentiation of human bone marrow-derived mesenchymal stem cells. *PLoS One* 9:e114627. doi: 10.1371/journal.pone.0114627

Yang, L., Xie, G., Fan, Q., and Xie, J. (2010). Activation of the hedgehog-signaling pathway in human cancer and the clinical implications. *Oncogene* 29, 469–481. doi: 10.1038/onc.2009.392

Yang, M., Guo, Q., Peng, H., Xiao, Y. Z., Xiao, Y., Huang, Y., et al. (2019). Krüppel-like factor 3 inhibition by mutated lncRNA results in human high bone mass syndrome. *J. Exp. Med.* 216, 1944–1964. doi: 10.1084/jem.20181554

Yoshida, M., Satoh, A., Lin, J. B., Mills, K. F., Sasaki, Y., Rensing, N., et al. (2019). Extracellular vesicle-contained enampt delays aging and extends lifespan in mice. *Cell Metab.* 30, 329–342. doi: 10.1016/j.cmet.2019.05.015

Yu, B., Kim, H. W., Gong, M., Wang, J., Millard, R. W., Wang, Y., et al. (2015). Exosomes secreted from GATA-4 overexpressing mesenchymal stem cells serve as a reservoir of anti-apoptotic microRNAs for cardioprotection. *Int. J. Cardiol.* 182, 349–360. doi: 10.1016/j.ijcard.2014.12.043

Yu, Y., Newman, H., Shen, L., Sharma, D., Hu, G., Mirando, A. J., et al. (2019). Glutamine Metabolism Regulates Proliferation and Lineage Allocation in Skeletal Stem Cells. *Cell Metab.* 29, 966.e4–978.e4. doi: 10.1016/j.cmet.2019.01.016

Zhang, H., and Lyden, D. (2019). Asymmetric-flow field-flow fractionation technology for exomere and small extracellular vesicle separation and characterization. *Nat. Protoc.* 14, 1027–1053. doi: 10.1038/s41596-019-0126-x

Zhang, J., Guan, J., Niu, X., Hu, G., Guo, S., Li, Q., et al. (2015). Exosomes released from human induced pluripotent stem cells-derived MSCs facilitate cutaneous wound healing by promoting collagen synthesis and angiogenesis. *J. Transl. Med.* 13:49. doi: 10.1186/s12967-015-0417-0

Zhang, J., Liu, X., Li, H., Chen, C., Hu, B., Niu, X., et al. (2016). Exosomes/tricalcium phosphate combination scaffolds can enhance bone regeneration by activating the PI3K/Akt signaling pathway. *Stem Cell Res. Ther.* 7:136. doi: 10.1186/s13287-016-0391-3

Zhang, W. B., Zhong, W. J., and Wang, L. (2014). A signal-amplification circuit between miR-218 and Wnt/β-catenin signal promotes human adipose tissue-derived stem cells osteogenic differentiation. *Bone* 58, 59–66. doi: 10.1016/j.bone.2013.09.015

Zhao, C., Irie, N., Takada, Y., Shimoda, K., Miyamoto, T., Nishiwaki, T., et al. (2006). Bidirectional ephrinB2-EphB4 signaling controls bone homeostasis. *Cell Metab.* 4, 111–121. doi: 10.1016/j.cmet.2006.05.012

Zhao, C., Sun, W., Zhang, P., Ling, S., Li, Y., Zhao, D., et al. (2015). miR-214 promotes osteoclastogenesis by targeting Pten/PI3k/Akt pathway. *RNA Biol.* 12, 343–353. doi: 10.1080/15476286.2015.1017205

Zhu, W., Huang, L., Li, Y., Zhang, X., Gu, J., Yan, Y., et al. (2012). Exosomes derived from human bone marrow mesenchymal stem cells promote tumor growth in vivo. *Cancer Lett.* 315, 28–37. doi: 10.1016/j.canlet.2011.10.002

Zou, W., Greenblatt, M. B., Brady, N., Lotinun, S., Zhai, B., de Rivera, H., et al. (2013). The microtubule-associated protein DCAMKL1 regulates osteoblast function via repression of Runx2. *J. Exp. Med.* 210, 1793–1806. doi: 10.1084/jem.20111790

# 13

# A Novel Variant in *CLCN7* Regulates the Coupling of Angiogenesis and Osteogenesis

*Hui Peng[1], Hong-Bo He[2] and Ting Wen[2]**

[1] *Department of Endocrinology, Endocrinology Research Center, Xiangya Hospital of Central South University, Changsha, China,* [2] *Department of Orthopedic, Xiangya Hospital of Central South University, Changsha, China*

***Correspondence:***
*Ting Wen*
*tingwen163@126.com*

Autosomal dominant osteopetrosis type II (ADO II), characterized by increased bone mass and density, is caused by mutations in the chloride channel 7 (*CLCN7*) gene. In this study, a novel missense variant in *CLCN7* (c.1678A > G; p.Met560Val) was identified in three symptomatic subjects and one carrier of a Chinese family with ADO II. Notably, bone formation markers, including osteocalcin and total procollagen type N-terminal propeptide, have increased or presented at the upper limit of the normal range in the three patients. Serum factors secreted by osteoclast lineage cells and affecting the CD31$^{hi}$EMCN$^{hi}$ vessel formation, such as tartrate-resistant acid phosphatase 5b, platelet-derived growth factor-BB, vascular endothelial growth factor, and SLIT3, had a higher expression in three ADO II subjects than in 15 healthy age-matched and sex-matched controls. Moreover, the conditioned medium was obtained from preosteoclast induced from the ADO II patients' peripheral blood mononuclear cells. It was found to promote the CD31$^{hi}$EMCN$^{hi}$ vessel formation of human microvascular endothelial cells and osteogenic differentiation of bone marrow-derived stem cells. Taken together, our finding revealed a novel *CLCN7* variant associated with ADO II and suggested that the sclerotic bone was potentially associated with the increase of the CD31$^{hi}$EMCN$^{hi}$ vessel formation and bone formation.

**Keywords: autosomal dominant osteopetrosis type II, *CLCN7*, variant, CD31$^{hi}$Emcn$^{hi}$ vessel formation, bone formation**

## INTRODUCTION

Autosomal dominant osteopetrosis type II (ADO II; OPTA2, Online Mendelian Inheritance in Man: 166600), also known as "Albers Schönberg disease," is the most common type of osteopetrosis with an estimated prevalence of 2.5/100,000 (Bénichou et al., 2000; Del Fattore et al., 2008). It is characterized by segmentary osteosclerosis, predominantly involving in the vertebral endplates ("rugger-jersey spine"), iliac wings ("bone within bone" sign), and the skull base. Previous studies revealed that ADO II was a phenotypically heterogeneous disease whose clinical spectrums ranged from unaffected radiography mutation carriers to affected skeletal patients yet asymptomatic to severe manifestations including fracture, osteomyelitis, visual loss, and bone marrow failure (Bénichou et al., 2000; Waguespack et al., 2007).

The bone homeostasis was maintained by balancing osteoclast-mediated resorption and osteoblast-mediated formation (Wang et al., 2018; Hayashi et al., 2019; Rodriguez-Laguna et al., 2019). The disrupted bone mass and structure of osteopetrosis resulted from the impaired osteoclast-mediated bone resorption caused by genetic factors (Tolar et al., 2004; Sobacchi et al., 2013). Bénichou et al. (2001) previously considered that ADO II was genetically homogeneous with a single disease-causing gene on 16p13.3. Accumulated studies showed that roughly 70% of patients harbored heterozygous missense mutations of the *CLCN7* gene in a dominant-negative form (Cleiren et al., 2001). To date, more than 40 mutations in *CLCN7* has been identified in different osteopetrosis families (Leisle et al., 2011; Pang et al., 2016). *CLCN7* (Online Mendelian Inheritance in Man: 602727) is a multi-pass membrane protein that acts as a Cl-/H + exchanger by voltage gate (Leisle et al., 2011). It mainly resides in the late endosomes, lysosomes, and the ruffled membrane of osteoclasts. In osteoclasts, the ruffled border contains Cl-channels that are inserted by exocytotic fusion together with the H + -ATPase to ensure the acidification of extracellular resorption lacuna. Pathogenic mutations in *the CLCN7* gene impairing acidification of extracellular resorption lacuna were assumed to prevent degradation of the calcified and organic matrix of bone (Weinert et al., 2010). Furthermore, some studies suggested that chloride channels could be a drug target for osteopetrosis (Capulli et al., 2015). Mattia et al. demonstrated that *CLCN7* mutant-specific small interfering RNAs silenced dominant-negative *CLCN7* transcripts and subsequently ameliorated the bone phenotype in ADO II (Verkman and Galietta, 2009). Recent research also demonstrated that the specific small interfering RNA therapy normalized extra-skeletal manifestations on the ADO II mouse (Maurizi et al., 2019).

Some studies suggested that *CLCN7* mutations regulate bone formation in patients with osteopetrosis (Barvencik et al., 2014; Coudert et al., 2014). The vessels in the bone niche were reported to play great roles in bone formation (Abarrategi et al., 2018; Hao et al., 2019). A specific endothelium in the murine skeletal system, termed type H, strongly positive for CD31 and endomucin, is crucial in bone formation and regeneration (Kusumbe et al., 2014; Ramasamy et al., 2014; Langen et al., 2017). Accumulated evidence suggests that the type H vessels exert on bone formation in many aspects, ranging from mediating local growth of the vasculature, to providing a necessary microenvironment for perivascular osteoprogenitors, and coupling angiogenesis to osteogenesis (Yang et al., 2017). Previous findings revealed that platelet-derived growth factor-BB (PDGF-BB) secreted by preosteoclast could induce $CD31^{hi}Emcn^{hi}$ vessels subtype subsequently prevented bone loss in osteoporosis and bone-loss diseases (Xie et al., 2014). Furthermore, we recently found a mutation in *Reg1cp* involved in high bone mass syndrome through promoting angiogenesis (Yang et al., 2019). However, whether the bone accrual is associated with the coupling between angiogenesis and osteogenesis or not remains unclear.

Here, we ascertained a missense variant in *CLCN7* in a Chinese family. This is the first description genetically confirmed with this heterozygous missense mutation (c.1678A > G; p. Met560Val) responsible for ADO II. Additionally, these results indicated that the mutation might be associated with the dysfunction of the angiogenesis and osteogenesis, which further explained the elevated bone formation markers in this ADO II family.

# MATERIALS AND METHODS

## Family Collection

The Chinese family who suffered from ADO II was recruited from Xiangya Hospital Central South University. There were three affected individuals (II3, II7, and III2 in **Figure 1A**) in this family, and all of the affected subjects were not born of consanguineous parents. The patients underwent a series of clinical evaluation including laboratory and radiography examination in Xiangya Hospital, such as blood route, liver function test, renal function test, serum calcium (Ca), phosphate (P), alkaline phosphatase (ALP), β-Cross Laps of type I collagen containing cross-linked C-telopeptide, osteocalcin (OC), total procollagen type N-terminal propeptide (TPINP), and intact parathyroid hormone (PTH). Additionally, the patients were carried out with bone mineral density of the total body measured by a dual-energy X-ray absorptiometry densitometer and X-ray of bilateral hip joints and lumbar. The study was approved by the Ethics Committee of Xiangya Hospital Central South University. All subjects involved in this study signed informed consent documents before participating in the project.

## Whole-Genome Sequence

Genomic DNA was collected and extracted from peripheral whole blood samples using Qiagen DNA kits. The genomic DNA met the sequencing requirements of the purity (optical density 260/280 > 1.8) and concentration (50 ng/ml) of each sample. Whole-genome sequencing was conducted by Annoroad Gene Technology by using Illumina/TruSeq Nano DNA HT Library Preparation Kit for capture and Illumina sequencing platforms for data generation (150-bp paired-end, 300 cycles). Sequencing was performed with 150-bp paired-end reads on the Illumina NovaSeq 6000 sequencing platform. The mean coverage was 40×.

## Variant Filtering and Analysis

Sequence alignment was performed with the Burrows–Wheeler Aligner mem using human genome assembly hg19 as the reference, then produce called variants with RTG tools Hyplotype Caller. Annotation of gene context was carried out with annovar using Single Nucleotide Polymorphism Database, Refseq gene as the reference.

## Sanger Sequence

The variant was amplified by using DNA polymerase [MIX (GREEN), TSINGKE, China], and the former and reverse primers are CTTGAGGAGTCCACACCCAC and CTGGGAGCAGGTGGATGG, respectively. Forward and reverse sequencing reactions were performed with the Big Dye Terminator Cycle Sequencing Ready Reaction Kit (PE Applied Biosystems), and the products were analyzed on an ABI 3730XL automated sequencer (PE Applied Biosystems).

## Enzyme-Linked Immunosorbent Assay

Serum was obtained from peripheral blood using 4,000 rpm for 5 min. Then, we used the ELISA kits to test the expression of tartrate-resistant acid phosphatase 5b (TRAP-5b), PDGF-BB, vascular endothelial growth factor (VEGF; R&D Systems), and

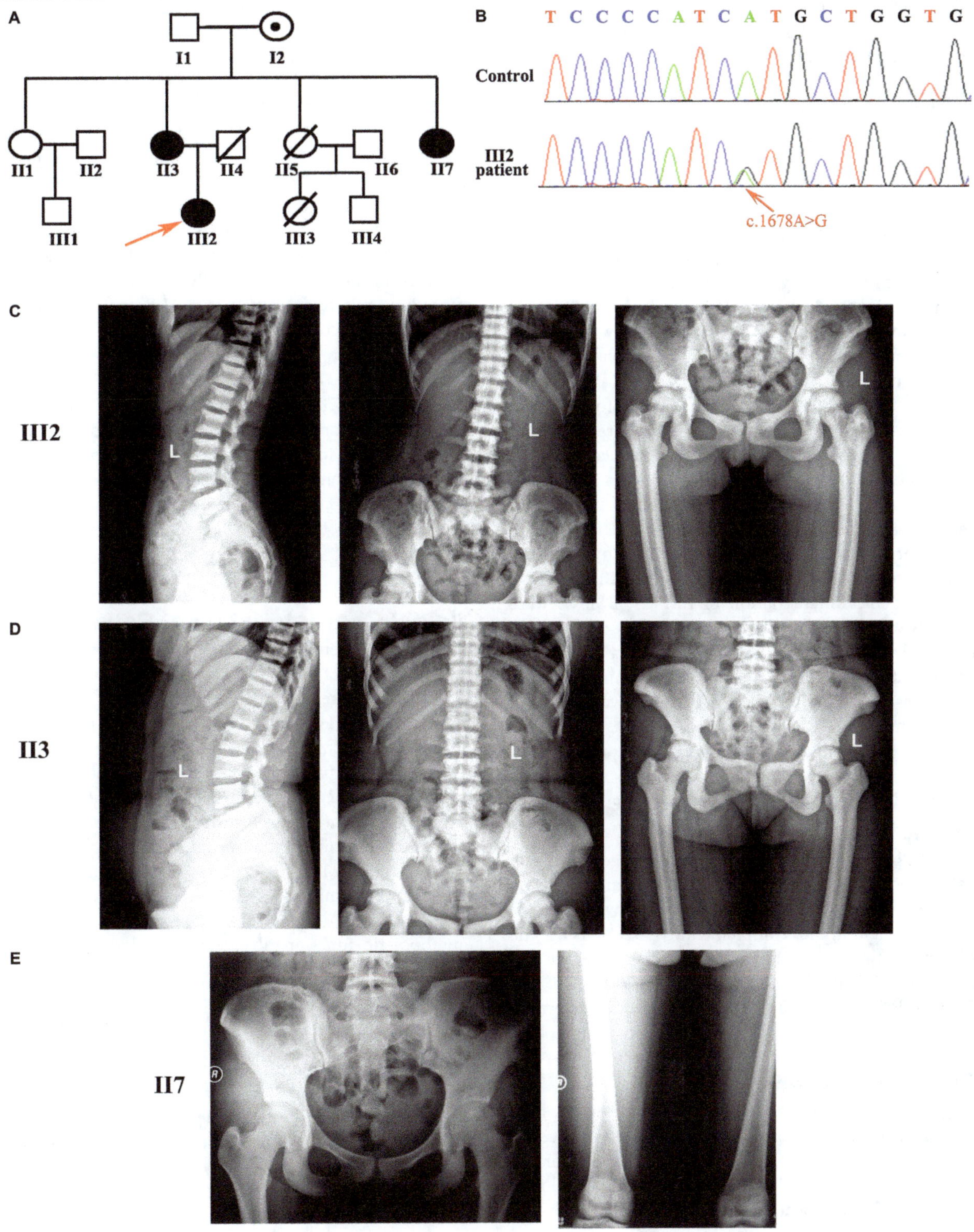


**FIGURE 1 |** Pedigree of the osteopetrosis family was associated with the mutation in *CLCN7*. **(A)** Pedigree of a Chinese family with osteopetrosis. Squares represent males, and circles represent females. Red arrow indicates the proband in this family. White symbols represent unaffected subjects, and black symbols indicate affected subjects. Symbols with an embedded black dot represent asymptomatic carriers. Symbols with a diagonal line represent deceased subjects. **(B)** Sanger sequence chromatograms from the proband and unaffected II1. c.1678A > G transition is indicated by the red arrow. **(C–E)** Radiographic image reveals osteosclerosis in three affected patients (radiographic images of III2 in the top row, images of II3 in the second row, and images of II7 in the bottom row). Images showed vertebral endplates ("rugger-jersey spine"; III2 and II3) and osteosclerosis of the pelvis and femoral (III2, II3, and II7).

SLIT3 (SED353Mi) in serum according to the manufacturers' instructions. The ELISA was replicated three times for the affected patients, and the mean values were used.

## Cell Culture

A total of 15 ml of heparin anti-coagulated peripheral blood was obtained from every subject, including all members of this family and healthy age- and sex-matched controls. Then, peripheral blood mononuclear cells (PBMCs) were washed using phosphate-buffered saline twice and cultured in minimum essential medium Eagle-α containing 10% fetal bovine serum, 100 U $ml^{-1}$ penicillin, 100 μg $ml^{-1}$ streptomycin sulfate, and 50 ng $ml^{-1}$ macrophage colony-stimulating factor (M-CSF; R&D Systems Inc.). Non-adherent cells were incubated with M-CSF (50 ng $ml^{-1}$) to obtain pure monocytes and macrophages. Then, PBMCs were cultured in 24-well plates at $1 \times 10^5$ cells per well with 50 ng $ml^{-1}$ of M-CSF and 100 ng $ml^{-1}$ receptor activator of nuclear factor-kappa-B ligand. Cells became preosteoclasts after a 3-day culture. We collected serum-containing conditioned medium from the preosteoclasts. After centrifugation (2,500 rpm for 10 min at 4°C), we aliquoted conditioned media and stored them at −80°C. Human BMSCs (HUXMA-0100; Cyagen Biosciences) were cultured in a human mesenchymal stem cell growth medium (HUXMA-90011; Cyagen Biosciences). To induce osteogenic differentiation of BMSCs, BMSCs were cultured in 48-well using the serum-containing conditioned medium. Then, we collected protein to test ALP activity on day 2, RNA on the 3rd day, and performed the ALP staining on day 7. Human microvascular endothelial cells (HMECs) were cultured with MCDB131 medium (Gibco) supplemented 10% fetal bovine serum, 100 U $ml^{-1}$ penicillin, and 100 μg $ml^{-1}$ streptomycin.

## Real-Time Quantitative Polymerase Chain Reaction

Quantitative PCR analysis was performed as described previously (Xiao et al., 2020). Briefly, we extracted RNA from cells using Trizol reagent (Takara). Then, 1,000-ng RNA was reverse-transcribed into first-strand complementary DNA using the Reverse Transcription Kit (Takara). Quantitative PCR was performed using SYBR Green PCR Master Mix (Takara), and messenger RNA expression was normalized to reference genes *GAPDH*.

## Tube Formation Assay

The Matrigel (BD Biosciences) was plated in 48-well plates and then incubated at 37°C for 45 min. HMECs were seeded in 48-well plates at $5 \times 10^4$ cells per well on polymerized Matrigel. The cells were cultured in the preosteoclast-conditioned medium collected from patients or control individuals for 4 h incubation at 37°C. Then, the tube formation was observed through microscopy, and the number of tube branches was quantified in four random microscope visual fields of each well.

## Alkaline Phosphatase Activity

On the second day of osteogenic differentiation, the cell lysates were homogenized for ALP activity assay by spectrophotometric measurement of *p*-nitrophenol release using an ALP Assay Kit (P0321S, Beyotime) according to the manufacturer's instructions.

## Alkaline Phosphatase Staining

The cells were washed using phosphate-buffered saline for three times, followed by 10% paraformaldehyde for 5 min. Then, cells were incubated in ALP incubation buffer (0.2-*g* barbital sodium, 0.4-*g* magnesium sulfate, 0.2-*g* calcium chloride, and 0.3-*g* beta-glycerophosphate) at 37°C for 2 h. Next, cells were washed with 2% calcium chloride and incubated with 2% cobaltous nitrate for 5 min. Finally, cells were incubated in 1:80 ammonium sulfate for 10 s. The ALP staining was observed through a microscope.

## Statistical Analysis

Data were imported into Excel and scaled and normalized to appropriate controls. Unpaired, two-tailed Student's *t*-tests were performed for the comparisons of two groups. Critical *P*-values were Bonferroni corrected and expressed as follows: $^{*}P < 0.05$. $^{**}P < 0.01$.

# RESULTS

## Clinical Characteristics of Patients

A Chinese patient, aged 22 years, was admitted to the Department of Endocrinology with a history of bone pain for 6 years. There was a family history of a similar disease of her mother (II3) and aunt (II7) shown in **Figure 1A**. All these three patients had a mild phenotype of osteopetrosis only with bone pain on hip joints and back. The proband also had a history of fracture in the hip. On examination, we did not find poor nutritional status, short stature, malformed craniofacial appearance, hepatosplenomegaly, and intellectual disability in the proband and other affected patients in this family.

Laboratory findings of the three patients showed that the hematopoietic function, liver function, kidney function, total serum calcium, and total serum phosphorus were within the normal ranges except for a slight increase of aspartate transaminase of II3 (**Table 1**). For bone turnover markers, β cross-linked C-telopeptide of type 1 collagen and ALP have not detected any abnormalities in this family (**Table 2**). However, markers of bone formation in the proband, such as OC and TPINP, were both found at the upper limit of the normal range (**Table 2**). Moreover, the levels of OC, TPINP, and PTH (parathormone) were found to be elevated in her mother (II3). The level of OC in her aunt (II7) also slightly increased. Thus, we hypothesized that bone formation in these patients had been elevated (**Table 2**).

The total bone mineral density values of the three patients at lumbar and hip sites, measured by dual-energy X-ray absorptiometry, are shown in **Table 3**. The three affected patients were all with regular menstruation. The *Z* values at different sites of the three patients were significantly higher than the those of the sex-matched and age-matched

**TABLE 1** | Hematopoietic, hepatorenal, and serum electrolytic data of ADO II subjects.

| Parameters | III2 | II3 | II7 | Normal range |
|---|---|---|---|---|
| WBC ($10^9 \cdot L^{-1}$) | 4.2 | 5.3 | 5.46 | 3.5–9.5 |
| Hb ($g \cdot L^{-1}$) | 124 | 126 | 126 | 115–150 |
| RBC ($10^{12} \cdot L^{-1}$) | 4.52 | 4.34 | 4.19 | 3.80–5.10 |
| PLT ($10^9 \cdot L^{-1}$) | 295 | 240 | 146 | 125–350 |
| ALT (μ/L) | 9.3 | 21.6 | 20.4 | 7.0–40.0 |
| AST (μ/L) | 32.4 | 46.5 | 22.5 | 13.0–35.0 |
| BUN (mmol/L) | 4.58 | 5.56 | 6.95 | 2.60–7.50 |
| Cre (μmol/L) | 55 | 69 | 53 | 41.0–111.0 |
| UA (μmol/L) | 287.5 | 289.5 | 246 | 155.0–357.0 |
| Na (mmol/L) | 140 | 142.8 | 142 | 137.0–147.0 |
| K (mmol/L) | 4.54 | 4.22 | 3.6 | 3.50–5.30 |
| Cl (mmol/L) | 103.4 | 107.8 | 105.6 | 99.0–110.0 |
| Ca (mmol/L) | 2.45 | 2.28 | 2.22 | 2.00–2.60 |
| Mg (mmol/L) | 0.91 | 0.84 | 0.98 | 0.66–1.07 |
| P (mmol/L) | 1.41 | 1.45 | 1.25 | 0.86–1.78 |

*WBC, white blood cells; RBC, red blood cells; Hb, hemoglobin; PLT, platelet; ALT, alanine transaminase; AST, aspartate transaminase; BUN, blood urea nitrogen; Cre, creatinine; and UA, uric acid.*

**TABLE 2** | Bone biomarker of ADO II subjects.

| | III2 | II3 | II7 | Normal range |
|---|---|---|---|---|
| ALP (μ/L) | 55.3 | 64.5 | 46.8 | 45.0–125.0 |
| OC (ng/ml) | 20.44 | 26.79 | 45 | 4.11–21.87 |
| TPINP (ng/ml) | 58.37 | 131.4 | NA | 8.53–64.32 |
| PTH (pg/ml) | 44.8 | 83.8 | 59.85 | 15.0–68.3 |
| β-CTX (pg/ml) | 290.5 | 243.5 | 572 | 68–680 |

*ALP, alkaline phosphatase; OC, osteocalcin; TPINP, total procollagen type N-terminal propeptide; PTH, parathormone; β-CTX, β cross-linked C-telopeptide of type 1 collagen; and NA, not available.*

**TABLE 3** | Bone mass density of the ADO II subjects.

| Subjects | Age | Total | | Lumbar | | Left hip | |
|---|---|---|---|---|---|---|---|
| | | Total BMD (g/cm²) | Z value | Total BMD (g/cm²) | Z value | Total BMD (g/cm²) | Z value |
| III2 | 21 | 1.611 | 5.8 | 2.221 | 12.1 | 1.591 | 6.9 |
| II 3 | 42 | 2.063 | 8.0 | 2.304 | 12.7 | 1.918 | 9.6 |
| II7 | 29 | 1.973 | 7.6 | 2.245 | 11.2 | 1.855 | 8.3 |

*BMD, Bone mineral density.*

controls (**Table 3**). Radiological features of the three patients revealed diffused osteosclerosis, predominantly at the vertebral endplates ("rugger-jersey spine"). The superior ramus of the pubis, sacral vertebrae, femoral head, and greater trochanter of femur also presented diffuse osteosclerosis. The boundaries among cancellous bone, cortical bone, and bone medullary disappeared (**Figures 1C–E**). Based on their clinical and radiological assessment, the family was diagnosed with ADO II.

## Genetic Analysis With Whole-Genome Sequencing and Identification of the Pathogenic Variant

We performed the whole-genome sequence in the three affected patients. Firstly, we filtered the common variants, which were unlikely to cause the rare heritable disorder (allele frequency greater than 0.1% in the 1000 Genomes database and Exome Variant Server). Then, we excluded the variants with low confidence and the putative impact. Next, we tried to find the shared variant in the three patients. Interestingly, a heterozygous missense variant (c.1678A > G, p.Met560Val) in *CLCN7* segregated with osteopetrosis among three affected patients. We then performed the Sanger sequence in all members of this family and found the variant occurred in three patients and a non-penetrant carrier (I2 in **Figure 1A** was asymptomatic and did not present abnormal bone phenotype as well as laboratory findings; **Figure 1B**).

Various mutations in *CLCN7* have been reported to be involved in the pathogenesis of osteopetrosis (**Figure 2**). In gnomAD database, the PopMax Allele Frequency and allele count of this variant were 0.00000900058 and 1, respectively, (the total Allele number was 245442). Moreover, this variant was not found in East Asian with 17228 Allele number in total. Pro560 in *CLCN7*, which is substituted to a Valine in three patients, is phylogenetically highly conserved among both vertebrates and invertebrates (**Figure 3**) [Phylop] score of 6.111 and [PhastCons] score of 1. *CLCN7* gene was also predicted to be intolerant whose Residual Variation Intolerance Score is 7.0381% (**Table 4**). Furthermore, the effect of missense mutation Met560Val in *CLCN7* was predicted by different variant effect prediction software (PolyPhen-2, MutationTaster, CADD, MPC). It suggested that the Met560Val substitution is likely to be deleterious (PolyPhen score of 0.991, probably damaging; MutationTaster score of 0.999, disease-causing; CADD score of 24.3, damaging; MPC score of 1.0788, possibly damaging; **Table 4**). Based on the genetic analysis, this study revealed that the heterozygous missense mutation was possibly responsible for the ADO II.

## *CLCN7* Mutation Induces the Type H Vessel Formation and Osteogenic Differentiation *in vitro*

The cross-talks between osteoclasts and other cells, including osteoblasts, endothelium cells, have been well established (Phan et al., 2004; Ramasamy et al., 2014; Xie et al., 2014; Yang et al., 2017, 2019; Chen et al., 2018; Li et al., 2019). Additionally, PDGF-BB secreted by preosteoclasts could result in elevated bone mass through inducing angiogenesis during coupling with osteogenesis (Xie et al., 2014). To investigate if the osteosclerotic bone of these patients was associated with the coupling between angiogenesis and osteogenesis, we collected the serum from ADO II individuals and 15 normal controls for further studies. TRAP-5b is well-established to be secreted by osteoclasts, and PDGF-BB, VEGF, and SLIT3 can also be secreted by osteoclasts/preosteoclasts, which were reported to be

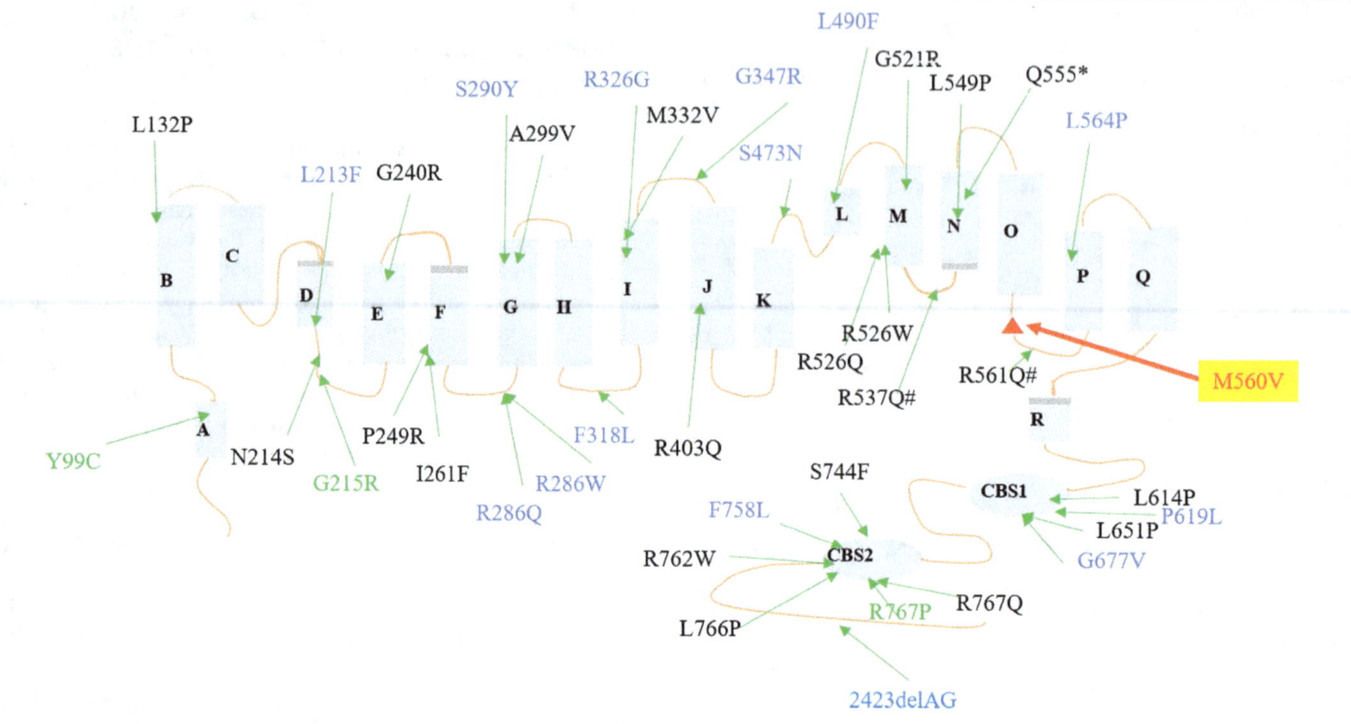


**FIGURE 2 |** Reported mutations of *CLCN7* in osteopetrosis family. Red mutation was found in this family. Black mutations were reported to cause osteopetrosis autosomal recessive 4, blue mutations were reported to cause ADO II, and green mutations were reported to cause different types of osteopetrosis.

```
H.sapiens    G V I K A T M L V L M I P F G Y T V N S T
M.mulatta    G V I K A T M L V L M I P F G Y T V N S T
M.musculus   G V I K A T M L V L M I P F G Y T V N S T
C.familiaris G V I K A T M L V L M I P F G Y T V N S T
Rattus       G V I K A T M L V L M I P F G Y T V N S T
G.gallus     G V I K A T M L V L M I P F G Y T V N S T
D.rerio      G V I K A T M L V L M I P F G Y T V N S T
```

p. Met560Val

**FIGURE 3 |** Conservation of the mutated amino acids. Alignment of the *CLCN7* proteins, showing the conservation of the mutated residues among different species. p. Met560Val transition is indicated by the red arrow.

**TABLE 4 |** Summary of the *CLCN7* mutation in this family with ADO II.

| Variant (Missense) | Numbers | | Rarity in gnomAD | | Conservation (Extremely conserved) | | Pathogenic prediction (Damaging) | | | |
|---|---|---|---|---|---|---|---|---|---|---|
| | Patients | Carrier | PopMax AF | Allele count | Phylop score | PhastCon score | MutationTaster score | MPC | CADD score Phred | RVIS% |
| c.1678A > G p.Met560Val | 3 | 1 | 9.00058E-06 | 1 | 6.111 | 1 | 0.999 | 1.0788 | 24.3 | 7.04% |

*PopMax AF, Maximum allele frequency in any one population; MPC, mutant prevention concentration; CADD, Combined Annotation Dependent Depletion; and RVIS, Residual Variation Intolerance Score.*

involved in the type H formation (Bollerslev et al., 2013; Sivaraj and Adams, 2016; Kim et al., 2018; Peng et al., 2020). Thus, we selected them to see if they have been altered in ADO II patients. Surprisingly, the level of TRAP-5b, PDGF-BB, VEGF, and SLIT3 showed a remarkable increase in ADO II patients compared with the 15 control groups with matched age and sex (**Figures 4A–D**). To further confirm the possible effect of type H vessels in this kindred, we purified the PBMCs from the patients and control normal subjects. Then, the collected preosteoclast condition medium from osteoclastic-induced PBMCs has been

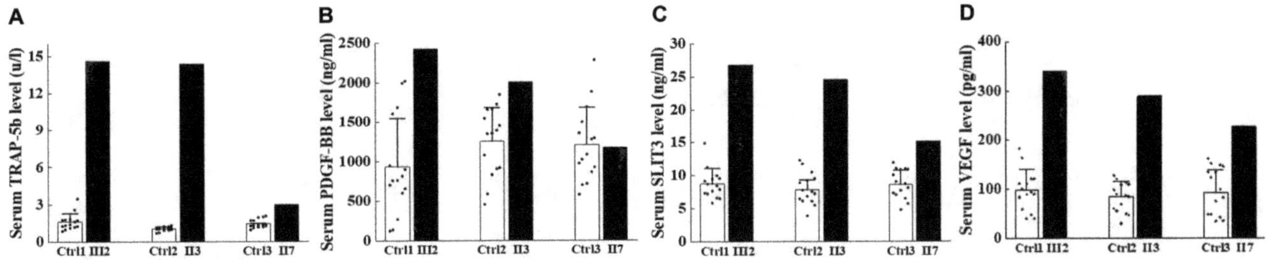


**FIGURE 4 |** Expression of factors secreted by osteoclast lineage cells elevated in the affected patients. Serum analysis of ADO II subjects and age-matched and sex-matched. **(A)** Expression of serum TRAP-5b. **(B)** Expression of serum PDGF-BB. **(C)** Expression of serum SLIT3. **(D)** Expression of serum VEGF. Number of controls = 15. Data are shown as mean ± SD.

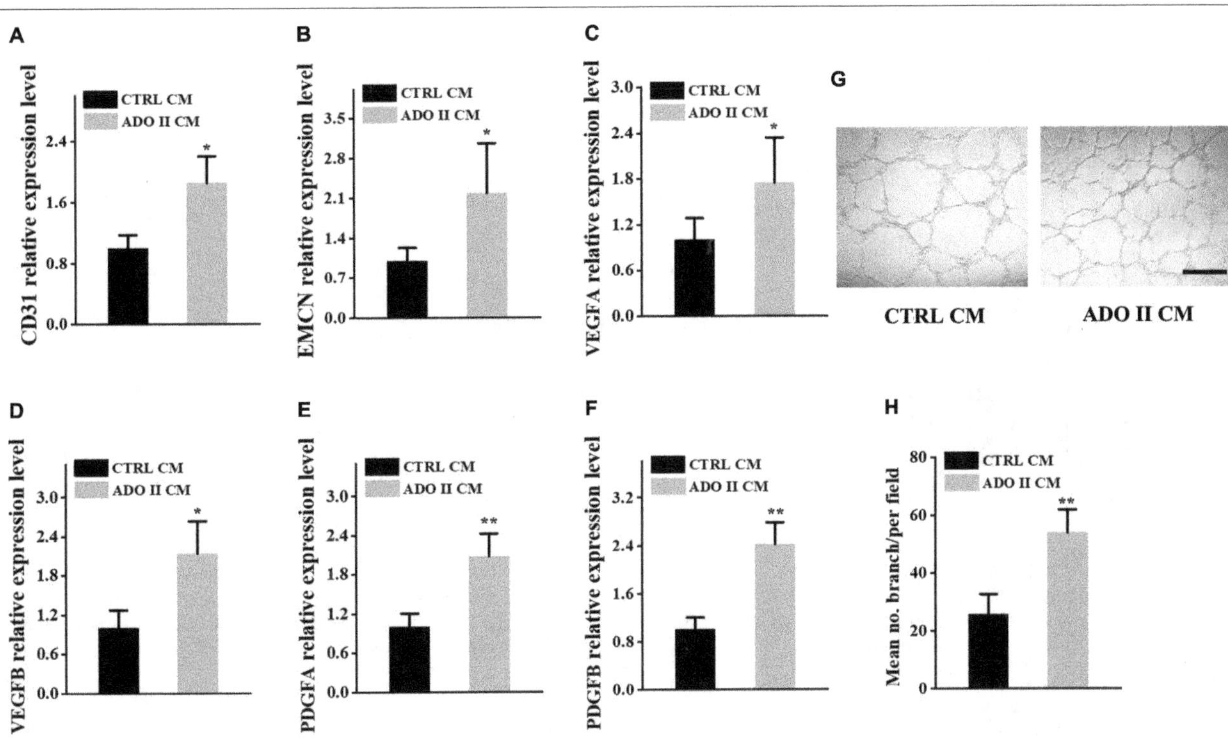


**FIGURE 5 |** Preosteoclast-conditioned medium from ADO II patients promotes vessel formation *in vitro*. HMECs were treated with a preosteoclast-conditioned medium from ADO II patients or control groups. **(A,B)** qRT-PCR analysis of the relative levels of *CD31* **(A)**, *EMCN* **(B)**, *VEGFA* **(C)**, *VEGFB* **(D)**, *PDGFA* **(E)**, and *PDGFB* **(F)** in HMECs. **(G)** Representative images of tube formation. **(H)** Quantification of tube branch numbers per field. CTRL CM, control conditioned medium; ADO II CM, ADO II conditioned medium. These experiments were replicated three times. Data are shown as mean ± SD. $^{*}P < 0.05$ and $^{**}P < 0.01$.

used to culture the HMECs. As expected, the expression of *CD31*, *EMCN*, and vessel growth factors, including *VEGFA*, *VEGFB*, *PDGFA*, and *PDGFB*, has increased in the cells treated with preosteoclast-conditioned medium from ADO II cells compared with the cells from control individuals (**Figures 5A–F**). Moreover, the tube formation also has been promoted by the ADO II-conditioned medium (**Figures 5G,H**). Even the expression of *RUNX2* was not altered by the conditioned medium from patients; other osteogenic markers in hBMSCs, such as *ALPL* and *SP7*, elevated (**Figures 6A–C**). Consistent with these results, both ALP activity and ALP staining showed a significant difference between the two groups (**Figures 6D,E**). Together, these data suggested that the *CLCN7* mutation might cause the bone accrual partially because of the elevated coupling of bone formation with type H formation.

## DISCUSSION

Osteopetrosis is a rare genetic condition of increased bone mass and density generally due to a defect of bone resorption. The common complications are confined to the skeleton, including bone fracture, bone pain, osteomyelitis, and rare bone marrow failure (Bénichou et al., 2000). Bone pain on the back was described in three affected patients and fracture on the hip of the proband. Their prominent radiographic signatures of vertebral

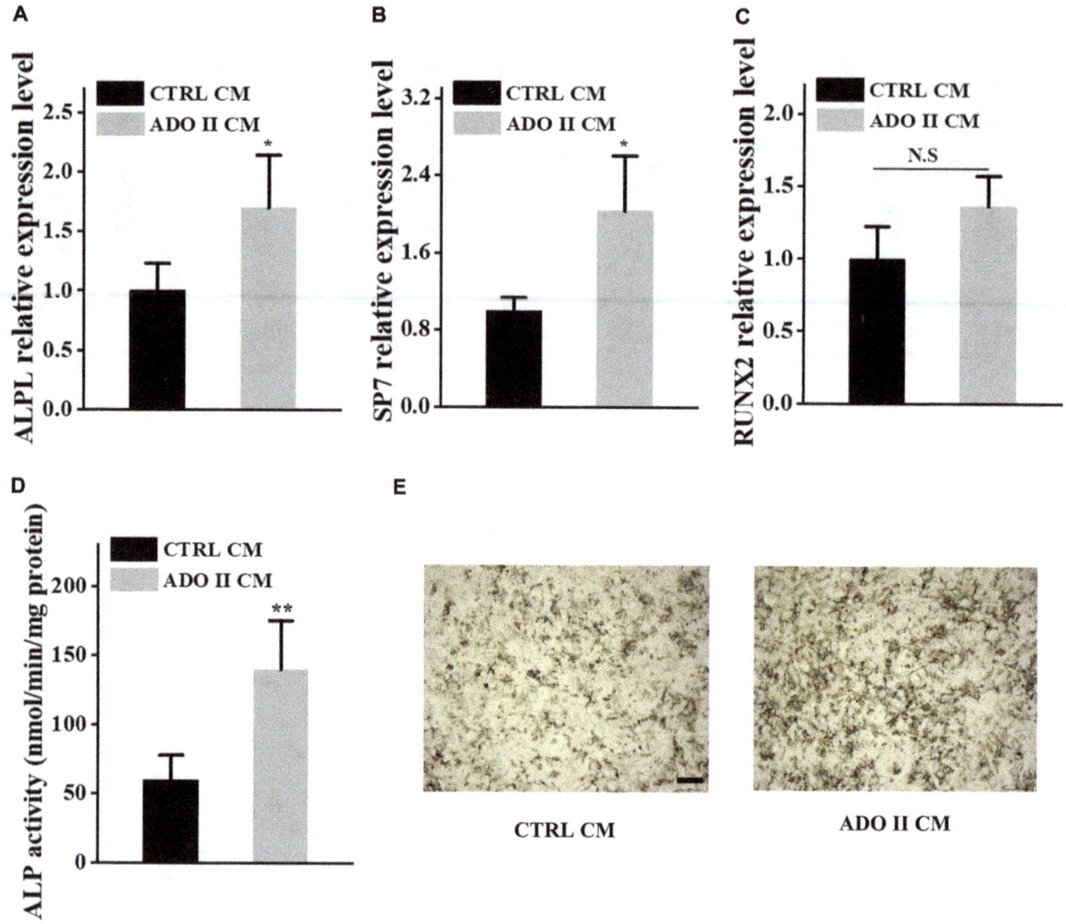


**FIGURE 6 |** Preosteoclast-conditioned medium from ADO II patients enhances osteoblastic differentiation *in vitro*. BMSCs were treated with a preosteoclast-conditioned medium from ADO II patients or control groups. **(A–C)** qRT–PCR analysis of the relative levels of *ALPL* **(A)**, *SP7* **(B)**, and *RUNX2* **(C)** in BMSCs. **(D)** ALP activity in BMSCs. **(E)** Representative images of ALP staining in BMSCs. Scale bar = 300 μm. These experiments were replicated three times. Data are shown as mean ± SD. $^{*}P < 0.05$ and $^{**}P < 0.01$.

endplates ("rugger-jersey spine") and diffused bone sclerosis were found in three affected patients.

The mutation analysis in this family was in agreement with the clinical diagnosis of ADO-II. Previous studies that reported several mutations in *CLCN7* could result in severe recessive, dominant, and intermediate osteopetrosis (Frattini et al., 2003). Currently, genetic and molecular diagnoses were available for patients with ADO II, especially to the missense mutations in the *CLCN7* gene (Bollerslev et al., 2013). Above 70% of patients harbored heterozygous dominant-negative mutations of the *CLCN7* gene (Cleiren et al., 2001). These *CLCN7*-related mutations are usually located in different structures of its protein, such as intramembrane α helices, extracellular loops, Cl-binding sites, and CBS domains (Pang et al., 2016; Jentsch and Pusch, 2018). We identified a heterozygous variant p.Met560Val located in the loop between helix N and helix O in three patients and an unaffected carrier. There was only one allele of the identified mutation in gnomAD and was not presented in East Asian populations. Additionally, Steven et al. have estimated the penetrance of ADO II to be approximately 66% (62 clinically affected individuals/94 subjects with the gene mutation), which means among the individuals with *CLCN7* mutations, one third were asymptomatic gene carriers without osteopetrosis-related signs in clinical, biochemical, and radiological results (Waguespack et al., 2003). Thus, the carrier did not present the related osteosclerotic bone associated with the incomplete penetrance. The phenotypical and genetic heterogeneity and incomplete penetrance remain unclear in skeletal dysplasia (Alam et al., 2017; Chen et al., 2020). It is likely to be related to the environmental factors, methylated gene modification, the complex interaction between other genes and *CLCN7*, and even some unidentified loci (Zhang et al., 2009; Leisle et al., 2011; Boudin et al., 2016), which need more further studies to elucidate.

The previous investigation indicated that ADO was one of the osteoclast-rich forms of osteopetrosis (Bollerslev et al., 2013). The bone biopsies from patients with ADO showed increased size and number of osteoclasts (Bollerslev et al., 1993). Chen et al. revealed that c.1856C > T mutation in *CLCN7* identified in an ADO II case resulted in enhanced but hypofunctional osteoclastogenesis (Chen et al., 2016). Besides, previous studies showed that the serum TRAP-5b was significantly elevated in osteoclast-rich ADO II mice and patients (Chen et al., 2016; Alam et al., 2017). Consistent with these studies, the elevated serum TRAP-5b was also found in these patients with ADO II (Alatalo et al., 2004). The prominently elevated biochemical measurements of TRAP-5b suggested that the variant affected the function of osteoclast and indicated the molecular feature to be osteoclast-rich osteopetrosis in this family.

Osteopetrosis is a clinically heterogenetic disorder. In this Chinese family with the *CLCN7* variant, the serum bone formation markers (OC, TPINP, and PTH) were at the upper limit range in the proband. They also elevated in the proband's mother (II3), and the level of OC increased remarkably in the aunt (II7). The variable level of bone formation markers in the three affected patients might be associated with the characterization of clinical heterogeneity or some factors, such as age, lifestyle, and other environmental stimulus (Lundberg et al., 2018; Chevalier et al., 2020). Taken together, the upregulated or upper limit range of serum bone formation markers implied that the bone formation increased. It is extensively reported that the coupling of angiogenesis with osteogenesis plays a great role in bone modeling and remodeling (Phan et al., 2004; Ramasamy et al., 2014; Xie et al., 2014; Yang et al., 2017, 2019; Chen et al., 2018; Li et al., 2018). Previous findings revealed that PDGF-BB secreted by preosteoclasts could stimulate angiogenesis during coupling with osteogenesis (Xie et al., 2014). Furthermore, we demonstrated that *Reg1cp* mutation potentially caused high bone mass syndrome by regulating the coupling of angiogenesis with osteogenesis (Yang et al., 2019). Other studies revealed that the secret factors, including VEGF and SLIT3 by osteoclast lineage cells, could regulate type H formation during bone regeneration (Xu et al., 2018; Peng et al., 2020). Based on these findings, we investigated if this *CLCN7* mutation contributed to the increased bone mass by regulating the process of angiogenesis and osteogenesis. Intriguingly, we found that the levels of PDGF-BB, VEGF, and SLIT3 were increased in ADO II individuals. Of note, the conditioned medium from PBMCs of ADO II patients promoted vessel formation of HMECs as well as osteogenic differentiation of hBMSCs. These results gave some new insights into the pathogenesis in this family.

In this study, we identified a novel missense variant (p.Met560Val) in *CLCN7* through whole-genome sequencing and detected it in all affected family members by Sanger sequence. The rarity, conservation, and pathogenic predication all supported that this *CLCN7* mutation might be a disease-causing one. Furthermore, the *in vitro* experiments showed that the variant promoted the vessel formation and osteogenic differentiation in this family. To conclude, we presented a novel heterozygous mutation (p.Met560Val) in *CLCN7* segregated with ADO II in this Chinese family and revealed that it might be associated with the increased type H vessel formation and bone formation.

## ETHICS STATEMENT

The studies involving human participants were reviewed and approved by Ethics Committee of the Xiangya Hospital of Central South University. The patients/participants provided their written informed consent to participate in this study. Written informed consent was obtained from the individual(s) for the publication of any potentially identifiable images or data included in this article.

## AUTHOR CONTRIBUTIONS

HP designed the experiments, performed whole-genome sequencing analysis, carried out most of the experiments, and drafted the manuscript. TW and H-BH recruited the patients. TW supervised the experiments, analyzed results, and proofread the manuscript. All authors were involved in the final approval of the submitted version.

## ACKNOWLEDGMENTS

The authors would like to thank the family for their participation in this study. The authors gratefully acknowledge Prof. Stephen P. Robertson at the University of Otago, providing the platform and the method of genetic analysis.

## REFERENCES

Abarrategi, A., Mian, S. A., Passaro, D., Rouault-Pierre, K., Grey, W., and Bonnet, D. (2018). Modeling the human bone marrow niche in mice: from host bone marrow engraftment to bioengineering approaches. *J. Exp. Med.* 215, 729–743. doi: 10.1084/jem.20172139

Alam, I., McQueen, A. K., Acton, D., Reilly, A. M., Gerard-O'Riley, R. L., Oakes, D. K., et al. (2017). Phenotypic severity of autosomal dominant osteopetrosis type II (ADO2) mice on different genetic backgrounds recapitulates the features of human disease. *Bone* 94, 34–41. doi: 10.1016/j.bone.2016.10.016

Alatalo, S. L., Ivaska, K. K., Waguespack, S. G., Econs, M. J., Väänänen, K., and Halleen, J. M. (2004). Osteoclast-derived serum tartrate-resistant acid phosphatase 5b in Albers-Schonberg disease (type II autosomal dominant osteopetrosis). *Clin. Chem.* 50, 883–890. doi: 10.1373/clinchem.2003.029355

Barvencik, F., Kurth, I., Koehne, T., Stauber, T., Zustin, J., Tsiakas, K., et al. (2014). CLCN7 and TCIRG1 mutations differentially affect bone matrix mineralization in osteopetrotic individuals. *J. Bone Miner. Res.* 29, 982–991. doi: 10.1002/jbmr.2100

Bénichou, O., Cleiren, E., Gram, J., Bollerslev, J., de Vernejoul, M.-C., and Van Hul, W. (2001). Mapping of autosomal dominant osteopetrosis type II (Albers-Schönberg disease) to chromosome 16p13.3. *Am. J. Hum. Genet.* 69, 647–654. doi: 10.1086/323132

Bénichou, O. D., Laredo, J. D., and de Vernejoul, M. C. (2000). Type II autosomal dominant osteopetrosis (Albers-Schönberg disease): clinical and radiological manifestations in 42 patients. *Bone* 26, 87–93. doi: 10.1016/S8756-3282(99)00244-6

Bollerslev, J., Henriksen, K., Frost Nielsen, M., Brixen, K., and Van Hul, W. (2013). Autosomal dominant osteopetrosis revisited: lessons from recent studies. *Eur. J. Endocrinol.* 169, R39–R57. doi: 10.1530/EJE-13-0136

Bollerslev, J., Marks, S. C. Jr., Pockwinse, S., Kassem, M., and Brixen, K. (1993). Ultrastructural investigations of bone resorptive cells in two types of autosomal dominant osteopetrosis. *Bone* 14, 865–869. doi: 10.1016/8756-3282(93)90316-3

Boudin, E., Fijalkowski, I., Hendrickx, G., and Van Hul, W. (2016). Genetic control of bone mass. *Mol. Cell. Endocrinol.* 432, 3–13. doi: 10.1016/j.mce.2015.12.021

Capulli, M., Maurizi, A., Ventura, L., Rucci, N., and Teti, A. (2015). Effective small interfering RNA therapy to treat CLCN7-dependent autosomal dominant osteopetrosis type 2. *Mol. Ther. Nucleic Acids* 4:e248. doi: 10.1038/mtna.2015.21

Chen, X., Wang, Z., Duan, N., Zhu, G., Schwarz, E. M., and Xie, C. (2018). Osteoblast–osteoclast interactions. *Connect. Tissue Res.* 59, 99–107. doi: 10.1080/03008207.2017.1290085

Chen, X., Zhang, K., Hock, J., Wang, C., and Yu, X. (2016). Enhanced but hypofunctional osteoclastogenesis in an autosomal dominant osteopetrosis type II case carrying a c.1856C>T mutation in CLCN7. *Bone Res.* 4:16035. doi: 10.1038/boneres.2016.35

Chen, Y.-H., Grigelioniene, G., Newton, P. T., Gullander, J., Elfving, M., Hammarsjö, A., et al. (2020). Absence of GP130 cytokine receptor signaling causes extended Stüve-Wiedemann syndrome. *J. Exp. Med.* 217:e20191306. doi: 10.1084/jem.20191306

Chevalier, C., Kieser, S., Çolakoğlu, M., Hadadi, N., Brun, J., Rigo, D., et al. (2020). Warmth prevents bone loss through the gut microbiota. *Cell Metab.* 32, 575.e7–590.e7. doi: 10.1016/j.cmet.2020.08.012

Cleiren, E., Bénichou, O., Van Hul, E., Gram, J., Bollerslev, J., Singer, F. R., et al. (2001). Albers-Schonberg disease (autosomal dominant osteopetrosis, type II) results from mutations in the ClCN7 chloride channel gene. *Hum. Mol. Genet.* 10, 2861–2867. doi: 10.1093/hmg/10.25.2861

Coudert, A. E., Del Fattore, A., Baulard, C., Olaso, R., Schiltz, C., Collet, C., et al. (2014). Differentially expressed genes in autosomal dominant osteopetrosis type II osteoclasts reveal known and novel pathways for osteoclast biology. *Lab. Investig.* 94, 275–285. doi: 10.1038/labinvest.2013.140

Del Fattore, A., Cappariello, A., and Teti, A. (2008). Genetics, pathogenesis and complications of osteopetrosis. *Bone* 42, 19–29. doi: 10.1016/j.bone.2007.08.029

Frattini, A., Pangrazio, A., Susani, L., Sobacchi, C., Mirolo, M., Abinun, M., et al. (2003). Chloride channel ClCN7 mutations are responsible for severe recessive, dominant, and intermediate osteopetrosis. *J. Bone Miner. Res.* 18, 1740–1747. doi: 10.1359/jbmr.2003.18.10.1740

Hao, X., Gu, H., Chen, C., Huang, D., Zhao, Y., Xie, L., et al. (2019). Metabolic imaging reveals a unique preference of symmetric cell division and homing of leukemia-initiating cells in an endosteal niche. *Cell Metab.* 29, 950.e6–965.e6. doi: 10.1016/j.cmet.2018.11.013

Hayashi, M., Nakashima, T., Yoshimura, N., Okamoto, K., Tanaka, S., and Takayanagi, H. (2019). Autoregulation of osteocyte sema3a orchestrates estrogen action and counteracts bone aging. *Cell Metab.* 29, 627.e5–637.e5. doi: 10.1016/j.cmet.2018.12.021

Jentsch, T. J., and Pusch, M. (2018). CLC chloride channels and transporters: structure, function, physiology, and disease. *Physiol. Rev.* 98, 1493–1590. doi: 10.1152/physrev.00047.2017

Kim, B. J., Lee, Y. S., Lee, S. Y., Baek, W. Y., Choi, Y. J., Moon, S. A., et al. (2018). Osteoclast-secreted SLIT3 coordinates bone resorption and formation. *J. Clin. Invest.* 128, 1429–1441. doi: 10.1172/JCI91086

Kusumbe, A. P., Ramasamy, S. K., and Adams, R. H. (2014). Coupling of angiogenesis and osteogenesis by a specific vessel subtype in bone. *Nature* 507, 323–328. doi: 10.1038/nature13145

Langen, U. H., Pitulescu, M. E., Kim, J. M., Enriquez-Gasca, R., Sivaraj, K. K., Kusumbe, A. P., et al. (2017). Cell-matrix signals specify bone endothelial cells during developmental osteogenesis. *Nat. Cell Biol.* 19, 189–201. doi: 10.1038/ncb3476

Leisle, L., Ludwig, C. F., Wagner, F. A., Jentsch, T. J., and Stauber, T. (2011). ClC-7 is a slowly voltage-gated 2Cl−/1H+-exchanger and requires Ostm1 for transport activity. *EMBO J.* 30, 2140–2152. doi: 10.1038/emboj.2011.137

Li, C., Xiao, Y., Yang, M., Su, T., Sun, X., Guo, Q., et al. (2018). Long noncoding RNA Bmncr regulates mesenchymal stem cell fate during skeletal aging. *J. Clin. Invest.* 128, 5251–5266. doi: 10.1172/JCI99044

Li, X., Sun, X., and Carmeliet, P. (2019). Hallmarks of endothelial cell metabolism in health and disease. *Cell Metab.* 30, 414–433. doi: 10.1016/j.cmet.2019.08.011

Lundberg, J. O., Carlström, M., and Weitzberg, E. (2018). Metabolic effects of dietary nitrate in health and disease. *Cell Metab.* 28, 9–22. doi: 10.1016/j.cmet.2018.06.007

Maurizi, A., Capulli, M., Curle, A., Patel, R., Ucci, A., Côrtes, J. A., et al. (2019). Extra-skeletal manifestations in mice affected by Clcn7-dependent autosomal dominant osteopetrosis type 2 clinical and therapeutic implications. *Bone Res.* 7:17. doi: 10.1038/s41413-019-0055-x

Pang, Q., Chi, Y., Zhao, Z., Xing, X., Li, M., Wang, O., et al. (2016). Novel mutations of CLCN7 cause autosomal dominant osteopetrosis type II (ADO-II) and intermediate autosomal recessive osteopetrosis (IARO) in Chinese patients. *Osteoporos. Int.* 27, 1047–1055. doi: 10.1007/s00198-015-3320-x

Peng, Y., Wu, S., Li, Y., and Crane, J. L. (2020). Type H blood vessels in bone modeling and remodeling. *Theranostics* 10, 426–436. doi: 10.7150/thno.34126

Phan, T. C. A., Xu, J., and Zheng, M. H. (2004). Interaction between osteoblast and osteoclast: impact in bone disease. *Histol. Histopathol.* 19, 1325–1344. doi: 10.14670/HH-19.1325

Ramasamy, S. K., Kusumbe, A. P., Wang, L., and Adams, R. H. (2014). Endothelial Notch activity promotes angiogenesis and osteogenesis in bone. *Nature* 507, 376–380. doi: 10.1038/nature13146

Rodriguez-Laguna, L., Agra, N., Ibañez, K., Oliva-Molina, G., Gordo, G., Khurana, N., et al. (2019). Somatic activating mutations in PIK3CA cause generalized lymphatic anomaly. *J. Exp. Med.* 216, 407–418. doi: 10.1084/jem.20181353

Sivaraj, K. K., and Adams, R. H. (2016). Blood vessel formation and function in bone. *Development* 143, 2706–2715. doi: 10.1242/dev.136861

Sobacchi, C., Schulz, A., Coxon, F. P., Villa, A., and Helfrich, M. H. (2013). Osteopetrosis: genetics, treatment and new insights into osteoclast function. *Nat. Rev. Endocrinol.* 9, 522–536. doi: 10.1038/nrendo.2013.137

Tolar, J., Teitelbaum, S. L., and Orchard, P. J. (2004). Osteopetrosis. *N. Engl. J. Med.* 351, 2839–2849. doi: 10.1056/NEJMra040952

Verkman, A. S., and Galietta, L. J. V. (2009). Chloride channels as drug targets. *Nat. Rev. Drug Discov.* 8, 153–171. doi: 10.1038/nrd2780

Waguespack, S. G., Hui, S. L., DiMeglio, L. A., and Econs, M. J. (2007). Autosomal dominant osteopetrosis: clinical severity and natural history of 94 subjects with a chloride channel 7 gene mutation. *J. Clin. Endocrinol. Metab.* 92, 771–778. doi: 10.1210/jc.2006-1986

Waguespack, S. G., Koller, D. L., White, K. E., Fishburn, T., Carn, G., Buckwalter, K. A., et al. (2003). Chloride channel 7 (ClCN7) gene mutations and autosomal dominant osteopetrosis, type II. *J. Bone Miner. Res.* 18, 1513–1518. doi: 10.1359/jbmr.2003.18.8.1513

Wang, C., Hockerman, S., Jacobsen, E. J., Alippe, Y., Selness, S. R., Hope, H. R., et al. (2018). Selective inhibition of the p38α MAPK–MK2 axis inhibits inflammatory cues including inflammasome priming signals. *J. Exp. Med.* 215, 1315–1325. doi: 10.1084/jem.20172063

Weinert, S., Jabs, S., Supanchart, C., Schweizer, M., Gimber, N., Richter, M., et al. (2010). Lysosomal pathology and osteopetrosis upon loss of H+-driven lysosomal Cl-accumulation. *Science* 328, 1401–1403. doi: 10.1126/science.1188072

Xiao, Y.-Z., Yang, M., Xiao, Y., Guo, Q., Huang, Y., Li, C.-J., et al. (2020). Reducing hypothalamic stem cell senescence protects against aging-associated physiological decline. *Cell Metab.* 31, 534.e5–548.e5. doi: 10.1016/j.cmet.2020.01.002

Xie, H., Cui, Z., Wang, L., Xia, Z., Hu, Y., Xian, L., et al. (2014). PDGF-BB secreted by preosteoclasts induces angiogenesis during coupling with osteogenesis. *Nat. Med.* 20, 1270–1278. doi: 10.1038/nm.3668

Xu, R., Yallowitz, A., Qin, A., Wu, Z., Shin, D. Y., Kim, J.-M., et al. (2018). Targeting skeletal endothelium to ameliorate bone loss. *Nat. Med.* 24, 823–833. doi: 10.1038/s41591-018-0020-z

Yang, M., Guo, Q., Peng, H., Xiao, Y.-Z., Xiao, Y., Huang, Y., et al. (2019). Krüppel-like factor 3 inhibition by mutated lncRNA Reg1cp results in human high bone mass syndrome. *J. Exp. Med.* 216, 1944–1964. doi: 10.1084/jem.2018 1554

Yang, M., Li, C.-J., Sun, X., Guo, Q., Xiao, Y., Su, T., et al. (2017). MiR-497 195 cluster regulates angiogenesis during coupling with osteogenesis by maintaining endothelial Notch and HIF-1α activity. *Nat. Commun.* 8, 1–11. doi: 10.1038/ncomms16003

Zhang, Z., He, J., Zhang, H., Hu, W., Fu, W., Gu, J., et al. (2009). Identification of the CLCN7 gene mutations in two Chinese families with autosomal dominant osteopetrosis (type II). *J. Bone Miner. Metab.* 27, 444–451. doi: 10.1007/s00774-009-0051-0

14

# Construction of a Five-Super-Enhancer-Associated-Genes Prognostic Model for Osteosarcoma Patients

*Zhanbo Ouyang[1], Guohua Li[1], Haihong Zhu[1], Jiaojiao Wang[1], Tingting Qi[1], Qiang Qu[2], Chao Tu[3], Jian Qu[1]* and Qiong Lu[1]**

*[1] Department of Pharmacy, The Second Xiangya Hospital, Central South University; Institute of Clinical Pharmacy, Central South University, Changsha, China, [2] Department of Pharmacy, Xiangya Hospital, Central South University, Changsha, China, [3] Department of Orthopaedics, The Second Xiangya Hospital, Central South University, Changsha, China*

***Correspondence:**
*Jian Qu*
*qujianstanley@csu.edu.cn*
*Qiong Lu*
*christy_luq@csu.edu.cn*

Osteosarcoma is a malignant tumor most commonly arising in children and adolescents and associated with poor prognosis. In recent years, some prognostic models have been constructed to assist clinicians in the treatment of osteosarcoma. However, the prognosis and treatment of patients with osteosarcoma remain unsatisfactory. Notably, super-enhancer (SE)-associated genes strongly promote the progression of osteosarcoma. In the present study, we constructed a novel effective prognostic model using SE-associated genes from osteosarcoma. Five SE-associated genes were initially screened through the least absolute shrinkage and selection operator (Lasso) penalized Cox regression, as well as univariate and multivariate Cox regression analyses. Meanwhile, a risk score model was constructed using the expression of these five genes. The excellent performance of the five-SE-associated-gene-based prognostic model was determined via time-dependent receiver operating characteristic (ROC) curves and Kaplan–Meier curves. Inferior outcome of overall survival (OS) was predicted in the high-risk group. A nomogram based on the polygenic risk score model was further established to validate the performance of the prognostic model. It showed that our prognostic model performed outstandingly in predicting 1-, 3-, and 5-year OS of patients with osteosarcoma. Meanwhile, these five genes also belonged to the hub genes associated with survival and necrosis of osteosarcoma according to the result of weighted gene co-expression network analysis based on the dataset of GSE39058. Therefore, we believe that the five-SE-associated-gene-based prognostic model established in this study can accurately predict the prognosis of patients with osteosarcoma and effectively assist clinicians in treating osteosarcoma in the future.

**Keywords: osteosarcoma, super-enhancer, prognostic model, Lasso, weighted gene co-expression network analysis, overall survival**

**Abbreviations:** AIC, Akaike information criterion; AUC, area under the ROC; C-index, concordance index; GEO, Gene Expression Omnibus; GS, gene significance; HR, hazard ratio; IGV, Integrative Genomics Viewer; K–M, Kaplan–Meier; Lasso, least absolute shrinkage and selection operator; MM, module membership; OS, overall survival; ROC, receiver operating characteristic; SE, super-enhancer; TCGA, The Cancer Genome Atlas; WGCNA, weighted gene co-expression network analysis.

## INTRODUCTION

Osteosarcoma, the most common primary bone tumor, is most commonly arising in children and adolescents (Bielack et al., 2009). The survival rate of patients with osteosarcoma is markedly low due to the tendency of osteosarcoma for early metastasis and rapid progression (Kempf-Bielack et al., 2005). The overall 5-year survival rate of patients with non-metastatic osteosarcoma is approximately 60–70%, while the survival rate of osteosarcoma patients with metastatic symptoms is only 20–30% (Kempf-Bielack et al., 2005; Luetke et al., 2014; Meazza and Scanagatta, 2016). Moreover, high-grade patients comprise nearly 80–90% of those diagnosed with osteosarcoma; the treatment of these patients is challenging (Bielack et al., 2009). Furthermore, despite advancements in treatment in recent years, the therapeutic outcomes remain unsatisfactory. Although numerous traditional predictive factors, such as age, necrosis, recurrence, and clinical stage, are important contributors to clinical outcome, they are less effective in predicting the survival status due to the complex molecular mechanisms of osteosarcoma progression. Thus, it is urgent to investigate novel effective molecular biomarkers for the more precise prediction of the prognosis of patients with osteosarcoma.

Super-enhancer is a large cluster of *cis*-regulatory DNA elements densely bound by transcription factors and cofactors, playing vital roles in defining cell fate and identity (Hnisz et al., 2013). Histone marks (H3K27ac, H3K4me1, and H3K4me3), cofactor (p300), and mediators (CDK7 and BRD4) are common biomarkers used to define SE (Lovén et al., 2013; Hnisz et al., 2015; Ma et al., 2019); among them, H3K27ac is the most efficient biomarker for identifying SE (Creyghton et al., 2010; Hnisz et al., 2013; Whyte et al., 2013). Therefore, we used H3K27ac, H3K4me1, and H3K4me3 as SE biomarkers in this study based on the ChIP–seq profiles data from Cistrome. Moreover, SE plays a critical role in the progression of osteosarcoma through activating the expression of its downstream target oncogenes, such as *MYC*, *LIF*, and *STAT3* (Chen et al., 2018; Lu et al., 2020; Zhang et al., 2020). Furthermore, SE inhibitors (e.g., JQ1, THZ1, and THZ2), which were developed for the treatment of osteosarcoma, could restore the expression levels of these genes (Lee et al., 2015; Chen et al., 2018; Zhang et al., 2020). Thus, screening and identifying hub oncogenes driven by SE will provide novel insights into the diagnosis, prognosis, and treatment of osteosarcoma.

The Lasso penalized Cox regression analysis, designed by Tibshirani (1997), is an accurate statistical method frequently used for the selection of variables in the Cox regression model. It can remarkably improve the accuracy of the model it generates compared with the stepwise regression method, as it involves fewer variables and produces more interpretable models (Tibshirani, 1997; Xiong et al., 2019). The reason for Lasso screening fewer variables is that it can regularize the impact of some variables by shrinking their coefficients to zero (Zhang et al., 2018). Nowadays, Lasso is widely used in constructing prognostic models for the prediction of survival based on complicated high-throughput genomic data (Zhang et al., 2013; Lu et al., 2019; Wang et al., 2019; Wu et al., 2019). Based on this advantage, we applied the Lasso regression method to the construction of a prognostic model of osteosarcoma.

Weighted gene co-expression network analysis (WGCNA) is a system bioinformatics method involving molecular interaction mechanism analysis and construction of correlation gene networks (Zhang and Horvath, 2005). WGCNA has been frequently utilized in identifying probable oncogenes and in screening candidate targets for various cancers (Udyavar et al., 2013). Using WGCNA, Tian et al. (2018) showed that the insulin-like growth factor-binding-associated genes may play a critical role in osteosarcoma metastasis progression. Guan et al. (2020) defined four key genes (*ALOX5AP*, *HLA-DMB*, *HLA-DRA*, and *SPINT2*) as prognostic markers for osteosarcoma metastasis. We adapted WGCNA to identify the five screened genes from SE-associated genes that were crucial hub genes of osteosarcoma. Prognostic models based on some cancer-related genes (Long et al., 2018; Zuo et al., 2019), long non-coding RNAs (Liu et al., 2020; Yang et al., 2020; Zhang et al., 2020), or other biomarkers (Park et al., 2017; Elwood et al., 2018) for improving patient prognosis attract considerable attention. For instance, Zhu et al. (2020) constructed a seven-gene signature associated with osteosarcoma energy metabolism for predicting the prognosis of osteosarcoma through WGCNA and Lasso Cox regression analysis. Dong et al. (2019) constructed a risk score model based on eight genes for predicting the metastasis of osteosarcoma mainly through Lasso logistic regression analysis. Thus, we attempted to perform WGCNA for osteosarcoma and screen hub genes related to clinical traits of this disease. Nomograms are interactive tools developed in recent years, which have been widely used to predict the probability of survival (Wang et al., 2018; Yap et al., 2018; Pan et al., 2019; Xiao et al., 2019; Zhang et al., 2019). Similarly, we constructed a prognostic model and a visualized nomogram based on this model to improve the prognosis of patients with osteosarcoma.

In this study, Lasso penalized Cox regression analysis was initially performed using 349 selected SE-associated genes. A gene cluster containing five SE-associated genes, namely, *AMN1*, *LIMS1*, *SAMD4A*, *SPARC*, and *ZP3*, was screened. Subsequently, a risk score model based on these five genes was constructed and verified using training and validation datasets. Meanwhile, univariate and multivariate Cox regression analyses and ROC curve analysis were also used to assess the predictive ability of the model. We further screened module genes related to clinical traits of patients with osteosarcoma via WGCNA. The five SE-associated genes were also part of the module genes linked to survival and recurrence of osteosarcoma. Finally, an interactive nomogram was constructed based on the risk score model including the five-gene risk group and clinical traits. The five-SE-associated-gene-based prognostic model developed in this study will provide promising inspiration for the clinical therapy of patients with osteosarcoma.

# MATERIALS AND METHODS

## Data Collection and Expression Matrix Preparation

We downloaded the osteosarcoma dataset GSE39058 as training data from the National Center for Biotechnology Information GEO[1]. The 20,819 genes in 42 samples of osteosarcoma were annotated according to the probe information from Illumina HumanHT-12 WG-DASL V4.0 R2 Expression BeadChip (GPL14951) (Kelly et al., 2013). We processed the raw data of the expression matrix by transformation of log2– via the R package "limma." The clinical information was organized into a matrix and is shown in **Table 1**. One sample (GSM954821) was excluded due to the lack of information on the survival status. The validation dataset Target-osteosarcoma (Target-OS) was downloaded from the publicly available database of TCGA[2]. The 434 SE-associated genes from the osteosarcoma cell line U2OS were obtained from the website of the SE database (version 1.03[3]). Following the intersection of SE-associated genes and 20,819 genes from GSE39058, 349 SE-associated genes were used for the subsequent analysis. Chromatin immunoprecipitation (ChIP) signals of H3K27ac-seq, H3K4me1-seq, and H3K4me3-seq in U2OS were also downloaded from Cistrome[4] and visualized using the IGV (Thorvaldsdottir et al., 2013).

## Lasso Penalized Cox Proportional Hazard Regression Model

Lasso penalized Cox regression analysis was performed to screen important prognostic genes for predicting the OS of patients with osteosarcoma using R package "glmnet" (Friedman et al., 2010; Simon et al., 2011; Tibshirani et al., 2012). The shrinking penalty was identified based on the tuning parameter lambda (λ), which was identified based on 10-fold cross-validation. Two optimal λ values ($\lambda_{min}$ and $\lambda_{lse}$) were highlighted by the vertical lines with a minimizing mean-square error. To determine the optimal λ value, we performed the Wilcoxon test and ROC curve analysis for the comparison of $\lambda_{min}$ and $\lambda_{lse}$ values. These two λ values were used to construct a new fitted Lasso model, and two lists of genes were generated.

[1]https://www.ncbi.nlm.nih.gov/geo/

[2]https://cancergenome.nih.gov/

[3]http://www.licpathway.net/sedb

[4]http://cistrome.org/db/#/

**TABLE 1** | The clinical information of 41 OS patients from dataset GSE39058.

| Variable | | Number |
|---|---|---|
| Gender | Male | 21 |
| | Female | 20 |
| Necrosis | Low | 14 |
| | High | 27 |
| Recurrence | No | 21 |
| | Yes | 20 |
| Death | No | 29 |
| | Yes | 12 |

## Cox Proportional Hazard Regression Model

Univariate and multivariate Cox proportional hazard regression analyses were performed to validate the associations between the expression levels of selected genes and OS of the patients via the R package "survival" and "survminer." The regression coefficient (β-value) and HR were predicted. Harrell's C-index, likelihood ratio test, and Wald test were also calculated, and the results are presented in the forest plot. Survival analysis of the single gene in the prognostic model was performed using the K–M survival curve and log-rank test via the R package "survival" and "survminer." Time-dependent ROC curve analysis was calculated to evaluate the predictive capability of OS of the prognostic model via the R package "timeROC."

## Polygenic Risk Score Model for Prognostic Prediction

To further investigate the prognostic model based on the gene group, a polygenic risk score model was constructed used the following forum RiskScore = $\Sigma\beta i * Xi$. Xi is the level of gene expression and βi is the regression coefficient. The risk score model was defined as the linear combination of the expression levels of selected genes. The patients with osteosarcoma in the two datasets were divided into high- and low-risk groups according to the risk score. We verified the power of the polygenic risk score model through single-gene expression status analysis, event distribution analysis, K–M survival analysis, and time-dependent ROC curve analysis.

## Predictive Nomogram for Prognostic Prediction

A nomogram based on independent prognostic factors of clinical traits and the polygenic risk score was constructed to predict the probability of 1-, 3-, and 5-year OS of patients with osteosarcoma. Subsequently, the discrimination of the nomogram was verified using the C-index obtained through a bootstrap method with 1,000 resamples. Calibration curves were plotted to compare the nomogram-predicted and ideal probabilities against the observed rates. Total points were calculated according to the parameters of prognostic factors using the R package "nomogramEx." Each variable of the nomogram yields points, and their sum represents the total points that a patient receives. Finally, we developed the interactive nomogram for predicting the probability of OS of patients with osteosarcoma using the R package "replot."

## WGCNA

Weighted gene co-expression network analysis was performed to screen SE-associated hub genes linked to clinical traits using the dataset GSE39058. The analysis was performed as previously described (Ma et al., 2019). The optimal soft-thresholding value was estimated based on scale independence and mean connectivity analysis. Clinical traits-related genes were clustered into different modules. Moreover, the correlation between modules and clinical traits was highlighted in the heatmap. The relationship between the clinically significant MM and GS was displayed in the scatter plots.

## Protein–Protein Interaction Analysis and Pathway Enrichment Analysis

Eigengenes within clinically significant modules and SE-associated genes were intersected using the Venn plot and produced a list of hub genes. An interaction network between hub genes and drugs was also constructed to identify some drugs related with these hub genes via "NetworkAnalyst 3.0" (Zhou et al., 2019). Subsequently, Kyoto Encyclopedia of Genes and Genomes (KEGG) pathway analysis was performed using these hub genes. The top 10 items of the enriched pathway were selected and shown in the dot plot.

# RESULTS

## Establishment and Validation of the Lasso Penalized Cox Regression Model

The flowchart shows our analysis procedures for the construction of the SE-associated gene-based prognostic model of osteosarcoma (**Figure 1**). The 349 SE-associated genes based on the dataset of GSE39058 were selected to perform the Lasso penalized Cox regression analysis. Firstly, to identify the best-fit parameter of the $\lambda$ parameter, two important optional $\lambda$ values ($\log\lambda_{min} = -1.91$ and $\log\lambda_{lse} = -1.48$) were calculated from the vertical lines with a minimizing mean-square error and further used to select two groups of genes (**Figures 2A–C**). Moreover, Lasso models were reconstructed according to the $\lambda_{min}$ and $\lambda_{lse}$, and survival probabilities were further estimated based on two gene lists (**Figure 2D**). As shown in **Figure 2D**, the use of the five gene-based prognostic model based on the $\lambda_{min}$ (Wilcoxon test, $p = 1.4e{-}05$) facilitated the obvious distinction of survival probabilities between samples obtained from living and expired patients. However, when a two-gene-based prognostic model was used based on the $\lambda_{lse}$, there was no statistically significant difference observed (Wilcoxon test, $p > 0.05$). Similarly, the outcome of ROC curve analysis showed that the area under the curve minimum ($AUC_{min}$) was 0.92, implying that the five-gene-based Lasso model performed well in predicting the probability of OS of patients with osteosarcoma (**Figure 2E**).

## Validation of Independent Prognostic Factors by the Cox Regression Model

For the validation of the Lasso penalized Cox regression model, we performed univariate and multivariate Cox regression analyses to determine whether these genes were independent

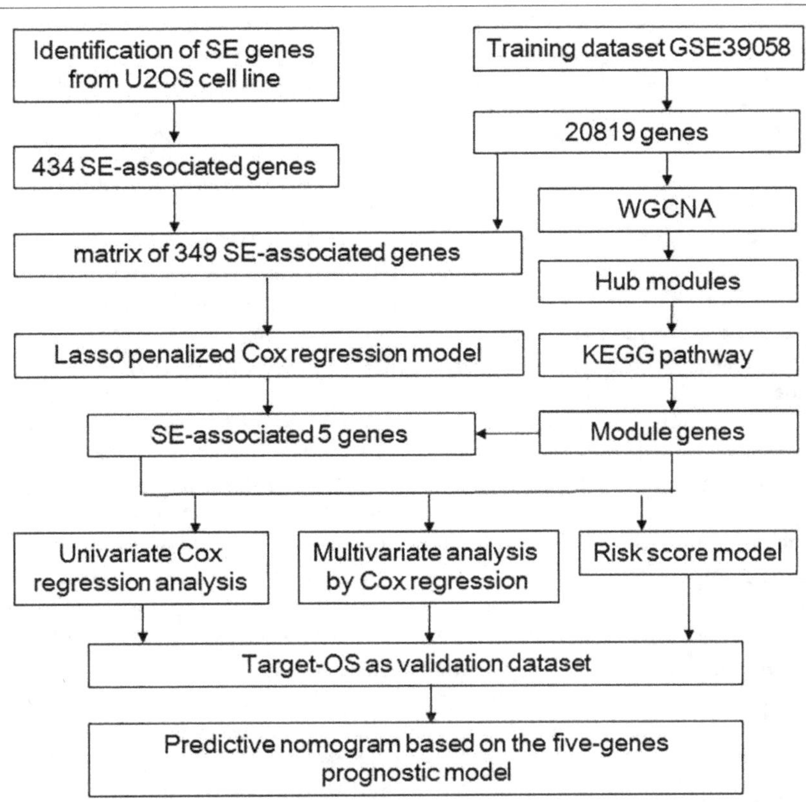


**FIGURE 1** | The procedure workflow used to establish and certify the SE-associated gene-based prognostic model for patients with osteosarcoma. KEGG, Kyoto Encyclopedia of Genes and Genomes; Lasso, least absolute shrinkage and selection operator; Target-OS, Target-osteosarcoma; SE, super-enhancer; WGCNA, weighted gene co-expression network analysis.

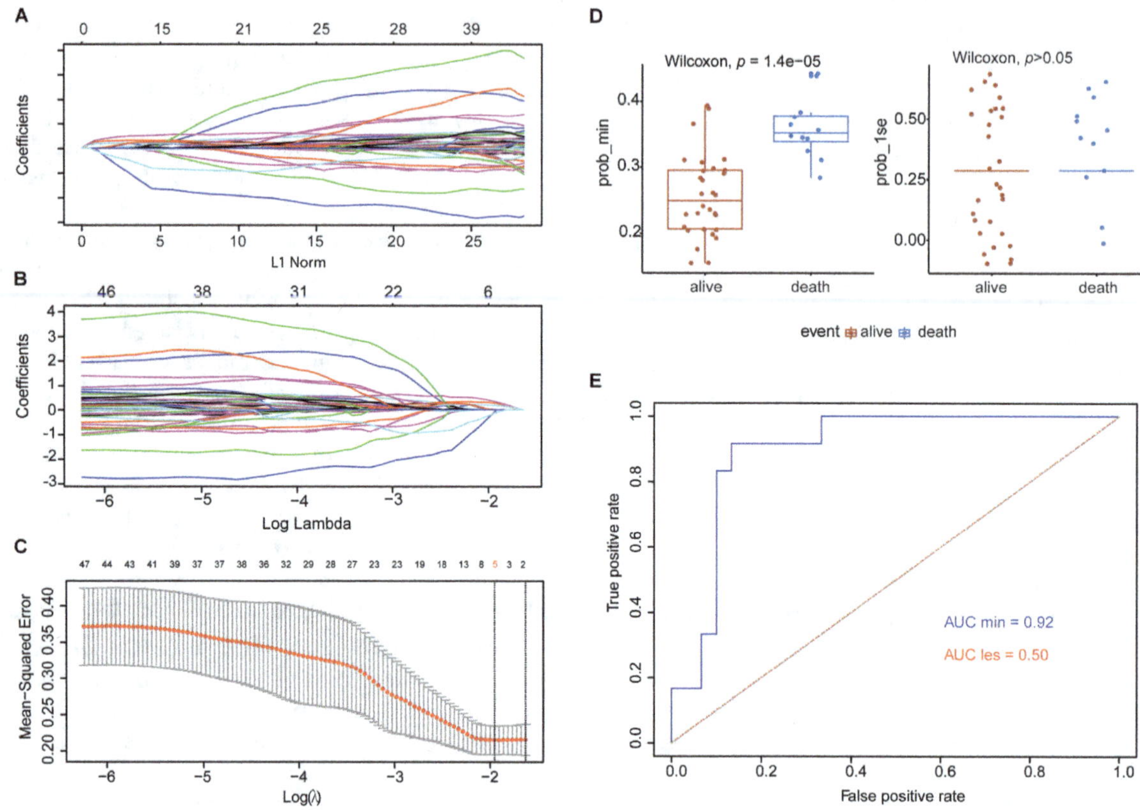


**FIGURE 2 |** Establishment of the five-gene prognostic model by Lasso regression analysis based on the 349 SE-associated genes from data downloaded from SEdb. **(A,B)** Lasso coefficient profiles of the 349 SE-associated genes. **(C)** Two optimal lambda (λ) values ($\lambda_{min}$ and $\lambda_{lse}$) were estimated according to the vertical lines with a minimizing mean-square error. The vertical axis represents the mean-square error, while the horizontal axis represents the value of log(λ). **(D)** The scatter plot of survival status of patients with osteosarcoma based on the five-gene model (left, $\lambda_{min}$, $p = 1.4e{-}05$) or two-gene model (right, $\lambda_{lse}$, $p > 0.05$) using the Wilcoxon test. **(E)** ROC curves of the two prognostic models based on $\lambda_{min}$ and $\lambda_{lse}$. The values of AUC were included in the figure. AUC, area under the curve; Lasso, least absolute shrinkage and selection operator; ROC, receiver operating characteristic; SE, super-enhancer; SEdb, super-enhancer database.

prognostic factors for the OS of patients with osteosarcoma. In the univariate Cox regression analysis, all log-rank *p*-values of these five genes were <0.05 (**Figure 3A**). Following multivariate Cox regression analysis, the global *p*-value (log-rank test) of the five-gene prognostic model was only 0.000171 (**Figure 3B**). The AIC was 59.74, and the C-index was 0.89, indicating that these five genes may be favorable prognostic factors for the OS of patients with osteosarcoma. Moreover, the outcome of K–M survival analysis was consistent with that of the univariate Cox regression analysis (**Figure 3C**). Furthermore, *AMN1* and *ZP3* may be protective factors in osteosarcoma (HR: 1.26e−36 and 1.13e−07, respectively), whereas *LIMS1*, *SAMD4A*, and *SPARC* appear to be harmful factors in this setting (HR: 699.2, 167, and 298.7, respectively). Thus, a Lasso penalized Cox regression model including five SE-associated genes may be used to predict the OS of patients with osteosarcoma.

## Establishment and Validation of the Polygenic Risk Score Model

We integrated the expression data of the five genes and corresponding coefficient derived from the above multivariate regression analysis to establish the risk score model. All patients in the training dataset of GSE39058 ($N = 41$) were divided into high-risk (risk score > 0) and low-risk groups (risk score < 0) (**Figure 4A**). As shown in **Figure 4B**, survival was more commonly observed in the low-risk group, whereas death was more frequent in the high-risk group. *LIMS1*, *SAMD4A*, and *SPARC* tended to upregulated, whereas *AMN1* and *ZP3* were downregulated in patients of the high-risk group (**Figure 4C**). The K–M OS analysis predicted an inferior outcome of OS in the high-risk group (log-rank test, $p = 0.0006$) (**Figure 4D**). Meanwhile, the AUCs of a time-dependent ROC curve calculated using the five-gene-based risk score model were >0.8 (**Figure 4E**), indicating that the forecast model had high sensitivity and specificity.

The Target-OS dataset was further used to verify the predictive values of the polygenic risk score. Following the multivariate Cox regression analysis, the global *p*-value (log-rank test) of the five-gene prognostic model for the Target-OS dataset was <0.05 (**Supplementary Figure S1A**). A total of 88 patients were classified into the low- and high-risk groups using the optimal cutoff value of the risk score (**Supplementary Figures S1B–D**). The K–M curves of two groups based on risk scores were

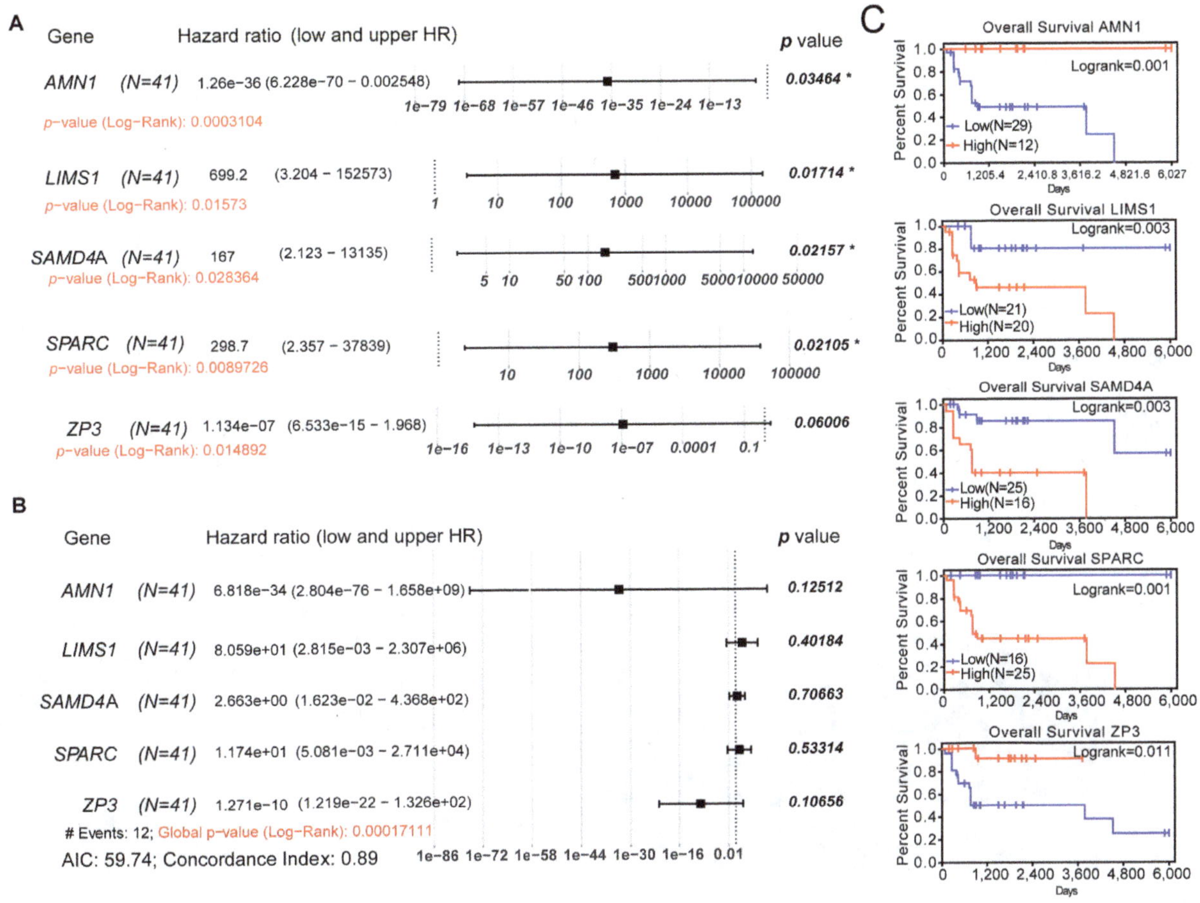


**FIGURE 3 |** Univariate and multivariate Cox regression analyses and K–M survival analysis of the five-gene prognostic model. **(A)** Univariate Cox regression analysis of each gene of the model. **(B)** Multivariate Cox regression analysis of the five-gene model. **(C)** K–M survival curves showing the difference in OS between the relative high- and low-expression groups for each gene according to the median of expression levels. K–M, Kaplan–Meier; AIC, Akaike information criterion; OS, overall survival.

significantly different (log-rank test, $p < 0.05$), and AUCs of time-dependent ROC curves also showed that the five-gene risk model could be a favorable approach to predicting the OS of patients with osteosarcoma (**Supplementary Figures S1E,F**).

## Construction of the Predictive Nomogram Based on the Risk Score Model for Prognostic Prediction

To visualize the Cox regression model, a nomogram was constructed for predicting the 1-, 3-, and 5-year OS probability for patients with osteosarcoma in the GSE39058 dataset ($N = 41$). The predictors of the nomogram included age, sex, necrosis, recurrence, and risk group (**Figure 5A**). The calibration plot shown in **Figure 5B** illustrates the performance of the nomogram. The calibration plots were close to the ideal prediction gray line (45° line), indicating that our nomogram performed well in predicting survival probability (**Figure 5B**). To assess the predictive effect of the risk group as an indicator of OS, we applied the nomogram to a specific patient (GSM954850) in GSE39058 (**Figures 5C,D**). The patient GSM954850 expired at 750 days. According to the model containing the risk group, the predicted probability of death at 1,095 days was 0.815; this value was markedly higher than that obtained for the model lacking the risk group (0.659). This finding implies that the predictive model containing the risk group as a parameter is more accurate than that lacking the risk group.

## Identification of SE-Related Hub Genes in Osteosarcoma Using WGCNA and a Protein–Protein Interaction Network

Weighted gene co-expression network analysis is another bioinformatics method for the analysis of clinical traits linked to the levels of gene expression. Cluster analysis was performed to display the heatmap of clinical traits (**Figure 6A**). As shown in **Figure 6B**, $\beta = 9$ was selected as the best soft-thresholding value via prediction of the scale independence and mean connectivity (**Figure 6B**) to construct the gene co-expression network. Subsequently, eigengenes were divided into different colored modules, producing 17 different modules. A module–trait relationship heatmap was developed according to Pearson's

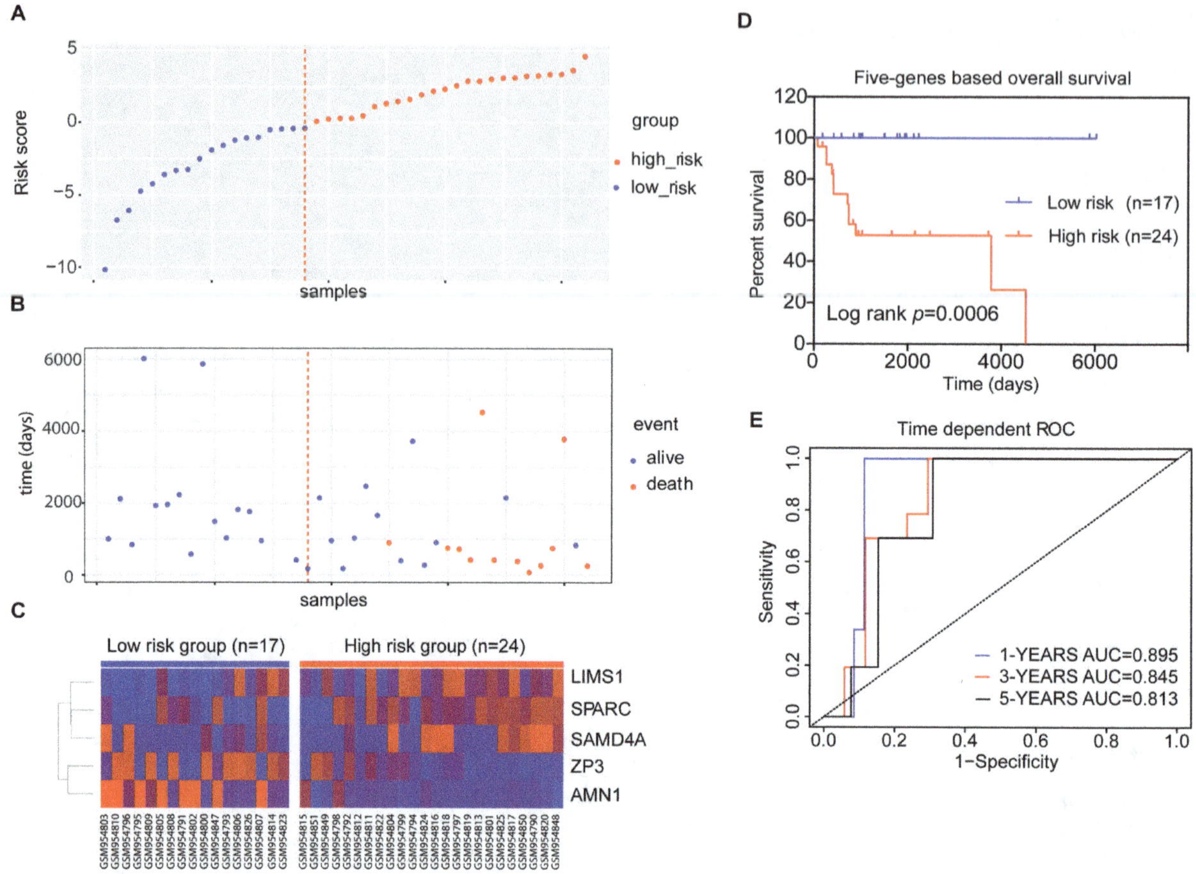


**FIGURE 4 |** The five-gene risk score model for the GSE39058 dataset ($N = 41$). **(A)** Scatter plot displaying the risk score of each patient in the GSE39058 dataset. Patients were divided into high- or low-risk groups according to the risk score. The blue plots represent the patients in the low-risk group (risk score $\leq 0$), while the red plots represent patients in the high-risk group (risk score $> 0$). **(B)** The survival status distribution of patients with osteosarcoma in the high- or low-risk groups. **(C)** The expression status of the five prognostic genes in 41 patients with osteosarcoma in the GSE39058 dataset. **(D)** K–M survival curves showing the difference in OS between high- and low-risk patients (41 patients) (log-rank test, $p = 0.0006$). **(E)** Time-dependent ROC curve analysis for the prediction of survival using the five-gene prognostic model. The AUCs of 1-, 3-, and 5-year OS are shown in the figure. AUC, area under the curve; K–M, Kaplan–Meier; OS, overall survival; ROC, receiver operating characteristic.

correlation coefficient (**Figure 6C**). Three modules presented higher correlation with clinical traits: MEgray60 with recurrence ($r = 0.37$, $p = 0.01$); MEblue with death ($r = 0.33$, $p = 0.03$); and MEpink with survival time ($r = 0.47$, $p = 0.002$) (**Figure 6C**). A scatter plot also showed that the MM of these three modules was positively correlated with GS (**Figure 6D**). A Venn plot of SE-associated genes derived from the SE-associated gene matrix was drawn, and the genes within three modules were intersected (**Figure 6E**). There were 13, 70, and 16 interaction genes between module gray60, blue, pink, and SE-associated genes. The interaction genes were enriched in numerous cancer-related pathways, such as proteoglycans in cancer and transcriptional misregulation in cancer (**Figure 6F**). In addition, we constructed a gene–drug interaction network using the five genes and related drugs (**Supplementary Figure S2**). All five genes interacted with JQ1 (an established SE inhibitor). The network depicted that these five genes were probably regulated by SE to a certain extent. Finally, we displayed the signal tracks for the H3K27ac, H3K4me1, and H3K4me3 ChIP–seq profiles of the five genes (**Figure 7**). We observed five predicted SEs near these five genes. These data suggest that the expression of the five genes is regulated by SE. In addition, the SE inhibitor JQ1 may regulate the expression pattern in U2OS cells.

## DISCUSSION

Notably, there is a lack of effective target treatment regimens in clinical practice, except for the traditional method of surgical resection. Recently, prognostic models based on some disease-related genes or other biomarkers for improving the prognosis of osteosarcoma have attracted considerable attention. The Lasso regression Cox model, gene risk score model, and univariate and multivariate Cox regression models are widely used for the screening and mining of hub genes related to survival and other clinical characteristics. Particularly, the Lasso model can be applied to solve "curse of dimensionality" (small sample size combined with a very large number of genes) when large amounts

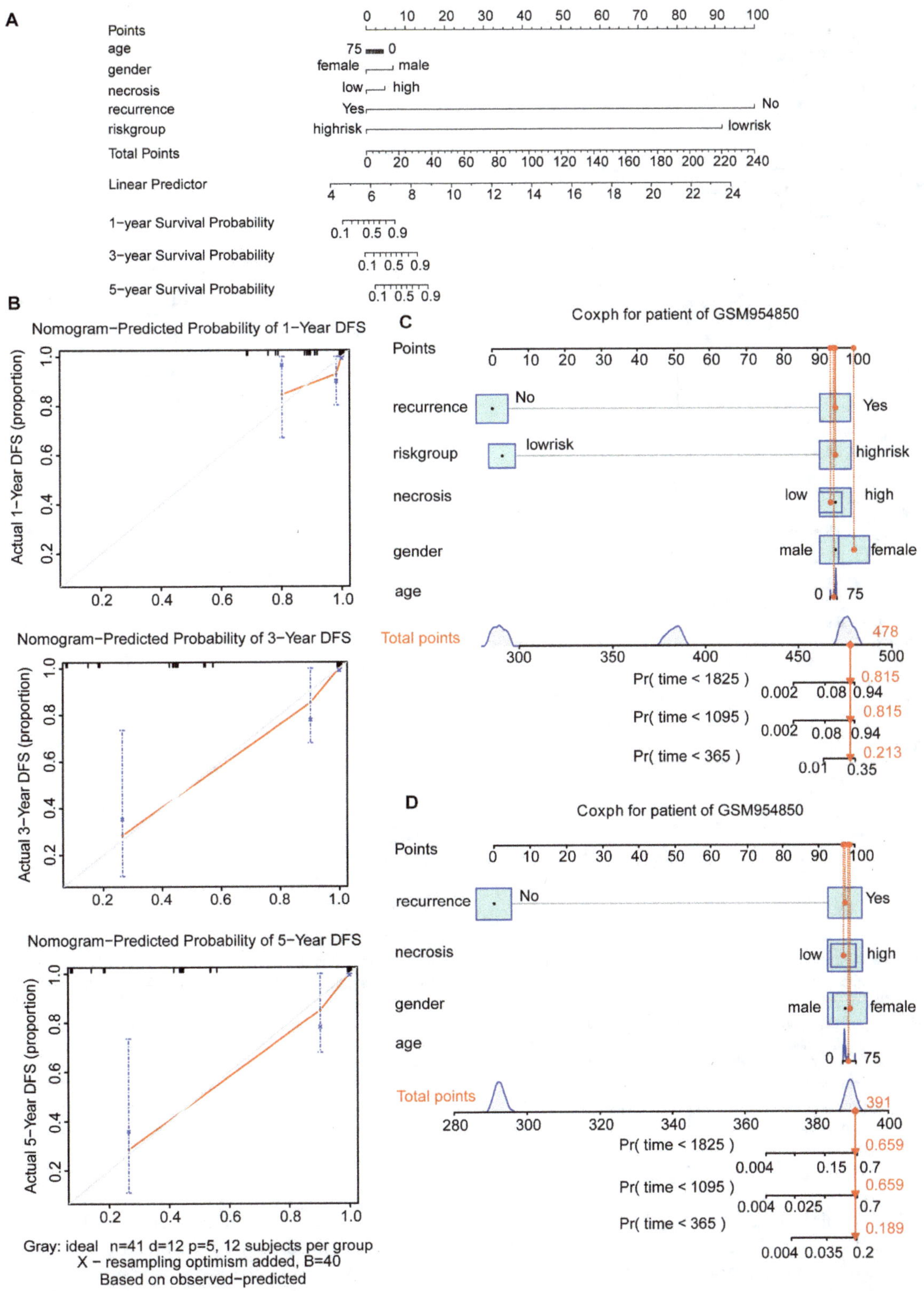


**FIGURE 5 |** Nomogram predicting the probability of 1-, 3-, and 5-year OS in patients with osteosarcoma. **(A)** Nomogram adding up the points identified on the points scale (the upward line) for each variable. The total points projected on the bottom scales indicate the probability of 1-, 3-, and 5-year OS. **(B)** Calibration plot for predicting the 1-, 3-, and 5-year OS. The gray line represents the ideal condition. **(C,D)** The nomograms predicting the probability of 1-, 3-, and 5-year OS for the specific patient GSM954850 based on the model containing or not containing the risk group in the GSE39058 dataset. OS, overall survival; DFS, disease-free survival.

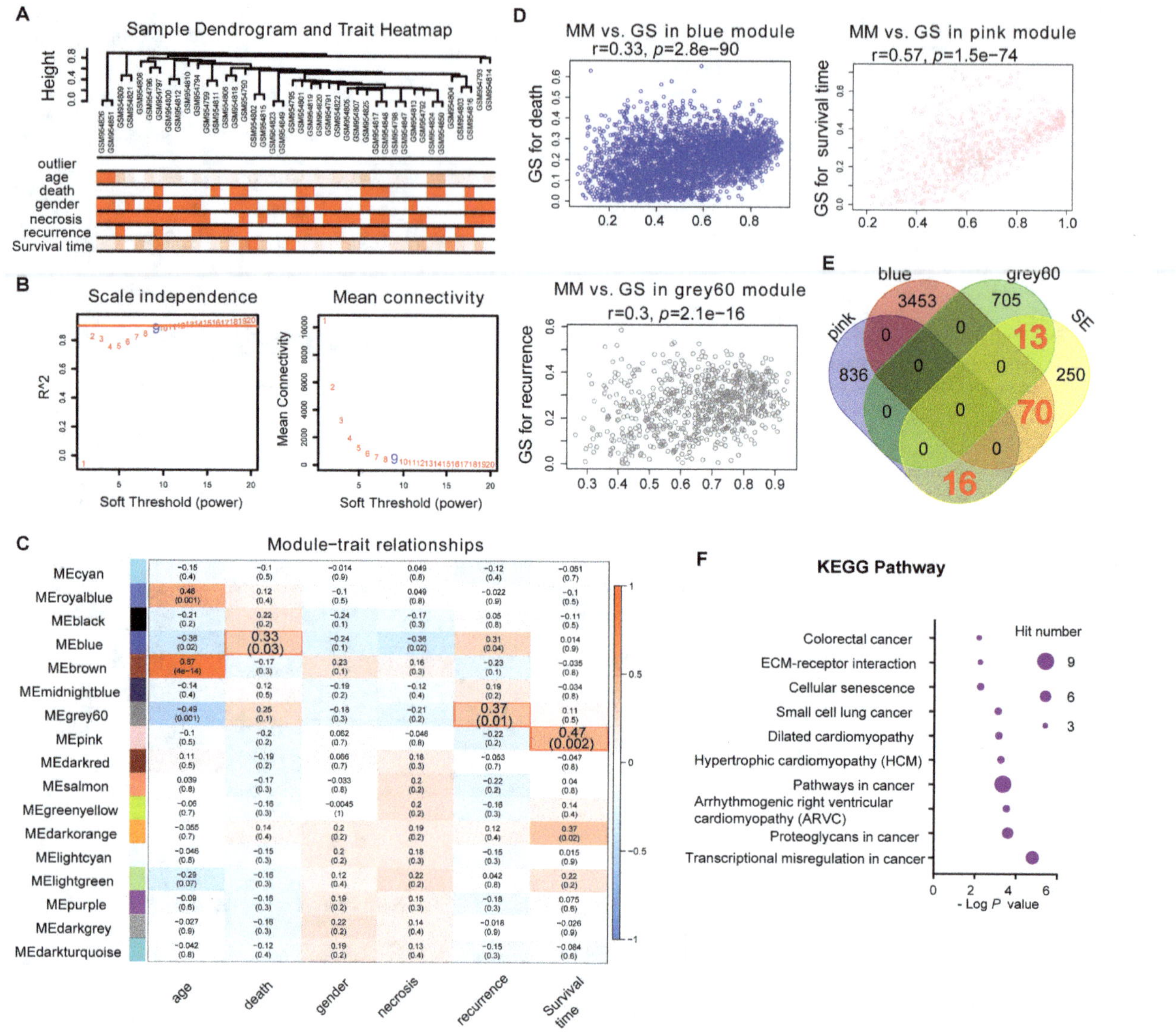


**FIGURE 6 |** Identification of SE-related hub genes in osteosarcoma based on the GSE39058 dataset through WGCNA analysis. **(A)** Cluster analysis between the gene expression in the GSE39058 dataset and sample outliers or clinical traits. Color intensity was proportional to sample outliers, age, gender, necrosis, recurrence, and survival time. **(B)** Analysis of the scale independence and mean connectivity (vertical axis) for various soft-thresholding powers (β value of horizontal axis). **(C)** Heatmap of the correlation between modules and clinical traits of osteosarcoma; *p*-values in the table specify the correlation between modules and clinical traits. Three modules had high correlation with clinical traits: MEgray60 with recurrence ($r = 0.37$, $p = 0.01$); MEblue with death ($r = 0.33$, $p = 0.03$); and MEpink with survival time ($r = 0.47$, $p = 0.002$). **(D)** Scatterplot showing the MM versus GS of module genes related to death in the blue module, recurrence in the gray60 module, or survival time in the pink module (horizontal axis: MM means module membership, vertical axis: GS means gene significance). **(E)** Venn plot of SE-related genes and eigengenes in the blue, gray60, and pink modules. There are 70, 13, and 16 correlated genes, respectively. **(F)** KEGG pathway analysis of the above-correlated genes in the Venn plot. KEGG, Kyoto Encyclopedia of Genes and Genomes; SE, super-enhancer; WGCNA, weighted gene co-expression network analysis.

of throughput biological data are processed. Recently, Lasso and WGCNA were used to construct a nomogram of radiomics of diagnostic computed tomography for predicting the survival of patients with high-grade osteosarcoma, which showed favorable performance (Wu et al., 2018). Another study also identified a seven-gene signature as a predictive biomarker for energy metabolism in osteosarcoma by Lasso and multivariate Cox regression (Zhu et al., 2020). Lasso coefficient profiles of the genes associated with the metastasis of osteosarcoma were established. These profiles were used to construct a risk score model for the prediction of metastasis of osteosarcoma (Dong et al., 2019). These findings imply that prognostic models based on different clinical traits and gene expression levels may help to potentiate the personalized treatment of patients with osteosarcoma.

In the present study, we constructed a five-SE-associated-gene-based nomogram prognostic model to improve the prognosis of patients with osteosarcoma. We first constructed an SE-associated gene expression matrix based on the 349

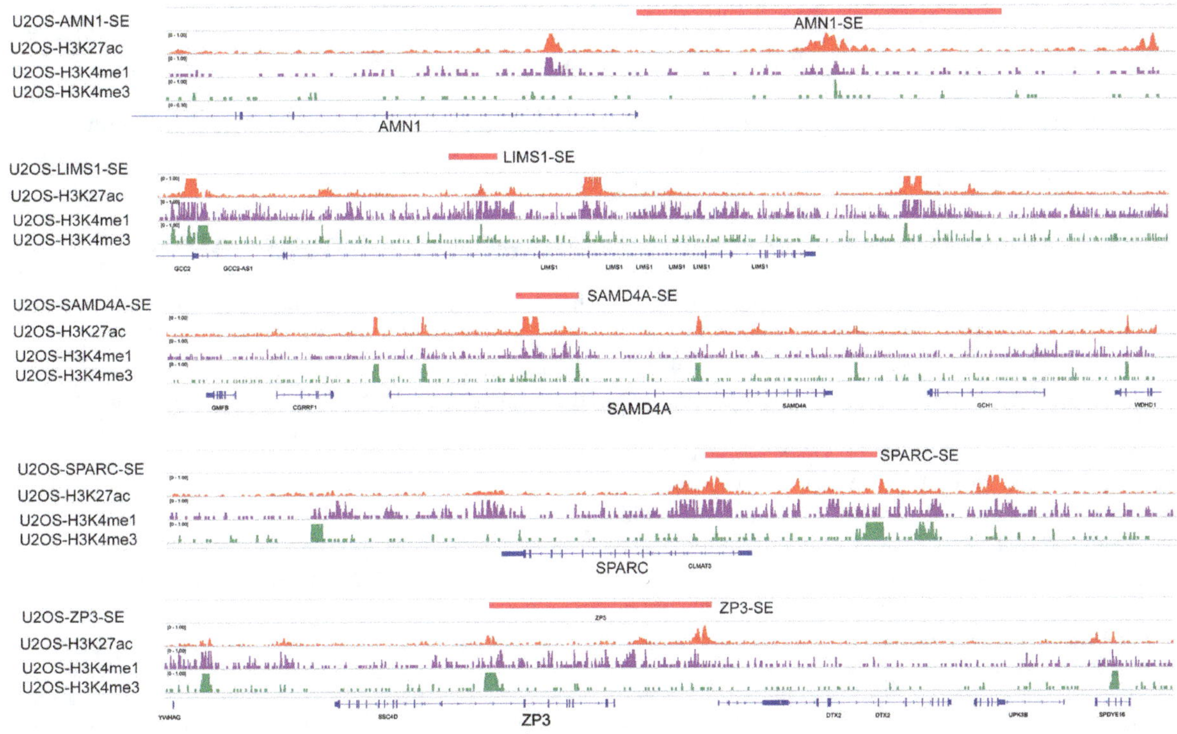


**FIGURE 7 |** Signal tracks for H3K27ac (red), H3K4me1 (purple), and H3K4me3 (green) ChIP–seq profiles of the five-SE-associated hub genes visualized using IGV. The regions of SE are shown in a pink bar upon the signal tracks. ChIP–seq, chromatin immunoprecipitation–sequencing; SE, super-enhancer; IGV, Integrative Genomics Viewer.

genes derived from the intersection of SE-associated genes and 20,819 genes from the GSE39058 dataset. According to this expression matrix, Lasso penalized Cox regression analysis was performed to screen a gene cluster containing *AMN1*, *LIMS1*, *SAMD4A*, *SPARC*, and *ZP3*, which was used to construct the risk score model based on the expression levels of five genes. Considering the group risk score as an independent indicator for prognosis, the K–M curve and log-rank test showed that a high risk score was correlated to augmented death ratio. We assessed the capability of the five-gene prognostic model in the GSE39058 dataset and also in the validation dataset Target-OS via univariate and multivariate Cox regression analyses and ROC curve analysis. The AUCs of the prognostic model for predicting the 1-, 3-, and 5-year OS were 0.895, 0.845, and 0.813, respectively, for the GSE39058 dataset and 0.549, 0.721, and 0.724, respectively, for the Target-OS dataset. The AUCs and C-index also showed that the five-gene prognostic model had a great performance for the prediction of survival and could be a robust and efficient model of prognosis. An interactive nomogram based on the risk score model and other clinical traits was constructed and identified using the calibration plots. To determine the predictive effect of the risk group as an indicator of OS, we also applied the nomogram to a specific patient (GSM954850) in the GSE39058 dataset. The predictive model containing the risk group as a parameter is more accurate compared with the nomogram model lacking the risk group. Through this approach, the prognosis of patients in the high-risk group may improve following the adjustment of individual treatment regimens for these patients.

The WGCNA of the 20,819 genes from the GSE39058 dataset revealed that the above five SE-associated genes also belonged to module genes. The KEGG analysis showed that the module genes associated with SE were enriched in numerous cancer-related pathways, such as proteoglycans in cancer and transcriptional misregulation in cancer. *LIMS1* functions as an oncogene to promote the survival of pancreatic cancer cells under oxygen–glucose deprivation conditions (Huang et al., 2019). The protein LIMS1 (also known as PINCH1) encoded by LIMS1 acts as an adaptor protein which contains five LIM domains or double zinc fingers (Hobert et al., 1999). LIMS1 can be involved in integrin signaling through interacting with integrin-linked kinase mediated by its LIM domain. Besides, LIMS1 can bind to integrin-linked kinase and parvin, which forms a protein complex, which is critical for the cell extracellular matrix adhesion (Ito et al., 2010). High expression of LIMS1 is associated with poor prognosis in human laryngeal carcinomas (Tsinias et al., 2018). Inhibition of LIMS1 through knockdown of LIMS1 can inhibit cell proliferation of neuroblastoma cells (Saeki et al., 2018). Thus, *LIMS1* may be considered as a biomarker for osteosarcoma. Secreted protein acidic and rich in cysteine (*SPARC*) encodes a cysteine-rich acidic matrix-associated protein, which is essential for extracellular matrix synthesis and epithelial–mesenchymal transition that promotes migration and invasion of many cancers (Sun et al., 2018; Jiang et al., 2019; López-Moncada et al., 2019). In particular, overexpression of *SPARC*, which was critical for the growth and maintenance of osteosarcoma, was found in 51 of 55 osteosarcoma tumor samples (Dalla-Torre et al., 2006). Overexpression of *SPARC* also mediated the suppressing effect of *TP53INP1* on the migration of pancreatic cancer cells and promoted the progression of malignant cancers (Seux et al., 2011). Therefore, it is convincing that *SPARC* can serve as a biomarker or treatment target for osteosarcoma. SAMD4A, encoded by the sterile alpha motif domain containing 4A (*SAMD4A*), was reported to involve in processes such as maternal RNA destabilization, translational repression, and early embryo development in the role of a posttranscriptional regulator (Smibert et al., 1996; Baez et al., 2011). Although studies about the function of *SAMD4A* in cancer are still rare, we believe that *SAMD4A* will become a novel biomarker for predicting the prognosis of osteosarcoma based on the findings of this study. Antagonist of the mitotic exit network 1 (*AMN1*) is essential for mitotic checkpoints and chromosome stability; the protein encoded by AMN1 is involved in the progression of cell cycle (Wang et al., 2003; Xie et al., 2019). Although there are no relative studies about the role of *ZP3* in osteosarcoma, even if in cancer, combined with the findings of our study, we should also pay attention to *AMN1* and *ZP3* in osteosarcoma in a certain extent. In the present study, the gene–drug interaction network of the five genes showed that all genes interacted with JQ1 (an established SE inhibitor). Moreover, according to the ChIP–seq signal of H3K27ac, H3K4me1, and H3K4me3, we detected strong signals of SEs around these five genes. These data support that the expression of the five genes may be regulated by SE, while JQ1 as an SE inhibitor probably regulated the expression pattern in U2OS cells. Further molecular mechanism studies are warranted to recover the relationship between expression and SE in the future.

In conclusion, this was the first study that used the Lasso model to screen prognostic indicators from the profile of SE-associated genes. The five-gene-based interactive nomogram may be used as a clinical tool for improving the prognosis of patients with osteosarcoma, offering novel insights into personalized therapy in this setting.

## AUTHOR CONTRIBUTIONS

JQ and QL conceived and designed the theme of this study. ZO drafted the manuscript. TQ, GL, HZ, JW, and CT provided some helpful advice in several statistic methods. JQ and QQ revised the manuscript. The manuscript was revised critically by all authors involving in this study and all authors approved the final version with one accord.

## SUPPLEMENTARY MATERIAL

**Supplementary Figure 1 |** Multivariate Cox regression analysis and risk score model analysis of the validation dataset Target-OS ($N = 88$). **(A)** Multivariate Cox regression analysis of dataset Target-OS based on the five-gene model. **(B)** Scatterplot displaying the risk score of each patient in the Target-OS dataset. The patients were divided into the high- or low-risk groups according to the risk score. The blue plots represent the patients in the low-risk group (risk score $\leq 0$), while the red plots represent those in the high-risk group (risk score $> 0$). **(C)** Survival status distribution of the high- or low-risk groups in the Target-OS dataset. **(D)** The expression status of the five prognostic genes for patients in the Target-OS dataset. **(E)** K–M survival curves showing the difference in OS between high- and low-risk patients in the Target-OS dataset (log-rank test, $p = 0.0438$). **(F)** Time-dependent ROC curves analysis of survival prediction for patients in the Target-OS dataset using the five-gene prognostic model. The AUCs for 1-, 3-, and 5-year OS are shown in the figure. AUC, area under curve; K–M, Kaplan–Meier; ROC, receiver operating characteristic; Target-OS, Target-osteosarcoma, OS, overall survival; AIC, Akaike information criterion.

**Supplementary Figure 2 |** Gene–drug interaction network analysis of the five genes and drugs.

## REFERENCES

Baez, M. V., Luchelli, L., Maschi, D., Habif, M., Pascual, M., Thomas, M. G., et al. (2011). Smaug1 mRNA-silencing foci respond to NMDA and modulate synapse formation. *J. Cell. Biol.* 195, 1141–1157. doi: 10.1083/jcb.201108159

Bielack, S., Carrle, D., and Casali, P. G. (2009). Osteosarcoma: ESMO clinical recommendations for diagnosis, treatment and follow-up. *Ann. Oncol.* 20(Suppl. 4), 137–139. doi: 10.1093/annonc/mdp154

Chen, D., Zhao, Z., Huang, Z., Chen, D.-C., Zhu, X.-X., Wang, Y.-Z., et al. (2018). Super enhancer inhibitors suppress MYC driven transcriptional amplification and tumor progression in osteosarcoma. *Bone Res.* 6:11.

Creyghton, M. P., Cheng, A. W., Welstead, G. G., Kooistra, T., Carey, B. W., Steine, E. J., et al. (2010). Histone H3K27ac separates active from poised enhancers and predicts developmental state. *Proc. Natl. Acad. Sci. U.S.A.* 107, 21931–21936. doi: 10.1073/pnas.1016071107

Dalla-Torre, C. A., Yoshimoto, M., Lee, C. H., Joshua, A. M., de Toledo, S. R., Petrilli, A. S., et al. (2006). Effects of THBS3, SPARC and SPP1 expression on biological behavior and survival in patients with osteosarcoma. *BMC Cancer* 6:237. doi: 10.1186/1471-2407-6-237

Dong, S., Huo, H., Mao, Y., Li, X., and Dong, L. (2019). A risk score model for the prediction of osteosarcoma metastasis. *FEBS Open Biol.* 9, 519–526. doi: 10.1002/2211-5463.12592

Elwood, J. M., Tawfiq, E., TinTin, S., Marshall, R. J., Phung, T. M., Campbell, I., et al. (2018). Development and validation of a new predictive model for breast cancer survival in New Zealand and comparison to the Nottingham prognostic index. *BMC Cancer* 18:897. doi: 10.1186/s12885-018-4791-x

Friedman, J., Hastie, T., and Tibshirani, R. (2010). Regularization paths for generalized linear models via coordinate descent. *J. Stat. Softw.* 33, 1–22.

Guan, X., Guan, Z., and Song, C. (2020). Expression profile analysis identifies key genes as prognostic markers for metastasis of osteosarcoma. *Cancer Cell. Int.* 20:104.

Hnisz, D., Abraham, B. J., Lee, T. I., Lau, A., Saint-André, V., Sigova, A. A., et al. (2013). Super-enhancers in the control of cell identity and disease. *Cell* 155, 934–947. doi: 10.1016/j.cell.2013.09.053

Hnisz, D., Schuijers, J., Lin, C. Y., Weintraub, A. S., Abraham, B. J., Lee, T. I., et al. (2015). Convergence of developmental and oncogenic signaling pathways at transcriptional super-enhancers. *Mol. Cell.* 58, 362–370. doi: 10.1016/j.molcel. 2015.02.014

Hobert, O., Moerman, D. G., Clark, K. A., Beckerle, M. C., and Ruvkun, G. (1999). A conserved LIM protein that affects muscular adherens junction integrity and mechanosensory function in *Caenorhabditis elegans*. *J. Cell. Biol.* 144, 45–57. doi: 10.1083/jcb.144.1.45

Huang, C., Li, Y., Li, Z., Xu, Y., Li, N., Ge, Y., et al. (2019). LIMS1 promotes pancreatic cancer cell survival under oxygen-glucose deprivation conditions by enhancing HIF1A protein translation. *Clin. Cancer Res.* 25, 4091–4103. doi: 10.1158/1078-0432.ccr-18-3533

Ito, S., Takahara, Y., Hyodo, T., Hasegawa, H., Asano, E., Hamaguchi, M., et al. (2010). The roles of two distinct regions of PINCH-1 in the regulation of cell attachment and spreading. *Mol. Biol. Cell.* 21, 4120–4129. doi: 10.1091/mbc. E10-05-0459

Jiang, X., Liu, F., Wang, Y., and Gao, J. (2019). Secreted protein acidic and rich in cysteine promotes epithelial-mesenchymal transition of hepatocellular carcinoma cells and acquisition of cancerstem cell phenotypes. *J. Gastroenterol. Hepatol.* 34, 1860–1868. doi: 10.1111/jgh.14692

Kelly, A. D., Haibe-Kains, B., Janeway, K. A., Hill, K. E., Howe, E., Goldsmith, J., et al. (2013). MicroRNA paraffin-based studies in osteosarcoma reveal reproducible independent prognostic profiles at 14q32. *Genome Med.* 5:2. doi: 10.1186/gm406

Kempf-Bielack, B., Bielack, S. S., Jurgens, H., Branscheid, D., Berdel, W. E., Exner, G. U., et al. (2005). Osteosarcoma relapse after combined modality therapy: an analysis of unselected patients in the cooperative osteosarcoma study group (COSS). *J. Clin. Oncol.* 23, 559–568. doi: 10.1200/jco.2005.04.063

Lee, D. H., Qi, J., Bradner, J. E., Said, J. W., Doan, N. B., Forscher, C., et al. (2015). Synergistic effect of JQ1 and rapamycin for treatment of human osteosarcoma. *Int. J. Cancer* 136, 2055–2064. doi: 10.1002/ijc.29269

Liu, Y., Gou, X., Wei, Z., Yu, H., Zhou, X., and Li, X. (2020). Bioinformatics profiling integrating a four immune-related long non-coding RNAs signature as a prognostic model for papillary renal cell carcinoma. *Aging* 12, 15359–15373. doi: 10.18632/aging.103580

Long, J., Zhang, L., Wan, X., Lin, J., Bai, Y., Xu, W., et al. (2018). A four-gene-based prognostic model predicts overall survival in patients with hepatocellular carcinoma. *J. Cell. Mol. Med.* 22, 5928–5938. doi: 10.1111/jcmm.13863

López-Moncada, F., Torres, M. J., Castellón, E. A., and Contreras, H. R. (2019). Secreted protein acidic and rich in cysteine (SPARC) induces epithelial-mesenchymal transition, enhancing migration and invasion, and is associated with high Gleason score in prostate cancer. *Asian J. Androl.* 21, 557–564. doi: 10.4103/aja.aja_23_19

Lovén, J., Hoke, H. A., Lin, C. Y., Lau, A., Orlando, D. A., Vakoc, C. R., et al. (2013). Selective inhibition of tumor oncogenes by disruption of super-enhancers. *Cell* 153, 320–334. doi: 10.1016/j.cell.2013.03.036

Lu, B., He, Y., He, J., Wang, L., Liu, Z., Yang, J., et al. (2020). Epigenetic profiling identifies LIF as a super-enhancer-controlled regulator of stem cell-like properties in osteosarcoma. *Mol. Cancer Res.* 18, 57–67. doi: 10.1158/1541-7786.mcr-19-0470

Lu, L., Wu, Y., Feng, M., Xue, X., and Fan, Y. (2019). A novel seven-miRNA prognostic model to predict overall survival in head and neck squamous cell carcinoma patients. *Mol. Med. Rep.* 20, 4340–4348. doi: 10.3892/mmr.2019. 10665

Luetke, A., Meyers, P. A., Lewis, I., and Juergens, H. (2014). Osteosarcoma treatment - where do we stand? A state of the art review. *Cancer Treat. Rev.* 40, 523–532. doi: 10.1016/j.ctrv.2013.11.006

Ma, H., Qu, J., Luo, J., Qi, T., Tan, H., Jiang, Z., et al. (2019). Super-enhancer-associated hub genes in chronic myeloid leukemia identified using weighted gene co-expression network analysis. *Cancer Manag. Res.* 11, 10705–10718. doi: 10.2147/CMAR.S214614

Meazza, C., and Scanagatta, P. (2016). Metastatic osteosarcoma: a challenging multidisciplinary treatment. *Expert Rev. Anticancer Ther.* 16, 543–556. doi: 10.1586/14737140.2016.1168697

Pan, X., Yang, W., Chen, Y., Tong, L., Li, C., and Li, H. (2019). Nomogram for predicting the overall survival of patients with inflammatory breast cancer: a SEER-based study. *Breast* 47, 56–61. doi: 10.1016/j.breast.2019.05.015

Park, H. S., Park, J. S., Chun, Y. J., Roh, Y. H., Moon, J., Chon, H. J., et al. (2017). Prognostic factors and scoring model for survival in metastatic biliary tract cancer. *Cancer Res. Treat.* 49, 1127–1139. doi: 10.4143/crt.2016.538

Saeki, N., Saito, A., Sugaya, Y., Amemiya, M., Ono, H., Komatsuzaki, R., et al. (2018). Chromatin immunoprecipitation and DNA sequencing identified a LIMS1/ILK pathway regulated by LMO1 in neuroblastoma. *Cancer Genomics Proteomics* 15, 165–174. doi: 10.21873/cgp.20074

Seux, M., Peuget, S., Montero, M. P., Siret, C., Rigot, V., Clerc, P., et al. (2011). TP53INP1 decreases pancreatic cancer cell migration by regulating SPARC expression. *Oncogene* 30, 3049–3061. doi: 10.1038/onc.2011.25

Simon, N., Friedman, J., Hastie, T., and Tibshirani, R. (2011). Regularization paths for Cox's proportional hazards model via coordinate descent. *J. Stat. Softw.* 39, 1–13. doi: 10.18637/jss.v039.i05

Smibert, C. A., Wilson, J. E., Kerr, K., and Macdonald, P. M. (1996). smaug protein represses translation of unlocalized nanos mRNA in the *Drosophila embryo*. *Genes Dev.* 10, 2600–2609. doi: 10.1101/gad.10.20.2600

Sun, W., Feng, J., Yi, Q., Xu, X., Chen, Y., and Tang, L. (2018). SPARC acts as a mediator of TGF-β1 in promoting epithelial-to-mesenchymal transition in A549 and H1299 lung cancer cells. *Biofactors* 44, 453–464. doi: 10.1002/biof. 1442

Thorvaldsdottir, H., Robinson, J. T., and Mesirov, J. P. (2013). Integrative Genomics Viewer (IGV): high-performance genomics data visualization and exploration. *Brief. Bioinform.* 14, 178–192. doi: 10.1093/bib/bbs017

Tian, H., Guan, D., and Li, J. (2018). Identifying osteosarcoma metastasis associated genes by weighted gene co-expression network analysis (WGCNA). *Medicine* 97:e10781. doi: 10.1097/md.0000000000010781

Tibshirani, R. (1997). The lasso method for variable selection in the Cox model. *Stat. Med.* 16, 385–395. doi: 10.1002/(sici)1097-0258(19970228)16:4<385::aid-sim380>3.0.co;2-3

Tibshirani, R., Bien, J., Friedman, J., Hastie, T., Simon, N., Taylor, J., et al. (2012). Strong rules for discarding predictors in lasso-type problems. *J. R. Stat. Soc. Ser. B Stat. Methodol.* 74, 245–266. doi: 10.1111/j.1467-9868.2011.01004.x

Tsinias, G., Nikou, S., Papadas, T., Pitsos, P., Papadaki, H., and Bravou, V. (2018). High PINCH1 expression in human laryngeal carcinoma associates with poor prognosis. *Anal. Cell. Pathol.* 2018:2989635. doi: 10.1155/2018/2989635

Udyavar, A. R., Hoeksema, M. D., Clark, J. E., Zou, Y., Tang, Z., Li, Z., et al. (2013). Co-expression network analysis identifies spleen tyrosine kinase (SYK) as a candidate oncogenic driver in a subset of small-cell lung cancer. *BMC Syst. Biol.* 7(Suppl. 5):S1. doi: 10.1186/1752-0509-7-S5-S1

Wang, L., Shi, J., Huang, Y., Liu, S., Zhang, J., Ding, H., et al. (2019). A six-gene prognostic model predicts overall survival in bladder cancer patients. *Cancer Cell. Int.* 19:229. doi: 10.1186/s12935-019-0950-7

Wang, S., Yang, L., Ci, B., Maclean, M., Gerber, D. E., Xiao, G., et al. (2018). Development and validation of a nomogram prognostic model for SCLC patients. *J. Thorac. Oncol.* 13, 1338–1348. doi: 10.1016/j.jtho.2018.05.037

Wang, Y., Shirogane, T., Liu, D., Harper, J. W., and Elledge, S. J. (2003). Exit from exit: resetting the cell cycle through Amn1 inhibition of G protein signaling. *Cell* 112, 697–709. doi: 10.1016/s0092-8674(03)00121-1

Whyte, W. A., Orlando, D. A., Hnisz, D., Abraham, B. J., Lin, C. Y., Kagey, M. H., et al. (2013). Master transcription factors and mediator establish super-enhancers at key cell identity genes. *Cell* 153, 307–319. doi: 10.1016/j.cell.2013. 03.035

Wu, M., Li, X., Zhang, T., Liu, Z., and Zhao, Y. (2019). Identification of a nine-gene signature and establishment of a prognostic nomogram predicting overall survival of pancreatic cancer. *Front. Oncol.* 9:996. doi: 10.3389/fonc.2019.00996

Wu, Y., Xu, L., Yang, P., Lin, N., Huang, X., Pan, W., et al. (2018). Survival prediction in high-grade osteosarcoma using radiomics of diagnostic computed tomography. *EBioMedicine* 34, 27–34. doi: 10.1016/j.ebiom.2018.07.006

Xiao, Z., Shi, Z., Hu, L., Gao, Y., Zhao, J., Liu, Y., et al. (2019). A new nomogram from the SEER database for predicting the prognosis of gallbladder cancer patients after surgery. *Ann. Transl. Med.* 7, 738. doi: 10.21037/atm.2019.11.112

Xie, B., Becker, E., Stuparevic, I., Wery, M., Szachnowski, U., Morillon, A., et al. (2019). The anti-cancer drug 5-fluorouracil affects cell cycle regulators and potential regulatory long non-coding RNAs in yeast. *RNA Biol.* 16, 727–741. doi: 10.1080/15476286.2019.1581596

Xiong, Y., Ling, Q. H., Han, F., and Liu, Q. H. (2019). An efficient gene selection method for microarray data based on LASSO and BPSO. *BMC Bioinformatics* 20(Suppl. 22):715. doi: 10.1186/s12859-019-3228-0

Yang, S., Wang, Y., Ren, J., Zhou, X., Cai, K., Guo, L., et al. (2020). Identification of diagnostic and prognostic lncRNA biomarkers in oral squamous carcinoma by integrated analysis and machine learning. *Cancer Biomark.* [Epub ahead of print]. doi: 10.3233/cbm-191215

Yap, W. K., Shih, M. C., Kuo, C., Pai, P. C., Chou, W. C., Chang, K. P., et al. (2018). Development and validation of a nomogram for assessing survival in patients with metastatic lung cancer referred for radiotherapy for bone metastases. *JAMA Netw. Open* 1:e183242. doi: 10.1001/jamanetworkopen.2018.3242

Zhang, B., and Horvath, S. (2005). A general framework for weighted gene co-expression network analysis. *Stat. Appl. Genet. Mol. Biol.* 4:17.

Zhang, D., Zeng, S., and Hu, X. (2020). Identification of a three-long noncoding RNA prognostic model involved competitive endogenous RNA in kidney renal clear cell carcinoma. *Cancer Cell. Int.* 20:319. doi: 10.1186/s12935-020-01423-4

Zhang, F., Tapera, T. M., and Gou, J. (2018). Application of a new dietary pattern analysis method in nutritional epidemiology. *BMC Med. Res. Methodol.* 18:119. doi: 10.1186/s12874-018-0585-8

Zhang, J., Fan, J., Yin, R., Geng, L., Zhu, M., Shen, W., et al. (2019). A nomogram to predict overall survival of patients with early stage non-small cell lung cancer. *J. Thorac. Dis.* 11, 5407–5416. doi: 10.21037/jtd.2019.11.53

Zhang, J., Liu, W., Zou, C., Zhao, Z., Lai, Y., Shi, Z., et al. (2020). Targeting super-enhancer-associated oncogenes in osteosarcoma with THZ2, a covalent CDK7 inhibitor. *Clin. Cancer Res.* 26, 2681–2692. doi: 10.1158/1078-0432.CCR-19-1418

Zhang, J. X., Song, W., Chen, Z. H., Wei, J. H., Liao, Y. J., Lei, J., et al. (2013). Prognostic and predictive value of a microRNA signature in stage II colon cancer: a microRNA expression analysis. *Lancet Oncol.* 14, 1295–1306. doi: 10.1016/s1470-2045(13)70491-1

Zhou, G., Soufan, O., Ewald, J., Hancock, R. E. W., Basu, N., and Xia, J. (2019). NetworkAnalyst 3.0: a visual analytics platform for comprehensive gene expression profiling and meta-analysis. *Nucleic Acids Res.* 47, W234–W241. doi: 10.1093/nar/gkz240

Zhu, N., Hou, J., Ma, G., Guo, S., Zhao, C., and Chen, B. (2020). Co-expression network analysis identifies a gene signature as a predictive biomarker for energy metabolism in osteosarcoma. *Cancer Cell. Int.* 20:259. doi: 10.1186/s12935-020-01352-2

Zuo, S., Wei, M., Zhang, H., Chen, A., Wu, J., Wei, J., et al. (2019). A robust six-gene prognostic signature for prediction of both disease-free and overall survival in non-small cell lung cancer. *J. Transl. Med.* 17:152. doi: 10.1186/s12967-019-1899-y

# 15

# Moderate Fluid Shear Stress Regulates Heme Oxygenase-1 Expression to Promote Autophagy and ECM Homeostasis in the Nucleus Pulposus Cells

*Sheng Chen[1,2], Lei Qin[2], Xiaohao Wu[2], Xuekun Fu[2], Sixiong Lin[2,3], Di Chen[4], Guozhi Xiao[2], Zengwu Shao[1]* and Huiling Cao[2]**

*[1] Department of Orthopaedics, Union Hospital, Tongji Medical College, Huazhong University of Science and Technology, Wuhan, China, [2] Guangdong Provincial Key Laboratory of Cell Microenvironment and Disease Research, Shenzhen Key Laboratory of Cell Microenvironment, and Department of Biology, Southern University of Science and Technology, Shenzhen, China, [3] Guangdong Provincial Key Laboratory of Orthopedics and Traumatology, Orthopedic Research Institute and Department of Spinal Surgery, The First Affiliated Hospital of Sun Yat-sen University, Guangzhou, China, [4] Department of Orthopedic Surgery, Rush University Medical Center, Chicago, IL, United States*

***Correspondence:**
*Zengwu Shao*
*szwpro@163.com*
*Huiling Cao*
*caohl@sustech.edu.cn;*
*xizi20042093@hotmail.com*

In vertebrate, the nucleus pulposus (NP), which is an essential component of the intervertebral disk, is constantly impacted by fluid shear stress (FSS); however, molecular mechanism(s) through which FSS modulates the NP homeostasis is poorly understood. Here we show that FSS regulates the extracellular matrix (ECM) homeostasis in NP cells. A moderate dose of FSS (i.e., 12 dyne/cm$^2$) increases the sulfated glycosaminoglycan (sGAG) content and protein levels of Col2a1 and Aggrecan and decreases those of matrix metalloproteinase 13 (MMP13) and a disintegrin and metalloproteinase with thrombospondin motif 5 (ADMATS5) in rat NP cells, while a higher dose of FSS (i.e., 24 dyne/cm$^2$) displays opposite effects. Results from RNA sequencing analysis, quantitative real-time RT-PCR analysis and western blotting establish that the heme oxygenase-1 (HO-1) is a key downstream mediator of the FSS actions in NP cells. HO-1 knockdown abolishes FSS-induced alterations in ECM protein production and sGAG content in NP cells, which is reversed by HO-1 induction. Furthermore, FSS activates the autophagic pathway by increasing the LC3-II/LC3-I ratio, Beclin-1 protein level, and formation of autophagosome and autolysosome and thereby regulates ECM protein and sGAG production in a HO-1 dependent manner. Finally, we demonstrate that the intraflagellar transport (IFT) 88, a core trafficking protein of primary cilia, is critically involved in the HO-1-mediated autophagy activation and ECM protein and sGAG production in FSS-treated NP cells. Thus, we for the first time demonstrate that FSS plays an important role in maintaining ECM homeostasis through HO-1-dependent activation of autophagy in NP cells.

**Keywords: nucleus pulposus cell, fluid shear stress, autophagy, heme oxygenase-1, intraflagellar transport (IFT) 88**

## INTRODUCTION

Low back pain is a common and frequently recurring musculoskeletal disorder, which causes heavy financial burden worldwide (Chen et al., 2017; Clouet et al., 2018; Ma et al., 2019). Epidemiological investigations show that over 80% of the world population will experience LBP at some point in their life, and LBP has become the leading cause of years lived with disability and the second most common reason for hospital visits (Maher et al., 2017; Henry et al., 2018; Chen et al., 2019). In the United States, the annual cost of LBP is over $100 billion, which is even more than the total cost of stroke, coronary artery disease, diabetes, rheumatoid disease and respiratory infection (Katz, 2006). Intervertebral disk degeneration is considered to be the main cause of LBP (Frapin et al., 2019), thus, it is of great importance to understand the pathophysiology of IVD.

The IVD is an avascular and fibrocartilaginous tissue, which lies between the vertebral bodies and functions as a shock absorber by distributing biomechanical loads along the spinal column (Priyadarshani et al., 2016). Each IVD can be roughly divided into three distinct regions: in the center was the gelatinous NP, encompassed by outer fibrocartilaginous AF, bordered superiorly and inferiorly by CEP (Sakai and Grad, 2015). Under normal physiological condition, although there is low cellularity in both NP and AF tissues, the resident cells, especially NP cells, synthesize and secrete the complex ECM molecules to maintain ECM homeostasis and resist the mechanical stresses, which plays a key role in the protection against IVD degeneration (Hu et al., 2016; Silagi et al., 2018; Bonnevie et al., 2019). In healthy NP tissues, ECM contains three major components: collagen type II (Col2), glycosaminoglycan (GAG) and PGs. Aggrecan, bound by massive sGAG side chains, is the most abundant PG in NP. During the process of IVD degeneration, the degradation of these ECM proteins by catabolic proteinases, such as a disintegrin and metalloproteinase with thrombospondin motif 5 (ADMATS5) and matrix metalloproteinase 13 (MMP13), is accelerated, while their biosynthesis is decreased, leading to an imbalance between the anabolic and catabolic metabolism of ECM.

Increasing evidence suggests that mechanical stresses, including FSS, hydrostatic pressure, compressive stress, tensile stress and other mechanical stresses, play a pivotal role in the regulation of ECM homeostasis in IVD (Neidlinger-Wilke et al., 2014; Chou et al., 2016). To maintain erect posture, the IVD is under compressive stress, which can induce deformation and produce hydrostatic pressure in NP. The hydrostatic pressure is then transferred to AF and induces the generation of tensile stress. During body motion and spine movement, tissue fluid within the NP flows in and out to accommodate the change of these stresses. Consequently, NP cells are constantly exposed to FSS (**Figure 1A**; Ye et al., 2018). However, whether and how FSS regulates ECM homeostasis in NP cells is poorly understood.

Autophagy is a highly conserved and adaptive process involving selectively eliminating and recycling bulk harmful cytoplasmic materials, such as misfolded proteins and damaged intracellular organelles, thereby acting as a main cytoprotective system to maintain cellular homeostasis (Towers and Thorburn, 2016; Dikic and Elazar, 2018). Generally, cells exhibit a low and basal level of autophagy. But the level of autophagy can significantly increase in response to external environment stress, including mechanical stress and nutrient deprivation, in order to provide nutrients for essential cellular functions (Gross and Graef, 2019). The HO-1, which has been identified in many tissues and organs as well as different pathophysiological scenarios, is the rate-limiting enzyme in the metabolism of heme into biliverdin, carbon monoxide and iron, and can exert cytoprotective effects against various external environment stress-induced oxidative stress, inflammation and cell death (Otterbein et al., 2016; Chiang et al., 2018). Using our recently established rat NP cell line and a Flexcell Streamer System, in the present study we demonstrate that moderate FSS maintains ECM homeostasis by promoting cell autophagy through modulation of HO-1.

## MATERIALS AND METHODS

### NP Cell Line Culture and FSS Experiments

An immortalized rat NP cell line used in this study was described in Oh et al. (2016). The cells were cultured in Dulbecco's Modification of Eagle's Medium (10-013-CVR; Corning, United States) containing 10% FBS (10099-141; Gibco, Australia) supplemented with 1% penicillin-streptomycin (SV30010; Hyclone, United States) at 37°C with 5% $CO_2$. FSS experiments were conducted as previously described (Yang et al., 2019). Cells were seeded onto collagen I-coated culture slips (75 mm × 25 mm × 1 mm; FFCS-C; Flexcell, United States) at a density of $3.0 \times 10^4/cm^2$ and incubated in a 5% $CO_2$ incubator at 37°C. When cells reached up to 85% confluence, the slips were then placed in a parallel plate flow chamber of Streamer® System (STR-4000; Flexcell, United States) (**Figure 1B**) and cells are exposed to 12 or 24 dyne/cm$^2$ FSS for 0, 1, 2, 3, and 4 h. For certain experiments, NP cells were pre-treated with 10 μM CoPP (Sigma, United States, C1900) for 1 h or 500 nM rapamycin (Selleck, United States, S1039) for 12 h before exposure to FSS.

### RNA Sequencing Analysis

Total RNA was isolated from NP cells with or without FSS stimulation using a TransZol Up Plus RNA Kit (ER501-01; Transgen, China) and 3 μg RNA per sample was used as input material for the RNA sample preparations. Sequencing libraries were generated using NEBNext® UltraTM RNA Library Prep Kit (Illunina, NEB, United States) and the library quality

**Abbreviations:** ADAMTS5, A disintegrin and metalloproteinase with thrombospondin motif 5; AF, annulus fibrosus; CEP, cartilage endplate; Col2, collagen type II; CoPP, cobalt protoporphyrin IX; CS, chondroitin sulfate; ECM, extracellular matrix; FSS, fluid shear stress; HA, hyaluronic acid; HO-1, heme oxygenase-1; IFT, intraflagellar transport; IVD, intervertebral disk; KS, keratin sulfate; LBP, low back pain; MMP13, matrix metalloproteinase 13; NP, nucleus pulposus; PGs, proteoglycans; RAP, rapamycin; sGAG, sulfated glycosaminoglycan.

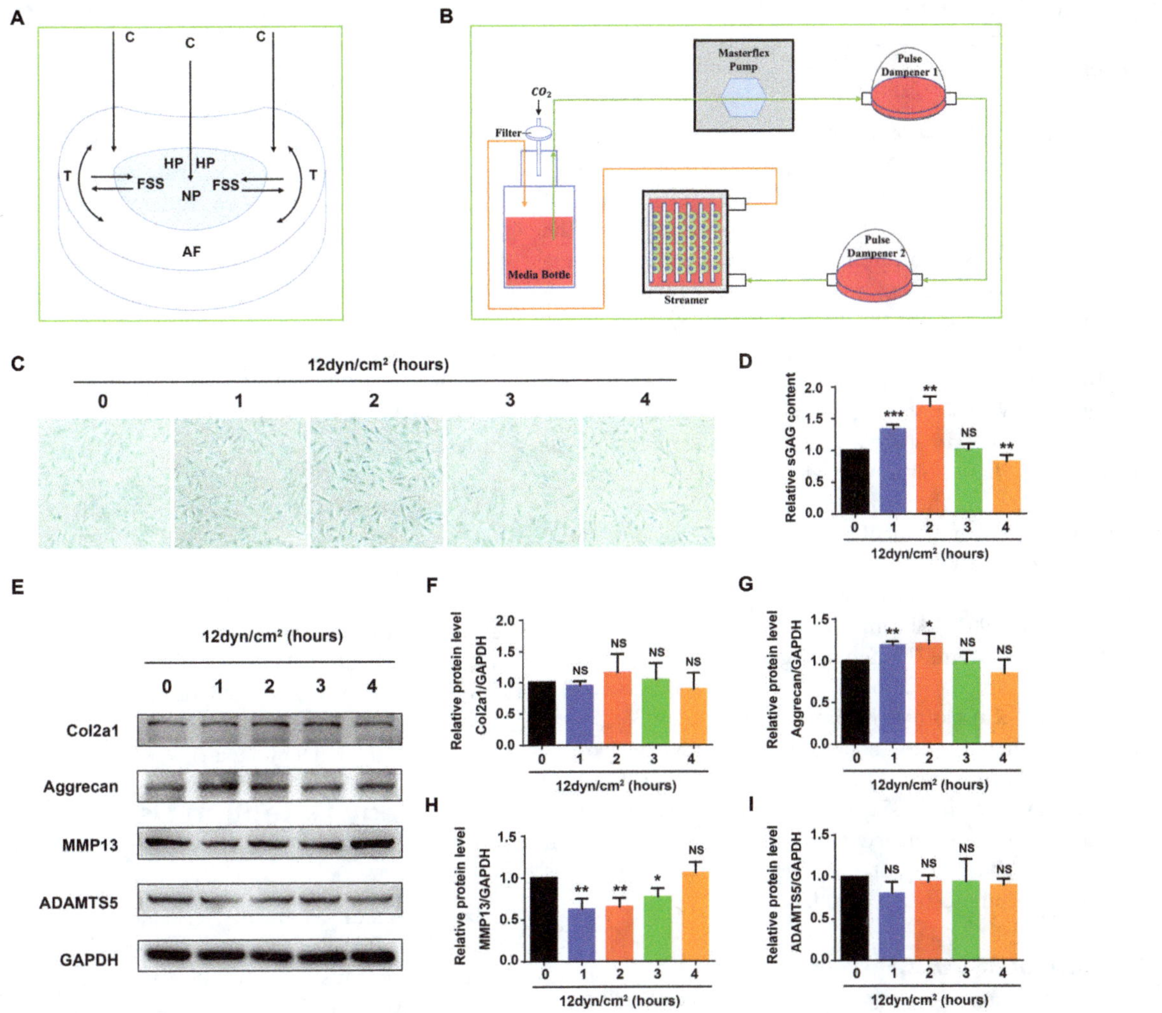


**FIGURE 1 |** Fluid shear stress regulates expression of ECM proteins and sGAG content in nucleus pulposus cells. **(A)** The formation of fluid shear stress (FSS) in nucleus pulposus cells (NP). Compressive stress (C), hydrostatic pressure (HP), and tensile stress (T) are indicated. **(B)** Schematic diagram of the Flexcell Streamer System. **(C)** Alcian blue staining. NP cells were treated with 12 dyne/cm$^2$ FSS for the indicated times. Bar, 100 $\mu$m. **(D)** sGAG content. NP cells were treated as in panel **(B)**, followed by the Blyscan Sulfated Glycosaminoglycan Assay. **(E–I)** Western blotting. NP cells were treated as in panel **(C)**, followed by Western blotting analyses for expression of Col2a1, aggrecan, MMP13, and ADAMTS5. Quantitative data from three independent experiments **(D,F–I)**. Results are expressed as mean ± standard deviation (s.d.). NS, no statistical significance, $^*P < 0.05$, $^{**}P < 0.01$, and $^{***}P < 0.001$ vs. un-treated group (0 h).

was assessed on the Agilent Bioanalyzer 2100 system. After cluster generation, the library preparations were sequenced on an Illumina Hiseq platform and 150 bp paired-end reads were generated. After quality control, reads mapping to the reference genome and quantification of gene expression level, differential expression analysis was performed by using the DESeq2 R package (1.16.1), and GO and KEGG enrichment analyses were performed by using the cluster Profiler R package. The RNASeq data have been deposited in Sequence Read Archive (SRA, PRJNA587407).

## Analysis of sGAG Content

After fixed with 4% paraformaldehyde, NP cells were dehydrated by different concentrations of ethanol and xylol. The cells were then stained with alcian blue. To measure the sGAG content, cells were digested with papain extraction reagent and then the sGAG content was quantified by Blyscan Sulfated Glycosaminoglycan Assay (B1000; Biocolor, United Kingdom) according to the manufacturer's instructions.

## Quantitative Real-Time Polymerase Chain Reaction (qRT-PCR) Analysis

Total RNA was extracted from NP cells using Tripure Isolation Reagent (11667165001; Roche, Germany). Reverse transcription (RT) and qRT-PCR analyses were performed as we described previously (Cao et al., 2010). Briefly, RNA was reverse transcribed into cDNA using PrimeScript$^{TM}$ RT Master Mix (RR036A; Takara, Japan) according to the manufacturer's protocol. After reverse transcription, qRT-PCR was performed using iTaq$^{TM}$ Universal SYBR® Green Supermix (172-5121; Bio-Rad).

The $2^{-\Delta\Delta CT}$ method was used to analyze the data, and GAPDH was used as an internal control. Primer sequences are shown in **Supplementary Table S1**.

## Western Blotting Analyses

Nucleus pulposus cells were lysed with Tripure Isolation Reagent (11667165001; Roche, Germany). After centrifugation at 12,000 × *g* for 10 min at 4°C, protein pellet was isolated from the lower red organic phase by alcohol precipitation steps. Wash the protein pellet with 0.3 M guanidine hydrochloride/95% ethanol for three times and dissolve the protein pellet by adding 1% sodium dodecyl sulfate. The protein content was detected by Pierce™ BCA Protein Assay Kit (23225; ThermoFisher Scientifc, United States). Western blot analyses were performed as previously described (Cao et al., 2020). Proteins were loaded on sodium dodecyl sulfate-polyacrylamide gel for electrophoresis. After protein transfer, the membranes were blocked by 5% skimmed milk and then incubated overnight at 4°C with antibody against Col2a1 (1:1000, A1560; Abclonal Technology, China), Aggrecan (1:1000, ab36861; Abcam, United Kingdom), MMP13 (1:3000, ab39012; Abcam, United Kingdom), ADAMTS5 (1:500, ab41037; Abcam, United Kingdom), HO-1 (1:1000, 10701-1-AP; Proteintech, China), LC3-I/II (1:1000, ab62721; Abcam, United Kingdom), Beclin-1 (1:1000, 3738s; Cell Signaling Technology, United States), IFT 88 (1:500, 13967-1-AP; Proteintech, China) and GAPDH (1:2000, TA-08; ZSGB-Bio, China). After washing with TBST for three times, the membranes were incubated with secondary antibodies for 1 h at room temperature. Finally, the proteins were detected using the enhanced chemiluminescence method.

## Immunofluorescence

Immunofluorescence staining was performed according to the method we previously used (Cao et al., 2020). After fixation in 4% paraformaldehyde at room temperature for 10 min, cells were permeabilized in 0.1% triton-100 for 15 min and blocked with 1% bovine serum albumin for 1 h at room temperature. Subsequently, cells were incubated overnight at 4°C with antibody against HO-1 (1:200, 10701-1-AP; Proteintech, China) and acetylated-tubulin (1:400, T6793; Sigma, United States), and then incubated for 1 h at room temperature with AlexaFluor 488-conjugated rabbit and mouse secondary antibodies (1:500, A11008 and A11001; ThermoFisher Scientifc, United States). After stained with DAPI, the cells were examined with a confocal microscope (A1R; Nikon, Japan) and analyzed with ImageJ software (Version 1.50; National Institutes of Health, United States).

## Cilium Length and Prevalence Measurements

A Nikon A1R confocal microscope with an oil immersion × 100 objective was used to create maximum projection of confocal z-stacks from which cilia length was measured by ImageJ software (Version 1.50; National Institutes of Health, United States). Confocal z maximum projection was also used to determine the cilium prevalence and DAPI nuclear staining.

## Transfection of Small Interfering RNA (siRNA)

The rat HO-1-siRNAs and IFT88-siRNAs were designed and manufactured by GenePharma (GenePharma Co.,Ltd., China). Transfection was performed as previously described (Cao et al., 2013). Briefly, NP cells were transfected with negative control (NC) siRNA and three independent HO-1-siRNAs and IFT88-siRNAs, respectively, the sequences are shown in **Supplementary Table S1**. The most effective target sequences for HO-1-siRNA (#2) and IFT88-siRNA (#1) were used. Cells were transfected with siRNAs at a concentration of 50 pmol/$10^5$ cell using Lipofectamine™ RNAiMAX Transfection Reagent (13778150; ThermoFisher Scientific, United States). 24 h later, the transfected cells were digested and seeded onto collagen I-coated culture slips for further study.

## Transmission Electron Microscopy (TEM)

Harvested NP cells were washed in PBS and deionized water, and then pelleted by centrifugation. Cells were fixed with 2.5% glutaraldehyde for 2 h and 1% osmium tetroxide for 2 h, respectively. The cells were then dehydrated in ethanol and infiltrated and embedded in Embed 812. Ultrathin sections were stained with UranyLess (22409; EMS, United Kingdom) and Lead Citrate (22410; EMS, United Kingdom) and examined with a TEM (HT7700; Hitachi, Japan).

## Autophagy Detection Using mRFP-GFP-LC3 Lentiviral Vector

Nucleus pulposus cells were seeded in 24 well plates (1 × $10^5$/plate). 24 h later, cells were infected with lentiviral vector (HanBio Technology Co.,Ltd., China) according to the manufacturer's instructions. 48 h after infection, puromycin was used to screen stable NP cell line expressing mRFP-GFP-LC3. The transfected cells were then used for autophagy detection. Autophagy was determined by confocal microscope (A1R; Nikon, Japan). Autophagic flux was detected by evaluating the number of GFP and mRFP puncta. Free red dots indicated autolysosomes and yellow dots indicated autophagosomes.

## Statistical Analysis

Statistical analysis was performed using GraphPad Prism 6 software (GraphPad Software Inc., United States). All experiments were carried out at least three independent experiments and the data were presented as mean ± standard deviation (s.d.). For analysis of two-group parameters, Student's *t*-tests were used. Statistical significance was set at a level of $P < 0.05$.

# RESULTS

## FSS Regulates ECM Protein Expression and sGAG Content in Rat NP Cells

As an initial step to explore mechanism(s) through which mechanical force regulates the homeostasis of IVD, we performed experiments to determine the effects of FSS on expression of

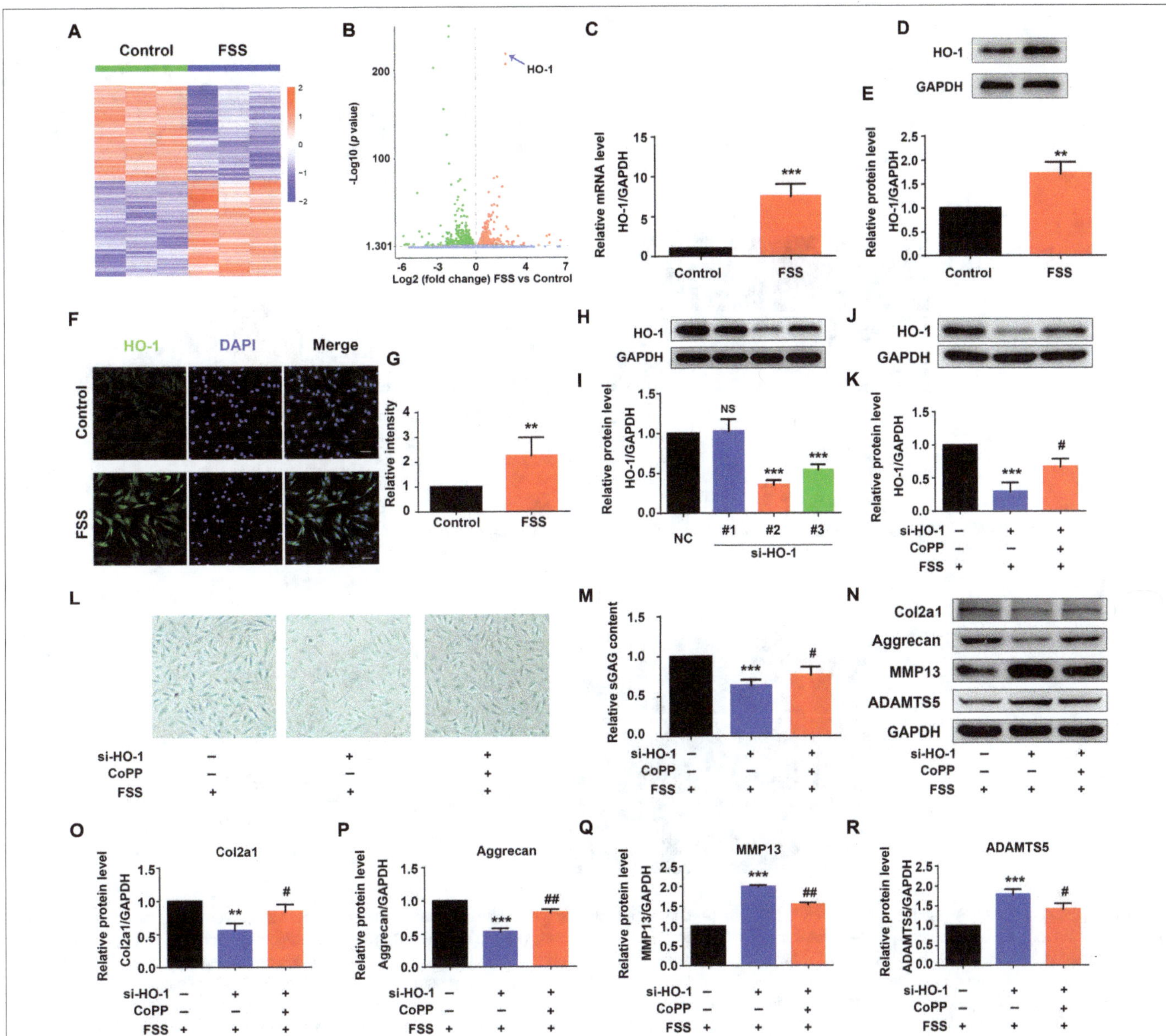


**FIGURE 2 |** Heme oxygenase-1 regulates FSS-mediated ECM production in NP cells. **(A)** The heat map of RNA-seq data. NP cells were treated with or without 12 dyne/cm$^2$ FSS for 2 h, followed by RNA-seq analysis as described in Materials and Methods. **(B)** Volcano plot of RNA-seq data. Blue arrow indicates heme oxygenase-1 (HO-1). **(C)** Quantitative real-time reverse transcriptase-polymerase chain reaction (qRT-PCR) analysis. NP cells were treated with or without 12 dyne/cm$^2$ FSS for 2 h, followed by qRT-PCR analysis. **(D,E)** Western blotting. NP cells were treated as in panel **(C)**, followed by western blotting. Quantitative data from three independent experiments **(E)**. **(F,G)** Immunofluorescence (IF) staining. NP cells were treated as in panel **(C)**, followed by IF staining **(E)**. Bar, 50 μm. Quantitative data from three independent experiments **(G)**. **(H,I)** HO-1 siRNA knockdown. NP cells were transfected with negative control siRNA (NC-siRNA) and three HO-1-siRNA (#1, #2, #3). Then, cells were subjected to western blotting for HO-1 **(H)**. Quantitative data from three independent experiments **(I)**. Note: #2 HO-1-siRNA showed the best knocking down effect and was used for all following experiments in this study. **(J,K)** Western blotting. NP cells were transfected with negative control siRNA (NC-siRNA) and HO-1-siRNA (#2). Then, cells were pretreated with or without HO-1 inducer cobalt protoporphyrin IX (CoPP) (10 μM) and subjected to 12 dyne/cm$^2$ FSS for 2 h, followed by western blotting for HO-1 **(J)**. Quantitative data from three independent experiments **(K)**. **(L,M)** sGAG content. NP cells were treated as in panel **(J)**, followed by alcian blue staining and Blyscan Sulfated Glycosaminoglycan Assay. Bar,100 μm. Quantitative data of sGAG content from three independent experiments **(M)**. **(N–R)** Western blotting. NP cells were treated as in panel **(J)**, followed by western blotting for expression of the indicated proteins. Quantitative data from three independent experiments **(O–R)**. Results are expressed as mean ± standard deviation (s.d.). NS, no statistical significance, $^{**}P < 0.05$, $^{***}P < 0.001$ vs. control, NC or FSS + NC-siRNA group; $^{\#}P < 0.01$ and $^{\#\#}P < 0.01$ vs. FSS + HO-1-siRNA group.

ECM proteins in rat NP cells. The NP cells were subjected to FSS treatment at a dose of 12 dyne/cm$^2$ for the indicated times (**Figure 1B**), followed by assays for sGAG content and expression of several key ECM proteins. The results showed that sGAG content and aggrecan protein level were significantly increased at 1 and 2 h of FSS treatment, and

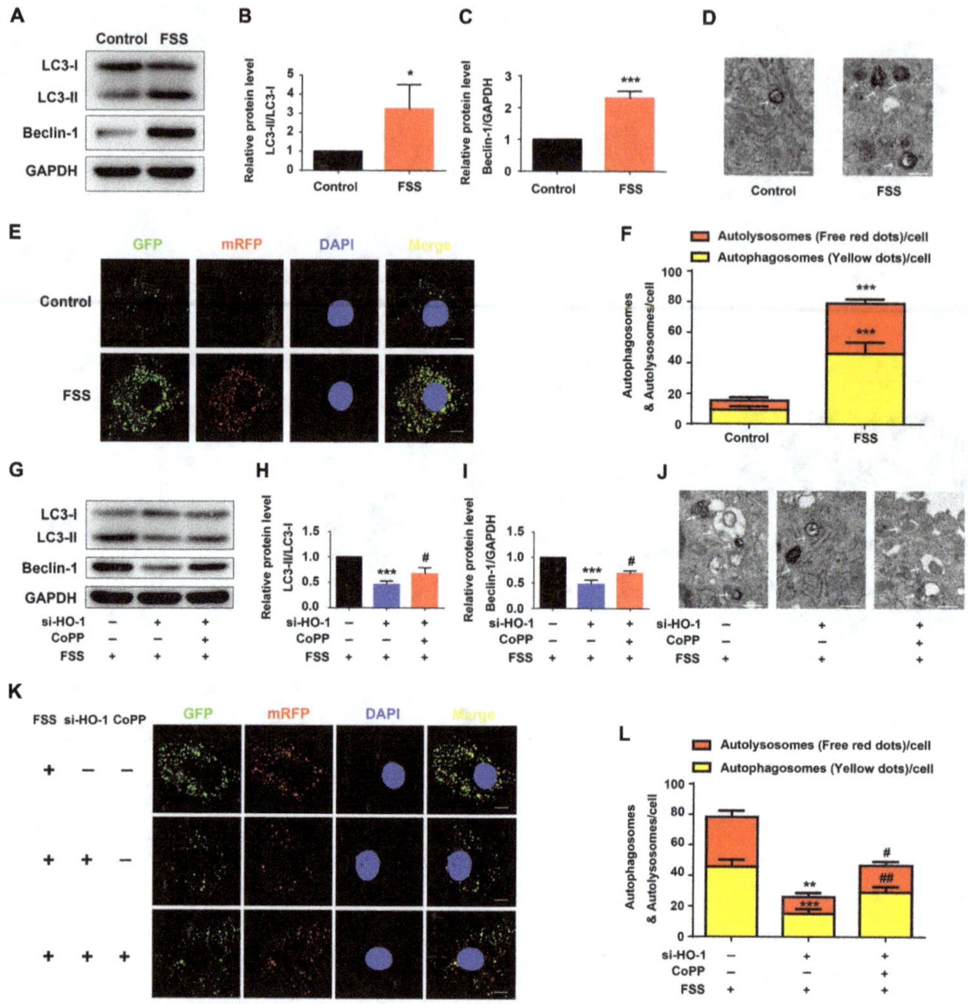


**FIGURE 3** | HO-1 mediates FSS-induced autophagy in NP cells. **(A–C)** Western blotting. NP cells were treated with or without 12 dyne/cm$^2$ FSS for 2 h, followed by western blotting for expression of the indicated proteins. Quantification of LC3-II/LC3-I ratio **(B)** and Beclin-1 **(C)**. **(D)** Transmission Electron Microscopy (TEM). NP cells were treated as in panel **(A)**. TEM images are shown. Arrows indicate double-membrane autophagosomes and autolysosomes at various stages. Bar, 500 nm. **(E,F)** Measurements of autophagosomes and autolysosomes. NP cells were infected with lentivirus expressing a tandem mRFP-GFP-LC3 construct and treated with or without 12 dyne/cm$^2$ FSS for 2 h. Fluorescence images were obtained. Bar, 5 μm. Quantification of autophagosomes (yellow dots) and autolysosomes (free red dots) **(F)**. **(G–I)** Western blotting. NP cells were first treated with and without HO-1 siRNA knockdown and in the presence and absence of CoPP. Then, cells were pretreated with or without HO-1 inducer cobalt protoporphyrin IX (CoPP) (10 μM) and subjected to 12 dyne/cm$^2$ FSS for 2 h, followed by western blotting for expression of the indicated proteins. Quantification of LC3-II/LC3-I ratio and Beclin-1 from three independent experiments **(H,I)**. **(J)** TEM. NP cells were treated as in panel **(G)**. TEM images are shown. The arrows indicate double-membrane autophagosomes and autolysosomes. Bar, 500 nm. **(K,L)** Measurements of autophagosomes and autolysosomes. NP cells were transduced with lentivirus expressing a tandem mRFP-GFP-LC3 construct and treated as in panel **(G)**. Fluorescence images were obtained. Bar, 5 μm. Quantification of autophagosomes (yellow dots) and autolysosomes (free red dots) from three independent experiments **(L)**. $^*P < 0.05$, $^{**}P < 0.01$, and $^{***}P < 0.001$ vs. control; $^{\#}P < 0.05$ and $^{\#\#}P < 0.01$ vs. FSS + HO-1-siRNA group.

MMP13 protein level was significantly decreased at 1, 2 and 3 h of FSS treatment (**Figures 1C–E,G,H**). FSS treatment slightly increased Col2a1 expression and decreased ADAMTS5 expression (**Figures 1F,I**). However, when NP cells were exposed to 24 dyne/cm$^2$ FSS treatment, sGAG content and the protein levels of Col2a1 and aggrecan were decreased, while the levels of MMP13 and ADAMTS5 were increased in a time-dependent manner (**Supplementary Figure S1**). These results suggest that moderate FSS upregulates sGAG content and anabolic ECM proteins (Col2a1 and aggrecan), and downregulates catabolic ECM proteins (MMP13 and ADAMTS5) in NP cells, while high FSS exerts opposite effects. We focused our next studies to determine potential mechanism(s) through which moderate FSS (i.e., 12 dyne/cm$^2$ for 2 h) regulates expression of key ECM proteins and sGAG content in NP cells.

## HO-1 Is Largely Upregulated by Moderate FSS in NP Cells

To identify genes that were regulated by moderate FSS treatment, NP cells were treated with or without FSS

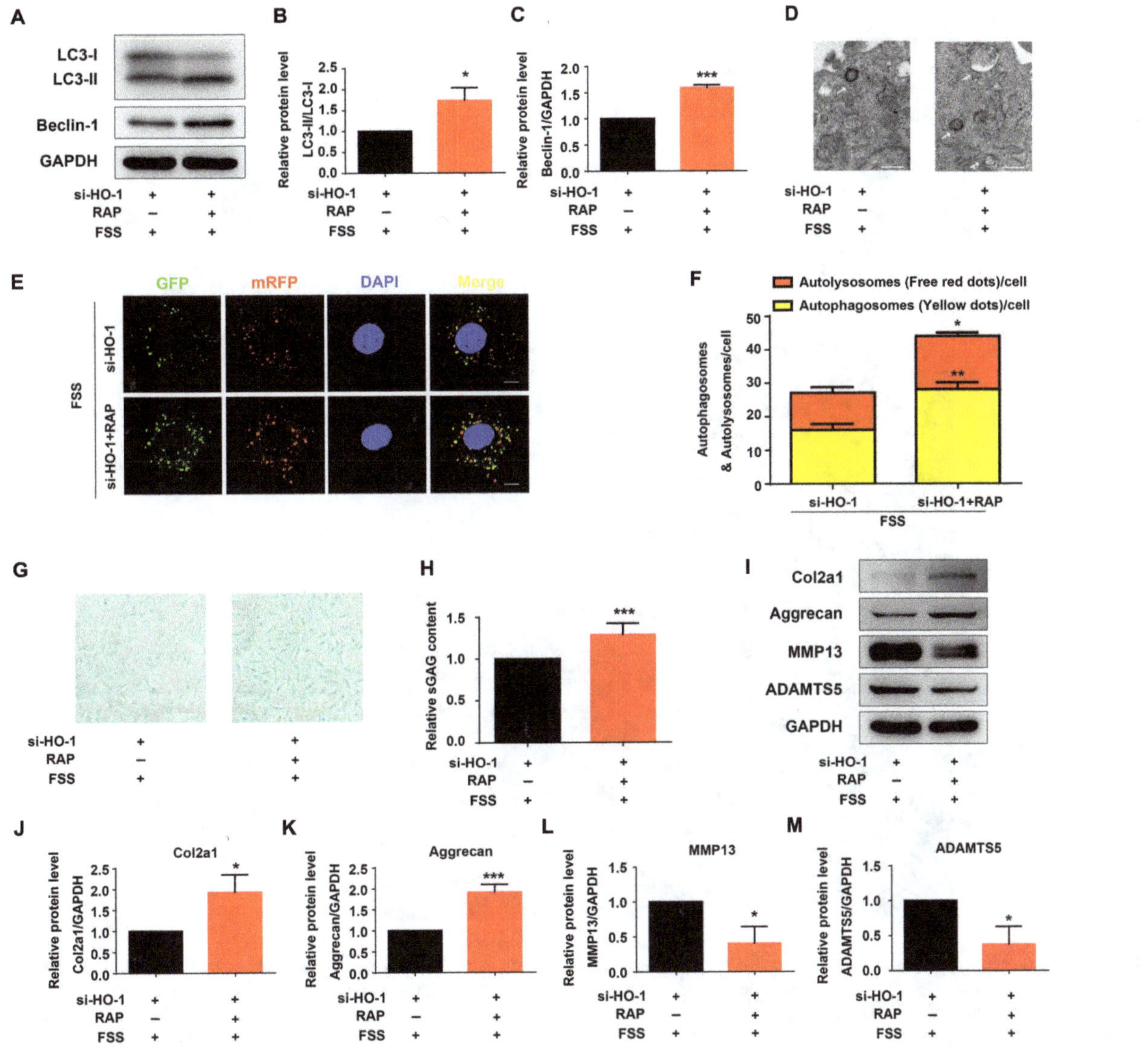


**FIGURE 4 |** Rapamycin regulates autophagy and ECM in NP cells. **(A–C)** Western blotting. NP cells were first transfected with HO-1 siRNA and treated with autophagy activator rapamycin (RAP, 500 nM) for 12 h. Cells were then treated with 12 dyne/cm$^2$ FSS for 2 h, followed by western blotting for expression of the indicated proteins. Quantification of LC3-II/LC3-I ratio and Beclin-1 from three independent experiments **(B,C)**. **(D)** Transmission Electron Microscopy (TEM). NP cells were treated as in panel **(A)**. TEM images are shown. The arrows indicate double-membrane autophagosomes and autolysosomes. Bar, 500 nm. **(E,F)** Measurements of autophagosomes and autolysosomes. NP cells were transduced with lentivirus expressing a tandem mRFP-GFP-LC3 construct and treated as in panel **(A)**. Fluorescence images were obtained. Bar, 5 μm. Quantification of autophagosomes (yellow dots) and autolysosomes (free red dots) from three independent experiments **(F)**. **(G,H)** sGAG content. NP cells were treated as in panel **(A)**, followed by alcian blue staining **(G)** and Blyscan Sulfated Glycosaminoglycan Assay **(H)**. Bar, 100 μm. **(I–M)** Western blotting. NP cells were treated as in panel **(A)**, followed by western blotting for expression of the indicated proteins **(I)**. Quantification of Col2a1, aggrecan, MMP13 and ADAMTS5 from three independent experiments **(J–M)**. Results are expressed as mean ± standard deviation (s.d.). *$P < 0.05$ and ***$P < 0.001$ vs. FSS + HO-1-siRNA group.

(12 dyne/cm$^2$ for 2 h). Total RNAs from both groups were isolated and subjected to RNA sequencing analysis as described in Materials and Methods. Genes upregulated (1463) or downregulated (1467) were presented in **Supplementary Table S2**. Among the upregulated genes, we found that HO-1 was significantly upregulated by FSS treatment with the lowest *p* value (**Figures 2A,B**). Results from qRT-PCR analysis, western blotting and immunofluorescence staining further verified that the levels of HO-1 mRNA and protein were dramatically increased by FSS treatment (**Figures 2C–G**).

## HO-1 Is Critical for Moderate FSS Regulation of ECM in NP Cells

Since HO-1 was reported to regulate ECM metabolism in NP cells (Hu et al., 2016), we next determined whether HO-1 is involved in FSS regulation of ECM proteins in NP cells. To do this, NP

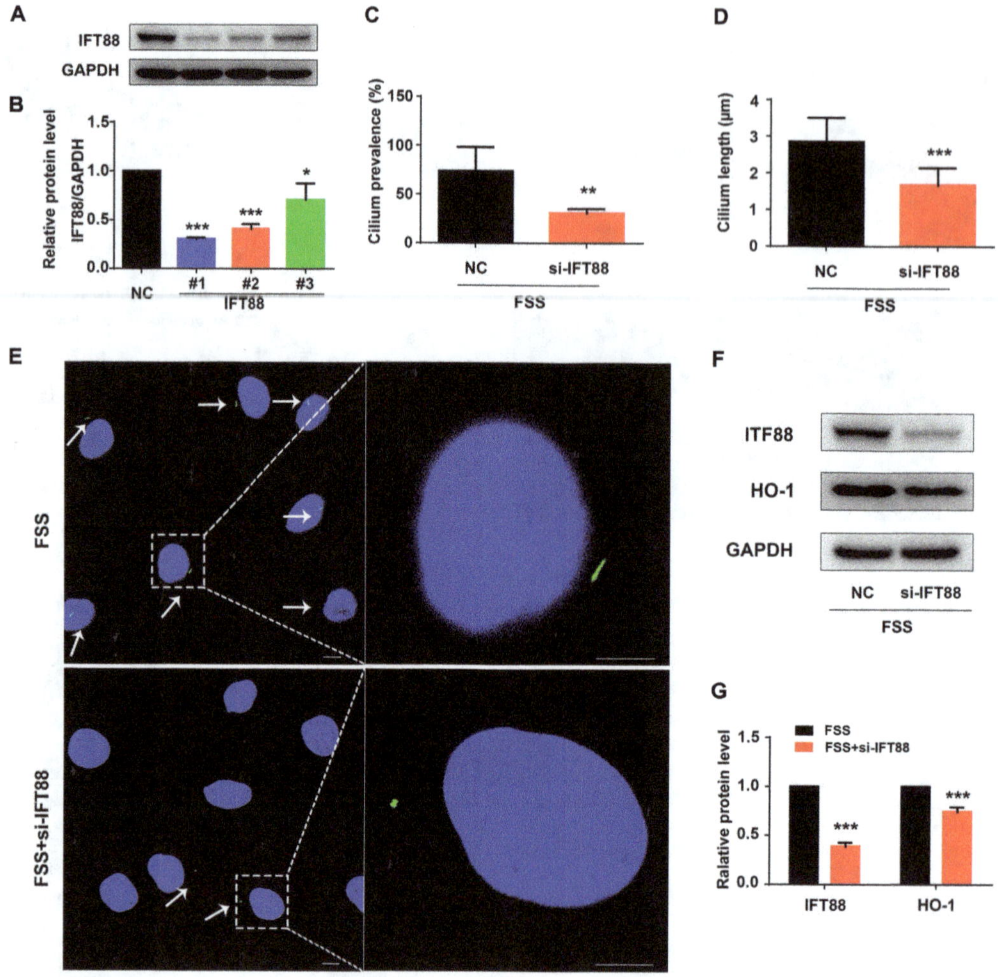


**FIGURE 5 |** Knockdown of IFT88 impairs cilium function and decreases expression of HO-1 in FSS-treated NP cells. **(A)** IFT88 Knockdown. NP cells were transfected with negative control siRNA (NC-siRNA) and three different IFT88-siRNA (#1, #2, #3). Then, cells were subjected to western blotting for expression of IFT88 **(A)**. Quantitative data from three independent experiments **(B)**. The #1 IFT88-siRNA was used for the following experiments in this study. **(C,D)** Qualification of cilium prevalence **(C)** and cilium length **(D)** in NP cells from three independent experiments. NP cells were transfected with negative control siRNA (NC-siRNA) and IFT88 siRNA. Then, cells were treated with 12 dyne/cm$^2$ FSS for 2 h. **(E)** Fluorescence images of primary cilia. Left bar, 10 μm; right bar, 5 μm. White arrows represent primary cilia. **(F,G)** Western blotting. NP cells were transfected with NC-siRNA or IFT88-siRNA (#1) and subjected to 12 dyne/cm$^2$ FSS for 2 h, followed by western blotting for expression of IFT88 and HO-1 **(F)**. Quantification of data from three independent experiments **(G)**. Results are expressed as mean ± standard deviation (s.d.). $^*P < 0.05$, $^{**}P < 0.01$, and $^{***}P < 0.001$ vs. NC or FSS + NC-siRNA group).

cells were transfected with negative control siRNA (NC-siRNA) and three different HO-1 siRNAs (#1, #2, and #3). We chose the #2 HO-1 siRNA for HO-1 knocking down in this study since the #2 HO-1 siRNA showed the best knocking down efficiency (**Figures 2H,I**). To determine whether HO-1 is involved in FSS regulation of ECM, NP cells were first transfected with control siRNA or HO-1-siRNA (#2). Then, cells were pretreated with or without HO-1 inducer cobalt protoporphyrin IX (CoPP) (10 μM) for 1 h and subjected to 12 dyne/cm$^2$ FSS for 2 h. As expected, HO-1 siRNA dramatically decreased the level of HO-1 protein, which was markedly reversed by treatment of CoPP treatment (**Figures 2J,K**). Furthermore, HO-1 siRNA significantly reduced the synthesis of sGAG, which was partially reversed by CoPP treatment (**Figures 2L,M**). Similarly, results from western blot analyses revealed that HO-1 siRNA downregulated the levels of anabolic ECM proteins (Col2a1 and aggrecan) and upregulated the levels of catabolic ECM proteins (MMP13 and ADAMTS5), which could be reversed by CoPP treatment (**Figures 2N–R**).

## FSS Promotes Autophagy in NP Cells

Fluid shear stress activates autophagy in multiple cell types (Zhang et al., 2018; Yang et al., 2019). Thus, we determined whether FSS activates autophagy in NP cells. Results showed that NP cells treated with FSS displayed increased autophagy compared to untreated cells, as demonstrated by dramatic increases in the LC3-II/LC3-I ratio and Beclin-1 protein level (**Figures 3A–C**). Likewise, TEM analyses showed a marked increase in the numbers of autophagosome and autolysosome in FSS-treated cells relative to untreated cells (**Figure 3D**). Furthermore, immunofluorescence confocal microscopy analyses

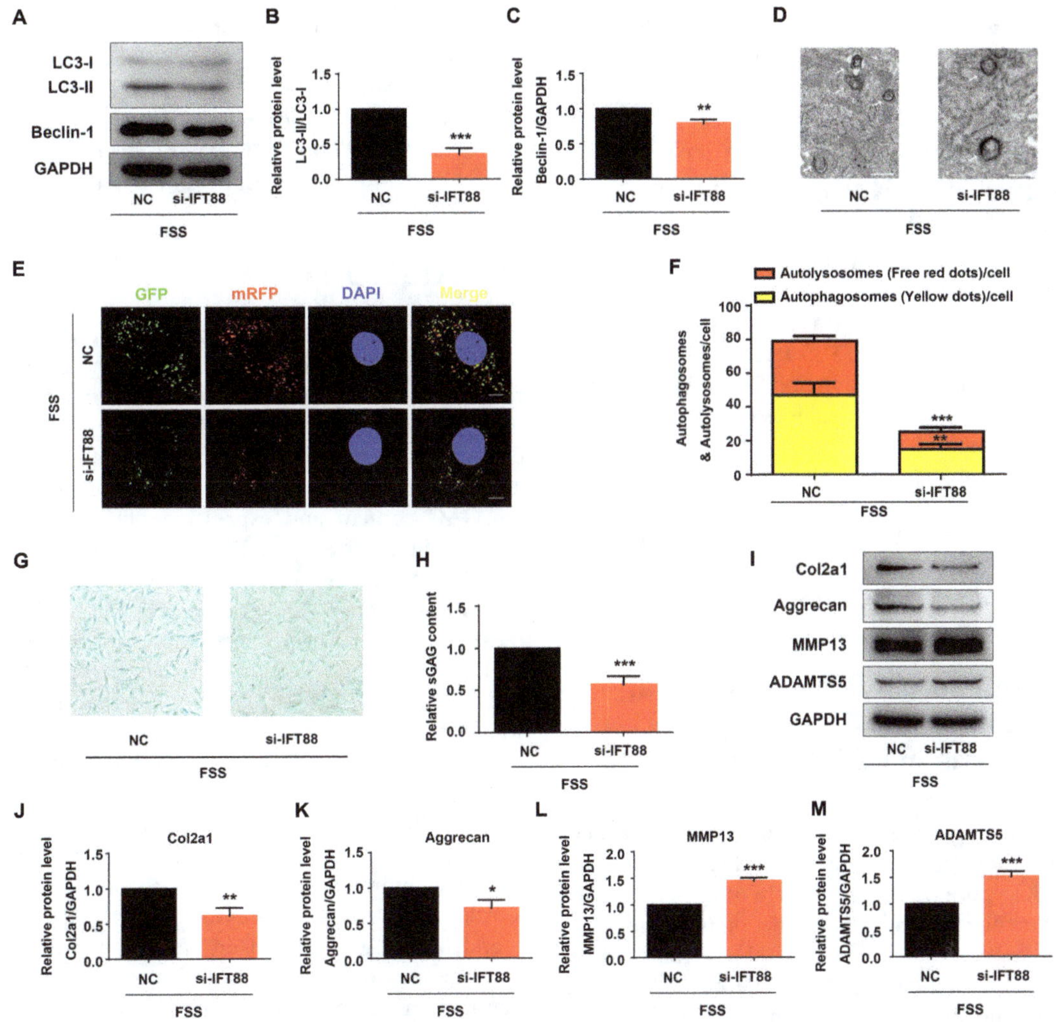


**FIGURE 6 |** IFT88 loss reduces autophagy and impairs ECM homeostasis in FSS-treated NP cells. **(A–C)** Western blotting. NP cells were transfected with negative control siRNA (NC-siRNA) or IFT88-siRNA (#1). Then, cells were subjected to 12 dyne/cm$^2$ FSS for 2 h, followed by western blotting for expression of LC3-I, LC3-II, and Beclin-1 **(A)**. Quantification of LC3-I/LC3-II ratio and Beclin-1 from three independent experiments **(B,C)**. **(D)** Transmission Electron Microscopy (TEM). NP cells were treated as in PANEL **(A)**. TEM images are shown. The arrows indicate double-membrane autophagosomes and autolysosomes. Bar, 500 nm. **(E,F)** Measurements of autophagosomes and autolysosomes. NP cells were transduced with lentivirus expressing a tandem mRFP-GFP-LC3 construct and treated as in panel **(A)**. Fluorescence images were obtained. Bar, 5 μm. Quantification of autophagosomes (yellow dots) and autolysosomes (free red dots) from three independent experiments **(F)**. **(G,H)** sGAG content. NP cells were treated as in panel **(A)**, followed by alcian blue staining **(G)** and Blyscan Sulfated Glycosaminoglycan Assay **(H)**. Bar, 100 μm. **(I–M)** Western blotting. NP cells were treated as in panel **(A)**, followed by western blotting for expression of the indicated proteins **(I)**. Quantification of expression of Col2a1, aggrecan, MMP13 and ADAMTS5 from three independent experiments **(J–M)**. Results are expressed as mean ± standard deviation (s.d.). *$P < 0.05$, **$P < 0.01$, and ***$P < 0.001$ vs. FSS + NC-siRNA group.

revealed that the numbers of both autophagosome (yellow dots) and autolysosome (free red dots) were dramatically increased in FSS-treated NP cells compared to those in untreated cells (**Figures 3E,F**).

## HO-1 Regulates the FSS-Induced Autophagy in NP Cells

Heme oxygenase-1 was reported to activate autophagy in NP cells (Hu et al., 2016). Thus, we next determined whether HO-1 plays a role in mediation of the FSS-induced autophagy in NP cells. NP cells were treated with FSS, with or without CoPP treatment, in the presence or absence of HO-1 knockdown by siRNA. The results showed that HO-1 knockdown dramatically reduced the increases of LC3-II/LC3-I ratio and Beclin-1 expression in NP cells induced by FSS treatment, which was markedly reversed by CoPP treatment (**Figures 3G–I**). TEM analyses showed that HO-1 siRNA significantly reduced the numbers of autophagosome and autolysosome in FSS-treated NP cells compared to control siRNA/FSS-treated cells, which was largely reversed by CoPP treatment (**Figure 3J**). Similarly, immunofluorescence confocal microscopy analyses showed that the numbers of both autophagosome (yellow dots) and autolysosome (free red dots) were dramatically decreased in HO-1 siRNA/FSS-treated NP cells compared to those in control siRNA/FSS-treated cells, which was reversed by CoPP treatment (**Figures 3K,L**).

## Rapamycin Reverses HO-1 Knockdown-Induced Alterations in Autophagy and ECM Homeostasis in FSS-Treated NP Cells

Rapamycin activates autophagy in multiple cell types (Spang et al., 2014; Lopez de Figueroa et al., 2015). We next determined the effect of rapamycin treatment on autophagy suppression induced by HO-1 knockdown in FSS-treated NP cells. NP cells were first transfected with HO-1 siRNA and then pretreated with or without rapamycin for 12 h and subjected to FSS treatment for 2 h. The results showed that rapamycin treatment of the NP cells significantly increased the LC3-II/LC3-I ratio, expression level of Beclin-1 protein and formation of autophagosome and autolysosome (**Figures 4A–F**). Furthermore, rapamycin treatment also reversed the decrease of sGAG content and alterations in expression of ECM proteins induced by HO-1 knockdown in the FSS-treated NP cells (**Figures 4G–M**).

## Primary Cilium Protein IFT88 Is Critical for HO-1 Regulation of Autophagy and ECM Homeostasis in FSS-Treated NP Cells

Primary cilium was reported to function as a mechano-sensor and plays an important role in mechanotransduction (He et al., 2016). As a core trafficking protein of primary cilium, IFT88 is critical for ciliary assembly and function (Coveney et al., 2018; Fu et al., 2019). We used IFT88-siRNA to knock down its expression in NP cells (**Figures 5A,B**). The #1 IFT88 siRNA displayed the best knocking down efficiency and was used in the following experiments (**Figures 5A,B**). Results showed that IFT88 knockdown significantly reduced the cilium prevalence and cilium length in FSS-treated NP cells (**Figures 5C–E**). Interestingly, IFT88 knockdown decreased the protein level of HO-1 in FSS-treated NP cells (**Figures 5F,G**). Moreover, IFT88 knockdown inhibited the autophagy activation by decreasing the LC3-II/LC3-I ratio, expression of Beclin-1 protein and formation of autophagosome and autolysosome in FSS-treated NP cells (**Figures 6A–F**). Furthermore, IFT88 knockdown decreased sGAG content and expression of anabolic proteins (Col2a1 and aggrecan) and increased expression of catabolic proteins (MMP13 and ADAMTS5) (**Figures 6G–M**).

## CoPP or Rapamycin Largely Reverses IFT88 Loss-Induced Alterations in Autophagy and ECM Homeostasis in FSS-Treated NP Cells

Finally, we determined whether rapamycin or upregulation of HO-1 by CoPP can reverse the alterations in autophagy and ECM protein expression induced by IFT88 knockdown in FSS-treated NP cells. NP cells were first transfected with IFT88-siRNA. Then, cells were pretreated with CoPP (10 μM) or rapamycin (500 nM) and then subjected to FSS treatment. The results showed that both CoPP or rapamycin treatment largely reversed the IFT88 knockdown-induced alterations in LC3-II/LC3-I ratio and Beclin-1 protein level (**Figures 7A–C**), formation of autophagosome and autolysosome (**Figures 7D–F**), sGAG content (**Figures 7G,H**) and expression of anabolic and catabolic ECM proteins (**Figures 7I–M**).

# DISCUSSION

In the present study, we demonstrate the effect of FSS on the regulation of ECM homeostasis in NP cells. We find that FSS regulates ECM metabolism in a loading magnitude- and time-dependent manner. When NP cells are subjected to the 24 dyne/cm$^2$ FSS treatment, the balance between ECM anabolism and catabolism is disrupted, as demonstrated by decreases in sGAG content and expression of Col2 and aggrecan and increase in expression of ECM-degrading proteinases MMP13 and ADAMTS5. However, when NP cells are exposed to the relatively moderate FSS (12 dyne/cm$^2$ for 1–2 h), FSS maintains the ECM homeostasis by promoting the ECM anabolism and inhibiting the ECM catabolism. The observed pro-anabolism and anti-catabolism effects of moderate FSS are consistent with previous studies in various cell types exposed to different mechanical stimuli. In rat fibrochondrocytes, Deschner et al. (2006) reported that dynamic tensile strain could significantly abrogate IL-1β-induced upregulation of MMPs (MMP3, MMP7, MMP8, MMP9, MMP13, MMP16, MMP17, and MMP19). In human chondrocytes, He et al. (2016) found that moderate cyclic tensile strain could reduce the protein expressions of MMP-1 and MMP-13 and exert an anti-catabolism effect to protect cartilage integrity. Results from Dai et al. (2014) demonstrated that dynamic compression could promote the synthesis of Col2 and aggrecan in adipose-derived stem cells. Our results suggested that NP cells could start an early ECM synthesis process to maintain ECM homeostasis in response to moderate FSS, and a deeper understanding of the specific mechanism by which moderate FSS regulates ECM homeostasis in NP cells might help us to seek for novel and early preventive and therapeutic targets for IVD degeneration.

Increasing evidence have revealed that HO-1 could attenuate inflammation- and oxidative stress-induced imbalance between ECM anabolism and catabolism in NP cells and chondrocytes (Guillen et al., 2008; Hu et al., 2016; An et al., 2018). In this study, we performed RNA sequencing analysis and focused on HO-1, which was significantly upregulated in NP cells exposed to moderate FSS. We found that HO-1 inhibition decreased sGAG content, downregulated ECM anabolism related proteins (Col2a1, aggrecan) and upregulated ECM catabolism related proteins (MMP13, ADAMTS5) in NP cells exposed to moderate FSS, which could be reversed by HO-1 inducer CoPP. These results suggest that HO-1 plays a critical role in the maintenance of ECM homeostasis induced by moderate FSS.

Results from different research groups indicated that FSS could induce protective autophagy in osteocytes, chondrocytes and hepatocellular carcinoma cells (Wang et al., 2018;

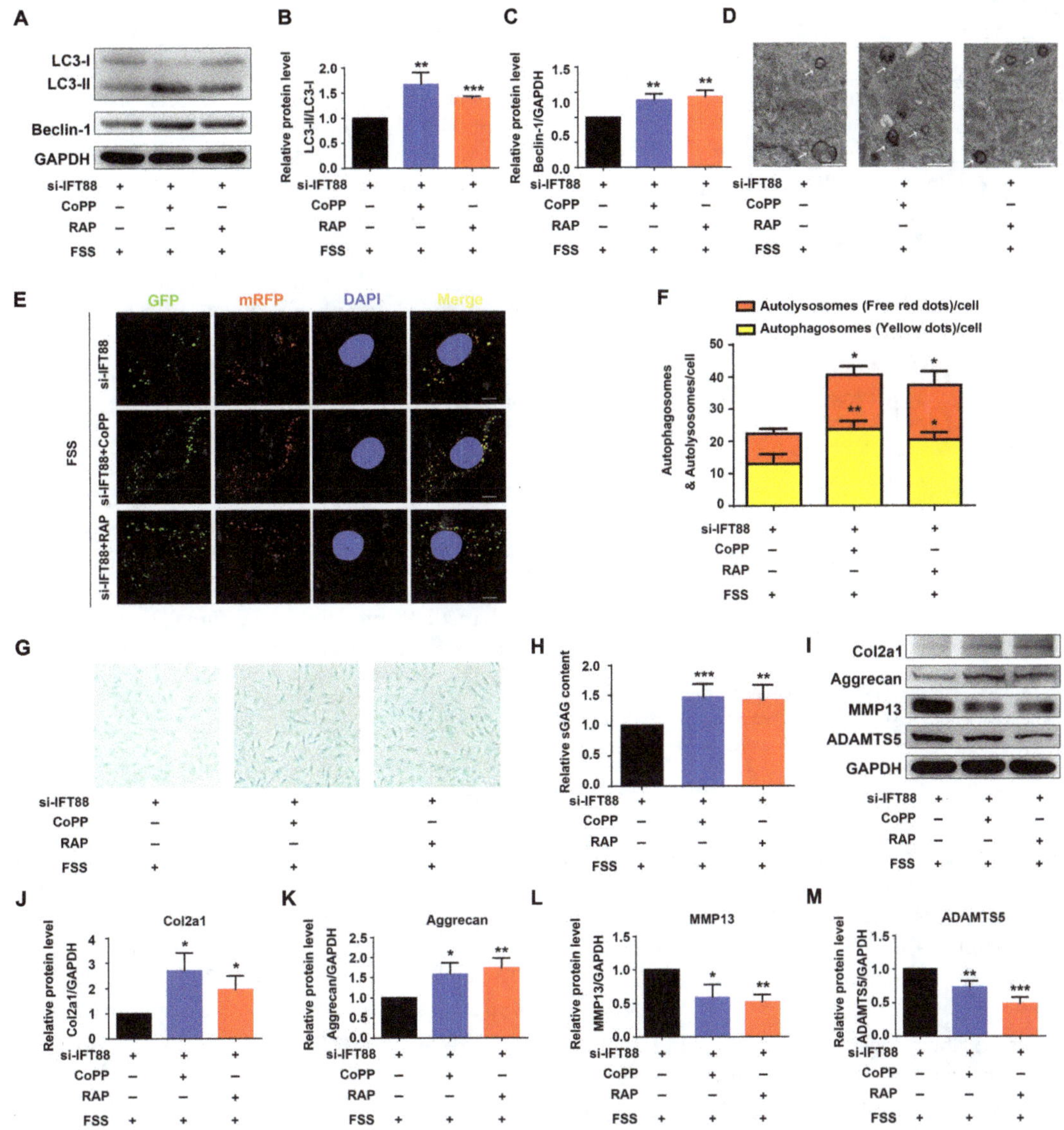


**FIGURE 7 |** HO-1 upregulation or rapamycin reverses IFT88 loss-induced alterations in autophagy and ECM production in FSS-treated NP cells. **(A–C)** Western blotting. NP cells were transfected with IFT88-siRNA. Then, cells were pretreated with CoPP (10 μM) or rapamycin (RAP, 500 nM) and subjected to 12 dyne/cm$^2$ FSS for 2 h, followed by western blotting for expression of LC3-I, LC3-II, and Beclin-1 **(A)**. Quantification of LC3-I/LC3-II ratio and Beclin-1 from three independent experiments **(B,C)**. **(D)** Transmission Electron Microscopy (TEM). NP cells were treated as in panel **(A)**. TEM images are shown. The arrows indicate double-membrane autophagosomes and autolysosomes. Bar, 500 nm. **(E,F)** Measurements of autophagosomes and autolysosomes. NP cells were transduced with lentivirus expressing a tandem mRFP-GFP-LC3 construct and treated as in panel **(A)**. Fluorescence images were obtained. Bar, 5 μm. Quantification of autophagosomes (yellow dots) and autolysosomes (free red dots) from three independent experiments **(F)**. **(G,H)** sGAG content. NP cells were treated as in panel **(A)**, followed by alcian blue staining **(G)** and Blyscan Sulfated Glycosaminoglycan Assay **(H)**. Bar, 100 μm. **(I–M)** Western blotting. NP cells were treated as in panel **(A)**, followed by western blotting for expression of the indicated proteins **(I)**. Quantification of expression of Col2a1, aggrecan, MMP13 and ADAMTS5 from three independent experiments **(J–M)**. Results are expressed as mean ± standard deviation (s.d). *$P < 0.05$, **$P < 0.01$, and ***$P < 0.001$ vs. FSS + IFT88-siRNA group.

Zhang et al., 2018; Yang et al., 2019). In line with previous studies, our data demonstrated that moderate FSS activated autophagy in NP cells by increasing the ratio of LC3-II to LC3-I, the protein expression of Beclin-1 and the number of autophagosomes and autolysosomes. HO-1 upregulation as a mean for autophagy induction has been reported in many diseases (Nakamura et al., 2018; Vasconcellos et al., 2018). For example, in a cadmium-induced emphysema mice model, Surolia et al. (2015) found that HO-1 mediated the activation of autophagy and protected against pulmonary endothelial cell apoptosis and development of emphysema. And in a diabetic nephropathy cell model, Dong et al. (2015) reported that HO-1 could enhance autophagy and inhibited high glucose-induced podocytes apoptosis. In this study, we demonstrated that HO-1 inhibition suppressed the FSS-induced autophagy activation, while HO-1 inducer CoPP reversed this process. Furthermore,

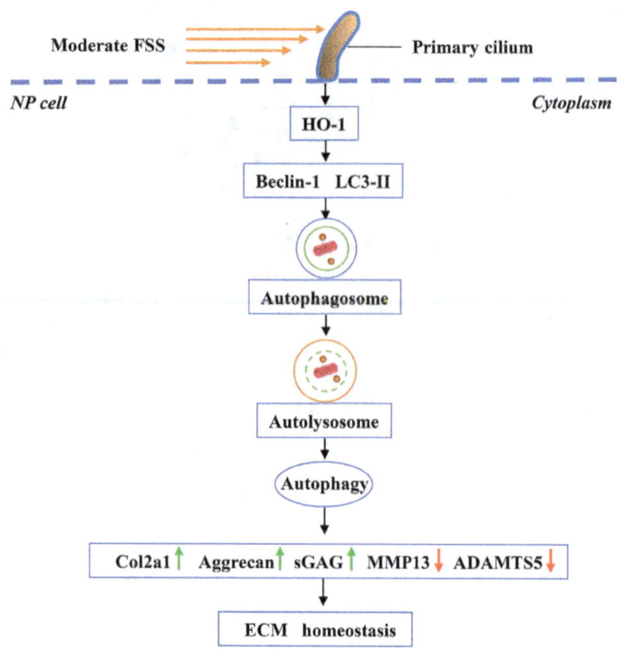


**FIGURE 8 |** Working model. Primary cilia sense and transmit extracellular FSS signal to NP cells, which activates HO-1 and thereby autophagy. Increased autophagy plays an important role in maintaining ECM homeostasis in NP cells.

autophagy activator rapamycin attenuated HO-1 inhibition induced disruption of FSS-induced autophagy activation and ECM homeostasis in NP cells. Collectively, these results suggest that moderate FSS maintains ECM homeostasis in NP cells, at least in part, through HO-1-mediated autophagy.

Although our results above revealed that FSS could regulate ECM homeostasis through HO-1-mediated autophagy in NP cells, how the cells sense FSS and convert it into downstream molecular signals remained unclear. Primary cilium is a microtubule-based organelle, which extends as a solitary protrusion from the surface of most mammalian cell types, including NP cells (Zheng et al., 2018; Anvarian et al., 2019). It can sense and transmit extracellular mechanical and chemical signals, to regulate various cellular processes and maintain tissue homeostasis (Hua and Ferland, 2018; Kim and Kim, 2019). Because primary cilium cannot synthesize proteins, cilium-associated trafficking proteins, such as IFT88, are therefore critical for cilium biogenesis, maintenance and function (Wang et al., 2016). Recent studies have demonstrated that hypomorphic mutation of IFT88 can result in severely stunted primary cilia and abolish the suppression effects of cyclic tensile strain on the inflammatory response to IL-1β in chondrocytes (Fu et al., 2019). Results from He et al. (2016) showed that disruption of the primary cilia in chondrocytes by IFT88-siRNA attenuated the anti-catabolism effects of moderate cyclic tensile strain. Moreover, Orhon et al. (2016) reported that hypomorphic deletion of the IFT88 impaired ciliary assembly and inhibited the FSS-induced autophagy activation in epithelial cells. Hence, we speculated that primary cilia associated with IFT88 might play a pivotal role in the mechanotransduction when NP cells were exposed to FSS. As expected, NP cells transfected with IFT88-siRNA exhibited defective primary cilia, and the disruption of primary cilia downregulated the protein expression of HO-1, inhibited the autophagy activation and destroyed the ECM homeostasis in NP cells exposed to moderate FSS. Meanwhile, we found that both CoPP and RAP partially reversed the changes. Therefore, our data suggest that primary cilium could sense and mediate moderate FSS signal to regulate HO-1 mediated autophagy activation and then maintain ECM homeostasis in NP cells (**Figure 8**).

## CONCLUSION

Findings from our study indicate that moderate FSS could maintain ECM homeostasis in NP cells which requires HO-1-mediated autophagy activation in the presence of primary cilium. This study could lead us to a better understanding of moderate FSS-mediated maintenance of ECM homeostasis in NP cells, and may shed lights into developing novel strategies for early prevention and treatment of IVD degeneration.

## AUTHOR CONTRIBUTIONS

GX, ZS, SC, and HC designed the study. SC, HC, LQ, XW, XF, and SL conducted the study and collected the data. SC and GX analyzed the data. GX, ZS, SC, DC, and HC interpreted the data. SC, HC, and GX drafted the manuscript. SC, GX, LQ, XW, XF, SL, ZS, and HC took the responsibility for the integrity of the data analysis.

## REFERENCES


An, Q. D., Li, Y. Y., Zhang, H. X., Lu, J., Yu, X. D., Lin, Q., et al. (2018). Inhibition of bromodomain-containing protein 4 ameliorates oxidative stress-mediated apoptosis and cartilage matrix degeneration through activation of NF-E2-related factor 2-heme oxygenase-1 signaling in rat chondrocytes. *J. Cell Biochem.* 119, 7719–7728. doi: 10.1002/jcb.27122

Anvarian, Z., Mykytyn, K., Mukhopadhyay, S., Pedersen, L. B., and Christensen, S. T. (2019). Cellular signalling by primary cilia in development, organ function and disease. *Nat. Rev. Nephrol.* 15, 199–219. doi: 10.1038/s41581-019-0116-9

Bonnevie, E. D., Gullbrand, S. E., Ashinsky, B. G., Tsinman, T. K., Elliott, D. M., Chao, P. G., et al. (2019). Aberrant mechanosensing in injured intervertebral discs as a result of boundary-constraint disruption and residual-strain loss. *Nat. Biomed. Eng.* 3, 998–1008. doi: 10.1038/s41551-019-0458-4

Cao, H., Yan, Q., Wang, D., Lai, Y., Zhou, B., Zhang, Q., et al. (2020). Focal adhesion protein Kindlin-2 regulates bone homeostasis in mice. *Bone Res.* 8:2. doi: 10.1038/s41413-019-0073-8

Cao, H., Yu, S., Yao, Z., Galson, D. L., Jiang, Y., Zhang, X., et al. (2010). Activating transcription factor 4 regulates osteoclast differentiation in mice. *J. Clin. Invest.* 120, 2755–2766. doi: 10.1172/JCI42106

Cao, H., Zhu, K., Qiu, L., Li, S., Niu, H., Hao, M., et al. (2013). Critical role of AKT protein in myeloma-induced osteoclast formation and osteolysis. *J. Biol. Chem.* 288, 30399–30410. doi: 10.1074/jbc.M113.469973

Chen, S., Liu, S., Ma, K., Zhao, L., Lin, H., and Shao, Z. (2019). TGF-beta signaling in intervertebral disc health and disease. *Osteoarthr. Cartil.* 27, 1109–1117. doi: 10.1016/j.joca.2019.05.005

Chen, S., Zhao, L., Deng, X., Shi, D., Wu, F., Liang, H., et al. (2017). Mesenchymal stem cells protect nucleus pulposus cells from compression-induced apoptosis by inhibiting the mitochondrial pathway. *Stem Cells Int.* 2017, 9843120. doi: 10.1155/2017/9843120

Chiang, S. K., Chen, S. E., and Chang, L. C. (2018). A dual role of heme oxygenase-1 in cancer cells. *Int. J. Mol. Sci.* 20:39. doi: 10.3390/ijms20010039

Chou, P. H., Wang, S. T., Yen, M. H., Liu, C. L., Chang, M. C., and Lee, O. K. (2016). Fluid-induced, shear stress-regulated extracellular matrix and matrix metalloproteinase genes expression on human annulus fibrosus cells. *Stem Cell Res. Ther.* 7:34. doi: 10.1186/s13287-016-0292-5

Clouet, J., Fusellier, M., Camus, A., Le Visage, C., and Guicheux, J. (2018). Intervertebral disc regeneration: from cell therapy to the development of novel bioinspired endogenous repair strategies. *Adv. Drug Deliv. Rev.* 146, 306–324. doi: 10.1016/j.addr.2018.04.017

Coveney, C. R., Collins, I., Mc Fie, M., Chanalaris, A., Yamamoto, K., and Wann, A. K. T. (2018). Cilia protein IFT88 regulates extracellular protease activity by optimizing LRP-1-mediated endocytosis. *FASEB J.* 32:fj201800334. doi: 10.1096/fj.201800334

Dai, J., Wang, H., Liu, G., Xu, Z., Li, F., and Fang, H. (2014). Dynamic compression and co-culture with nucleus pulposus cells promotes proliferation and differentiation of adipose-derived mesenchymal stem cells. *J Biomech.* 47, 966–972. doi: 10.1016/j.jbiomech.2014.01.023

Deschner, J., Rath-Deschner, B., and Agarwal, S. (2006). Regulation of matrix metalloproteinase expression by dynamic tensile strain in rat fibrochondrocytes. *Osteoarthr. Cartil.* 14, 264–272. doi: 10.1016/j.joca.2005.09.005

Dikic, I., and Elazar, Z. (2018). Mechanism and medical implications of mammalian autophagy. *Nat. Rev. Mol. Cell Biol.* 19, 349–364. doi: 10.1038/s41580-018-0003-4

Dong, C., Zheng, H., Huang, S., You, N., Xu, J., Ye, X., et al. (2015). Heme oxygenase-1 enhances autophagy in podocytes as a protective mechanism against high glucose-induced apoptosis. *Exp. Cell Res.* 337, 146–159. doi: 10.1016/j.yexcr.2015.04.005

Frapin, L., Clouet, J., Delplace, V., Fusellier, M., Guicheux, J., and Le Visage, C. (2019). Lessons learned from intervertebral disc pathophysiology to guide rational design of sequential delivery systems for therapeutic biological factors. *Adv. Drug Deliv. Rev.* 14, 49–71. doi: 10.1016/j.addr.2019.08.007

Fu, S., Thompson, C. L., Ali, A., Wang, W., Chapple, J. P., Mitchison, H. M., et al. (2019). Mechanical loading inhibits cartilage inflammatory signalling via an HDAC6 and IFT-dependent mechanism regulating primary cilia elongation. *Osteoarthr. Cartil.* 27, 1064–1074. doi: 10.1016/j.joca.2019.03.003

Gross, A., and Graef, M. (2019). Mechanisms of autophagy in metabolic stress response. *J. Mol. Biol.* 432, 28–52. doi: 10.1016/j.jmb.2019.09.005

Guillen, M., Megias, J., Gomar, F., and Alcaraz, M. (2008). Haem oxygenase-1 regulates catabolic and anabolic processes in osteoarthritic chondrocytes. *J. Pathol.* 214, 515–522. doi: 10.1002/path.2313

He, Z., Leong, D. J., Zhuo, Z., Majeska, R. J., Cardoso, L., Spray, D. C., et al. (2016). Strain-induced mechanotransduction through primary cilia, extracellular ATP, purinergic calcium signaling, and ERK1/2 transactivates CITED2 and downregulates MMP-1 and MMP-13 gene expression in chondrocytes. *Osteoarthr. Cartil.* 24, 892–901. doi: 10.1016/j.joca.2015.11.015

Henry, N., Clouet, J., Le Bideau, J., Le Visage, C., and Guicheux, J. (2018). Innovative strategies for intervertebral disc regenerative medicine: from cell therapies to multiscale delivery systems. *Biotechnol. Adv.* 36, 281–294. doi: 10.1016/j.biotechadv.2017.11.009

Hu, B., Shi, C., Xu, C., Cao, P., Tian, Y., Zhang, Y., et al. (2016). Heme oxygenase-1 attenuates IL-1beta induced alteration of anabolic and catabolic activities in intervertebral disc degeneration. *Sci. Rep.* 6:21190. doi: 10.1038/srep21190

Hua, K., and Ferland, R. J. (2018). Primary cilia proteins: ciliary and extraciliary sites and functions. *Cell Mol. Life Sci.* 75, 1521–1540. doi: 10.1007/s00018-017-2740-5

Katz, J. N. (2006). Lumbar disc disorders and low-back pain: socioeconomic factors and consequences. *J. Bone Joint Surg. Am.* 88(Suppl. 2), 21–24. doi: 10.2106/JBJS.E.01273

Kim, Y. J., and Kim, J. (2019). Therapeutic perspectives for structural and functional abnormalities of cilia. *Cell Mol. Life Sci.* 76, 3695–3709. doi: 10.1007/s00018-019-03158-6

Lopez de Figueroa, P., Lotz, M. K., Blanco, F. J., and Carames, B. (2015). Autophagy activation and protection from mitochondrial dysfunction in human chondrocytes. *Arthritis Rheumatol.* 67, 966–976. doi: 10.1002/art.39025

Ma, K., Chen, S., Li, Z., Deng, X., Huang, D., Xiong, L., et al. (2019). Mechanisms of endogenous repair failure during intervertebral disc degeneration. *Osteoarthr. Cartil.* 27, 41–48. doi: 10.1016/j.joca.2018.08.021

Maher, C., Underwood, M., and Buchbinder, R. (2017). Non-specific low back pain. *Lancet* 389, 736–747. doi: 10.1016/s0140-6736(16)30970-9

Nakamura, K., Kageyama, S., Yue, S., Huang, J., Fujii, T., Ke, B., et al. (2018). Heme oxygenase-1 regulates sirtuin-1-autophagy pathway in liver transplantation: from mouse to human. *Am. J. Transplant.* 18, 1110–1121. doi: 10.1111/ajt.14586

Neidlinger-Wilke, C., Galbusera, F., Pratsinis, H., Mavrogonatou, E., Mietsch, A., Kletsas, D., et al. (2014). Mechanical loading of the intervertebral disc: from the macroscopic to the cellular level. *Eur. Spine J.* 23(Suppl. 3), S333–S343. doi: 10.1007/s00586-013-2855-9

Oh, C.-D., Im, H.-J., Suh, J., Chee, A., An, H., and Chen, D. (2016). Rho-associated kinase inhibitor immortalizes rat nucleus pulposus and annulus fibrosus cells: establishment of intervertebral disc cell lines with novel approaches. *Spine* 41, E255–E261. doi: 10.1097/BRS.0000000000001235

Orhon, I., Dupont, N., Zaidan, M., Boitez, V., Burtin, M., Schmitt, A., et al. (2016). Primary-cilium-dependent autophagy controls epithelial cell volume in response to fluid flow. *Nat. Cell Biol.* 18, 657–667. doi: 10.1038/ncb3360

Otterbein, L. E., Foresti, R., and Motterlini, R. (2016). Heme oxygenase-1 and carbon monoxide in the heart: the balancing act between danger signaling and pro-survival. *Circ. Res.* 118, 1940–1959. doi: 10.1161/CIRCRESAHA.116.306588

Priyadarshani, P., Li, Y., and Yao, L. (2016). Advances in biological therapy for nucleus pulposus regeneration. *Osteoarthr. Carti.* 24, 206–212. doi: 10.1016/j.joca.2015.08.014

Sakai, D., and Grad, S. (2015). Advancing the cellular and molecular therapy for intervertebral disc disease. *Adv. Drug. Deliv. Rev.* 84, 159–171. doi: 10.1016/j.addr.2014.06.009

Silagi, E. S., Shapiro, I. M., and Risbud, M. V. (2018). Glycosaminoglycan synthesis in the nucleus pulposus: dysregulation and the pathogenesis of disc degeneration. *Matrix Biol.* 7, 368–379. doi: 10.1016/j.matbio.2018.02.025

Spang, N., Feldmann, A., Huesmann, H., Bekbulat, F., Schmitt, V., Hiebel, C., et al. (2014). RAB3GAP1 and RAB3GAP2 modulate basal and rapamycin-induced autophagy. *Autophagy* 10, 2297–2309. doi: 10.4161/15548627.2014.994359

Surolia, R., Karki, S., Kim, H., Yu, Z., Kulkarni, T., Mirov, S. B., et al. (2015). Heme oxygenase-1-mediated autophagy protects against pulmonary endothelial cell death and development of emphysema in cadmium-treated mice. *Am. J. Physiol. Lung. Cell Mol. Physiol.* 309, L280–L292. doi: 10.1152/ajplung.00097.2015

Towers, C. G., and Thorburn, A. (2016). Therapeutic targeting of autophagy. *EBioMed.* 14, 15–23. doi: 10.1016/j.ebiom.2016.10.034

Vasconcellos, L. R., Siqueira, M. S., Moraes, R., Carneiro, L. A., Bozza, M. T., and Travassos, L. H. (2018). Heme Oxygenase-1 and Autophagy Linked for Cytoprotection. *Curr. Pharm. Des.* 24, 2311–2316. doi: 10.2174/1381612824666180727100909

Wang, X., Zhang, Y., Feng, T., Su, G., He, J., Gao, W., et al. (2018). fluid shear stress promotes autophagy in hepatocellular carcinoma cells. *Int. J. Biol. Sci.* 14, 1277–1290. doi: 10.7150/ijbs.27055

Wang, Z., Wann, A. K., Thompson, C. L., Hassen, A., Wang, W., and Knight, M. M. (2016). IFT88 influences chondrocyte actin organization and biomechanics. *Osteoarthri. Cartil.* 24, 544–554. doi: 10.1016/j.joca.2015.10.003

Yang, H., Wen, Y., Zhang, M., Liu, Q., Zhang, H., Zhang, J., et al. (2019). MTORC1 coordinates the autophagy and apoptosis signaling in articular chondrocytes in osteoarthritic temporomandibular joint. *Autophagy* 16, 271–288. doi: 10.1080/15548627.2019.1606647

Ye, D., Liang, W., Dai, L., and Yao, Y. (2018). Moderate fluid shear stress could regulate the cytoskeleton of nucleus pulposus and surrounding inflammatory mediators by activating the FAK-MEK5-ERK5-cFos-AP1 signaling pathway. *Dis. Markers* 2018:9405738. doi: 10.1155/2018/9405738

Zhang, B., Hou, R., Zou, Z., Luo, T., Zhang, Y., Wang, L., et al. (2018). Mechanically induced autophagy is associated with ATP metabolism and cellular viability in osteocytes in vitro. *Redox Biol.* 14, 492–498. doi: 10.1016/j.redox.2017.10.021

Zheng, L., Cao, Y., Ni, S., Qi, H., Ling, Z., Xu, X., et al. (2018). Ciliary parathyroid hormone signaling activates transforming growth factor-beta to maintain intervertebral disc homeostasis during aging. *Bone Res.* 6:21. doi: 10.1038/s41413-018-0022-y

16

# Positive Effect of Gushukang on Type-H Vessel and Bone Formation

**Wantao Li[1†], Xiaoqing Zhou[1†], Tiejian Jiang[1], Hongbo He[2] and Ting Wen[2*]**

[1] Department of Endocrinology, Endocrinology Research Center, Xiangya Hospital of Central South University, Changsha, China, [2] Department of Orthopedic, Xiangya Hospital of Central South University, Changsha, China

***Correspondence:**
*Ting Wen*
*tingwen163@126.com*

*† These authors have contributed equally to this work*

Gushukang (GSK) is a traditional herbal compound used in Chinese medicine for the treatment of osteoporosis. Numerous studies have been conducted to elucidate the effects of GSK, but the mechanisms underlying these effects remain unclear. In the present study, we cultured osteoblasts and osteoclasts with low and high doses of GSK, and also administered 3-month-old mice with 4 and 8 g/kg/day of GSK solution. Gushukang was found to promote osteoblast differentiation and inhibit osteoclast differentiation *in vitro*. *In vivo*, mice in the GSK treatment groups showed an increase in bone mass, as measured by micro-computed tomography (Micro-CT). Tartrate resistant acid phosphatase (TRAP) staining and osteocalcin (OCN) staining experiments revealed decreased bone resorption and increased bone formation in the GSK treatment groups. In addition, we found a novel effect of GSK—it could induce type-H vessel formation in mice. The underlying mechanisms of these actions were further explored at the molecular level to investigate whether these effects were due to an overexpression of the hypoxia inducible factor-1 (HIF-1α). Our findings indicate the utility of GSK as a therapeutic for the prevention of osteoporosis.

**Keywords: Gushukang, bone mass, bone formation, type-H vessel, HIF-1α**

## INTRODUCTION

Primary osteoporosis is a bone disease characterized by decreased bone mass and bone density, resulting from estrogen deficiency and aging (Ng et al., 2015; Wang et al., 2015; Su et al., 2019; Rendina-Ruedy and Rosen, 2020). The risk of fractures is increased in primary osteoporosis, with the potential for serious disability and increased mortality in afflicted patients (Schett and Bozec, 2014; Nevius et al., 2015; Yang et al., 2019). The current treatment for osteoporosis comprises antiresorptive and bone-forming medicines (Cao et al., 2018), including estrogens (Hayashi et al., 2019), parathyroid hormone (Fan et al., 2017), bisphosphonates (Wei et al., 2016), and drugs, which blockade follicular stimulating hormone (Sponton and Kajimura, 2017). Most of these treatments concentrate on a single aspect of the disease, and thorough assessments of their efficacy and safety is still needed (Rauch et al., 2010). Thus, an exploration of new safer and more effective therapies is warranted.

Traditional Chinese herbal medicines have recently gained interest among medical researchers due to their low cost and limited side effects, and this renewed interest includes Gushukang (GSK), a traditional medicine made up of several traditional herbs, including *Herba Epimedii, Rehmannia glutinosa*, and *Rhizoma Drynariae* (Li et al., 2015; Xiao et al., 2020). Gushukang has already been approved for listing in the Chinese Pharmacopeia for the prevention and treatment of osteoporosis.

In clinical experiments, GSK–*Herba Epimedii*, an important GSK-containing formulation, has been reported to demonstrate positive effects on bone health (Indran et al., 2016). In a pharmacological study, GSK was demonstrated to increase bone density and promote the healing of bone fractures (Wang et al., 2007). Additionally, bone loss was prevented in hens fed with GSK, and an improvement in egg production was observed (Zhou et al., 2009), which suggests that the anti-osteoporosis effect of GSK is across species. In recent studies aimed at understanding the specific mechanisms underlying this action, Li et al. (2019) revealed that GSK modulates calcium homeostasis in OVX mice and that it has a favorable effect on bone formation (Li et al., 2019). In another study, this favorable effect was demonstrated to be related to the BMP-2/Smads signaling pathway (Chai et al., 2019). In summary, GSK is beneficial for bone mass development, although details of the underlying mechanisms remain unclear. Here, we reveal a new mechanism of GSK action that may pave the way for future osteoporosis treatments.

## MATERIALS AND METHODS

### Experimental Animals

C57BL mice were purchased from the Experimental Animal Center of Central South University and raised in pathogen-free facilities, under a 12-h light/dark cycle as described previously (Li et al., 2018). The mice were provided with ample plastic bedding and clean water. All the experimental protocols were approved by the Subcommittee on Research and Animal Care (SRAC) of Central South University.

### Tissue Collection

Drugs were administered daily at 9:00–11:00 AM for 3 months as in the study by Kondegowda et al. (2015). Next, 24, 3-month-old mice were randomly divided into three groups: the control group, the low-dose group, and the high-dose GSK treatment group. Gushukang was dissolved in PBS and then administered. Mice in the low-dose group were administered 4 g/kg/day of GSK solution, whereas mice in the high-dose group were administered 8 g/kg/day of GSK solution intragastrically each day (Li et al., 2019). Three months later, the mice were killed by euthanasia. The femurs were collected and dissected free of soft tissue, fixed in 4% paraformaldehyde solution, and maintained in PBS until micro-computed tomography (Micro-CT) analysis, histomorphometry, and immunohistochemistry (Goldberg and Dixit, 2019).

### Osteoclast Differentiation

Bone marrow-derived macrophages (BMMs) were cultured as described by Schmitz et al. (2015). C57BL/6 mice aged 4 weeks were used to obtain BMMs. Cells from the bone marrow cavity were flushed with PBS and centrifuged at 1,000 rpm at 37°C. After centrifugation, the cells were cultured overnight with 100 ng/ml macrophage colony-stimulating factor (MCSF, 416-ML/CF, R&D, Minneapolis, MN, United States). Next, the unattached cells were gathered and further cultured for 48 h until sufficient BMMs were obtained. Gushukang serum was prepared as described previously (Zhao et al., 2019). Bone marrow-derived macrophages were cultured with 100 ng/ml macrophage colony-stimulating factor and 50 ng/ml receptor activator for nuclear factor-κB ligand (RANKL, 462-TR/CF, R&D, Minneapolis, MN, United States). Then, they were treated either with a low dose (20 μl/well) or a high dose (200 μl/well) of GSK serum. The osteoclasts were allowed to differentiate for 8 days, following which the effect of the GSK serum was evaluated by Tartrate resistant acid phosphatase (TRAP) staining. An osteoclast was defined as a positively stained cell with more than three nuclei (Berger et al., 2019).

### Osteoblast Differentiation

Osteoblasts were cultured as described in a previous study (Yu et al., 2019). The femurs were cut into small pieces and treated with 1 mg/ml collagenase solution, containing collagenase type I and collagenase type II at 1:3 ratio (Worthington, Newark, NJ, United States). Then, bone marrow-derived mesenchymal stem cells (BMSCs) were collected and cultured in Dulbecco's Modified Eagle's Medium (Invitrogen, Carlsbad, CA, United States), to which 10% fetal bovine serum (Invitrogen, New Zealand) and 100 U/ml penicillin and streptomycin (Invitrogen) were added. The cells were cultured with 50 μM ascorbic acid, 50 mM β-glycerophosphate, 50 nM dexamethasone (Sigma, St. Louis, MO, United States), and GSK serum (a low dose of 200 μl/well or a high dose of 2 ml/well) for 14 days. Next, the cells were fixed with 4% paraformaldehyde solution and then stained with 1% Alizarin red S (pH 4.2, Sigma-Aldrich, GmbH, Munich, Germany) for 10 min. After washing with PBS three times, four visual fields were randomly selected and from each slide and analyzed. The volume of mineralized bone nodules was quantified by image J software.

### Immunohistochemistry Staining

Immunohistochemical staining was performed as described in previous studies (Albrecht et al., 2011; Chen et al., 2020). Fresh femurs were obtained and fixed in 4% paraformaldehyde solution at 4°C for 24 h, and then they were placed in 10% ethylene diamine tetraacetic acid solution (pH 7.4) and decalcified for 21 days. Next, the bones were embedded in paraffin. Paraffin wax blocks were sliced into longitudinally oriented bone sections with a thickness of 4 μm. Osteocalcin staining was performed to determine the number of osteoblasts and study their surface characteristics. Tartrate resistant acid phosphatase staining was performed to determine the number of osteoclasts and study their surface characteristics. Both the staining kits were purchased from Sigma Company (St. Louis, MO, United States). The distal metaphysic area of each femur was chosen for counting the number of positive-stained cells in four random visual fields from five consecutive sections of each mouse. Then, they were normalized to the number per millimeter in the adjacent bone surface (N $mm^{-1}$).

### Immunofluorescence Staining

Immunofluorescence staining was conducted as described in previous studies (Rached et al., 2010; Yang et al., 2017).

Fresh bone tissues were collected and fixed immediately in 4% paraformaldehyde solution at 4°C for 4 h. Subsequently, the bone tissues were placed in 0.5 M ethylene diamine tetraacetic acid solution (pH 7.4) for decalcification at 4°C for 48 h, followed by dehydration with 20% sucrose and 2% polyvinylpyrrolidone (PVP) solution for 1 day until they descended to the bottom. Next, 8% gelatin (porcine; Sigma, G2500), 20% sucrose, and 2% PVP (Sigma, PVP360) were mixed and dissolved with PBS at 60°C. Finally, the tissues were embedded as described above. Forty-micrometer-thick, longitudinally oriented bone sections were sliced and stained with primary antibodies of mouse CD31 (Abcam, ab28364, 1:100) and endomucin (Santa Cruz, V.7C7, 1:50) overnight at 4°C. Next, the sections were incubated with secondary antibodies (Jackson ImmunoResearch, 415-605-166, 1:500; 315-545-003, 1:500) at 37°C for 1 h, away from light. Polyclonal goat IgG (R&D Systems, AB-108-C) and monoclonal rat IgG2A (R&D Systems, 54447) were used as negative controls. The specimens were observed using a confocal microscope (FLUOVIEW FV300, Olympus).

## Micro-Computed Tomography Analysis

Bone structure was measured by high-resolution micro-CT as described in Mills et al.'s (2016) study. The femurs were scanned at 0.5 mm under the growth plate with a voltage of 70 kV and a current of 154 mA. The following software packages were used for the three-dimensional analysis of bones: image reconstruction software (NRecon v1.6), three-dimensional model visualization software (mCTVol v2.0), and data analysis software (CTAn v1.9). Bone parameters were expressed as trabecular bone volume per tissue volume (Tb. BV/TV), trabecular number (Tb. N), trabecular thickness (Tb. Th), and trabecular separation (Tb. Sp).

## Western Blotting

Protein levels were measured as described in Stier et al.'s (2018) study. The femurs were ground in a mortar after adding liquid nitrogen. The powders obtained from each bone sample were treated with a 500 μl RIPA buffer for 20 min. After centrifugation, protein lysates were obtained, which were then transferred to SDS at a ratio of 4:1 and boiled at 100°C for 10 min. The lysates were separated by 10% SDS-PAGE and blotted onto a PVDF membrane. After being blocked with milk for 60 min, the membrane was treated with primary antibodies against HIF-1α (Cell Signaling Technology, Danvers, MA, United States) overnight at 4°C and then incubated with goat antirabbit immunoglobulin (1:2,000; Santa Cruz Biotechnology) for 1 h at 37°C. Finally the bands were developed using ELC reagents.

## QT-PCR

The femur and tibia were collected from each mice. mRNA levels were determined as described in Walter et al.'s (2014) study. Total RNA was extracted from bone tissues by using the TRIzol reagent (Invitrogen, Carlsbad, CA, United States); this was followed by complementary DNA (cDNA) synthesis using a cDNA Kit (Pharmacia, Piscataway, NJ, United States). QT-PCR was carried out by using a KAPA SYBR FAST qPCR Kit (KAPA Biosystems, Wilmington, MA, United States) and an ABI PRISM® 7900HT System (Applied Biosystems, Foster City, CA, United States). The primer sequence of HIF-1a was shown as follows: forward (5′–3′) TCTGGAAGGTATGTGGCATT, reverse (5′–3′) AGGGTGGGCAGAACATTTAT. mRNA expression was determined by using the $2^{-\Delta\Delta CT}$ method (Ouyang et al., 2018).

## Statistical Analysis

All data are shown as mean ± SD for each group. One-way ANOVA was used for analyzing differences among the three groups (groups of control, low-dose, and high-dose GSK treatment) with PRISM, version 7.0 (GraphPad), as described in Wei et al.'s (2014) study. All experiments were conducted more than three times. Differences were considered to be significant only when $P < 0.05$.

# RESULTS

## GSK Promoted Bone Formation in Mice

Micro-computed tomography is a commonly used method for the measurement of bone mass density (Hirose et al., 2014). We found that the GSK-treated mice had higher values of bone mineral density (BMD) than the control group mice (**Figure 1A**). Moreover, mice treated with a low dose of GSK had a lower BMD than mice treated with a high dose of GSK. Important 3D outcomes of micro-CT analysis including BV/TV, Tb.N, and Tb.Th were higher in the GSK treatment groups than in the control group (**Figure 1B**; $P < 0.05$). Moreover, these values were lower in the low-dose GSK treatment group than in the high-dose GSK group. In contrast, trabecular separation (Tb.Sp) was lower in the GSK treatment groups (**Figure 1B**; $P < 0.05$). These results indicate that GSK treatment had a positive effect on bone formation.

## GSK Increased Osteoblastogenesis *in vivo* and *in vitro*

To determine whether GSK increased bone mass by affecting the process of osteoblastogenesis, we cultured osteoblasts *in vitro*. Alizarin red staining demonstrated that formation of mineralized bone nodules was increased in cells treated with GSK compared to that in the control cells, and that the formation of additional mineralized bone nodules was dose dependent (**Figure 2A**). The optical density of the mineralized bone nodules was quantified as illustrated in **Figure 2B** ($P < 0.05$). The results obtained *in vivo* following GSK treatment are consistent with these *in vitro* results. Immunohistochemistry staining showed that the femurs from GSK-treated mice expressed a higher ratio of osteocalcin (OCN)-positive area surface to bone area than femurs from control mice. Moreover, the high-dose GSK group showed a higher ratio than the low-dose GSK group (**Figures 3A,B**; $P < 0.05$). As OCN is an important osteogenic differentiation biomarker (Li et al., 2009), the results indicate

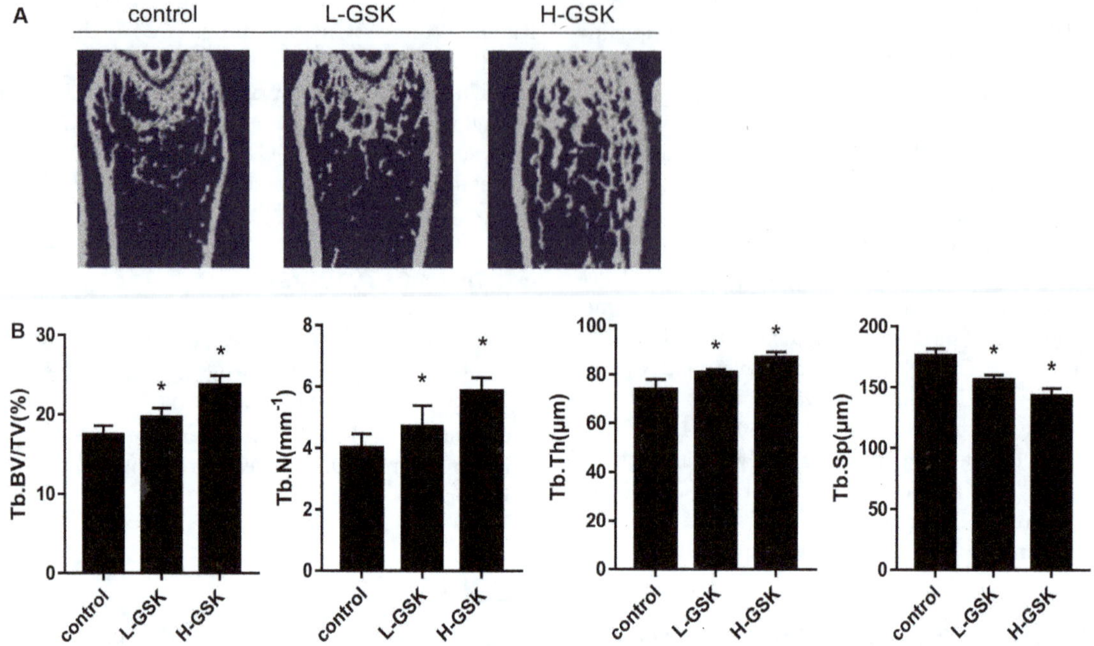


**FIGURE 1 |** GSK prevented bone loss in mice. **(A)** Representative μCT images of femurs collected from mice treated with low-dose (4 g/kg/day) and high-dose (8 g/kg/day) GSK or control. **(B)** Quantitation of Tb.BV/TV (trabecular bone volume per tissue volume); Tb.N (trabecular number); Tb.Th (trabecular thickness); and Tb.Sp (trabecular separation). Values were expressed as mean ± SD.*$P < 0.05$; all the assays were repeated more than three times.

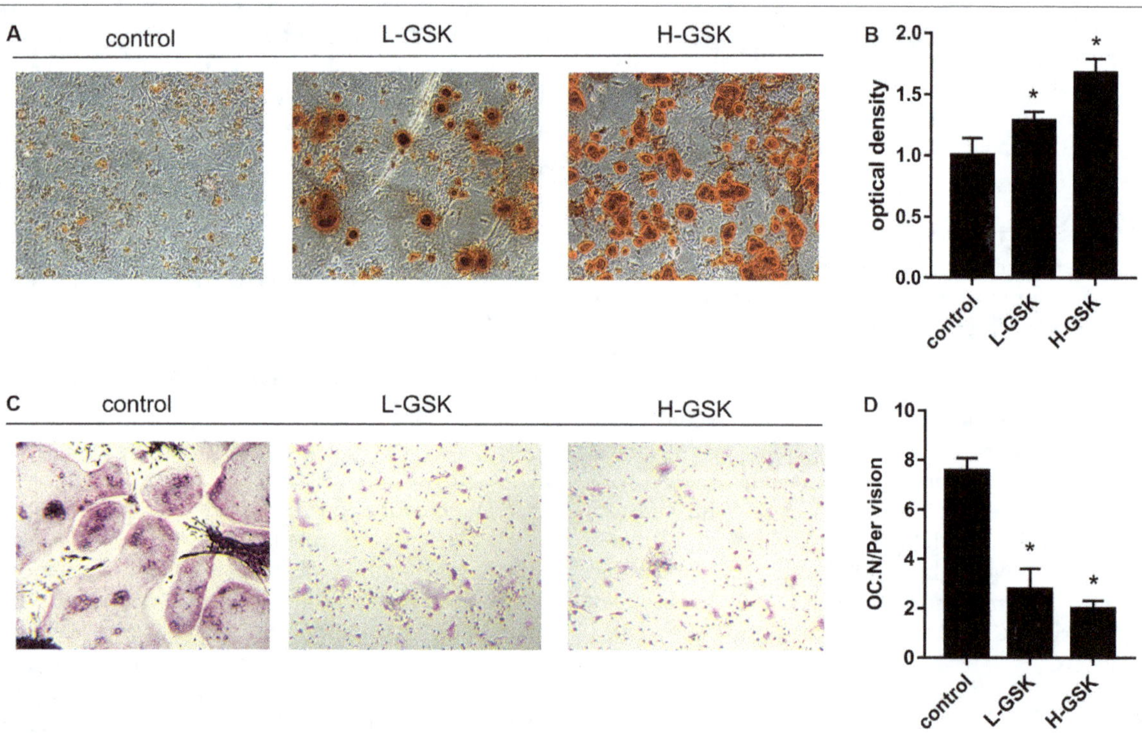


**FIGURE 2 |** GSK increases osteogenic differentiation and decreases osteoclast differentiation *in vitro*. **(A)** BMSCs were gathered from C57BL/6 mice (4 weeks) and cultured with GSK serum. Alizarin red staining was carried out at day 14 to assess osteogenic differentiation. Scale bar = 100 μm. **(B)** The Alizarin red staining optical density was quantified by ImageJ. *$P < 0.05$; the groups of GSK versus control. **(C)** BMMs were obtained from 4 weeks C57BL/6 mice and treated with M-CSF (100 ng/ml) and RANKL (50 ng/ml) (control), M-CSF, and RANKL added GSK serum. Osteoclast differentiation was evaluated at day 8 by TRAP staining. Scale bar = 100 μm. **(D)** The number of osteoclasts was quantified. Values were expressed as mean ± SD. *$P < 0.05$; all the assays were repeated more than three times.

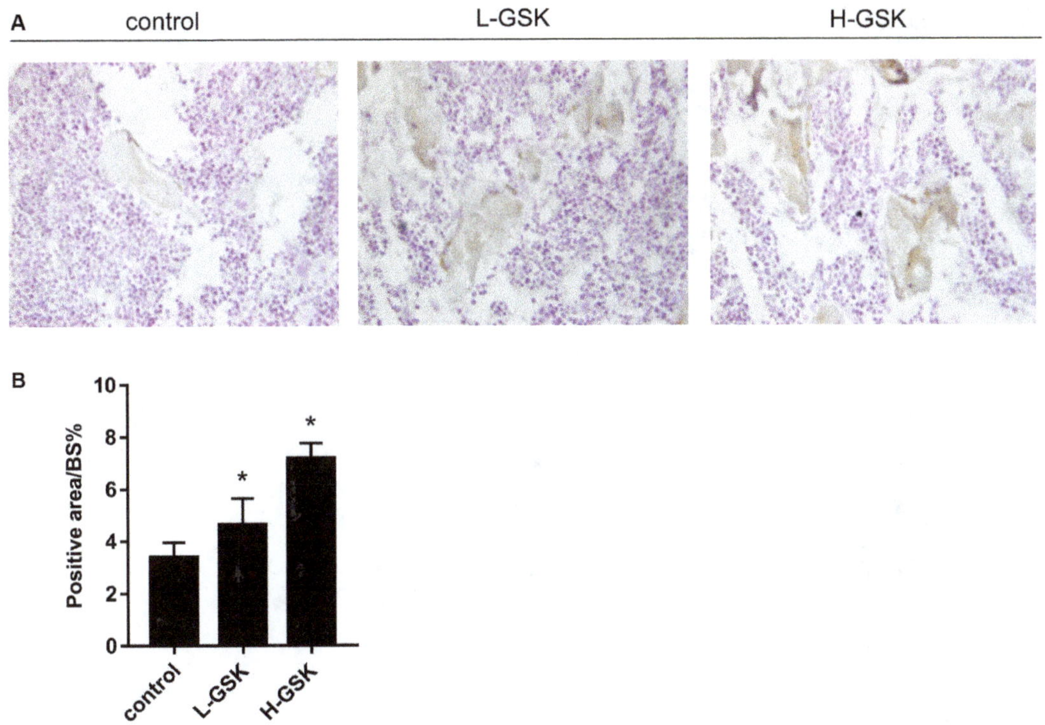


**FIGURE 3 |** GSK promoted the expressions of OCN in mice. **(A,B)** The protein expression of osteocalcin (OCN) of femurs gathered from mice treated with low-dose and high-dose GSK or control (saline) was determined by immunohistological staining. Scale bar = 100 μm. Values were expressed as mean ± SD. $^*P < 0.05$; all the assays were repeated more than three times.

that GSK could increase bone mass partly by inducing osteoblast differentiation.

## GSK Inhibited Osteoclastogenesis *in vivo* and *in vitro*

We next investigated the influence of GSK on the process of osteoclastogenesis. Osteoclasts were induced from BMMs and quantified as shown in **Figure 2D** ($P < 0.05$). We observed that the number of osteoclasts was significantly suppressed in the GSK treatment groups, and that this inhibitory capacity increased with increasing doses of GSK (**Figure 2C**). This observation was subsequently confirmed *in vivo*, since TRAP-positive osteoclasts were significantly decreased in GSK treatment groups, with high-dose GSK treatment groups showing fewer positive cells than the low-dose groups (**Figure 4A**). When the ratio of OCs to%BS and the absolute number of OCs were quantified, the GSK treatment groups showed fewer osteoclasts per area than the control groups (**Figures 4B,C**; $P < 0.05$). Thus, our findings provide evidence that GSK treatment also increases bone mass by inhibiting osteoclastogenesis.

## GSK Accelerated Type-H Vessels Formation in Mice

Type-H vessels are associated with the differentiation of perivascular osteoprogenitors and bone formation (Weber et al., 2015). The type-H vessels are characterized as CD31 positive and endomucin positive (Morrison et al., 2014). The GSK treatment groups had more type-H vessels, as revealed by the number of $CD31^{hi}Emcn^{hi}$ endothelial cells, than the control group, and the formation of type-H vessels was higher in the high-dose GSK treatment group than in the low-dose group (**Figure 5A**). The ratio of type-H vessels to BS% was quantified as shown in **Figure 5B** ($P < 0.05$).

## GSK Promoted the Activation of HIF-1a

The hypoxia inducible factor-1α (HIF-1α) is an important transcription factor that is activated under hypoxic conditions (Dai et al., 2019) and during the process of angiogenesis (Zhang et al., 2010). Hypoxia inducible factor-1α expression levels were increased in the GSK treatment groups, and HIF-1α expression was dependent on the GSK dose (**Figure 6A**; $P < 0.05$). These results suggest that GSK was able to upregulate the expression of HIF-1α protein. Moreover, when qRT-PCR was performed to assess the mRNA expression levels of *HIF-1α*, the GSK treatment groups showed higher levels of *HIF-1α* mRNA expression than the control group, and the high-dose group showed higher mRNA levels than the low-dose group (**Figure 6B**; $P < 0.05$). Thus, our data suggest that GSK can induce *HIF-1α* activation.

# DISCUSSION

Gushukang, a traditional Chinese herbal medicine, has been used for the treatment of osteoporosis for many years, and

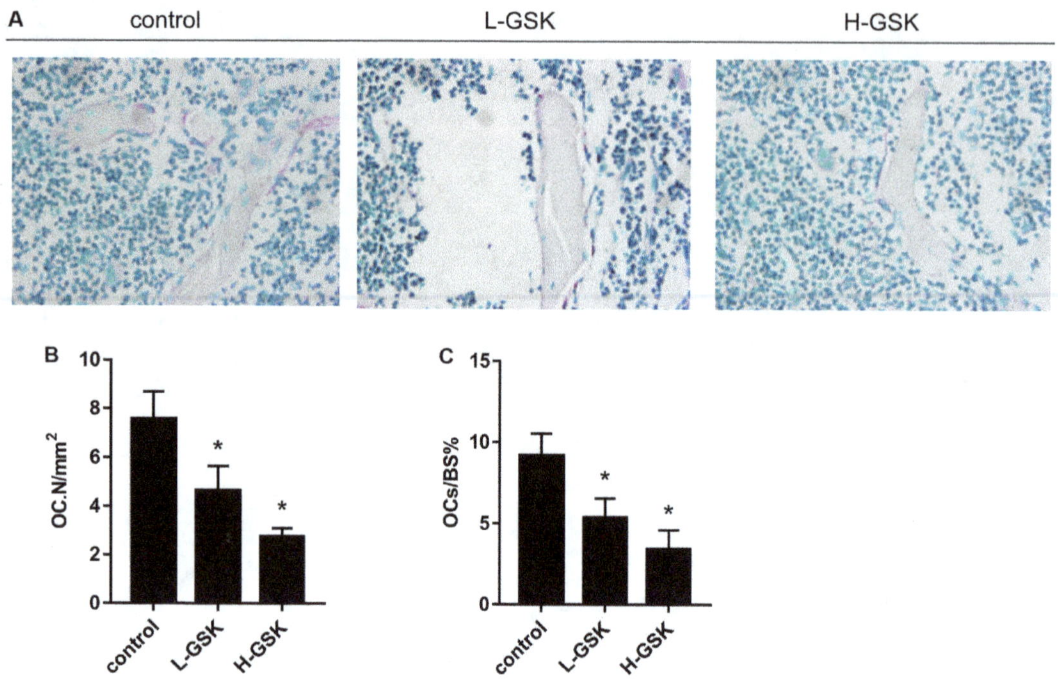


**FIGURE 4 |** GSK decreases the number of osteoclasts in mice. **(A)** TRAP staining was performed on femurs collected from the group of low-dose and high-dose GSK or control (saline). Scale bar = 100 μm. **(B)** Osteoclast-covered surface over bone surface (OCs/BS%) of each group was quantified. **(C)** Osteoclast number (OC.N). Values were expressed as mean ± standard deviation (SD). $^{*}P < 0.05$; all the assays were repeated more than three times.

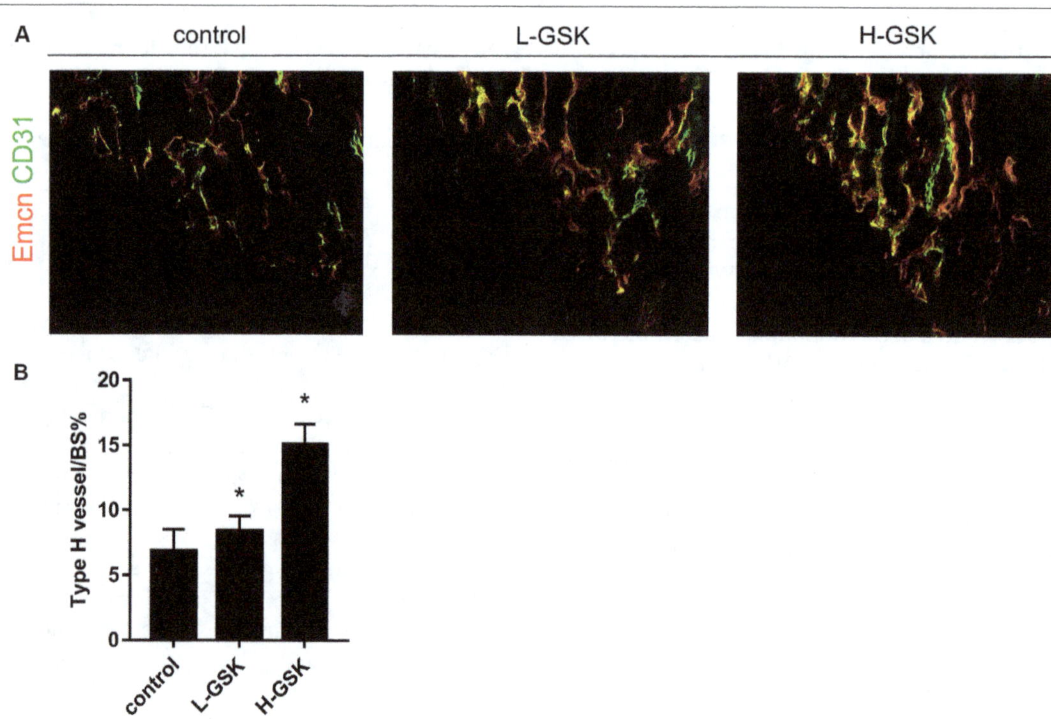


**FIGURE 5 |** GSK accelerated CD31hiEmcnhi vessels formation in mice. **(A)** Representative images of CD31 (green), Emcn (red) of femurs from the group of low-dose and high-dose GSK or control (saline) by immunofluorescence staining. Scale bar = 100 μm. **(B)** Type-H vessel surface was quantified. Values were expressed as mean ± SD. $^{*}P < 0.05$; all the assays were repeated more than three times.

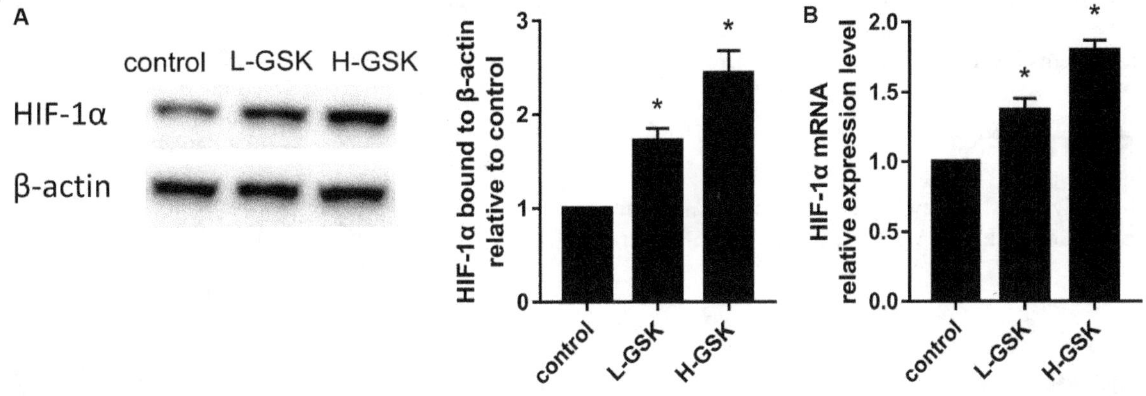


**FIGURE 6 |** GSK induced overexpression of HIF-1a. **(A)** Representative images of WB and quantification of the protein expression level of HIF-1a. **(B)** Quantification of the mRNA expression level of HIF-1a.Values were expressed as mean ± SD. $^{*}P < 0.05$; all the assays were repeated more than three times.

the significant effects of this compound have been certified by clinical practices and approved by patients. Li et al. (2001) selected 197 male and female osteoporosis patients, and GSK was either administered (GSK treatment group) or not administered (control group) to patients randomly assigned to these groups (Li et al., 2001). Six months after GSK treatment, while BMD had decreased in the control group, the BMD decrease was slowed, and BMD even increased in some cases, in the GSK-treated group.

Here, we explored the underlying mechanism of GSK action and found that cells in the GSK treatment group demonstrated enhanced osteoblastogenesis during the period of osteoblast differentiation from BMSCs. In addition, the number of osteoclasts in the GSK treatment groups was lower than in the control groups, suggesting that the osteoclastogenesis ability of BMMs was inhibited by GSK. These results were found to be consistent with previous research (Wang et al., 2018). Thus, we conclude that GSK increases osteoblastogenesis and suppresses osteoclastogenesis *in vitro*.

To further understand the role of GSK *in vivo*, we evaluated bone mass and bone biochemical markers in mice. Using micro-CT, increased cortical and cancellous bone mass in the GSK treatment group could be inferred from the higher BV/TV, Tb.N, and Tb.Th and the lower Tb.Sp values observed in this group than in the control group. These results suggest that bone anabolism is greater than bone catabolism after GSK treatment, confirming that GSK enhances bone density and bone mass. Tartrate-resistant acid phosphatase, produced by osteoclasts, and OCN, secreted by osteoblasts (Booth et al., 2016; Calvier et al., 2017), levels reflect the activity of osteoclasts and osteoblasts as well as the status of bone resorption and bone formation (Long et al., 2014; Yu et al., 2015; Huang et al., 2020). In our study, TRAP and OCN staining results suggest that GSK treatment increased bone mass by activating osteoblasts and suppressing osteoclasts. Thus, bone formation was promoted and bone resorption was inhibited. This result was consistent with the results we obtained in cells, verifying the osteogenesis activity of GSK *in vivo*.

Type-H vessels are a special subtype of vessel in bone characterized by high levels of endomucin and CD31 expression (Diebold et al., 2015). Type-H vessels have recently been shown to possess the ability to induce angiogenesis and bone formation (Peng et al., 2020). Our results show that GSK-treated mice have more $CD31^{hi}Emcn^{hi}$ vessels than control mice, which suggests that GSK may have increased the abundance of type-H vessels. These results are consistent with the notion that angiogenesis and bone formation are coupled. This is the first study to report a role for GSK in angiogenesis and specifically in the formation of type-H vessels. This newfound action of GSK may find additional application in other diseases.

The mechanism underlying the effect of GSK on type-H vessels and coupling with angiogenesis were further investigated. Previous studies have shown that GSK upregulated calcium-binding protein-28k and the vitamin D receptor (Li et al., 2019), and also Osteirx and Runx2 (Wang et al., 2018). In this study, we reveal that HIF-1α, a factor produced under hypoxic conditions (Baik et al., 2019), may also play a regulatory role, with its overexpression contributing to angiogenesis and osteogenesis (Stegen et al., 2016; Hulea et al., 2018). The results of our western blot analyses show that bones from the GSK treatment group expressed higher HIF-1α protein levels and that this increase was dependent on the GSK dose. Similarly, *HIF-1α* mRNA levels measured by qRT-PCR were higher in the GSK treatment group than in the control group. These data suggest that GSK treatment may induce formation of type-H vessels and bone formation by enhancing the expression of *HIF-1α*.

## CONCLUSION

In conclusion, GSK can increase bone mass by promoting bone formation and the formation of the type-H vessels, and by inhibiting bone resorption. These functions may be related to HIF-1α activity. The results of our study may advance new therapeutic treatments for the prevention of osteoporosis.

## ETHICS STATEMENT

The animal study was reviewed and approved by the Subcommittee on Research and Animal Care (SRAC) of Central South University.

## AUTHOR CONTRIBUTIONS

TW designed and guided the experiment. WL and XZ carried out the experiment. TJ analyzed the data. WL and HH wrote the manuscript. All authors contributed to manuscript revision and read and approved the submitted version.

## ACKNOWLEDGMENTS

Gushukang was provided by Liaoningkangchen of China.

## REFERENCES

Albrecht, S. C., Barata, A. G., Grosshans, J., Teleman, A. A., and Dick, T. P. (2011). In vivo mapping of hydrogen peroxide and oxidized glutathione reveals chemical and regional specificity of redox homeostasis. *Cell Metab.* 14, 819–829. doi: 10.1016/j.cmet.2011.10.010

Baik, S. H., Kang, S., Lee, W., Choi, H., Chung, S., Kim, J. I., et al. (2019). A Breakdown in Metabolic reprogramming causes microglia dysfunction in Alzheimers Disease. *Cell Metab.* 30, 493.e6–507.e6. doi: 10.1016/j.cmet.2019.06.005

Berger, J. M., Singh, P., Khrimian, L., Morgan, D. A., Chowdhury, S., Arteaga-Solis, E., et al. (2019). Mediation of the acute stress response by the skeleton. *Cell Metab.* 30, 890.e8–902.e8. doi: 10.1016/j.cmet.2019.08.012

Booth, F. W., Ruegsegger, G. N., and Olver, T. D. (2016). exercise has a bone to pick with skeletal muscle. *Cell Metab.* 23, 961–962. doi: 10.1016/j.cmet.2016.05.016

Calvier, L., Chouvarine, P., Legchenko, E., Hoffmann, N., Geldner, J., Borchert, P., et al. (2017). PPARgamma Links BMP2 and TGFbetal pathways in vascular smooth muscle cells, regulating cell proliferation and glucose metabolism. *Cell Metab.* 25, 1118.e7–1134.e7. doi: 10.1016/j.cmet.2017.03.011

Cao, Q., Chen, X., Wu, X., Liao, R., Huang, P., Tan, Y., et al. (2018). Inhibition of UGT8 suppresses basal-like breast cancer progression by attenuating sulfatide-alphaVbeta5 axis. *J. Exp. Med.* 215, 1679–1692. doi: 10.1084/jem.20172048

Chai, S., Wan, L., Wang, J. L., Huang, J. C., and Huang, H. X. (2019). Gushukang inhibits osteocyte apoptosis and enhances BMP-2/Smads signaling pathway in ovariectomized rats. *Phytomedicine* 64:153063. doi: 10.1016/j.phymed.2019.153063

Chen, H. J., Tas, S. W., and de Winther, M. (2020). Type-I interferons in atherosclerosis. *J. Exp. Med.* 217:e20190459. doi: 10.1084/jem.20190459

Dai, J., Escara-Wilke, J., Keller, J. M., Jung, Y., Taichman, R. S., Pienta, K. J., et al. (2019). Primary prostate cancer educates bone stroma through exosomal pyruvate kinase M2 to promote bone metastasis. *J. Exp. Med.* 216, 2883–2899. doi: 10.1084/jem.20190158

Diebold, I., Hennigs, J. K., Miyagawa, K., Li, C. G., Nickel, N. P., Kaschwich, M., et al. (2015). BMPR2 preserves mitochondrial function and DNA during reoxygenation to promote endothelial cell survival and reverse pulmonary hypertension. *Cell Metab.* 21, 596–608. doi: 10.1016/j.cmet.2015.03.010

Fan, Y., Hanai, J. I., Le, P. T., Bi, R., Maridas, D., DeMambro, V., et al. (2017). Parathyroid hormone directs bone marrow mesenchymal cell fate. *Cell Metab.* 25, 661–672. doi: 10.1016/j.cmet.2017.01.001

Goldberg, E. L., and Dixit, V. D. (2019). Bone marrow: an immunometabolic refuge during energy depletion. *Cell Metab.* 30, 621–623. doi: 10.1016/j.cmet.2019.08.022

Hayashi, M., Nakashima, T., Yoshimura, N., Okamoto, K., Tanaka, S., and Takayanagi, H. (2019). Autoregulation of osteocyte sema3a orchestrates estrogen action and counteracts bone aging. *Cell Metab.* 29, 627.e5–637.e5. doi: 10.1016/j.cmet.2018.12.021

Hirose, J., Masuda, H., Tokuyama, N., Omata, Y., Matsumoto, T., Yasui, T., et al. (2014). Bone resorption is regulated by cell-autonomous negative feedback loop of Stat5-Dusp axis in the osteoclast. *J. Exp. Med.* 211, 153–163. doi: 10.1084/jem.20130538

Huang, Y., Xiao, Y., Liu, Y., Guo, M., Guo, Q., Zhou, F., et al. (2020). MicroRNA-188 regulates aging-associated metabolic phenotype. *Aging Cell* 19:e13077. doi: 10.1111/acel.13077

Hulea, L., Gravel, S. P., Morita, M., Cargnello, M., Uchenunu, O., Im, Y. K., et al. (2018). Translational and HIF-1alpha-dependent metabolic reprogramming underpin metabolic plasticity and responses to kinase inhibitors and biguanides. *Cell Metab.* 28, 817.e8–832.e8. doi: 10.1016/j.cmet.2018.09.001

Indran, I. R., Liang, R. L., Min, T. E., and Yong, E. L. (2016). Preclinical studies and clinical evaluation of compounds from the genus Epimedium for osteoporosis and bone health. *Pharmacol. Ther.* 162, 188–205. doi: 10.1016/j.pharmthera.2016.01.015

Kondegowda, N. G., Fenutria, R., Pollack, I. R., Orthofer, M., Garcia-Ocana, A., Penninger, J. M., et al. (2015). Osteoprotegerin and denosumab stimulate human beta cell proliferation through inhibition of the receptor activator of NF-kappaB ligand pathway. *Cell Metab.* 22, 77–85. doi: 10.1016/j.cmet.2015.05.021

Li, C. J., Cheng, P., Liang, M. K., Chen, Y. S., Lu, Q., Wang, J. Y., et al. (2015). MicroRNA-188 regulates age-related switch between osteoblast and adipocyte differentiation. *J. Clin. Invest.* 125, 1509–1522. doi: 10.1172/JCI77716

Li, C. J., Xiao, Y., Yang, M., Su, T., Sun, X., Guo, Q., et al. (2018). Long noncoding RNA Bmncr regulates mesenchymal stem cell fate during skeletal aging. *J. Clin. Invest.* 128, 5251–5266. doi: 10.1172/JCI99044

Li, H., Xie, H., Liu, W., Hu, R., Huang, B., Tan, Y. F., et al. (2009). A novel microRNA targeting HDAC5 regulates osteoblast differentiation in mice and contributes to primary osteoporosis in humans. *J. Clin. Invest.* 119, 3666–3677. doi: 10.1172/JCI39832

Li, S. Q., Pei, Z. G., and Liu, Y. M. (2001). Clinical study on effect of gushukang granule in preventing and treating primary osteoporosis]. *Zhongguo Zhong Xi Yi Jie He Za Zhi* 21, 265–268.

Li, X. L., Wang, L., Bi, X. L., Chen, B. B., and Zhang, Y. (2019). Gushukang exerts osteopreserve effects by regulating vitamin D and calcium metabolism in ovariectomized mice. *J. Bone Miner. Metab.* 37, 224–234. doi: 10.1007/s00774-018-0924-1

Long, J. Z., Svensson, K. J., Tsai, L., Zeng, X., Roh, H. C., Kong, X., et al. (2014). A smooth muscle-like origin for beige adipocytes. *Cell Metab.* 19, 810–820. doi: 10.1016/j.cmet.2014.03.025

Mills, K. F., Yoshida, S., Stein, L. R., Grozio, A., Kubota, S., Sasaki, Y., et al. (2016). Long-Term administration of nicotinamide mononucleotide mitigates age-associated physiological decline in mice. *Cell Metab.* 24, 795–806. doi: 10.1016/j.cmet.2016.09.013

Morrison, A. R., Yarovinsky, T. O., Young, B. D., Moraes, F., Ross, T. D., Ceneri, N., et al. (2014). Chemokine-coupled beta2 integrin-induced macrophage Rac2-Myosin IIA interaction regulates VEGF-A mRNA stability and arteriogenesis. *J. Exp. Med.* 211, 1957–1968. doi: 10.1084/jem.20132130

Nevius, E., Pinho, F., Dhodapkar, M., Jin, H., Nadrah, K., Horowitz, M. C., et al. (2015). Oxysterols and EBI2 promote osteoclast precursor migration to bone surfaces and regulate bone mass homeostasis. *J. Exp. Med.* 212, 1931–1946. doi: 10.1084/jem.20150088

Ng, K. S., Kuncewicz, T. M., and Karp, J. M. (2015). Beyond hit-and-run: stem cells leave a lasting memory. *Cell Metab.* 22, 541–543. doi: 10.1016/j.cmet.2015.09.019

Ouyang, X., Han, S. N., Zhang, J. Y., Dioletis, E., Nemeth, B. T., Pacher, P., et al. (2018). Digoxin suppresses pyruvate kinase M2-promoted HIF-1alpha transactivation in steatohepatitis. *Cell Metab.* 27, :339.e3–350.e3. doi: 10.1016/j.cmet.2018.04.007

Peng, Y., Wu, S., Li, Y., and Crane, J. L. (2020). Type H blood vessels in bone modeling and remodeling. *Theranostics* 10, 426–436. doi: 10.7150/thno.34126

Rached, M. T., Kode, A., Xu, L., Yoshikawa, Y., Paik, J. H., Depinho, R. A., et al. (2010). FoxO1 is a positive regulator of bone formation by favoring protein synthesis and resistance to oxidative stress in osteoblasts. *Cell Metab.* 11, 147–160. doi: 10.1016/j.cmet.2010.01.001

Rauch, A., Seitz, S., Baschant, U., Schilling, A. F., Illing, A., Stride, B., et al. (2010). Glucocorticoids suppress bone formation by attenuating osteoblast differentiation via the monomeric glucocorticoid receptor. *Cell Metab.* 11, 517–531. doi: 10.1016/j.cmet.2010.05.005

Rendina-Ruedy, E., and Rosen, C. J. (2020). Lipids in the bone marrow: an evolving perspective. *Cell Metab.* 31, 219–231. doi: 10.1016/j.cmet.2019.09.015

Schett, G., and Bozec, A. (2014). Removing the bone brake. *Cell Metab.* 20, 394–395. doi: 10.1016/j.cmet.2014.08.009

Schmitz, F., Roscioni, S., and Lickert, H. (2015). Repurposing an osteoporosis drug for beta cell regeneration in diabetic patients. *Cell Metab.* 22, 58–59. doi: 10.1016/j.cmet.2015.05.024

Sponton, C. H., and Kajimura, S. (2017). Burning fat and building bone by FSH blockade. *Cell Metab.* 26, 285–287. doi: 10.1016/j.cmet.2017.07.018

Stegen, S., van Gastel, N., Eelen, G., Ghesquiere, B., D'Anna, F., Thienpont, B., et al. (2016). HIF-1alpha promotes glutamine-mediated redox homeostasis and glycogen-dependent bioenergetics to support postimplantation bone cell survival. *Cell Metab.* 23, 265–279. doi: 10.1016/j.cmet.2016.01.002

Stier, M. T., Zhang, J., Goleniewska, K., Cephus, J. Y., Rusznak, M., Wu, L., et al. (2018). IL-33 promotes the egress of group 2 innate lymphoid cells from the bone marrow. *J. Exp. Med.* 215, 263–281. doi: 10.1084/jem.20170449

Su, T., Xiao, Y., Xiao, Y., Guo, Q., Li, C., Huang, Y., et al. (2019). Bone Marrow mesenchymal stem cells-derived exosomal MiR-29b-3p regulates aging-associated insulin resistance. *ACS Nano* 13, 2450–2462. doi: 10.1021/acsnano.8b09375

Walter, K. M., Schonenberger, M. J., Trotzmuller, M., Horn, M., Elsasser, H. P., Moser, A. B., et al. (2014). Hif-2alpha promotes degradation of mammalian peroxisomes by selective autophagy. *Cell Metab.* 20, 882–897. doi: 10.1016/j.cmet.2014.09.017

Wang, Q., Zhao, Y., Sha, N., Zhang, Y., Li, C., Zhang, H., et al. (2018). The systemic bone protective effects of Gushukang granules in ovariectomized mice by inhibiting osteoclastogenesis and stimulating osteoblastogenesis. *J. Pharmacol. Sci.* 136, 155–164. doi: 10.1016/j.jphs.2018.01.007

Wang, X., Wei, W., Krzeszinski, J. Y., Wang, Y., and Wan, Y. (2015). A liver-bone endocrine relay by IGFBP1 promotes osteoclastogenesis and mediates fgf21-induced bone resorption. *Cell Metab.* 22, 811–824. doi: 10.1016/j.cmet.2015.09.010

Wang, X. J., Liang, R. X., and Zhao, L. (2007). [Progress of study on prevention and treatment of osteoporosis by compound Gushukang]. *Zhongguo Zhong Xi Yi Jie He Za Zhi* 27, 282–285.

Weber, E. W., Han, F., Tauseef, M., Birnbaumer, L., Mehta, D., and Muller, W. A. (2015). TRPC6 is the endothelial calcium channel that regulates leukocyte transendothelial migration during the inflammatory response. *J. Exp. Med.* 212, 1883–1899. doi: 10.1084/jem.20150353

Wei, W., Motoike, T., Krzeszinski, J. Y., Jin, Z., Xie, X. J., Dechow, P. C., et al. (2014). Orexin regulates bone remodeling via a dominant positive central action and a subordinate negative peripheral action. *Cell Metab.* 19, 927–940. doi: 10.1016/j.cmet.2014.03.016

Wei, W., Schwaid, A. G., Wang, X., Wang, X., Chen, S., Chu, Q., et al. (2016). Ligand activation of ERRalpha by cholesterol mediates statin and bisphosphonate effects. *Cell Metab.* 23, 479–491. doi: 10.1016/j.cmet.2015.12.010

Xiao, Y. Z., Yang, M., Xiao, Y., Guo, Q., Huang, Y., Li, C. J., et al. (2020). Reducing hypothalamic stem cell senescence protects against aging-associated physiological decline. *Cell Metab* 31, 534.e5–548.e5. doi: 10.1016/j.cmet.2020.01.002

Yang, M., Guo, Q., Peng, H., Xiao, Y. Z., Xiao, Y., Huang, Y., et al. (2019). Kruppel-like factor 3 inhibition by mutated lncRNA Reg1cp results in human high bone mass syndrome. *J. Exp. Med.* 216, 1944–1964. doi: 10.1084/jem.20181554

Yang, M., Li, C. J., Sun, X., Guo, Q., Xiao, Y., Su, T., et al. (2017). MiR-497 approximately 195 cluster regulates angiogenesis during coupling with osteogenesis by maintaining endothelial Notch and HIF-1alpha activity. *Nat. Commun.* 8:16003. doi: 10.1038/ncomms16003

Yu, V. W., Saez, B., Cook, C., Lotinun, S., Pardo-Saganta, A., Wang, Y. H., et al. (2015). Specific bone cells produce DLL4 to generate thymus-seeding progenitors from bone marrow. *J. Exp. Med.* 212, 759–774. doi: 10.1084/jem.20141843

Yu, Y., Newman, H., Shen, L., Sharma, D., Hu, G., Mirando, A. J., et al. (2019). Glutamine metabolism regulates proliferation and lineage allocation in skeletal stem cells. *Cell Metab.* 29, 966.e4–978.e4. doi: 10.1016/j.cmet.2019.01.016

Zhang, N., Fu, Z., Linke, S., Chicher, J., Gorman, J. J., Visk, D., et al. (2010). The asparaginyl hydroxylase factor inhibiting HIF-1alpha is an essential regulator of metabolism. *Cell Metab.* 11, 364–378. doi: 10.1016/j.cmet.2010.03.001

Zhao, Y., Wang, Q., Liu, S., Wang, Y., Shu, B., and Zhao, D. (2019). Preparation Of Gushukang (GSK) granules for in vivo and in vitro experiments. *J. Vis. Exp.* 9:e59171. doi: 10.3791/59171

Zhou, Z. L., Deng, Y. F., Tao, Q. S., Hu, Y. F., and Hou, J. F. (2009). Effects of Gushukang, a Chinese herbal medicine, on bone characteristics and osteoporosis in laying hens. *Poult Sci.* 88, 2342–2345. doi: 10.3382/ps.2009-00285

# 17

# Human Umbilical Mesenchymal Stem Cells Display Therapeutic Potential in Rheumatoid Arthritis by Regulating Interactions Between Immunity and Gut Microbiota *via* the Aryl Hydrocarbon Receptor

*Xiaoya Li[1,2,3†], Cheng Lu[4†], Danping Fan[2,3], Xiangchen Lu[2,5], Ya Xia[2,5], Hongyan Zhao[6], Huihui Xu[6], Yongliang Zhu[7], Jingtao Li[8], Honglin Liu[2*] and Cheng Xiao[1,2,3*]*

[1] Department of Emergency, China-Japan Friendship Hospital, Beijing, China, [2] Institute of Clinical Medical Sciences, China-Japan Friendship Hospital, Beijing, China, [3] Graduate School of Peking Union Medical College, Chinese Academy of Medical Sciences/Peking Union Medical College, Beijing, China, [4] Institute of Basic Research in Clinical Medicine, China Academy of Chinese Medical Sciences, Beijing, China, [5] School of Traditional Chinese Medicine, Beijing University of Chinese Medicine, Beijing, China, [6] Beijing Key Laboratory of Research of Chinese Medicine on Prevention and Treatment for Major Diseases, Experimental Research Center, China Academy of Chinese Medical Sciences, Beijing, China, [7] Department of Plant and Microbial Biology, University of California, Berkeley, Berkeley, CA, United States, [8] Department of Gastroenterology, China-Japan Friendship Hospital, Beijing, China

***Correspondence:***
*Cheng Xiao*
*xc2002812@126.com*
*Honglin Liu*
*honglinl2003@163.com*

*† These authors have contributed equally to this work*

**Background:** Rheumatoid arthritis (RA) is an autoimmune disease that may be associated with gut microbiota *via* the aryl hydrocarbon receptor (AhR). Human umbilical mesenchymal stem cells (HUMSCs) have therapeutic potential against RA, but the underlying mechanism has not been fully elucidated. The purpose of this study was to explore the mechanism of action of HUMSCs in rats with collagen-induced arthritis (CIA).

**Method:** HUMSCs ($1 \times 10^6$) were transplanted into each rat with CIA. The tissue localization of HUMSCs and the therapeutic effects in the ankles were assessed. The immune status and expression of immune-related genes and proteins in related lymphoid tissues were subsequently tested. Furthermore, the levels of immune-related factors in serum and the changes in gut microbiota in the ileum were detected, and the levels of indole and their derivatives in plasma and the levels of AhR in the ileum were evaluated.

**Results:** HUMSCs homed to the popliteal lymph node (PLN), mesenteric lymph node (MLN), ankle cartilage, and ileum mucosa in rats with CIA. The transplantation of HUMSCs reduced the pathology scores and the degree of bone damage in the ankles. The immune status of T regulatory cells (Tregs) and T helper (Th)17 cells and the gene expression levels of interleukin (IL)-10, transforming growth factor (TGF)-β*1*, and IL-17A were altered in the PLN, which is the lymph tissue closest to the nidus, and the MLN, which is one of the gut-associated lymphoid tissues (GALTs). The proportion and function of B cells, Tregs, and Th17 cells were regulated in other GALTs, namely,

Peyer's patches and the lamina propria. The gene expression of TGF-β*1* and IL-17A and protein expression of IL-10, TGF-β*1*, IL-17A, IL-22, and immunoglobulin A (IgA) were modulated in the ileum, and the serum levels of IL-10, TGF-β1, IL-17A, IL-1β, and tumor necrosis factor (TNF)-α were regulated in the rats with CIA. The relative abundances of the genera *Bacteroides* and *Bacillus* were increased in the HUMSCs-treated rat with CIA; in addition, the levels of indole, indoleacetic acid, and indole-3-lactic acid were consistently upregulated, and this upregulation was accompanied by increases in AhR gene and protein expression.

**Conclusion:** Our study demonstrates that HUMSCs play a therapeutic role in rats with CIA by regulating the interactions between host immunity and gut microbiota *via* the AhR.

**Keywords: human umbilical mesenchymal stem cells, rheumatoid arthritis, host immunity, gut microbiota, aryl hydrocarbon receptor**

## INTRODUCTION

Rheumatoid arthritis (RA) is a systemic, inflammatory, and autoimmune disease characterized by immune disorders and bone dysmetabolism that ultimately leads to functional disability. RA, one of the most common autoimmune diseases, has an incidence of 0.5%–1% worldwide and is three times more common in women than in men (Smolen et al., 2016). Previous studies have revealed that the complex interplay among genotype, environmental triggers, and chance is involved in the pathogenesis and progression of RA (McInnes and Schett, 2011). In addition, in-depth research in microbiota has gradually revealed that the bidirectional influence between gut microbiota/their metabolites and host immunity might be related to RA, and alterations in the gut microbiota have been found to be involved in improving RA symptoms (Wu X. et al., 2016). RA is correlated with the inflammatory response mediated by $CD4^+$ T helper 1 (Th1) lymphocytes, T helper 17 (Th17) lymphocytes, and an imbalance between Th17 lymphocytes and T regulatory cells (Tregs) (Noack and Miossec, 2014).

Stem cells are cells with multidifferentiation capacity that exert immunomodulatory effects by modulating T and B cell proliferation and differentiation, dendritic cell maturation, and natural killer (NK) cell activity (Naik et al., 2018). In addition to their self-renewal ability, human umbilical mesenchymal stem cells (HUMSCs) exhibit minimal immune rejection and can be used for allogeneic transplantation (Ma et al., 2019). The abovementioned characteristics indicate the potential of using HUMSCs to treat autoimmune diseases (ADs), and this finding has been verified (Uccelli et al., 2008). Specifically, the use of HUMSCs in RA has shown promising results in clinical trials (Shadmanfar et al., 2018; Ghoryani et al., 2019). Basic studies have also suggested that HUMSCs can alleviate collagen-induced arthritis (CIA) partly by regulating Tregs and Th17 cells (Liu et al., 2010; Tong et al., 2015; Ma et al., 2019), but further research on the molecular mechanisms and interconnections between these different mechanisms remains rare.

The aryl hydrocarbon receptor (AhR) is a cytoplasmic receptor that responds to multiple exogenous and endogenous compounds from the diet, host metabolites, and the gut microbiota (Shinde and McGaha, 2018). Tryptophan metabolites are the main ligands of the gut microbiota (Gao et al., 2018). An increasing number of studies have shown that the AhR plays an indispensable role in the regulation of innate and adaptive immunity, including the regulation of the differentiation and function of Tregs and Th17 cells (Rothhammer and Quintana, 2019). Therefore, the AhR plays a key role in connecting immunity to the microenvironment. Although drugs that regulate Tregs and Th17 cells in CIA reportedly function through the AhR and the interaction between the AhR and the gut microbiota affects the disease status, no interaction among the gut microbiota, the AhR, Tregs/Th17 cells, and HUMSCs has been detected.

In this study, we detected the suppressive effect of HUMSCs on the differentiation of osteoclasts (OCs) in CIA. We also demonstrated that HUMSCs can regulate the immune status of the lymph tissue closest to the nidus—the popliteal lymph node (PLN). More importantly, the study showed that the immune status of gut-associated lymphoid tissues (GALTs) and the gut microbiota in the ileum were also altered by HUMSCs. In addition, the possible mechanisms underlying these effects were explored.

## MATERIALS AND METHODS

### Isolation and Culture of Human Umbilical Mesenchymal Stem Cells and Phenotype Identification

This study was approved by the Research Ethics Committee at the China-Japan Friendship Hospital (2019-124-K86). Fresh umbilical cord samples were obtained from the Obstetrics Department at the China-Japan Friendship Hospital after normal spontaneous full-term delivery, and written informed consent was provided by the mother. The umbilical tissue was transferred into Hanks' balanced salt solution (HBSS) (Gibco BRL Life Technologies, Grand Island, NY, United States) to remove aggregation and blood vessels. The remaining tissue was then dissected into cubes approximately 0.5 $cm^3$ in size and incubated with 0.25% trypsin (Gibco) in an incubator for 15 min. The tissue was transferred to culture vessels containing high-glucose Dulbecco's modified Eagle's medium (DMEM; Gibco) with 10% fetal bovine serum (FBS; Gibco) and antibiotics (100 IU/ml penicillin, 100 μg/ml streptomycin; Gibco) at 37°C in 5% $CO_2$ and left undisturbed for 2 to 4 weeks to allow the migration of HUMSCs from the tissues. Once many cells surrounded the tissue, the cells were refed and passaged. After the third passage, the cells were harvested for phenotype identification through staining with antibodies against CD34, CD45, CD11b, CD19, HLA-DR, CD73, CD90, and CD105 (BD Pharmingen, San Diego, CA, United States) and analyzed with a FACS Canto II flow cytometer (FACS Canto II, Becton, Dickinson, Co., Franklin Lakes, NJ, United States). HUMSCs after the third to fifth passages were used for the experiments.

## Induction of Arthritis and Arthritis Assessment

Forty male Sprague-Dawley rats (190 ± 10 g) were purchased from the National Institutes for Food and Drug Control [animal license number: SCXK (Beijing) 2014-0013]. The rats were maintained in a specific pathogen-free animal laboratory with an environment with a constant temperature of 23°C (± 2°C) and an alternating 12-h light/12-h dark cycle at the Experimental Animal Center of the Institute of Clinical Medical Sciences, China-Japan Friendship Hospital [Experiment Animal Center license number: SYXK (Beijing) 2016-0043]. Two to three rats were housed in each cage with free access to standard rodent chow and water. All the experimental procedures were examined and approved by the Institute of Clinical Medical Sciences, China-Japan Friendship Hospital, Beijing, China (No. 180207).

After the rats were subjected to adjustable feeding for 7 days, arthritis was induced as previously described (Zhao et al., 2018). Briefly, the rats were immunized on day 0 with 100 μg of bovine type II collagen (Chondrex, Inc., Redmond, WA, United States) emulsified in isopyknic incomplete Freund's adjuvant (Chondrex) *via* intradermal injection at one side of the base of the tail while avoiding the tail vein and administered booster immunization with the same preparation on day 7 on the other side of the base of the tail. The arthritis severity was examined every 3 days starting on day 1 and expressed through an arthritic index (AI) ranging from 0 to 4 points each hind leg according to conventional criteria (Zhao et al., 2018) as follows: 0 = no change, 1 = red or slight swelling, 2 = mild swelling, 3 = pronounced swelling, 4 = limb deformity and inability.

## Experimental Groups and Treatments

After the onset of arthritis, the CIA model rats with no change in their AI score were excluded, and the remaining rats were randomly divided into the following three groups and started to undergo treatment on day 10: (1) normal control rats (Control group), (2) rats with CIA (CIA group), (3) CIA rats with methotrexate (MTX, Xinyi, Shanghai, China) (MTX group), and (4) CIA rats transplanted with HUMSCs (HUMSCs group). The rats in the HUMSCs group were administered $1 \times 10^6$ HUMSCs suspended in 200 μl of a 0.9% NaCl solution, and the rats belonging to the other groups were administered an equal solution of 0.9% NaCl solution *via* tail vein injection. The rats in MTX group were intragastrically administered MTX (1.5 mg/kg twice a week), and the rats in the control, CIA, and HUMSCs groups were treated with the same volume of pure water as MTX group.

## Immunohistochemistry and Immunofluorescence

The rats were sacrificed on day 38 (after 28 days of treatment). For immunohistochemistry (IHC) assessment, paraffin-embedded sections (5-μm-thick) of the spleen, PLN, mesenteric lymph node (MLN), ileum, and knee joints after decalcification with 10% EDTA-$Na_2$ were heated in a water bath for antigen retrieval using citrate buffer (pH 6.0) or ethylenediaminetetraacetic acid (EDTA; pH 9.0) depending on the primary antibody. The sections were then incubated with 3% hydrogen peroxide ($H_2O_2$) for 15 min away from light. The ileum sections were incubated with the following primary antibodies: rabbit anti-rat interleukin (IL)-10 (Abcam, Cambridge, MA, United States; 1:400), rabbit anti-rat transforming growth factor (TGF)-*β1* (Abcam; 1:100), rabbit anti-rat IL-17A (Absin, Shanghai, China; 1:100), rabbit anti-rat IL-22 (Absin; 1:500), goat anti-rat immunoglobulin A (IgA; Abcam; 1:400), and rabbit anti-rat AhR (Proteintech, Rosemont, IL, United States; 1:200). Sections of the spleen, PLN, MLN, ileum, and knee joints of the HUMSCs group were incubated with primary mouse anti-human nuclear mitotic apparatus (NuMA) (Santa Cruz Biotechnology; 1:200) (a human cell-specific nuclear antigen) in antibody diluent overnight at 4°C and then with horseradish peroxidase (HRP)-linked species-specific antibodies for 20 min. The sections were subsequently stained with 3,3′-diaminobenzidine (DAB) and counterstained with hematoxylin at room temperature. Images were randomly captured using a ZEISS Axio Observer 3 microscope, and Image Pro-Plus was used to determine the positive staining area and the integral optical density of each index, which was calculated with the following formula: mean optical density = integral optical density/positive staining area. The immunofluorescence (IF) experiments involved the use of primary mouse anti-human NuMA antibody and no incubation with secondary antibody. Specifically, in the IF experiments, the samples were incubated with Alexa Fluor 555-conjugated species-specific antibodies (Cell Signaling Technology, Boston, MA, United States) for 1 h at room temperature in the dark and then sealed with mounting medium containing 4′,6-diamidino-2-phenylindole (DAPI; Invitrogen, Carlsbad, CA, United States). Images were captured randomly using a laser scanning confocal microscope (Zeiss, LSM 800).

## Histopathological Evaluation and Tartrate-Resistant Acid Phosphatase Staining of Ankle Bones

The left ankle bones were decalcified and used to prepare 5-μm-thick slices, and the slices were then stained with Hematoxylin-Eosin staining (H&E). The mean inflammation score was assessed microscopically on a scale of 0–3 according to the degree of lymphocyte infiltration, synovial hyperplasia, pannus, cartilage damage, and joint destruction (0 = normal, 1 = weak, 2 = moderate, and 3 = severe). The OCs of the ankle joints were counted by staining slices of the ankle samples with tartrate-resistant acid phosphatase (TRACP; Sigma, St. Louis, MO, United States) and were identified by the presence of multinucleated cells that stained positive for TRACP and contained at least three nuclei.

## Micro-CT Analysis

A Skyscan 1174 micro-CT scanner (Bruker, Belgium) was used to scan the left ankle joints and paws of the rats, and three-dimensional (3D) images were reconstructed with the corresponding software, N-Recon, to obtain the 3D model. The corresponding CT-AN software was then used for 3D analysis to detect the following indices: bone volume (BV), bone surface (BS), and ratio of bone surface to bone volume (BS/BV).

## Flow Cytometry

PLN, MLN, Peyer's patch (PP), and lamina propria lymphocyte (LPL) were evaluated according to the manufacturer's recommended protocol. Briefly, the lymph nodes and PPs of the four groups were isolated, placed in sterile normal saline solution and then ground with a 300-mesh sieve. The cell suspension was centrifuged, suspended in RPMI medium containing 10% FBS and filtered through 70-μm cell sieve. LPL was isolated as previously reported (Xiao et al., 2006), and antibodies against $CD4^+$ and IL-$17^+$ were then used to identify Th17 cells. However, cytoplasmic IL-17 was easily secreted into the extracellular space, and the concentration of IL-17 was low. Therefore, a cell stimulation cocktail with protein transport inhibitors (eBioscience, San Diego, CA, United States) was used for IL-17 stimulation overnight at 37°C prior to antibody staining. Antibodies against $CD4^+$, $CD25^+$, and $Foxp3^+$ were used to stain Tregs, and antibodies against Foxp3 were added to the cells after fixation and permeabilization using a Foxp3/Transcription Factor Staining Buffer Set (eBioscience). B cells were identified as $CD45RA^+$ and $CD3^-$ cells. The Tregs and Th17 cells in the PLN, MLN, and PP and among the LPL and the B cells in the MLN and PP and among the LPL were analyzed using a FACS Canto II flow cytometer.

## Quantitative Real-Time PCR

The mRNA expression of IL-10, TGF-β1, and IL-17A in both the PLN and MLN and the mRNA expression of IL-10, TGF-β1, IL-17A, and AhR in the ileum were evaluated by quantitative real-time PCR (Q-PCR). Total RNA was extracted from the four groups using the TRIzol reagent (Invitrogen) according to the manufacturer's recommended procedure, and gDNA elimination and cDNA synthesis were then performed using a PrimeScript RT Reagent Kit with gDNA Eraser (TaKaRa, Tokyo, Japan). PCR was performed using SYBR Premix Ex Taq (Tli RNaseH Plus) (TaKaRa) with a Quant Studio 5 Real-Time PCR System (Thermo Fisher Scientific, Waltham, MA, United States). Amplification was performed using the following steps: initial denaturation at 95°C for 30 s and 40 cycles of 95°C for 15 s and 60°C for 34 s. All the experiments were performed in duplicate, and the relative mRNA expression levels were determined by the $2^{-\Delta\Delta Ct}$ method. The primers used in this analysis are shown in **Table 1**.

**TABLE 1** | Specific primers used for PCR.

| Gene | Forward primer | Revised primer |
|---|---|---|
| IL-10 | 5′-GATCCAGAGATCTTAGCTA-3′ | 5′-CTGAGGTATCAGAGGTAA-3′ |
| TGF-β1 | 5′-ATCGACATGGAGCTGGTGA-3′ | 5′-TTGGCATGGTAGCCCTTGG-3′ |
| IL-17A | 5′-GGAGAATTCCATCCATGTGC-3′ | 5′-CAGAGTCCAGGGTGAAGTGG-3′ |
| AhR | 5′-CGCGGGCACCATGAGCAG-3′ | 5′-CTGTAACAAGAACTCTCC-3′ |
| β-Actin | 5′-CACCCGCGAGTACAACCTTC-3′ | 5′-CCCATACCCACCATCACACC-3′ |

*IL, interleukin; TGF, transforming growth factor; AhR, aryl hydrocarbon receptor.*

## Quantitation of Serum Cytokines

The quantifications were performed according to the manufacturer's instructions. The serum levels of the inflammatory and immune-related factors IL-10, TGF-β1, IL-17A, IL-1β, and tumor necrosis factor (TNF)-α were determined by Shanghai Laizee Biotech Co., Ltd. (China) using serological Luminex multiplex cytokine analysis technology. A Bio-Plex 200 system (Bio-Rad Laboratories, Hercules, CA, United States) was used to acquire the data.

## Microbiota Analysis by 16S rRNA Gene Sequencing

The ileum intestinal contents were harvested, immediately shock-frozen in liquid nitrogen, and then transferred to −80°C. A QIAamp PowerFecal DNA Kit (Qiagen, Valencia, CA, United States) was used to extract microbial DNA from the digesta according to the manufacturer's instructions. The V3–V4 region of 16S rRNA was amplified by PCR using the 16S rRNA universal primer. The PCR products were purified using a QIAquick Gel Extraction Kit (Qiagen) and quantified with the Nanodrop and Qubit systems, respectively. The purified products underwent PE250 sequencing using HiSeq 2500 according to standard protocols. After quality inspection and sequence splicing, effective sequences were obtained for further analysis. Using the Greengenes database as a reference, sequences with 97% similarity into operational taxonomic units (OTUs) were classified using the usearch61 clustering method in QIIME (v1.9.1) software, and the OTUs were annotated according to reference taxonomy in the Ribosomal Database Project (RDP) database to obtain the taxonomic assignment. The alpha diversity was analyzed using QIIME and R to obtain indices of richness (the Chao1 diversity index) and diversity (the Shannon or Simpson index). The relative abundance was estimated in terms of the phylum, genus, and species. The intestinal microbial community was analyzed *via* partial least square discriminant analysis (PLS-DA). The differences between groups at different levels of taxonomy were obtained by Lefse analyses.

## Detection of Indole and Its Derivatives in Plasma

The levels of indole, indoleacetic acid (IAA), and indole-3-lactic acid (ILA) in the plasma were detected by liquid chromatography-tandem mass spectrometry (LC-MS/MS). A standard stock solution was gradient diluted into working standard solutions with different target concentrations. Subsequently, 80 μl of the plasma samples or working standard solutions was mixed with 240 μl of precipitating agent containing 2 μg/ml 3-methyl-d3-indole. The admixture was vortexed for 5 min and then centrifuged at 13,200 rpm and 4°C for 10 min, and the supernatant was the final solution used in the LC-MS/MS system.

Chromatographic separation was achieved with an Acquity UPLC BEH C8 (1.7 μm, 2.1 mm × 100 mm) column (Waters, Milford, MA, United States) using a mobile phase of (A) 0.01% formic acid and (B) acetonitrile at a flow rate of 0.3 ml/min. The gradient elution program was as follows: 0–2.0 min, 10% B; 3.0–4.0 min, 30% B; 5.0–7.0 min, 100% B; and 7.1–9.0 min, 10% B.

MS detection was performed using an Xevo TQ-S micro spectrometer (Waters) equipped with an electrospray ionization (ESI) source in the multiple reaction monitoring (MRM) mode. The optimized MS parameters were as follows: capillary voltage, 3,000.00 V; desolvation temperature, 550°C; cone gas flow, 10 L/h; desolvation gas flow, 10.00 L/h; and target column temperature, 45°C. TargetLynx (Waters) was used for data acquisition and quantitation.

## Statistical Analysis

The statistical analyses were performed with SPSS statistics 22.0 software. The significance of the differences was determined by unpaired *t*-tests (Mann–Whitney) or one-way analysis of variance (ANOVA) followed by the least significant difference (LSD) test. The non-parametric Kruskal–Wallis and Mann–Whitney *U* tests were used if the data were not normally distributed. Each data point was expressed as the mean ± *SEM* or median [interquartile range (IQR)]. $P < 0.05$ indicated significance.

# RESULTS

## Identification of Human Umbilical Mesenchymal Stem Cells

Cells were successfully isolated and cultured from fresh umbilical cord samples. HUMSCs were identified by harvesting cells at the third passage and analyzing them by flow cytometry. The cells were positive for the expression of CD105, CD90, and CD73 but negative for the expression of HLA-DR, CD11b, CD19, CD34, and CD45 (**Figure 1**). The results showed that the cells obtained from fresh

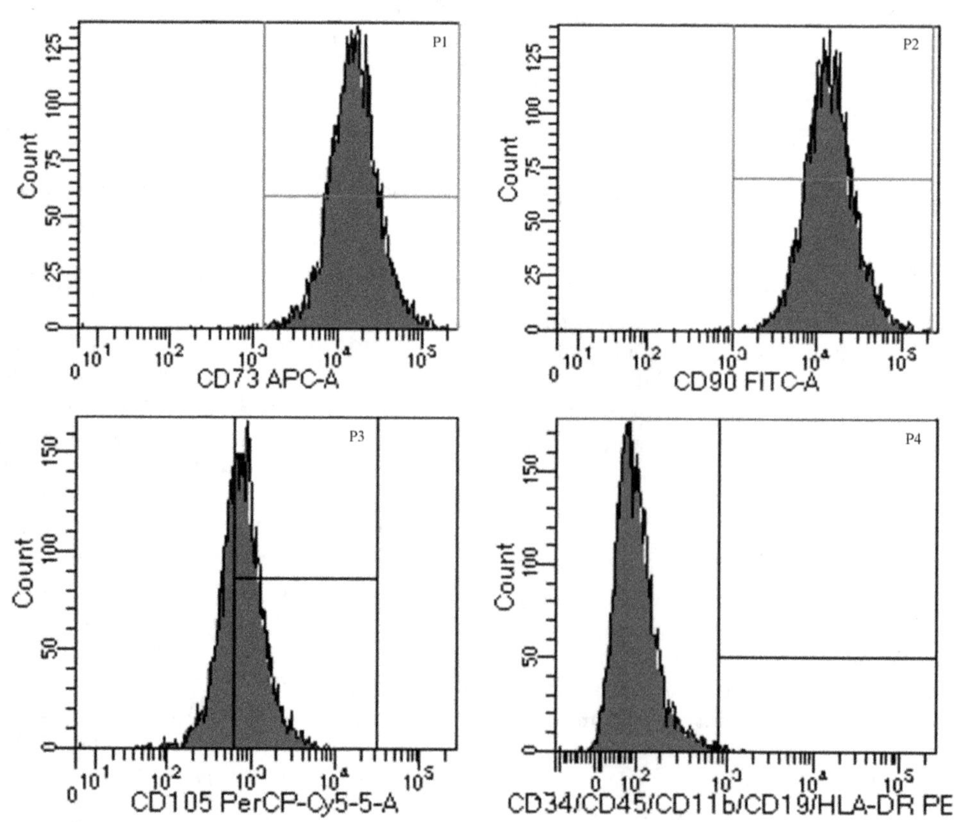


**FIGURE 1 |** Characteristics of human umbilical mesenchymal stem cells (HUMSCs). The cells were labeled with APC, Allophycocyanin; FITC, Fluoresein Isothiocyanate; PerCP-cy5-5, Peridinin-Chlorophyll-Protein Complex-Cyanin 5-5; PE, Phycoerythrin-conjugated anti-HUMSC surface markers and analyzed by flow cytometry.

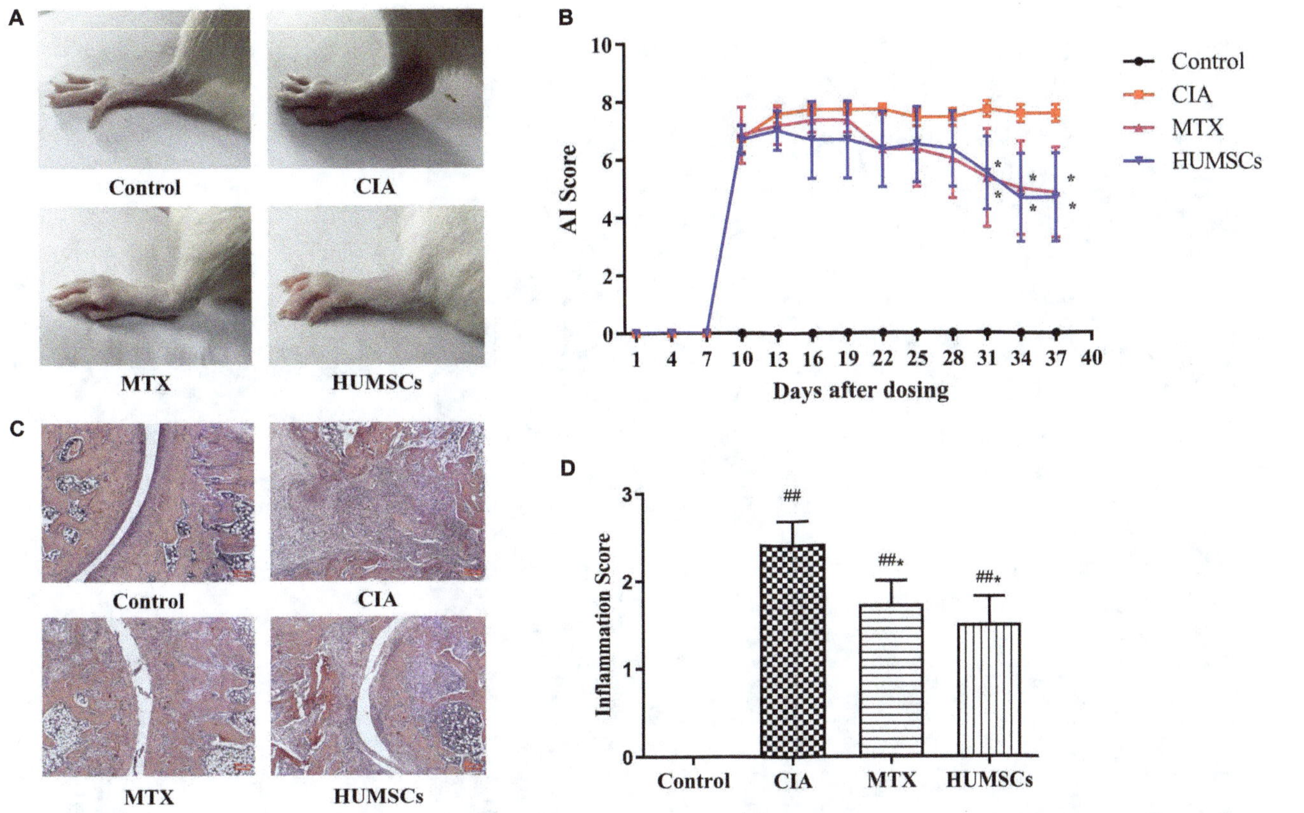


**FIGURE 2 |** Therapeutic effect of human umbilical mesenchymal stem cells (HUMSCs) transplantation on the rat model of collagen-induced arthritis (CIA). The rats were injected with HUMSCs *via* the tail vein ($1 \times 10^6$ cells/rat, only once) or orally administered methotrexate (MTX; 1.5 mg/kg, twice a week) or pure water (both the control and CIA groups) for 28 days beginning on day 10 after primary immunization, and the arthritic index (AI) and inflammation score were then evaluated. **(A)** Representative gross lesions of the ankle joints after model development and treatments. **(B)** The arthritis severity was assessed every 3 days. Line plots show the AI score of all the groups. **(C)** Representative pathological sections of the ankle joints subjected to H&E staining. Scale bar = 200 μm. **(D)** The degree of inflammation in the ankle joints was scored according to lymphocyte infiltration, synovial hyperplasia, pannus, cartilage damage, and joint destruction based on H&E staining $N = 8$. The data are presented as the mean ± *SEM*. $^{##}P < 0.01$ compared with the Control group, $^{*}P < 0.05$ compared with the CIA group. Control group = normal control group, CIA group = model group, MTX treatment group = positive control group, HUMSCs group = HUMSCs transplantation group.

umbilical cord were HUMSCs and could be used for subsequent experiments.

## Effects of Human Umbilical Mesenchymal Stem Cells in Arthritis

On day 38, the CIA group exhibited severe swelling and degeneration of the ankle joints, whereas these effects were alleviated 28 days after HUMSC transplantation (**Figure 2A**). In addition, the AI of the MTX and HUMSCs groups decreased over time compared with the CIA group, and the difference was statistically significant starting at day 31 ($P < 0.05$) (**Figure 2B**). H&E staining and inflammation score revealed severe pathological changes, including lymphocyte infiltration, synovial hyperplasia, cartilage damage, joint destruction, and excessive formation of pannus in the ankles of the rats belonging to the CIA group, and MTX and HUMSC treatment of rats with CIA significantly reduced CIA joint injury and inflammation ($P < 0.05$) (**Figures 2C,D**). These findings illustrated that HUMSCs arrested the development and progression of CIA in rats.

## Human Umbilical Mesenchymal Stem Cells Tissue Localization in Human Umbilical Mesenchymal Stem Cell-Transplanted Rats

To observe the homing of HUMSCs in the CIA rats, NuMA, a human cell-specific nuclear antigen, was used for the detection of HUMSCs in the PLN, MLN, ileum, and knee joints by IF and IHC. As shown in **Figures 3A,B**, extremely small numbers of protein-positive cells were found in all the observed tissues, which demonstrated that HUMSCs homed to the PLN, MLN, ankle cartilage, and ileum mucosa.

## Human Umbilical Mesenchymal Stem Cells Alleviated Bone Erosion and Bone Destruction in Arthritis

The ankle joints were reconstructed in 3D and are shown in **Figure 4A**. CIA caused simultaneous and severe bone erosion of the ankle, digital joints, and metatarsal joints, and treatment with MTX and HUMSCs transplantation significantly decreased

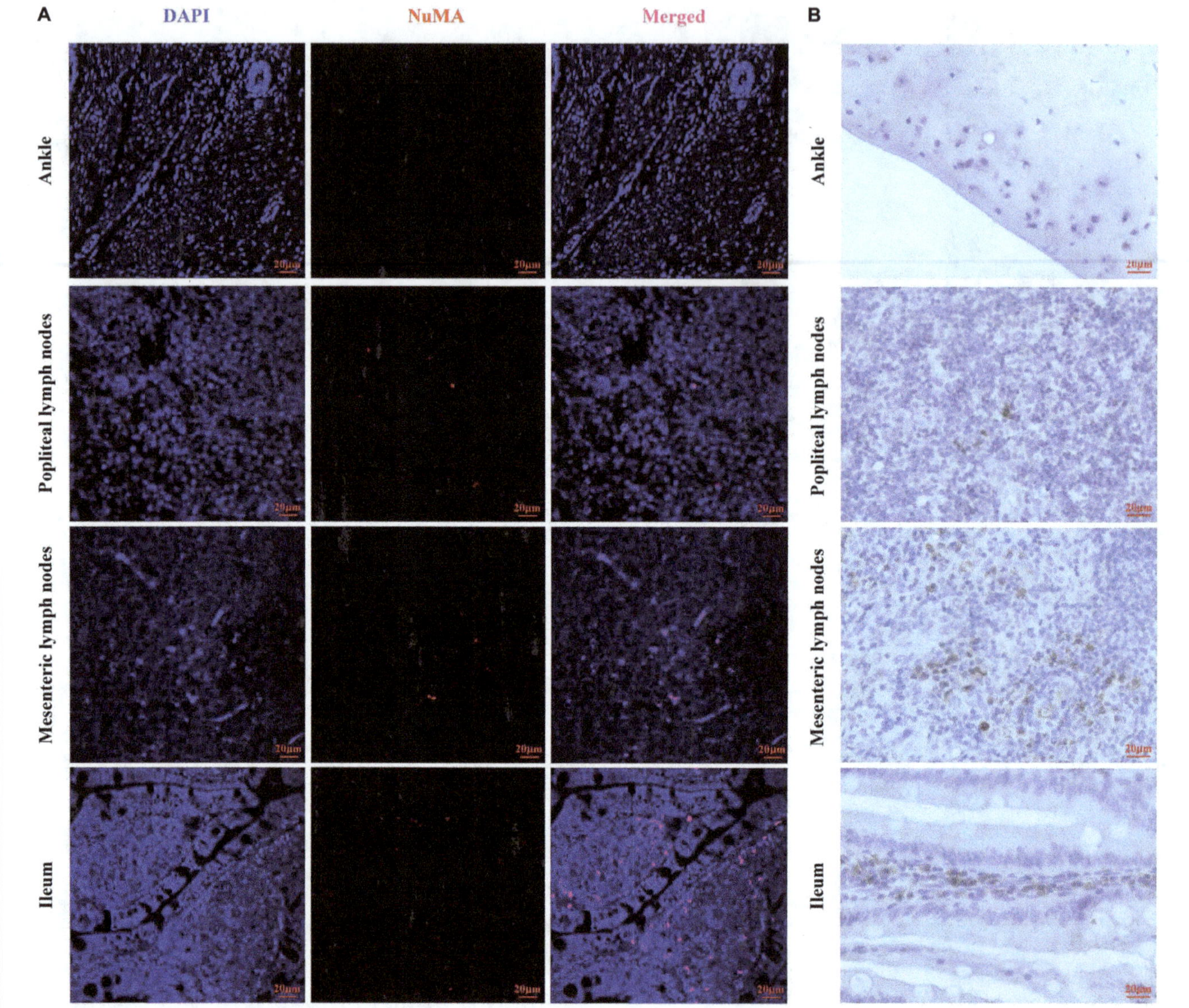


**FIGURE 3 |** Representative images of human umbilical mesenchymal stem cells (HUMSCs) in the different tissues examined. **(A)** Representative immunofluorescence images of NuMA protein expression in the ankle, popliteal lymph node (PLN), mesenteric lymph node (MLN), and ileum. **(B)** Representative immunohistochemical images of NuMA protein expression in the ankle, PLN, MLN, and ileum (magnification, 20×).

the degree of bone erosion in these joints. Furthermore, the BV, BS, and BS/BV were analyzed for the quantitative evaluation of bone destruction (**Figure 4B**). The BV did not differ among the Control, CIA, MTX, and HUMSC groups. In addition, the BS was obviously increased in the CIA compared with the Control group ($P < 0.01$), but MTX and HUMSCs had no effect on the BS. However, HUMSC transplantation significantly reduced the BS/BV ($P < 0.05$). The differentiation and function of OCs play a key role in bone erosion and bone destruction in both CIA and RA (Zhao et al., 2018). To determine whether the bone-protective effect of HUMSCs on joints was related to OC inhibition, TRACP staining was performed, and the ankle OCs were counted (**Figures 4C,D**). As expected, almost no OCs were found in the ankle joints in the Control group, whereas a large number of OCs were observed in the ankle joints of the CIA group. In addition, both MTX treatment and HUMSC transplantation significantly reduced the number of OCs in the ankle joints compared with those found in the CIA group ($P < 0.05$). These results suggested that the HUMSC-mediated improvement in CIA is related to inhibition of the differentiation of OCs to protect bone.

## Human Umbilical Mesenchymal Stem Cells Regulated Immune Status in the Popliteal Lymph Node

The immune status in the PLN was used to represent that of the lesion site as the PLN was the closest immune tissue to

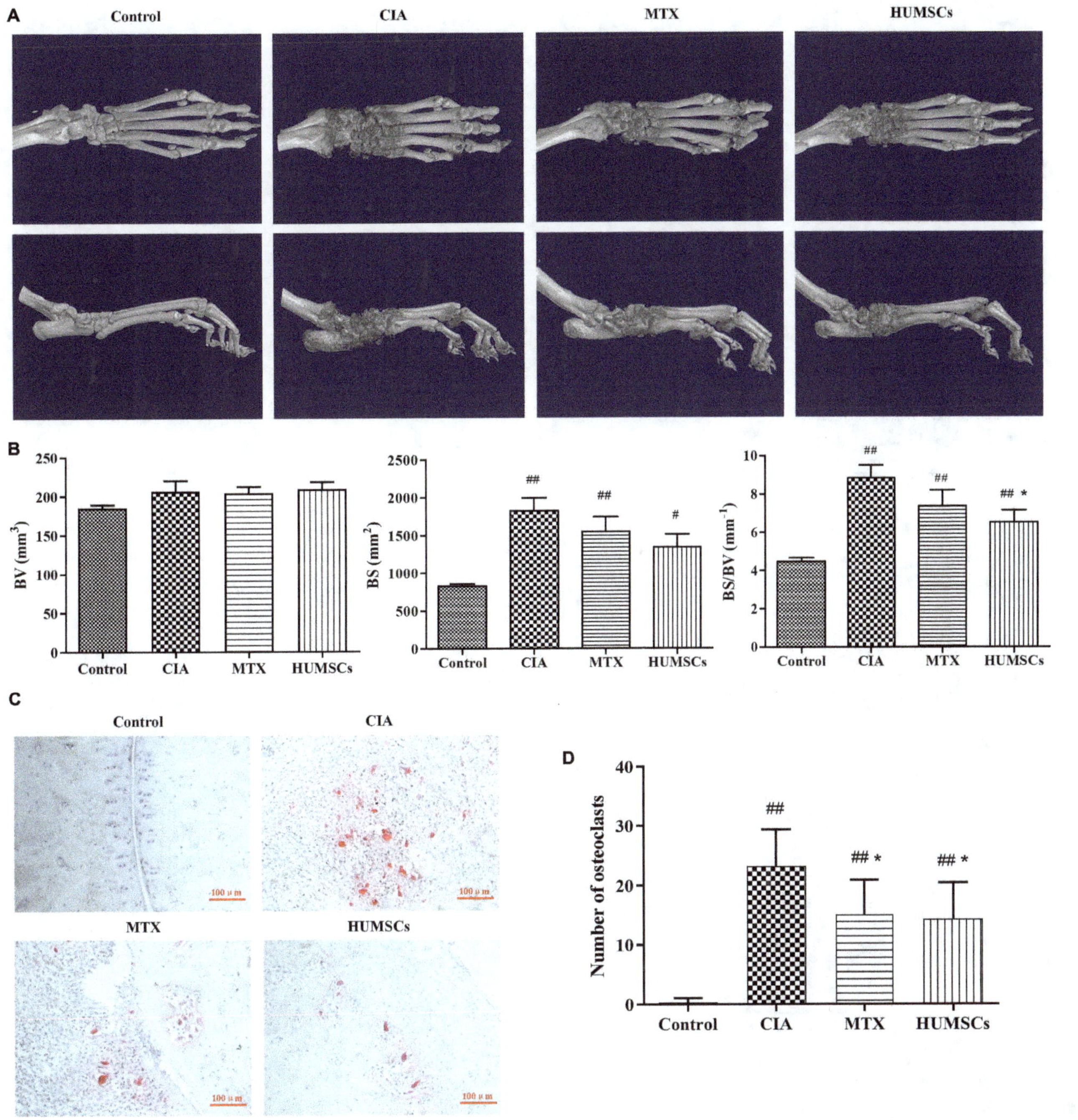


**FIGURE 4 |** Bone-protective effect of human umbilical mesenchymal stem cells (HUMSCs) transplantation in the ankle joints of rats with collagen-induced arthritis (CIA). Three-dimensional images of the left ankle joints and paws were reconstructed and analyzed based on micro-CT scans. The osteoclasts in the ankle joints were detected and counted after tartrate-resistant acid phosphatase (TRACP) staining. **(A)** Representative three-dimensional (3D) images of the ankle joints and paws taken from above and the side. **(B)** Bar plots showing bone volume (BV), bone surface (BS), and ratio of bone surface to bone volume (BS/BV). **(C)** Representative images of ankle joints osteoclasts detected by TRACP staining. **(D)** Bar plots showing the mean numbers of osteoclasts in the ankle joints. The data are presented as the mean ± *SEM N* = 8. $^{\#}P < 0.05$ compared with the Control group, $^{\#\#}P < 0.01$ compared with the Control group, $^{*}P < 0.05$ compared with the CIA group.

the lesion site. The percentages of Tregs and Th17 cells in the PLN were determined *via* flow cytometry (**Figures 5A,B**). The percentage of Tregs in the CIA group was lower than that in the Control group ($P < 0.05$). In contrast, the percentage of Tregs was higher in the HUMSC and MTX groups than in the CIA group ($P < 0.05$). The percentage of Th17 cells was higher in the CIA group than in the Control group ($P < 0.05$), while the percentage of Th17 cells in both the

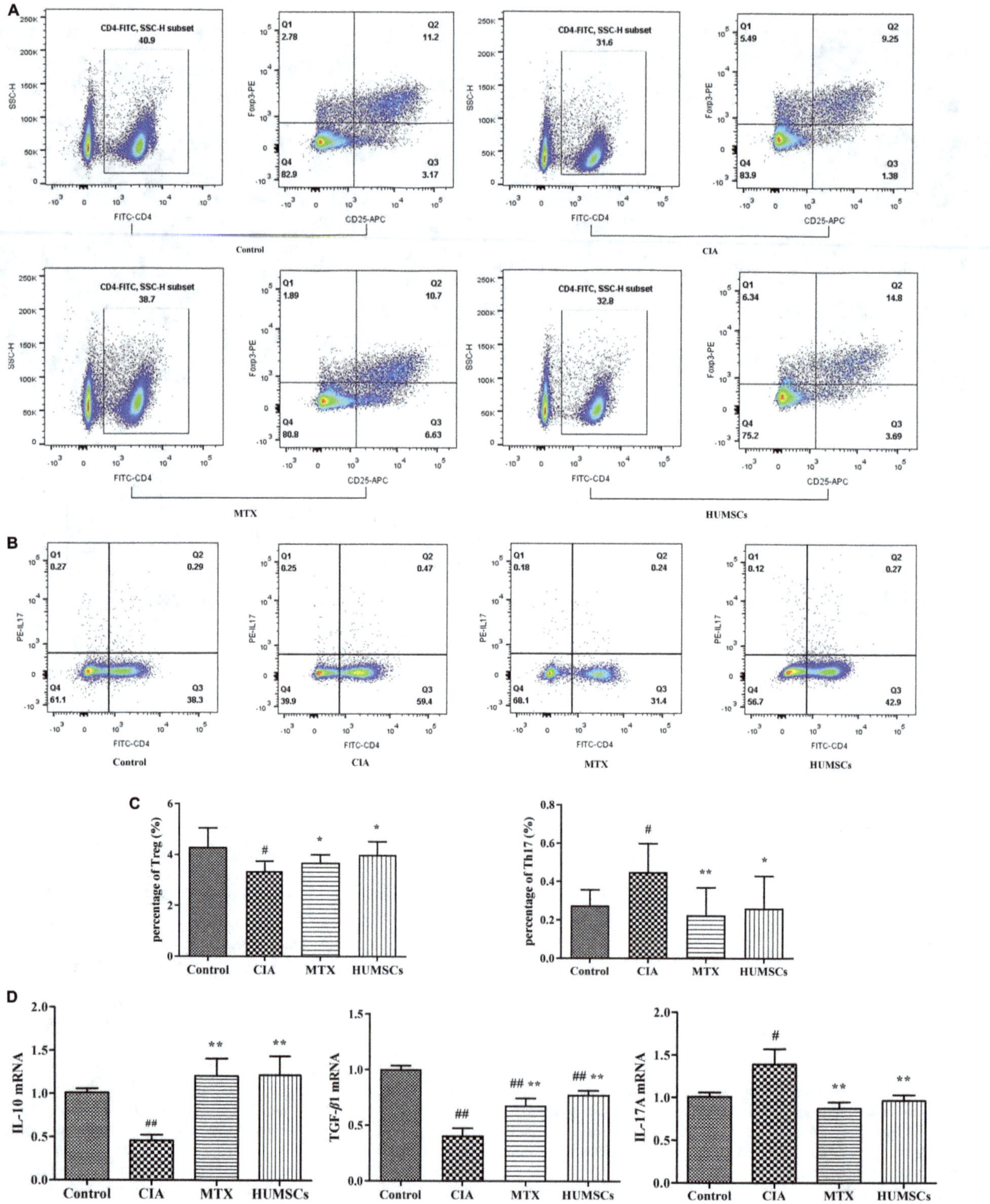


**FIGURE 5 |** Human umbilical mesenchymal stem cells (HUMSCs) transplantation-mediated regulation of the percentage of T regulatory cells (Tregs) and T helper (Th)17 cells and related gene expression in the popliteal lymph node (PLN) of rats with collagen-induced arthritis (CIA). The percentages of Tregs and Th17 cells were detected by flow cytometry, and the RNA expression levels of interleukin (IL)-10, transforming growth factor (TGF)-β1, and IL-17A were determined by quantitative real-time PCR (Q-PCR). **(A,B)** Representative flow cytometry images of Tregs and Th17 cells in the PLN. **(C)** Bar plots showing the percentages of Tregs and Th17 cells. **(D)** Bar plots showing the mean relative RNA expression levels of IL-10, TGF-β1, and IL-17A. The data are presented as the mean ± *SEM N* = 8. $^{\#}P < 0.05$ compared with the Control group, $^{\#\#}P < 0.01$ compared with the Control group, $^{*}P < 0.05$ compared with the CIA group, $^{**}P < 0.01$ compared with the CIA group.

HUMSC and MTX groups was decreased compared to that in the CIA group ($P < 0.01$, $P < 0.05$; **Figure 5C**). Additionally, as shown in **Figure 5D**, the mRNA expression of IL-10, TGF-β1, and IL-17A in the PLN was regulated by HUMSCs and MTX. The levels of both IL-10 and TGF-β1 in the CIA group were lower than those in the Control group, while the level of IL-17A was higher ($P < 0.01$, $P < 0.05$, respectively). HUMSCs and MTX enhanced the mRNA expression of IL-10 and TGF-β1 and reduced the level of IL-17A compared to those in the CIA group ($P < 0.05$). The results indicated that HUMSCs and MTX regulated the immune status and function of Tregs and Th17 cells.

## Human Umbilical Mesenchymal Stem Cells Regulated the Expression of Serum Cytokines

As shown in **Figure 6**, the CIA group exhibited downregulated expression of serum IL-10 and TGF-*β1* and upregulated levels of IL-17A, IL-1β, and TNF-α compared with the Control group ($P < 0.05$, $P < 0.01$, respectively). HUMSC transplantation increased the levels of IL-10 and TGF-*β1* and decreased the levels of IL-17A, IL-1β, and TNF-α compared with those found in the CIA group ($P < 0.05$). MTX also upregulated the expression of IL-10 and TGF-*β1* ($P < 0.05$) and downregulated the expression of IL-17A and IL-1β compared with those in the CIA group ($P < 0.05$). The MTX group also showed decreased TNF-α expression compared with the CIA group, but this difference was not statistically significant. The results showed that HUMSCs can regulate not only the local but also the systemic immune state.

## Human Umbilical Mesenchymal Stem Cells Modulated the Immune Status of Gut-Associated Lymphoid Tissues

To explore the effect of HUMSCs on the MLN and ileum, the percentages of Tregs and Th17 and B cells in the MLN and PP and among LPL were detected by flow cytometry (**Table 2**). CIA increased the percentage of Th17 cells in the MLN ($P < 0.05$). MTX treatment increased the percentage of only Tregs ($P < 0.05$), whereas HUMSC transplantation both increased the percentage of Tregs and decreased the percentage of Th17 cells ($P < 0.05$). Modeling and treatment did not appear to affect B cells. The proportions of the three cell subtypes in PP changed slightly with treatment, and no difference in the proportion of Tregs between the Control and CIA groups. Interestingly, the proportion of Tregs in MTX group was lower than those in the Control and CIA groups ($P < 0.05$), whereas the proportion of Tregs in the HUMSC group was higher than that in the CIA group ($P < 0.05$) and even higher than that in the Control group ($P < 0.01$). The change in the proportion of Th17 cells in PP was similar to that in the MLN, but MTX intervention also reduced the proportion of Th17 cells in PP ($P < 0.05$). Although the proportion of B cells in the MLN was not significantly different, the proportion of B cells in PP decreased after modeling ($P < 0.05$), and the proportions of B cells in the MTX and HUMSC groups increased after treatment and were higher than those in the rats belonging to the Control group ($P < 0.05$). The proportions of Tregs and Th17 cells among LPL were higher than those in the MLN and PP. The assessment of the variations in Tregs among LPL between the groups revealed a trend similar to that found in the MLN, whereas the variations

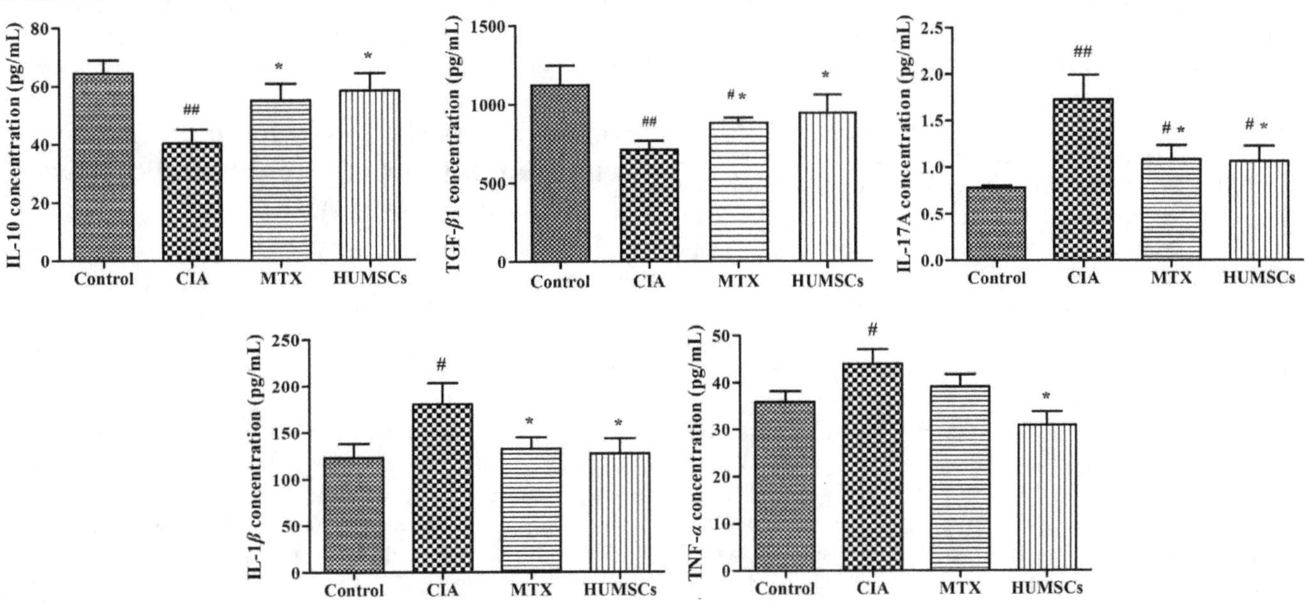


**FIGURE 6 |** Human umbilical mesenchymal stem cells (HUMSCs) transplantation-mediated regulation of cytokines in the collagen-induced arthritis (CIA) rats. The serum cytokine levels were measured by Luminex assays. Bar plots showing the mean levels of interleukin (IL)-10, transforming growth factor (TGF)-β1, IL-17A, IL-1β, and tumor necrosis factor (TNF)-α in all the groups $N = 8$. The data are presented as the mean ± *SEM*. $^{\#}P < 0.05$ compared with the Control group, $^{\#\#}P < 0.01$ compared with the Control group, $^{*}P < 0.05$ compared with the CIA group.

**TABLE 2 |** Percentages of Tregs, Th17, and B cells in gut-associated lymphoid tissues ($N$ = 8).

| Tissues | Group | Cell type | | |
|---|---|---|---|---|
| | | Tregs (%) | Th17 cells (%) | B cells (%) |
| Mesenteric lymph node | Control | 6.07 ± 2.21 | 0.20 ± 0.12 | 31.50 ± 3.34 |
| | CIA | 5.41 ± 1.31 | 0.34 ± 0.05# | 32.82 ± 4.18 |
| | MTX | 7.06 ± 0.80* | 0.32 ± 0.08 | 34.34 ± 3.73 |
| | HUMSCs | 7.27 ± 0.73* | 0.24 ± 0.05* | 35.20 ± 5.43 |
| Peyer's patch | Control | 10.77 ± 1.62 | 0.67 ± 0.39 | 44.80 ± 5.74 |
| | CIA | 10.86 ± 1.79 | 1.17 ± 0.90# | 30.23 ± 4.81# |
| | MTX | 8.29 ± 1.90#* | 0.46 ± 0.27* | 55.06 ± 4.63#** |
| | HUMSCs | 14.81 ± 3.09##* | 0.48 ± 0.18* | 54.12 ± 6.82#** |
| Lamina propria lymphocyte | Control | 27.98 ± 2.89 | 2.57 ± 1.46 | 37.37 ± 2.96 |
| | CIA | 21.03 ± 5.41# | 8.30 ± 2.02# | 31.92 ± 3.85# |
| | MTX | 31.08 ± 9.66* | 3.46 ± 0.89** | 46.26 ± 11.39* |
| | HUMSCs | 28.75 ± 4.15* | 3.04 ± 1.42** | 49.00 ± 15.89* |

*The data are presented as the mean ± SEM. #P < 0.05 compared with the Control group, ##P < 0.01 compared with the Control group, *P < 0.05 compared with the CIA group, **P < 0.01 compared with the CIA group. Tregs, T regulatory cells; Th17, T helper 17; CIA, collagen-induced arthritis; MTX, methotrexate; HUMSCs, human umbilical mesenchymal stem cells.*

in Th17 cells and B cells followed a trend similar to those found for Th17 cells and B cells in PP, respectively, with the only difference being that the proportion of B cells after treatment was between the proportions of B cells in the Control and CIA groups. The above-described results suggested that HUMSC therapy exerts extensive immunomodulatory effects on GALTs. The most affected tissues were those closest to the intestinal contents, and these effects might be induced by metabolites or antigens related to the gut microbiota.

Furthermore, various gene and protein expression levels were detected by Q-PCR and IHC, respectively (**Figure 7**). Modeling significantly decreased the IL-10 levels in the MLN and the TGF-β1 levels in the MLN and ileum ($P$ < 0.05), and treatment with MTX and HUMSC transplantation increased the expression of IL-10 and TGF-β1 to levels that were higher than that those found in the Control group ($P$ < 0.05 and $P$ < 0.01, respectively) (**Figures 7A,B**). The expression levels of IL-17A in the MLN and ileum were similar. The IL-17A gene expression levels were highest in the CIA group and decreased following intervention with MTX and HUMSCs ($P$ < 0.05 and $P$ < 0.01, respectively), and the lowest IL-17A gene level was found in the MTX group (**Figures 7A,B**). The *in situ* protein expression levels were similar to the corresponding gene expression levels (**Figures 7C,D**). Downregulated IL-10 and TGF-β1 expression and upregulated IL-17A expression were detected in the ileum of rats with CIA, and as expected, both MTX treatment and HUMSC transplantation increased the levels of IL-10 and TGF-β1 and decreased the expression of IL-17A ($P$ < 0.05 and $P$ < 0.01, respectively). The above-described results indicated that the levels of the major cytokines of Tregs and Th17 cells were abnormal in the MLN and ileum of rats with CIA and that MTX and HUMSCs effectively reversed Tregs and Th17 cell dysfunction. These results suggested that HUMSCs regulate the proportions and functions of Tregs and Th17 and B cells in GALTs.

We also tested the expression of IL-22 and IgA because IL-22 plays an important role in resisting pathogens and repairing the intestinal barrier by inducing intestinal epithelial cells (IECs) to produce antimicrobial peptides, and secretory IgA (SIgA) is known to regulate intestinal microorganisms. The IL-22 and IgA levels in the CIA group were significantly lower than those in the Control group ($P$ < 0.01), which suggested that CIA modeling affects the mucosal immune barrier in the ileum to a certain extent and decreased the clearance of pathogenic microorganisms. MTX treatment and HUMSC transplantation affected the IL-22 and IgA levels ($P$ < 0.05, $P$ < 0.01, respectively) (**Figures 7C,D**), which suggested that both treatments can reshape the immune barrier and restore the regulatory effect of the intestinal tract on intestinal bacteria.

## Human Umbilical Mesenchymal Stem Cells Regulated the Intestinal Microbial Community in Rats With Collagen-Induced Arthritis

The intestinal microbial diversity of the ileum was measured by determining the OTUs and the Chao1 and Shannon diversity indices (**Figures 8A–C**). The OTUs and Chao1 diversity indices in the CIA group were higher than those in the Control group ($P$ < 0.05), and both of these measures were lower in the MTX and HUMSCs groups compared with the Control and CIA groups ($P$ < 0.01). The analysis of the Shannon diversity index revealed no significant difference among the four groups. The results shown in **Figures 8A–C** indicated that CIA modeling and both treatments changed the rats' intestinal microbial species and the community richness but had no effect on the community diversity.

The similarity between the intestinal microbial communities was analyzed by PLS-DA. As shown in **Figure 8D**, the bacterial structures of the Control, CIA, MTX, and HUMSC groups were distributed in a counterclockwise direction. With the exception

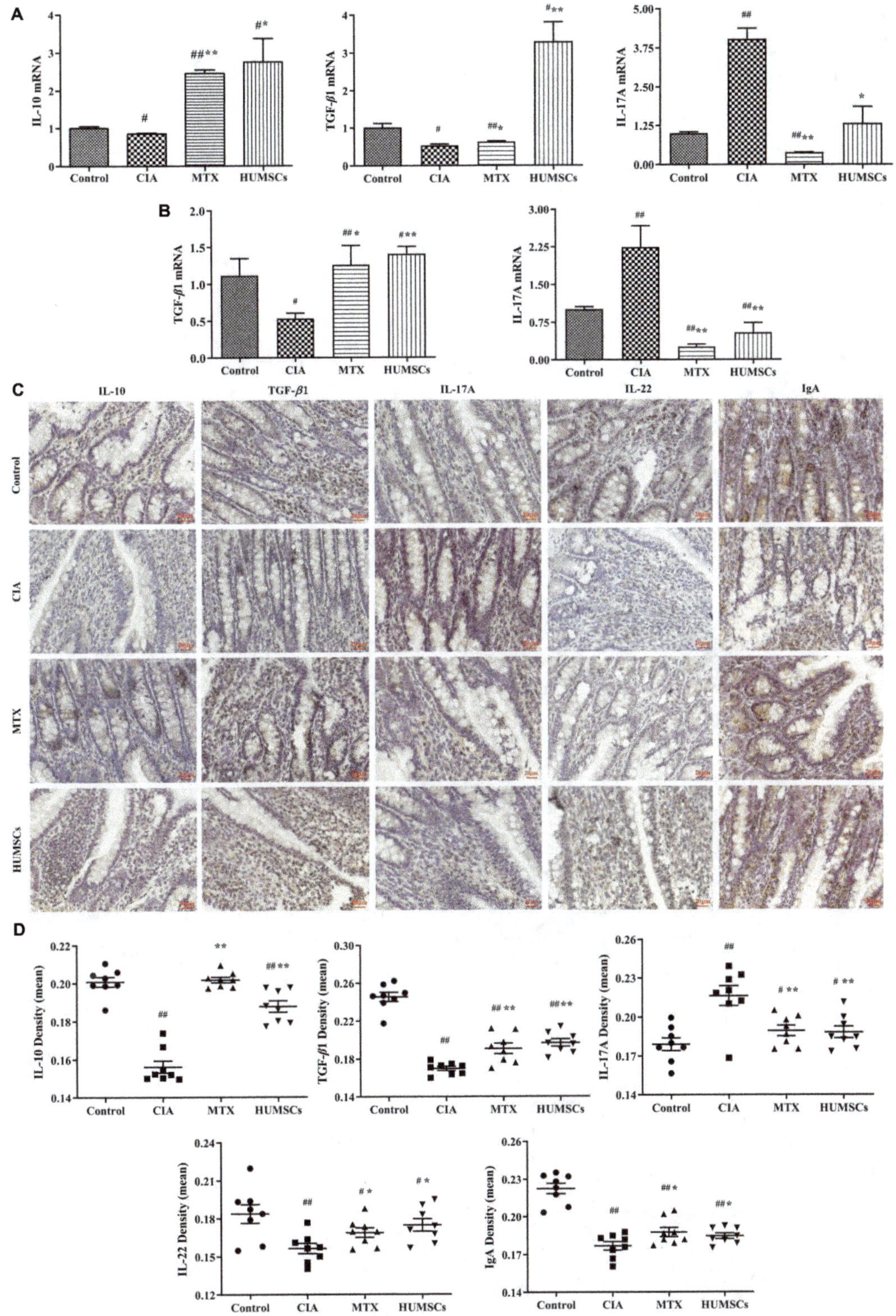


**FIGURE 7 |** Human umbilical mesenchymal stem cells (HUMSCs) modulate the immune status of the mesenteric lymph node (MLN) and ileum. The interleukin (IL)-10, IL-17A, and transforming growth factor (TGF)-β*1* mRNA expression levels in the MLN and the IL-17A and TGF-β*1* mRNA expression levels in the ileum were detected by quantitative real-time PCR (Q-PCR). The protein expression of IL-10, IL-17A, TGF-β*1*, IL-22, and immunoglobulin A (IgA) was determined by immunohistochemistry (IHC) assay. **(A)** Gene expression of IL-10, IL-17A, and TGF-β*1* in the MLN. **(B)** Gene expression of IL-17A and TGF-β*1* in the ileum. **(C)** Representative images of the ileum obtained by IHC (20×). **(D)** Protein expression of IL-10, IL-17A, TGF-β*1*, IL-22, and IgA in the ileum $N = 8$. The data are presented as the mean ± *SEM*. $^{\#}P < 0.05$ compared with the Control group, $^{\#\#}P < 0.01$ compared with the Control group, $^{*}P < 0.05$ compared with the CIA group, $^{**}P < 0.01$ compared with the CIA group.

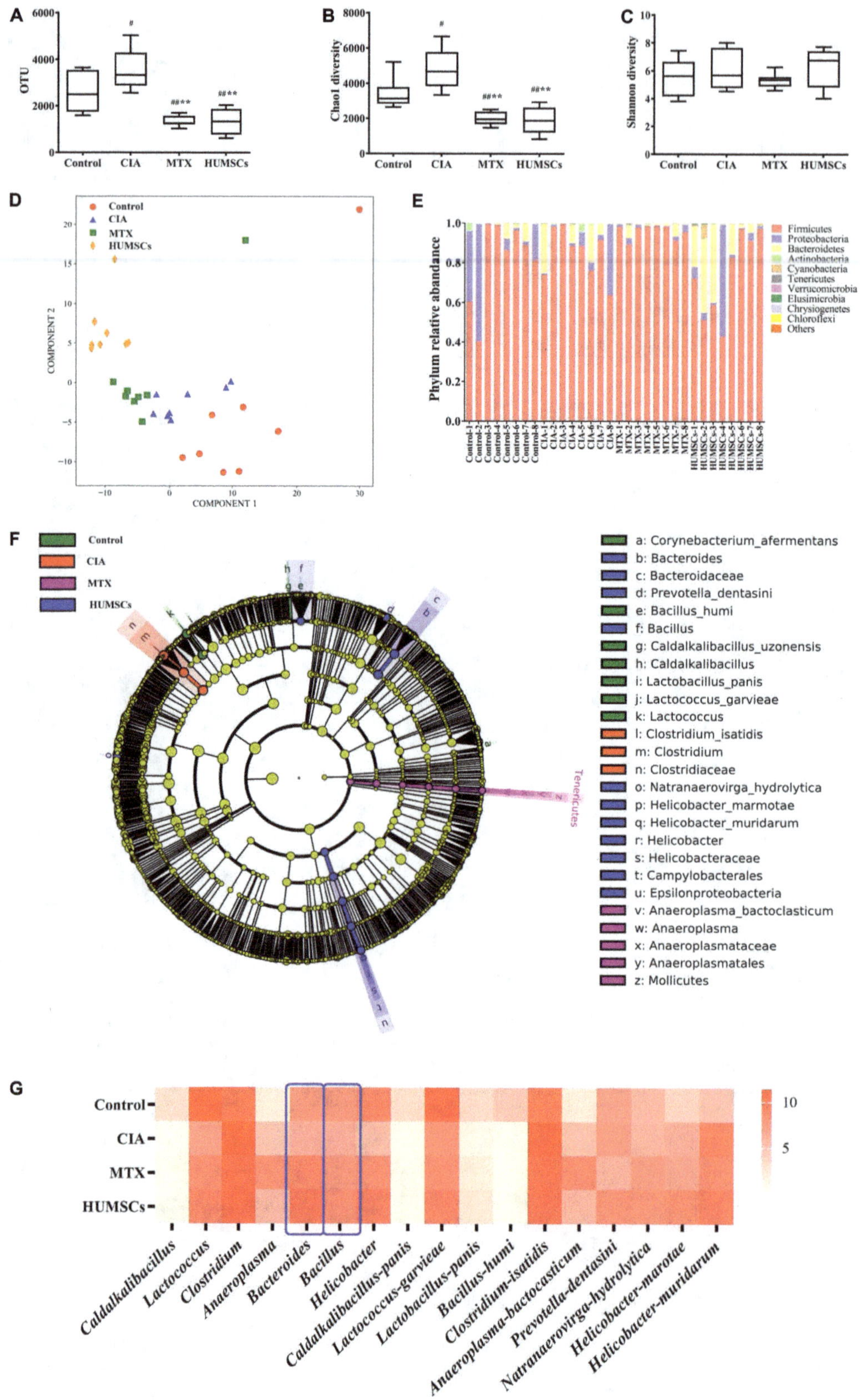


**FIGURE 8 |** Changes in the gut microbiota in collagen-induced arthritis (CIA), methotrexate (MTX), and human umbilical mesenchymal stem cells (HUMSCs) groups. The alpha diversity, beta diversity, and the typical bacterial genera and species were obtained by 16S sequencing. **(A–C)** Bar plots showing the mean Chao1 and

*(Continued)*

**FIGURE 8 |** Continued
Shannon diversity indices and the operational taxonomic units (OTUs) of all groups. **(D)** Relative abundance of the top 10 most abundant phyla in each sample. **(E)** The differences in the intestinal microbial communities among the groups were assessed by partial least square discriminant analysis (PLS-DA). **(F)** Taxonomical differences among the groups at the different levels. The dominant bacteria were determined by Lefse analyses. **(G)** Relative abundances among the groups at the genus and species levels $N = 8$. The data in panels **(A–C)** are presented as the medians [interquartile range (IQR)]. $^{\#}P < 0.05$ compared with the Control group, $^{\#\#}P < 0.01$ compared with the Control group, $^{*}P < 0.05$ compared with the CIA group, $^{**}P < 0.01$ compared with the CIA group.

of a few outliers, the microflora structures in each group were relatively similar, and the difference between the HUMSC rats and normal rats, between the HUMSC rats and CIA rats were the obvious, but the microbial communities of the CIA group were very similar to those of the MTX group. The results indicated that the therapeutic effect of MTX on CIA might only be slightly related to the gut microbiota, whereas the effect of HUMSCs might be largely mediated by the gut microbiota.

An overview of the gut microbiota in the four groups at the phylum level is shown in **Figure 8E**. Overall, the bacteria with the highest abundance belonged to the phylum *Firmicutes*, followed by the phyla *Proteobacteria* and *Bacteroidetes*. The abundances of the phyla *Proteobacteria* and *Bacteroidetes* among the rats varied considerably. The phyla *Chrysiogenetes* and *Chloroflexi* disappeared after treatment with MTX and HUMSCs.

The intestinal microbial species in the different groups were compared by Lefse analysis to characterize the changes in the intestinal microflora structure (**Figure 8F**). The relative abundances of two genera (*Caldalkalibacillus* and *Lactococcus*) and five species (*Caldalkalibacillus panis, Lactococcus garvieae, Lactobacillus panis, Bacillus humi,* and *Corynebacterium afermentans*) were highest in the control group. The dominant bacteria in the CIA group were relatively unitary: family *Clostridiaceae,* genus *Clostridium,* and species *Clostridium isatidis.* After MTX intervention, the relative abundance of one unit was higher than that of the other three groups from the phylum to the species level: phylum *Tenericutes*, class *Mollicutes*, order *Anaeroplasmatales*, family *Anaeroplasmataceae*, genus *Anaeroplasma*, and species *Anaeroplasma bactocasticum.* HUMSC therapy changed the most bacterial units: one class (*Epsilonproteobacteria*), one order (*Campylobacterales*), two families (*Bacteroidaceae* and *Helicobacteraceae*), three genera (*Bacteroides, Bacillus*, and *Helicobacter*), and four species (*Prevotella dentasini, Natranaerovirga hydrolytica, Helicobacter marotae*, and *Helicobacter muridarum*). The abovementioned results indicated that CIA modeling plays an important role in the changes in the gut microbiota and that HUMSCs had a greater influence on the flora than MTX.

The specific gut microbiota changes were further assessed at the genus and species levels (**Figure 8G**). CIA modeling significantly decreased the abundances of various genera, including *Caldalkalibacillus, Lactococcus, Bacteroides, Bacillus,* and others and various species, including *Caldalkalibacillus panis, Lactococcus garvieae, Lactobacillus panis,* and *Bacillus humi* and others, and treatment with MTX and HUMSCs increased the abundances of the genera *Lactococcus, Bacteroides,* and *Bacillus* and the species *Lactococcus garvieae* and *Lactobacillus panis* but did not affect the abundances of the genus *Caldalkalibacillus* and the species *Caldalkalibacillus panis* and *Bacillus humi.* Conversely, the relative abundance of the genus *Clostridium* and the species *Clostridium isatidis, Anaeroplasma bactocasticum, Helicobacter marotae,* and *Helicobacter muridarum* increased after modeling. In addition, treatment with MTX and/or HUMSCs slightly decreased the abundances of some genera and species (genus *Clostridium* and species *Clostridium isatidis* and *Helicobacter muridarum*) but increased the abundances of some bacteria (species *Anaeroplasma bactocasticum* and *Helicobacter marotae*). In addition, a few bacteria were not affected by CIA modeling but exhibited an altered abundance after treatment with MTX and HUMSCs (species *Prevotella dentasini* and *Natranaerovirga hydrolytica*). Collectively, these data indicate that although the major intestinal microbial communities exhibited differences after MTX and HUMSC treatment, the abundance of some bacteria still changed in a synchronous manner. These results indicated that MTX and HUMSCs might modulate mucosal immunity through a common mechanism involving the gut microbiota.

## Gut Microbiota Regulated the Aryl Hydrocarbon Receptor Pathway Through Indole Metabolism

Based on the above-described results and those obtained in other studies, we found that *Bacteroides* and *Bacillus* can metabolize dietary tryptophan to produce indole, IAA, or ILA (Amin and Latif, 2017; Roager and Licht, 2018). Interestingly, these metabolites are AhR ligands that can stimulate the AhR and regulate intestinal mucosal immunity (Shinde and McGaha, 2018). Therefore, we detected the levels of indole, IAA, and ILA in plasma by LC-MS/MS and the AhR gene and protein expression levels in the ileum by Q-PCR and IHC, respectively. As shown in **Figure 9A**, the levels of indole, IAA, and ILA in the CIA group were significantly lower compared with those in the Control group ($P < 0.05$ and $P < 0.01$, respectively). Treatment with HUMSCs increased the levels of these three metabolites compared with those in the CIA group, and this difference was significant ($P < 0.05$). The levels of the three metabolites in the MTX group were also increased, but only the indole and ILA levels were different from those in the rats with CIA ($P < 0.05$). This result was consistent with the results from the analysis of the gut microbiota because the bacteria found at higher abundances in the HUMSC group (mainly *Lactococcus* and *Bacteroides*) can metabolize tryptophan and produce indole and other metabolites that are absorbed into the blood through the small intestine.

The assessment of the AhR expression in the ileum (**Figures 9B–D**) revealed that the AhR gene and protein expression levels in the CIA group were consistent with changes

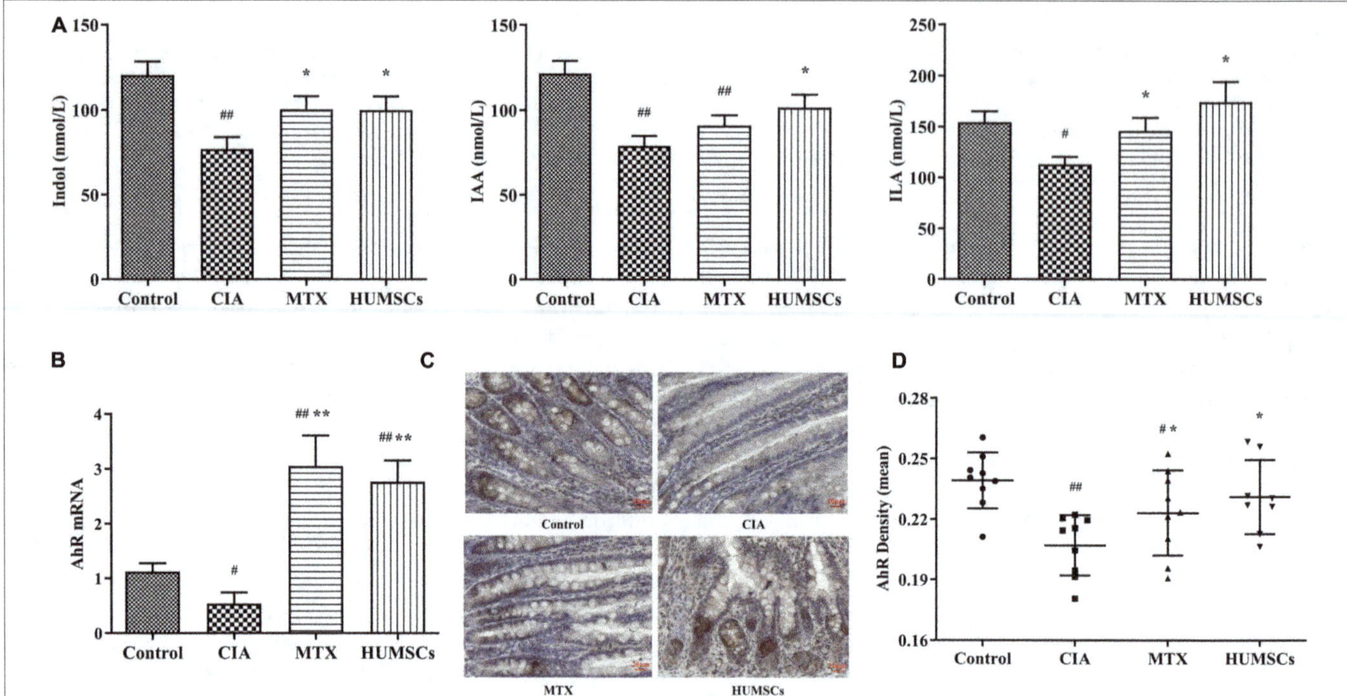


**FIGURE 9 |** Levels of indole and its derivatives in the plasma and aryl hydrocarbon receptor (AhR) expression in the ileum. The levels of indole, indoleacetic acid (IAA), and indole-3-lactic acid (ILA) in the plasma were detected by liquid chromatography-tandem mass spectrometry (LC-MS/MS), and the mRNA and protein expression levels of AhR were determined by quantitative real-time PCR (Q-PCR) and immunohistochemistry (IHC), respectively. **(A)** Bar plots showing the mean levels of indole, IAA, and ILA in all the groups. **(B)** AhR gene expression in the ileum. **(C)** Representative images of the ileum obtained by IHC (20×). **(D)** AhR protein expression in the ileum $N = 8$. The data are presented as the mean ± *SEM*. $^{\#}P < 0.05$ compared with the Control group, $^{\#\#}P < 0.01$ compared with the Control group, $^{*}P < 0.05$ compared with the CIA group, $^{**}P < 0.01$ compared with the CIA group.

in the levels of tryptophan metabolites, which were found at lower levels in this group compared with the Control group ($P < 0.05$ and $P < 0.01$, respectively). Treatment with MTX and HUMSCs upregulated the mRNA expression of AhR by 3-fold and more than 2-fold, respectively. However, the change in AhR protein expression was relatively minor compared with the change in its gene expression, and the AhR gene expression level in the treatment groups was between those in the Control and CIA groups but significantly differed from that in the CIA group ($P < 0.05$). These results confirms that indole, IAA, and ILA produced during bacterial decomposition activate the AhR. The regulatory effect of intestinal bacteria on mucosal immunity is likely dependent on activation of the AhR, a receptor that reportedly regulates the differentiation and function of Tregs and Th17 and B cells.

## DISCUSSION

Numerous studies have explored the therapeutic effects of HUMSCs that mediate the balance between Tregs and Th17 cells in RA (Ma et al., 2019). Several researchers have explored the effect and mechanism of other drugs on RA from the perspective of the gut microbiota (Bodkhe et al., 2019). However, no researchers have linked Tregs/Th17 cells with the gut microbiota to elucidate the therapeutic mechanism of HUMSCs. Based on the tissues to which HUMSCs home, we explored the influence of HUMSCs on bone destruction in the ankle joints and the proportions and functions of Tregs and Th17 cells in the nearest lymph node—the PLN. Furthermore, we focused on functions related to Tregs and Th17 cells and the functions through which B cells regulate the gut microbiota in GALTs: the MLN, PP, and LPL. We examined the changes in the gut microbiota in the ileum in depth and found changes in most bacteria involved in the metabolism of tryptophan to indole. To validate these results, we measured the plasma levels of indole and some of its derivatives and the AhR levels in the ileum, and the results showed a key link between indole metabolism and the immune system. Based on the current results, we can confirm that HUMSCs act as a therapeutic agent in CIA by regulating the interaction between host immunity and the gut microbiota and speculate that AhR is the key link between these factors.

Several clinical and experimental studies have investigated stem cell transplantation for the treatment of RA. A clinical trial conducted in Iran found that autologous bone marrow-derived mesenchymal stem cells ameliorated the clinical symptoms of refractory RA (Ghoryani et al., 2019). Another phase 1/2 clinical trial observed that autologous bone marrow-derived mesenchymal stromal cells increase the clinical efficacy of MTX and prednisolone and reduce their use (Shadmanfar et al., 2018). Animal experiments using relatively uniform methods have also shown that HUMSCs can be utilized to treat CIA (Cheng-Chi et al., 2012; Shin et al., 2016). Specifically, stem cells were injected at the same dose ($1 \times 10^6$ cells/rat or mouse) in most studies. However, the graft sites differed (tail vein, abdominal cavity, and articular cavity), and the observation time varied from half a month to a month. Our purpose was to observe the systemic regulatory effect of HUMSCs, and based on the treatment duration used in a previous experiment (Zhao et al., 2018), $1 \times 10^6$ cells/rat were injected *via* the tail vein for one month. Some researchers have tracked the entry of stem cells into the body. Liu et al. (2010) showed that intraperitoneally injected HUMSCs could not be detected in joints, but a positive signal for HUMSCs was found in the spleen on days 3 and 7 and disappeared on day 14 after injection. In addition, Wu C. C. et al. (2016) detected the expression of HLA-A protein, which is characteristic of HUMSCs, in knee cartilage and synovial tissue on day 14 after the injection of HUMSCs into the joint. In our study, positive NuMA signaling was simultaneously detected in the knee, PLN, MLN, and ileum mucosa on day 28 after HUMSC injection. The differences in the above-described results might be due to the different transplantation methods and transplantation durations used.

Because Tregs are immunosuppressive cells, their proportion and function are crucial in the suppression of ADs. Tregs act as cytotoxic agents through cell–cell interactions and function by secreting the cytokines IL-10 and TGF-β1 (Shevach, 2009). In the intestine, Tregs play an important role in the maintenance of immune tolerance to dietary antigens and the gut microbiota (Honda and Littman, 2016). Unlike Tregs, another cell subgroup, Th17 cells, induces immune activation by secreting IL-17A to promote inflammation (Patel and Kuchroo, 2015). However, the production of IL-17A and IL-22 by Th17 cells in the gut contributes to the defense against intestinal pathogens (Ubeda and Pamer, 2012). Tregs/Th17 cells are the most studied immune cells in the peripheral blood and spleen; although the immune statuses in these two tissues reflect the immune state of the system, they are not typical (Liu et al., 2010; Ma et al., 2019). More detailed studies of this mechanism have targeted tissues to reveal the local immune status, such as targeting Tregs/Th17 cells to the MLN and PP (Tong et al., 2015). However, the involvement of HUMSCs in influencing Tregs/Th17 cells in the PLN and among LPL in CIA has not been reported. We identified the distribution of HUMSCs in CIA through their localization and then specifically determined the proportions of these two cell subtypes in HUMSC-positive tissues, namely, the PLN, MLN, PP, and LPL. In addition, SIgA plays an important role in the resistance to intestinal bacterial adhesion and endotoxin neutralization (Iijima et al., 2001). Because precursor cells secrete SIgA, we also measured the proportion of B cells in the above-listed GALTs (Reboldi et al., 2016). Our results are generally consistent with those obtained in the limited number of previous reports. HUMSC therapy significantly increased the proportion of Tregs; significantly decreased the proportion of Th17 cells in the PLN, MLN, and PP and among the LPL compared with that found in the CIA group; and significantly increased the proportion of B cells in PP and among the LPL. The abovementioned results suggested that the immune status of intestinal-associated lymphoid tissues worsened after modeling and that the homing of HUMSCs partially reversed immune disorders, and the detection of Treg-, Th17 cell-, and B cell-related factors verified the above-described results.

The importance of the gut microbiome in RA has been reported in both human patients and mouse models. Alterations to the gut microbiota are related to the risk and severity of RA, and probiotic transplantation is beneficial for RA remission. Toivanen et al. (2002) showed that patients with early RA had on average only half as many bacteria belonging to the genera *Bacteroides*, *Prevotella*, and *Porphyromonas* compared with control subjects. Another study conducted by Vaahtovuo et al. (2008) similarly found that RA patients were characterized by a different fecal diversity with a decreased abundance of bacteria belonging to the *Bacteroides–Porphyromonas–Prevotella* group, the *Bacteroides fragilis* subgroup, and the *Eubacterium rectale–Clostridium coccoides* group compared with patients with fibromyalgia. *Lactobacillus casei* has been shown to be an effective probiotic in the treatment of RA. Alipour et al. (2014) treated 22 subjects with *L. casei* and compared them with 24 subjects treated with placebo. The C-reactive protein (CRP) level, number of inflamed and painful joints, and 28-joint disease activity score (DAS-28) were significantly decreased in the 22 subjects compared with the 24 controls. In animal models, both intestinal bacteria known to be correlated with arthritis and differences in the composition of the gut microbiota between animals with CIA and normal animals and even between arthritis-susceptible and healthy or arthritic hosts were consistently detected. In the K/BxN mouse, gut-residing segmented filamentous bacteria (SFB) were found to drive the rapid development of destructive arthritis (Doube and Collins, 1988). Liu et al. (2016) revealed that the genus *Lactobacillus* was the dominant genus in mice susceptible to CIA prior to the onset of arthritis. The development of the disease increased the abundances of the families *Bacteroidaceae*, *Lachnospiraceae*, and *S24-7* in CIA-susceptible mice. Notably, germ-free mice treated with the microbiota of CIA-susceptible mice showed a higher frequency of arthritis induction than those treated with the microbiota of CIA-resistant mice. Our results showed that CIA modeling decreased the abundances of the genera *Bacteroides*, *Lactococcus*, and species *Lactococcus garvieae* compared with those in the Control group, which was partly consistent with the above-described findings.

The gut serves as a bridge between intestinal microorganisms and their host. Intestinal bacteria synthesize and alter multiple compounds that impact physiology and immunity (Rooks and Garrett, 2016). Numerous studies have shown that Tregs and Th17 cells are simultaneously the target cells of intestinal commensal microbiota and the key to activating the host defense against pathogens, which could result in the avoidance of other immunopathologic consequences (Bennike et al., 2017). Under conventional conditions, *Lactobacillus bifidus* induces arthritis in IL-1ra$^{-/-}$ mice, which exhibit a decreased number of Tregs and an increased number of Th17 cells (Abdollahi-Roodsaz et al., 2008). In contrast, *Bifidobacterium infantis* can induce Tregs to play an anti-inflammatory role, and *B. fragilis* polysaccharide stimulates Tregs to produce IL-10

(Abdollahi-Roodsaz et al., 2008). A study conducted by Zhang et al. (2016) revealed that the supplementation of broiler diets with *Lactococcus garvieae B301* increased the body weight and exerted a positive effect on the serum levels of immune globulins. In addition, Wang et al. (2019) showed that recombinant *Bacillus subtilis* induces a mucosal SIgA response to pseudorabies and regulates the $CD3^{+}CD4^{+}$ T cell proliferative response by IL-10. Another study showed that a mixture of two *Clostridium* strains significantly reduces the Th17/Th1 balance (Lopez et al., 2016), and infection with *Clostridium perfringens* or *Clostridium difficile* induces a pro-inflammatory response related to Th17 cells (Yacyshyn et al., 2014; Yu et al., 2017). In the current study, regarding the relative abundances of the genera *Lactococcus*, *Bacillus*, and *Bacteroides* and the species *Lactococcus garvieae*, Tregs and the related cytokines and SIgA were increased in both MTX- and HUMSC-treated rats, whereas regarding the relative abundances of the genus *Clostridium*, Th17 cells and related cytokines were upregulated in rats with CIA and reduced after the treatments, as expected. Based on the discussion and results described above, we speculated that changes in the gut microbiota caused changes in immune regulation.

A review of the literature revealed that the bacterial genera *Bacillus* and *Bacteroides* are involved in the metabolism of tryptophan into indole and its derivatives

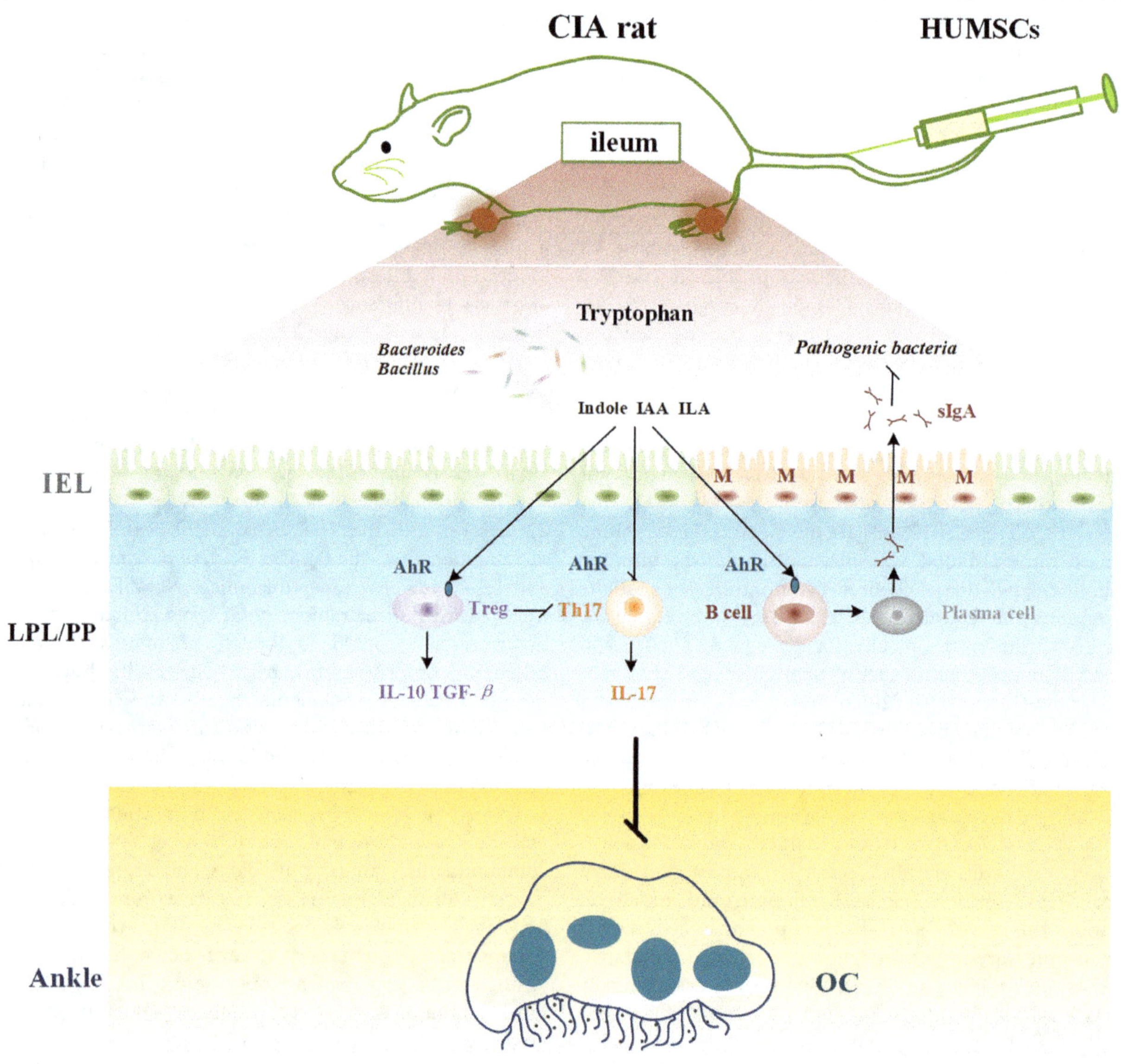


**FIGURE 10 |** Mechanism of HUMSCs therapy in CIA rat. CIA, collagen-induced arthritis; HUMSCs, Human umbilical mesenchymal stem cells; IAA, indoleacetic acid; ILA, indole-3-lactic acid; SIgA, secretory immunoglobulin A; MLN, mesenteric lymph node; AhR, aryl hydrocarbon receptor; Treg, T regulatory cell; Th17, T helper 17 cell; OC, osteoclast; PLN, popliteal lymph node.

(Shao et al., 2015; Roager and Licht, 2018). Interestingly, the components regulated by these bacteria, namely, indole, IAA, and ILA, are ligands of the AhR (Gao et al., 2018). The available evidence suggests that the AhR is a key sensor that allows immune cells to adapt to environmental conditions and that the inhibition of AhR activity is associated with ADs. Numerous studies have shown that activation of the AhR increases the differentiation and function of Tregs but inhibited inflammatory cytokines (Shinde and McGaha, 2018). Researchers have reported that sinomenine induces the generation of intestinal Tregs and attenuates arthritis *via* activation of the AhR even in CIA (Tong et al., 2016a). Some evidence suggests that AhR activation increases Th17 cell differentiation and the secretion of IL-17A and IL-22 (Shinde and McGaha, 2018). However, the results obtained after treatment of the CIA model consistently suggested that activation of the AhR inhibits the differentiation and function of Th17 cells (Tong et al., 2015, 2016b). This difference in results might be due to the type of ligand and animal species used and the disease type examined. In addition, Villa et al. (2017) demonstrated that intervention with 6-formylindolo[3,2-b]carbazole (FICZ), a natural agonist, increased AhR expression during B cell differentiation and the amount of AhR localized to the nucleus and significantly upregulated the expression of the downstream target gene CYP1A1 on B cells. These results imply that the AhR is involved in B cell proliferation and function. Our results demonstrated that the increased abundance of the genera *Bacteroides* and *Bacillus* might lead to increased levels of indole and its derivatives in the plasma, and these increases enhance AhR gene and protein expression in the ileum. Furthermore, activated AhR might regulate the gut microbiota by regulating Tregs and Th17 and B cells *via* a feedback loop. Although a few *Clostridium* strains, such as *Clostridium difficile* and *Clostridium sordellii*, can produce indole, IAA, or ILA (Roager and Licht, 2018), pathogenic bacteria species belonging to the genus *Clostridium* can produce toxins that induce clostridial disease. Our results showed that the genus *Clostridium* exhibited an increasing trend in the CIA group, which was in line with the function of this strain.

In summary, our results suggest that HUMSCs play a therapeutic role in CIA because these cells regulate immunity in rats with CIA and particularly immunity in GALTs. The underlying mechanism might be related to the crosstalk between immunity and the gut microbiota regulated by the AhR (**Figure 10**).

## ETHICS STATEMENT

The study involving human participants was reviewed and approved by the Research Ethics Committee at the China-Japan Friendship Hospital (2019-124-K86). The patients/participants provided their written informed consent to participate in this study. The animal study was reviewed and approved by the Institute of Clinical Medical Sciences, China-Japan Friendship Hospital, Beijing, China (No. 180207).

## AUTHOR CONTRIBUTIONS

CX and HL designed the conceptual framework of the study. XLi and CL designed the experiments and wrote the manuscript. XLi, CL, XLu, DF, YX, and JL performed the experiments. HZ, HX, and YZ analyzed the data.

## REFERENCES


Abdollahi-Roodsaz, S., Joosten, L. A., Koenders, M. I., Devesa, I., Roelofs, M. F., Radstake, T. R., et al. (2008). Stimulation of TLR2 and TLR4 differentially skews the balance of T cells in a mouse model of arthritis. *J. Clin. Invest.* 118, 205–216. doi: 10.1172/JCI32639

Alipour, B., Homayouni-Rad, A., Vaghef-Mehrabany, E., Sharif, S. K., Vaghef-Mehrabany, L., Asghari-Jafarabadi, M., et al. (2014). Effects of *Lactobacillus casei* supplementation on disease activity and inflammatory cytokines in rheumatoid arthritis patients: a randomized double-blind clinical trial. *Int. J. Rheum. Dis.* 17, 519–527. doi: 10.1111/1756-185X.12333

Amin, A., and Latif, Z. (2017). Screening of mercury-resistant and indole-3-acetic acid producing bacterial-consortium for growth promotion of *Cicer arietinum* L. *J. Basic Microbiol.* 57, 204–217. doi: 10.1002/jobm.201600352

Bennike, T. B., Ellingsen, T., Glerup, H., Bonderup, O. K., Carlsen, T. G., Meyer, M. K., et al. (2017). Proteome analysis of rheumatoid arthritis Gut Mucosa. *J. Proteome Res.* 16, 346–354. doi: 10.1021/acs.jproteome.6b00598

Bodkhe, R., Balakrishnan, B., and Taneja, V. (2019). The role of microbiome in rheumatoid arthritis treatment. *Ther. Adv. Musculoskelet. Dis.* 11:1759720X19844632. doi: 10.1177/1759720X19844632

Cheng-Chi, W., Tzu-Chin, W., Fei-Lan, L., Huey-Kang, S., and Deh-Ming, C. (2012). TNF-α inhibitor reverse the effects of human umbilical cord-derived stem cells on experimental arthritis by increasing immunosuppression. *Cell Immunol.* 273, 30–40. doi: 10.1016/j.cellimm.2011.11.009

Doube, A., and Collins, A. J. (1988). Is the gut intrinsically abnormal in rheumatoid arthritis? *Ann. Rheum. Dis.* 47, 617–619. doi: 10.1136/ard.47.8.617

Gao, J., Xu, K., Liu, H., Liu, G., Bai, M., Peng, C., et al. (2018). Impact of the gut microbiota on intestinal immunity mediated by Tryptophan metabolism. *Front. Cell Infect. Microbiol.* 8:13. doi: 10.3389/fcimb.2018.00013

Ghoryani, M., Shariati-Sarabi, Z., Tavakkol-Afshari, J., Ghasemi, A., Poursamimi, J., and Mohammadi, M. (2019). Amelioration of clinical symptoms of patients with refractory rheumatoid arthritis following treatment with autologous bone marrow-derived mesenchymal stem cells: a successful clinical trial in Iran. *Biomed. Pharmacother.* 109, 1834–1840. doi: 10.1016/j.biopha.2018.11.056

Honda, K., and Littman, D. R. (2016). The microbiota in adaptive immune homeostasis and disease. *Nature* 535, 75–84. doi: 10.1038/nature18848

Iijima, H., Takahashi, I., and Kiyono, H. (2001). Mucosal immune network in the gut for the control of infectious diseases. *Rev. Med. Virol.* 11, 117–133. doi: 10.1002/rmv.307

Liu, X., Zeng, B., Zhang, J., Li, W., Mou, F., Wang, H., et al. (2016). Role of the gut microbiome in modulating arthritis progression in mice. *Sci. Rep.* 6:30594. doi: 10.1038/srep30594

Liu, Y., Mu, R., Wang, S., Long, L., Liu, X., Li, R., et al. (2010). Therapeutic potential of human umbilical cord mesenchymal stem cells in the treatment of rheumatoid arthritis. *Arthrit. Res. Ther.* 12:R210. doi: 10.1186/ar3187

Lopez, P., de Paz, B., Rodriguez-Carrio, J., Hevia, A., Sanchez, B., Margolles, A., et al. (2016). Th17 responses and natural IgM antibodies are related to gut microbiota composition in systemic lupus erythematosus patients. *Sci. Rep.* 6:24072. doi: 10.1038/srep24072

Ma, D., Xu, K., Zhang, G., Liu, Y., Gao, J., Tian, M., et al. (2019). Immunomodulatory effect of human umbilical cord mesenchymal stem cells on T lymphocytes in rheumatoid arthritis. *Int. Immunopharmacol.* 74:105687. doi: 10.1016/j.intimp.2019.105687

McInnes, I. B., and Schett, G. (2011). The pathogenesis of rheumatoid arthritis. *N. Engl. J. Med.* 365, 2205–2219. doi: 10.1056/NEJMra1004965

Naik, S., Larsen, S. B., Cowley, C. J., and Fuchs, E. (2018). Two to tango: dialog between immunity and stem cells in health and disease. *Cell* 175, 908–920. doi: 10.1016/j.cell.2018.08.071

Noack, M., and Miossec, P. (2014). Th17 and regulatory T cell balance in autoimmune and inflammatory diseases. *Autoimmun. Rev.* 13, 668–677. doi: 10.1016/j.autrev.2013.12.004

Patel, D. D., and Kuchroo, V. K. (2015). Th17 cell pathway in human immunity: lessons from genetics and therapeutic interventions. *Immunity* 43, 1040–1051. doi: 10.1016/j.immuni.2015.12.003

Reboldi, A., Arnon, T. I., Rodda, L. B., Atakilit, A., Sheppard, D., and Cyster, J. G. (2016). IgA production requires B cell interaction with subepithelial dendritic cells in Peyer's patches. *Science* 352:f4822. doi: 10.1126/science.aaf4822

Roager, H. M., and Licht, T. R. (2018). Microbial tryptophan catabolites in health and disease. *Nat. Commun.* 9:3294. doi: 10.1038/s41467-018-05470-4

Rooks, M. G., and Garrett, W. S. (2016). Gut microbiota, metabolites and host immunity. *Nat. Rev. Immunol.* 16, 341–352. doi: 10.1038/nri.2016.42

Rothhammer, V., and Quintana, F. J. (2019). The aryl hydrocarbon receptor: an environmental sensor integrating immune responses in health and disease. *Nat. Rev. Immunol.* 19, 184–197. doi: 10.1038/s41577-019-0125-8

Shadmanfar, S., Labibzadeh, N., Emadedin, M., Jaroughi, N., Azimian, V., Mardpour, S., et al. (2018). Intra-articular knee implantation of autologous bone marrow-derived mesenchymal stromal cells in rheumatoid arthritis patients with knee involvement: results of a randomized, triple-blind, placebo-controlled phase 1/2 clinical trial. *Cytotherapy* 20, 499–506. doi: 10.1016/j.jcyt.2017.12.009

Shao, J., Li, S., Zhang, N., Cui, X., Zhou, X., Zhang, G., et al. (2015). Analysis and cloning of the synthetic pathway of the phytohormone indole-3-acetic acid in the plant-beneficial *Bacillus amyloliquefaciens* SQR9. *Microb. Cell Fact* 14:130. doi: 10.1186/s12934-015-0323-4

Shevach, E. M. (2009). Mechanisms of foxp3+ T regulatory cell-mediated suppression. *Immunity* 30, 636–645. doi: 10.1016/j.immuni.2009.04.010

Shin, T. H., Kim, H. S., Kang, T. W., Lee, B. C., Lee, H. Y., Kim, Y. J., et al. (2016). Human umbilical cord blood-stem cells direct macrophage polarization and block inflammasome activation to alleviate rheumatoid arthritis. *Cell Death Dis.* 7:e2524. doi: 10.1038/cddis.2016.442

Shinde, R., and McGaha, T. L. (2018). The Aryl hydrocarbon receptor: connecting immunity to the microenvironment. *Trends Immunol.* 39, 1005–1020. doi: 10.1016/j.it.2018.10.010

Smolen, J. S., Aletaha, D., and McInnes, I. B. (2016). Rheumatoid arthritis. *Lancet* 388, 2023–2038. doi: 10.1016/S0140-6736(16)30173-8

Toivanen, P., Vartiainen, S., Jalava, J., Luukkainen, R., Möttönen, T., Eerola, E., et al. (2002). Intestinal anaerobic bacteria in early rheumatoid arthritis (RA). *Arthrit. Res.* 4:5.

Tong, B., Dou, Y., Wang, T., Yu, J., Wu, X., Lu, Q., et al. (2015). Norisoboldine ameliorates collagen-induced arthritis through regulating the balance between Th17 and regulatory T cells in gut-associated lymphoid tissues. *Toxicol. Appl. Pharmacol.* 282, 90–99. doi: 10.1016/j.taap.2014.11.008

Tong, B., Yuan, X., Dou, Y., Wu, X., Chou, G., Wang, Z., et al. (2016a). Norisoboldine, an isoquinoline alkaloid, acts as an aryl hydrocarbon receptor ligand to induce intestinal Treg cells and thereby attenuate arthritis. *Int. J. Biochem. Cell Biol.* 75, 63–73. doi: 10.1016/j.biocel.2016.03.014

Tong, B., Yuan, X., Dou, Y., Wu, X., Wang, Y., Xia, Y., et al. (2016b). Sinomenine induces the generation of intestinal Treg cells and attenuates arthritis via activation of aryl hydrocarbon receptor. *Lab. Invest.* 96, 1076–1086. doi: 10.1038/labinvest.2016.86

Ubeda, C., and Pamer, E. G. (2012). Antibiotics, microbiota, and immune defense. *Trends Immunol.* 33, 459–466. doi: 10.1016/j.it.2012.05.003

Uccelli, A., Moretta, L., and Pistoia, V. (2008). Mesenchymal stem cells in health and disease. *Nat. Rev. Immunol.* 8, 726–736. doi: 10.1038/nri2395

Vaahtovuo, J., Munukka, E., Korkeamaki, M., Luukkainen, R., and Toivanen, P. (2008). Fecal microbiota in early rheumatoid arthritis. *J. Rheumatol.* 35, 1500–1505.

Villa, M., Gialitakis, M., Tolaini, M., Ahlfors, H., Henderson, C. J., Wolf, C. R., et al. (2017). Aryl hydrocarbon receptor is required for optimal B-cell proliferation. *EMBO J.* 36, 116–128. doi: 10.15252/embj.201695027

Wang, J., Wang, Y., Zhang, E., Zhou, M., Lin, J., and Yang, Q. (2019). Intranasal administration with recombinant *Bacillus subtilis* induces strong mucosal immune responses against pseudorabies. *Microb. Cell Fact* 18:103. doi: 10.1186/s12934-019-1151-8

Wu, C. C., Liu, F. L., Sytwu, H. K., Tsai, C. Y., and Chang, D. M. (2016). CD146+ mesenchymal stem cells display greater therapeutic potential than CD146- cells for treating collagen-induced arthritis in mice. *Stem Cell Res. Ther.* 7:23. doi: 10.1186/s13287-016-0285-4

Wu, X., He, B., Liu, J., Feng, H., Ma, Y., Li, D., et al. (2016). Molecular insight into gut microbiota and rheumatoid arthritis. *Int. J. Mol. Sci.* 17:431. doi: 10.3390/ijms17030431

Xiao, C., Lu, C., Zhao, L., Liu, Z., Zhang, W., He, Y., et al. (2006). The effects of triptolide on enteric mucosal immune responses of DBA/1 mice with collagen-induced arthritis. *Planta Med.* 72, 1268–1272. doi: 10.1055/s-2006-947240

Yacyshyn, M. B., Reddy, T. N., Plageman, L. R., Wu, J., Hollar, A. R., and Yacyshyn, B. R. (2014). Clostridium difficile recurrence is characterized by pro-inflammatory peripheral blood mononuclear cell (PBMC) phenotype. *J. Med. Microbiol.* 63, 1260–1273. doi: 10.1099/jmm.0.075382-0

Yu, H., Chen, K., Sun, Y., Carter, M., Garey, K. W., Savidge, T. C., et al. (2017). Cytokines are markers of the clostridium difficile-induced inflammatory response and predict disease severity. *Clin. Vacc. Immunol.* 24:e0037-17. doi: 10.1128/CVI.00037-17

Zhang, T., Xie, J., Zhang, M., Fu, N., and Zhang, Y. (2016). Effect of a potential probiotics *Lactococcus garvieae* B301 on the growth performance, immune parameters and caecum microflora of broiler chickens. *J. Anim. Physiol. Anim. Nutr.* 100, 413–421. doi: 10.1111/jpn.12388

Zhao, H., Xu, H., Zuo, Z., Wang, G., Liu, M., Guo, M., et al. (2018). Yi Shen Juan bi pill ameliorates bone loss and destruction induced by arthritis through modulating the balance of cytokines released by different subpopulations of T cells. *Front. Pharmacol.* 9:262. doi: 10.3389/fphar.2018.00262

# Permissions

All chapters in this book were first published by Frontiers; hereby published with permission under the Creative Commons Attribution License or equivalent. Every chapter published in this book has been scrutinized by our experts. Their significance has been extensively debated. The topics covered herein carry significant findings which will fuel the growth of the discipline. They may even be implemented as practical applications or may be referred to as a beginning point for another development.

The contributors of this book come from diverse backgrounds, making this book a truly international effort. This book will bring forth new frontiers with its revolutionizing research information and detailed analysis of the nascent developments around the world.

We would like to thank all the contributing authors for lending their expertise to make the book truly unique. They have played a crucial role in the development of this book. Without their invaluable contributions this book wouldn't have been possible. They have made vital efforts to compile up to date information on the varied aspects of this subject to make this book a valuable addition to the collection of many professionals and students.

This book was conceptualized with the vision of imparting up-to-date information and advanced data in this field. To ensure the same, a matchless editorial board was set up. Every individual on the board went through rigorous rounds of assessment to prove their worth. After which they invested a large part of their time researching and compiling the most relevant data for our readers.

The editorial board has been involved in producing this book since its inception. They have spent rigorous hours researching and exploring the diverse topics which have resulted in the successful publishing of this book. They have passed on their knowledge of decades through this book. To expedite this challenging task, the publisher supported the team at every step. A small team of assistant editors was also appointed to further simplify the editing procedure and attain best results for the readers.

Apart from the editorial board, the designing team has also invested a significant amount of their time in understanding the subject and creating the most relevant covers. They scrutinized every image to scout for the most suitable representation of the subject and create an appropriate cover for the book.

The publishing team has been an ardent support to the editorial, designing and production team. Their endless efforts to recruit the best for this project, has resulted in the accomplishment of this book. They are a veteran in the field of academics and their pool of knowledge is as vast as their experience in printing. Their expertise and guidance has proved useful at every step. Their uncompromising quality standards have made this book an exceptional effort. Their encouragement from time to time has been an inspiration for everyone.

The publisher and the editorial board hope that this book will prove to be a valuable piece of knowledge for researchers, students, practitioners and scholars across the globe.

# List of Contributors

**Qian Xiang, Liang Kang, Kangcheng Zhao, Juntan Wang, Wenbin Hua, Yu Song, Xiaobo Feng, Gaocai Li, Saideng Lu, Kun Wang, Cao Yang and Yukun Zhang**
Department of Orthopaedics, Union Hospital, Tongji Medical College, Huazhong University of Science and Technology, Wuhan, China

**Tenghui Tao, Danni Luo, Chenghao Gao, Hui Liu, Zehua Lei, Wenbin Liu, Chuankun Zhou, Dahu Qi, Xuying Sun and Jun Xiao**
Department of Orthopedics, Tongji Hospital, Tongji Medical College, Huazhong University of Science and Technology, Wuhan, China

**Zhenhan Deng**
Department of Sports Medicine, The First Affiliated Hospital of Shenzhen University, Shenzhen Second People's Hospital, Shenzhen, China

**Kaixuan Chen, Yurui Jiao, Ling Liu, Mei Huang, Chen He, Wenzhen He, Jing Hou and Mi Yang**
Department of Endocrinology, Endocrinology Research Center, The Xiangya Hospital of Central South University, Changsha, China

**Xianghang Luo and Changjun Li**
Department of Endocrinology, Endocrinology Research Center, The Xiangya Hospital of Central South University, Changsha, China
National Clinical Research Center for Geriatric Disorders, Xiangya Hospital, Changsha, China
Key Laboratory of Organ Injury, Aging and Regenerative Medicine of Hunan Province, Changsha, China

**Tie Liu**
Department of Oral Implantology, The Affiliated Hospital of Stomatology, School of Stomatology, Zhejiang University School of Medicine, Hangzhou, China
Key Laboratory of Oral Biomedical Research of Zhejiang Province, Hangzhou, China

**Wen Fang**
Key Laboratory of Oral Biomedical Research of Zhejiang Province, Hangzhou, China
Department of Periodontology, The Affiliated Hospital of Stomatology, School of Stomatology, Zhejiang University School of Medicine, Hangzhou, China

**Gang Wu and Yuelian Liu**
Department of Oral Implantology and Prosthetic Dentistry, Academic of Dentistry Amsterdam (ACTA), VU Universiteit Amsterdam and University of Amsterdam, Amsterdam, Netherlands

**Yining Li**
Key Laboratory of Oral Biomedical Research of Zhejiang Province, Hangzhou, China
Department of Oral Pathology, The Affiliated Hospital of Stomatology, School of Stomatology, Zhejiang University School of Medicine, Hangzhou, China

**Wenchao Zhang, Zhongyue Liu, Xiaolei Ren, Lin Qi, Lu Wan, Wanchun Wang, Chao Tu and Zhihong Li**
Department of Orthopedics, The Second Xiangya Hospital, Central South University, Changsha, China
Hunan Key Laboratory of Tumor Models and Individualized Medicine, The Second Xiangya Hospital, Central South University, Changsha, China

**Lile He**
Hunan Key Laboratory of Tumor Models and Individualized Medicine, The Second Xiangya Hospital, Central South University, Changsha, China
Department of Cardiovascular Surgery, The Second Xiangya Hospital, Central South University, Changsha, China

**Guo-dong Lu and Zhong Wang**
Department of Cardiology, The First Affiliated Hospital of Shihezi University Medical College, Shihezi, China

**Peng Cheng**
Division of Geriatric Endocrinology, The First Affiliated Hospital, Nanjing Medical University, Nanjing, China

**Ting Liu**
Department of Endocrinology, Changsha Central Hospital, Changsha, China

**Jian Qu, Zhanbo Ouyang, Guohua Li, Jiaojiao Wang and Qiong Lu**
Department of Pharmacy, The Second Xiangya Hospital, Central South University; Institute of Clinical Pharmacy, Central South University, Changsha, China
Hunan Key Laboratory of Tumor Models and Individualized Medicine, The Second Xiangya Hospital, Central South University, Changsha, China

**Wenqiang Wu**
Mathematical Engineering Academy of Chinese Medicine, Guangzhou University of Chinese Medicine, Guangzhou, China

**Lingli Zhang, Yu Yuan, Wei Wu, Zhongguang Sun, Le Lei and Jun Zou**
School of Kinesiology, Shanghai University of Sport, Shanghai, China

**Jing Fan and Bo Gao**
Institute of Orthopedic Surgery, Xijing Hospital, Fourth Military Medical University, Xi'an, China

**Liping Wang, Jing Zheng, Janak L. Pathak, Yunxin Chen, Dongliang Liang, Luxi Yang, Haobo Sun, Mei Zhong, Lihong Wu, Yongyong Yan, Dan Hou and Linhu Ge**
Guangzhou Key Laboratory of Basic and Applied Research in Oral Regenerative Medicine, Affiliated Stomatology Hospital of Guangzhou Medical University, Institute of Oral Disease, Guangzhou Medical University, Guangzhou, China

**Lijing Wang**
Guangzhou Key Laboratory of Basic and Applied Research in Oral Regenerative Medicine, Affiliated Stomatology Hospital of Guangzhou Medical University, Institute of Oral Disease, Guangzhou Medical University, Guangzhou, China
Vascular Biology Research Institute, School of Life Sciences and Biopharmaceutics, Guangdong Pharmaceutical University, Guangzhou, China

**Li Li, Shuhua Deng and Lingyun Zheng**
Vascular Biology Research Institute, School of Life Sciences and Biopharmaceutics, Guangdong Pharmaceutical University, Guangzhou, China

**Shangfu Li, Tianwei He, Depeng Wu, Liangming Zhang, Ruiqiang Chen, Bin Liu and Limin Rong**
Department of Spine Surgery, The Third Affiliated Hospital of Sun Yat-sen University, Guangzhou, China
Guangdong Provincial Center for Quality Control of Minimally Invasive Spine Surgery, Guangzhou, China
Guangdong Provincial Center for Engineering and Technology Research of Minimally Invasive Spine Surgery, Guangzhou, China

**Jinbo Yuan, Jennifer Tickner and Jiake Xu**
School of Biomedical Sciences, The University of Western Australia, Perth, WA, Australia

**An Qin**
Shanghai Key Laboratory of Orthopedic Implants, Department of Orthopedic Surgery, Shanghai Ninth People's Hospital, Shanghai Jiao Tong University School of Medicine, Shanghai, China

**Huili Lyu, Ye Xiao, Qi Guo and Yan Huang**
Endocrinology Research Center, Department of Endocrinology, Xiangya Hospital of Central South University, Changsha, China

**Hui Peng**
Department of Endocrinology, Endocrinology Research Center, Xiangya Hospital of Central South University, Changsha, China

**Hong-Bo He and Ting Wen**
Department of Orthopedic, Xiangya Hospital of Central South University, Changsha, China

**Haihong Zhu and Tingting Qi**
Department of Pharmacy, The Second Xiangya Hospital, Central South University; Institute of Clinical Pharmacy, Central South University, Changsha, China

**Qiang Qu**
Department of Pharmacy, Xiangya Hospital, Central South University, Changsha, China

**Zengwu Shao**
Department of Orthopaedics, Union Hospital, Tongji Medical College, Huazhong University of Science and Technology, Wuhan, China

**Sheng Chen**
Department of Orthopaedics, Union Hospital, Tongji Medical College, Huazhong University of Science and Technology, Wuhan, China
Guangdong Provincial Key Laboratory of Cell Microenvironment and Disease Research, Shenzhen Key Laboratory of Cell Microenvironment, and Department of Biology, Southern University of Science and Technology, Shenzhen, China

**Lei Qin, Xiaohao Wu, Xuekun Fu, Guozhi Xiao and Huiling Cao**
Guangdong Provincial Key Laboratory of Cell Microenvironment and Disease Research, Shenzhen Key Laboratory of Cell Microenvironment, and Department of Biology, Southern University of Science and Technology, Shenzhen, China

**Sixiong Lin**
Guangdong Provincial Key Laboratory of Cell Microenvironment and Disease Research, Shenzhen Key Laboratory of Cell Microenvironment, and Department of Biology, Southern University of Science and Technology, Shenzhen, China
Guangdong Provincial Key Laboratory of Orthopedics and Traumatology, Orthopedic Research Institute and Department of Spinal Surgery, The First Affiliated Hospital of Sun Yat-sen University, Guangzhou, China

**Di Chen**
Department of Orthopedic Surgery, Rush University Medical Center, Chicago, IL, United States

**Wantao Li, Xiaoqing Zhou and Tiejian Jiang**
Department of Endocrinology, Endocrinology Research Center, Xiangya Hospital of Central South University, Changsha, China

**Xiaoya Li and Cheng Xiao**
Department of Emergency, China-Japan Friendship Hospital, Beijing, China
Institute of Clinical Medical Sciences, China-Japan Friendship Hospital, Beijing, China
Graduate School of Peking Union Medical College, Chinese Academy of Medical Sciences/Peking Union Medical College, Beijing, China

**Honglin Liu**
Institute of Clinical Medical Sciences, China-Japan Friendship Hospital, Beijing, China

**Danping Fan**
Institute of Clinical Medical Sciences, China-Japan Friendship Hospital, Beijing, China
Graduate School of Peking Union Medical College, Chinese Academy of Medical Sciences/Peking Union Medical College, Beijing, China

**Cheng Lu**
Institute of Basic Research in Clinical Medicine, China Academy of Chinese Medical Sciences, Beijing, China

**Xiangchen Lu and Ya Xia**
Institute of Clinical Medical Sciences, China-Japan Friendship Hospital, Beijing, China
School of Traditional Chinese Medicine, Beijing University of Chinese Medicine, Beijing, China

**Hongyan Zhao and Huihui Xu**
Beijing Key Laboratory of Research of Chinese Medicine on Prevention and Treatment for Major Diseases, Experimental Research Center, China Academy of Chinese Medical Sciences, Beijing, China

**Yongliang Zhu**
Department of Plant and Microbial Biology, University of California, Berkeley, Berkeley, CA, United States

**Jingtao Li**
Department of Gastroenterology, China-Japan Friendship Hospital, Beijing, China

# Index


**A**

Acid Phosphatase, 112, 142, 173-174, 181, 211-212, 217, 222-223, 227

Adiponectin, 125-127, 130-133, 135-140

Alveolar Bone Loss, 109-110, 113-114, 120, 122

Angiogenesis, 40, 44-46, 74-83, 121, 123, 159, 161-167, 169-174, 177, 181-183, 215, 217, 219

Annulus Fibrosus, 2, 198, 209

Atherosclerosis, 59, 75, 80, 83, 137, 218

Autoimmune Disease, 220-221

Autosomal Dominant, 107, 173, 181-183

**B**

Bisphosphonates, 42, 211

Bone Defect Healing, 47-50, 52, 55-57

Bone Tissue Engineering, 48, 58-59, 156, 164, 167

**C**

Cardiomyoblast, 74, 83

Cartilage Dysplasia, 85-86, 89-90, 92

Cartilage Matrix, 68, 130, 209

Catabolism, 2-3, 26, 41, 206, 208, 217

Chondrocyte, 11, 18-21, 26, 30, 57, 72, 86, 90, 94, 130, 168, 170, 210

Cobalt Protoporphyrin, 198, 201-202, 204

Cortical Bone Area, 142, 145-146

**E**

Endogenous Bone, 57, 162, 169

Endomucin, 174, 213, 215, 217

Epithelial Cell, 124, 209

Estrogen Deficiency, 44, 160, 211

Ethylene Diamine, 213

Exosome, 30, 32, 38, 46, 75-80, 83, 156-158, 160, 162, 164-167, 169-171

Extracellular Matrix, 2, 16, 68, 83, 90, 130, 141-142, 147, 154-155, 163, 170, 193, 197-198, 209

**F**

Femoral Head Necrosis, 37, 159

Fibroblast Growth Factor, 37, 68, 137, 140

Fibrocartilaginous, 198

Fluid Shear Stress, 46, 97, 197-199, 204, 210

**G**

Gastric Carcinoma, 75, 79, 83, 154

Gingival Tissue, 109-110, 113-114, 124

Gushukang, 211-212, 215, 218-219

**H**

Hematopoiesis, 44, 64

Homeostasis, 2, 5, 15, 30, 32-33, 39, 44-46, 58, 61, 64, 72, 74, 97, 108, 110, 122, 127, 129, 142, 144, 154, 159, 163-164, 167, 170-173, 197-198, 200, 205-206, 208-210, 212, 218-219, 237

**I**

Immunoblotting, 63, 75

Immunoprecipitation, 1, 5-6, 12-14, 19-20, 23, 26, 63-64, 186, 193, 195

Intervertebral Disk Degeneration, 1

**K**

Knocking Down Efficiency, 204, 206

**L**

Lipotoxicity, 128, 135-136, 139

**M**

Mechanical Stress, 1-2, 4-7, 9, 12, 15, 106, 134, 169, 198

Metabolic Syndrome, 45, 129, 136-139

Microvascular, 83, 164, 173, 176

Morbidity, 1, 48, 59, 68

Multinucleated Cells, 55, 57, 143, 148, 159, 223

Musculoskeletal Disorder, 198

Myocardial Functions, 166

**N**

Neovascularization, 163-164, 167

Nephropathy, 128, 162, 166, 170, 207

Nucleotide, 4, 63-64, 71, 85, 90, 174

Nucleus Pulposus Cell, 1, 15, 197

**O**

Osteocalcin, 35, 78, 81, 96, 100, 107, 126, 138, 173-174, 177, 211-213, 215

Osteoclast, 18, 33-37, 39, 41, 43-45, 55, 57, 64-65, 71, 73, 82-83, 90, 94-95, 108, 126-127, 129, 134, 137, 141-143, 145-149, 154, 158-160, 168-171, 173-174, 179-182, 209, 211-212, 214, 216, 218, 236

Osteoclastogenesis, 18, 31, 43-46, 64, 82-83, 110, 113-114, 117, 120-123, 137, 139-140, 145-149, 151-155, 158, 160, 163, 171-172, 180, 182, 215, 217, 219

Osteoconductive, 48-49, 56

Osteopetrosis, 95, 145, 173-183

Osteosarcoma, 15, 32, 38, 40, 42, 44-46, 60-61, 66-67, 70-73, 84-89, 91-95, 121, 123, 161, 184-196

Ovariectomy, 44, 75, 127-128, 135-136, 155

**P**

Paraformaldehyde, 20, 100, 143, 176, 199-200, 212-213

Parathyroid Hormone, 43, 67-68, 82-83, 129, 140, 142, 155, 168, 174, 210-211, 218

Pathophysiology, 24, 45, 70, 110, 121-122, 131, 133, 140, 154, 198, 209

Periodontal Tissue, 109-114, 116-117, 120, 123

Phospholipid Bilayer, 37-38

Primary Cilium, 206, 208

Prostate Cancer, 46, 154, 157-158, 167-168, 195, 218

Protein Kinase, 17, 130, 141-142, 153-155, 168

**R**

Rheumatoid Arthritis, 18, 30, 32, 36, 41, 43-46, 60-61, 66-67, 70-72, 85-86, 89-90, 131, 135-139, 159, 220-221, 237-238

**S**

Saline Solution, 97, 223

Serum Cytokines, 223

Sexual Dimorphism, 152-154

**T**

Tartrate-resistant, 112, 142, 173-174, 181, 217, 222-223, 227

Tendon Cell, 37-38

Tetraacetic Acid Solution, 212-213

Thrombospondin, 2, 142, 153-154, 197-198

Trabecular Bone Mass, 78, 81

Transcription Factor, 67-68, 87-89, 94-95, 106, 130, 139, 170, 209, 215, 223

Tumorigenesis, 42, 66-67, 74, 86-88

**V**

Vertebral Bone, 126, 135, 138, 177

Vessel Formation, 80, 173, 177, 179, 181-182, 211

www.ingramcontent.com/pod-product-compliance
Lightning Source LLC
LaVergne TN
LVHW080953210926
848485LV00004B/829

* 9 7 8 1 6 3 9 2 7 9 3 9 5 *